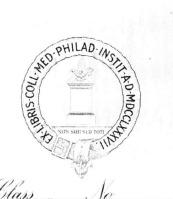

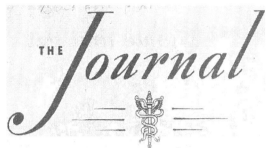

OF THE OKLAHOMA STATE MEDICAL ASSOCIATION

VOLUME XXXVI   •   OKLAHOMA CITY, OKLAHOMA, JANUARY, 1943   •   NUMBER 1

★ *Published Monthly at Oklahoma City, Oklahoma, Under Direction of the Council*

TABLE OF CONTENTS PAGE IV

Come and get it!

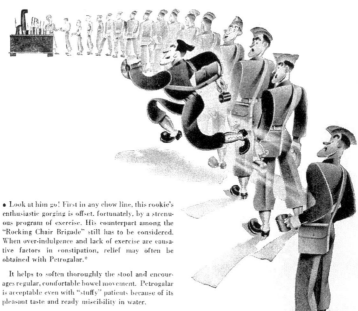

• Look at him go! First in any chow line, this rookie's enthusiastic gorging is offset, fortunately, by a strenuous program of exercise. His counterpart among the "Rocking Chair Brigade" still has to be considered. When over-indulgence and lack of exercise are causative factors in constipation, relief may often be obtained with Petrogalar.*

It helps to soften thoroughly the stool and encourages regular, comfortable bowel movement. Petrogalar is acceptable even with "stuffy" patients because of its pleasant taste and ready miscibility in water.

It may be taken directly from the spoon or from a glass. Consider Petrogalar for the treatment of constipation.

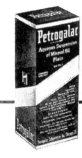

FOR THE TREATMENT OF CONSTIPATION

Petrogalar

*Reg. U. S. Pat. Off. Petrogalar is an aqueous suspension of pure mineral oil each 100 cc. of which contains 65 cc. pure mineral oil suspended in an aqueous jelly containing agar and acacia.

Petrogalar Laboratories, Inc. • 8134 McCormick Boulevard • Chicago, Illinois

THE JOURNAL
OF THE
OKLAHOMA STATE MEDICAL ASSOCIATION

| VOLUME XXXVI | OKLAHOMA CITY, OKLAHOMA, JANUARY, 1943 | NUMBER 1 |

Convulsions Encountered in General Practice

T. H. McCarley, A.B., M.D., F.A.C.P.

McALESTER, OKLAHOMA

The word "Encountered," as used in the caption of this paper, seems to me to be applicable, since it implies the necessity of overcoming an adversary when met. It must be the unusual doctor who can meet with temerity the child or adult patient in a generalized convulsion. This is the only type we shall consider, the many forms of tic and athetoid movements being beyond the limitations of this review.

He who has engaged in the general practice of medicine and surgery for a number of years has necessarily encountered a number of patients in convulsions. The family and friends of these patients, in most instances, regard a convulsion as a dire emergency. For this, they cannot be blamed because the spectacle of a loved one suddenly lapsing into unconsciousness, distorting himself with violent muscular contractions, cyanotic, breathing stertorously and "frothing at the mouth" (to use a favorite layman's expression) is sufficient to induce that panicky feeling in family, friends and possibly ever so slightly in the doctor himself.

It was only a few weeks after I had been licensed to practice the healing art that I encountered a patient in convulsions from a cause not again met in my thirty-four years of practice. I was doing my internship at a coal camp in southern Kentucky where I was the entire medical and surgical staff. A young miner had just gotten home from the day's work in the pit and while his face, hands and overalls were still grimey with lard oil and coal dust, was sitting in a chair leaning against the supporting post of the little porch of his shack. A shower with thunder and lightening came up. With a flash of lightening, a charge of electricity struck the porch and was grounded through the post against which the miner was sitting. Unconscious and in convulsions, he was thought to be dying by his family and the inhabitants of the village, all of whom were in the house that could get in and the rest were milling around on the outside in the rain. The convulsions were controlled by morphine and chloroform and after a few hours the patient aroused from his coma. The stock of the young doctor received a decided boost.

Not long after this experience, I met my first case of puerperal eclampsia. The night was cold and my entire corps of assistants was made up of grannies and neighbors. Following the teaching of the time, Norwood's Tr. Viratrum Viride was administered freely and chloroform cautiously. While discontinuing the chloroform for a time, the most severe convulsion, thus far, seized this young woman and the baby catapulted into the world. Hardly had I cut and tied the umbilical cord when I heard the hurried clatter of heavy boots on the frozen ground. A rap at the door and the messenger said, "Tell the doctor to come on up to my house. My wife needs him right away." After most of the night had worn away, baby number two was born and all was thought to be lovely. Suddenly, I heard a gushing as of falling water and I saw my patient pale and faint. While one fist was yet in her uterus and massage was being used to control the postpartum hemorrhage in this maternity patient number two, again the clank of boots on the frozen ground was heard, this time the messenger bringing the word that patient number one was having another fit. So the night was spent in hustling back and forth between my first case of eclampsia and my first case of postpartum hemorrhage.

My professional life has carried me

through the period when viratrum viride was the chief dependence in controlling convulsions of puerperal eclampsia, followed by the era when eclampsia at any stage of pregnancy in either primipara or multipara was considered an indication for immediate Cæsarean section. Succeeding this period, the more conservative plan of expectant treatment has evolved with a lessened morbidity and mortality. Better still, I have lived to see the public, and expectant mothers in particular, accept and demand careful prenatal care with the resulting decimation of the tragedy of puerperal convulsions.

We are interested in getting a conception of what alterations in cellular physiology occur to produce a convulsion. Every convulsion should be thought of as a manifestation of brain pathology. By this, I do not mean that the cause of the convulsion necessarily originates in the brain, but that the impulse causing the convulsion is transmitted to the brain, there producing an aberration of physiologic cellular activity. The head of the department of medicine of the medical school which I attended was wont to say that a convulsion was an "explosion of nerve force"— decidedly figurative you will say, but I doubt if we now have a much clearer concept of the alteration of function when a convulsion occurs.

Cobb lists fifty-six pathological states which give rise to fits and postulates thirteen different physiological mechanisms to explain their occurrence. The intrinsic nature of the subtle disturbance in brain-cell physiology constitutes the unsolved etiologic problem of convulsions. Certain observations are "suggestive," as that the factors which tend tto increase cell-membrane permeability are those recognized as favoring the occurrence of seizures; whereas, those which are associated with decrease in permeability are known to favor their cessation. To be more specific; excitation, brain trauma, alkalosis, superhydration, anoxemia and high serum lecithin over serum cholesterol increase membrane permeability and likewise increase the tendency to seizures; per contra, anaesthesia, sedation, acidosis, dehydration, ketosis and low serum lecithin over serum cholesterol decrease membrane permeability and likewise decrease the tendency to seizures.

We have long been taught, probably correctly so, that the convulsion in childhood corresponds to the chill in the adult at the onset of an acute infection.

The subject of convulsions in childhood from the standpoint of etiology has been most satisfactorily clarified by Dr. Peterman of Milwaukee. In 1939, he published the results of his study of convulsions in one thousand patients ranging in age from the neonatal period to sixteen years of age. The following table is a summary of his findings:

Convulsions in children, 1,000 cases.

(Peterman)

	Per cent
Acute Infection	34.0
Idiopathic Epilepsy	23.6
Cerebral birth injury or residue	15.5
Miscellaneous causes	12.7
Tetany	8.9
Cause not established	5.3

Peterman breaks down his findings according to age groups with interesting results. Cerebral birth injury is found to be responsible for 68 per cent of convulsions in infants under one month of age. Treatment of this condition is with sedation; spinal, cysternal or ventricular drainage and vitamin K.

In the age group from one month to 36 months, acute infection heads the list, emphasizing the necessity of preventive measures at this age. Tetany is third at this age (1 to 36 mo.) and is most satisfactorily treated with calcium—calcium chloride by mouth (gavage if necessary) and gluconate intravenously.

From three to 16 years of age, idiopathic epilepsy is the cause of as many convulsions as all other factors combined. The treatment in childhood does not differ essentially from that in adult age. I do not need to tell you that the treatment in most cases leaves much to be desired. The careful and intelligent use of the combined principles of fasting, ketogenic diet, acid-ash control and water restriction is worth the burdensome detail it demands of patient, nurse and doctor. Phenobarbital has been a boon to epileptics, but sodium dilantin has certain advantages over it.

Convulsions in adults differ from those in children in being less frequent and having a different significance. It is, perhaps, worthwhile to remember, as Cabot observes, that practically all causes of coma are also causes of convulsions. Notable exceptions are: opium and sunstroke cause coma, rarely if ever convulsions, strychnine and tetanus cause convulsions, rarely if ever coma. The same author, eliminating cases of alcoholism and cerebral hemorrhage as too numerous and indefinite to classify, lists the causes of convulsions in adults in order of frequency, Epilepsy, Uremia, Hysteria, Meningitis and Puerperal Eclampsia.

There is a tendency among neurologists, which seems to me to be commendable, to be slow to diagnose a case as idiopathic epilepsy. To place a patient in this category effectually brings him face to face with the inscription over the entrance to Dantes' Inferno, "All hope abandon, ye who enter here." Since there are those cases, though rare, amenable to treatment, as those of hyperinsulinism whose convulsions are stopped when more sugar is eaten; and the cases of hypothyroidism cured by thyroid extract, there is a ray of hope as long as they have not been seared with the brand "Epilepsy."

It may be worthwhile to enumerate the most important factors to be kept in mind as possible causative agents when confronted with a case of recurring generalized convulsions.

At least two-thirds of such cases have their beginning before the age of twenty. I should be slow to diagnose as epilepsy a case of recurring convulsions beginning after the age of forty.

Heredity, though difficult to evaluate as a factor, must be considered.

Brain injuries suffered at any age may produce organic brain lesions with resulting convulsions.

Congenital abnormalities of the brain as microcephalus hydrocephalus, etc., are possible causes.

Brain Tumor causes convulsions in adults more frequently than in children. In explanation of this, it has been pointed out that in children subtentorial tumors are frequent, while in adults, they are more frequently supratentorial.

Syphilis will, now and then, be found to be the explanation of convulsions occurring first at middle-age or beyond.

Toxic agents may be either endogenous as in uremia or exogenous as lead, strychnine and ergot.

Disturbances of intra-cranial circulation as in Stokes-Adams disease may cause convulsions.

The diagnosis is made in most cases on the age of the patient, history and physical examination. Of course, clinical, laboratory and x-ray examinations are helpful and often necessary. Electro-encephalography opens a promising and fascinating field. Possibly, it will add to our knowledge of cerebral function what the electro-cardiograph has added to that of the heart.

The treatment of convulsions is that of immediate symptomatic relief, (which is important) and that of the cause. While a patient rarely dies in a convulsion, it is reason-

able to believe that the more prolonged and numerous the convulsions, the greater the probability of permanent cerebral damage.

Curiosity prompted me, recently, to read the treatment on convulsions in childhood by eight different well-known pediatricists. They are unanimous only in their recommendation of enemas and bathing. Three advise morphine and one (Peterman) condems it whole-heartedly, stating that it should never be used because it "masks symptoms, depresses the respiratory center and diminishes or stops peristalsis." Holt mentions ether by inhalation while most of the others prefer chloroform. Chloral hydrate and spinal drainage are favored by a majority. Magnesium sulphate by rectum, intramuscularly and intravenously get the nod by about the same number. Other drugs listed are soluble phenobarbital salts, avertin, aspirin, calomel and castor oil.

Perhaps, I should add a word about convulsions resulting from trauma to the brain. We see most of them among the victims of car accidents. Sometimes, they are induced by the injudicious handing of these patients while being transported from the site of accident, or even in being moved in the course of x-ray or other examinations. Sedation with barbiturates, the use of magnesium sulphate intramuscularly or intravenously, hypertonic glucose intravenously and spinal drainage, are approved measures, one or more of which may be required.

BIBLIOGRAPHY

1. Peterman, M. G.: Convulsions in Childhood: A Review of One Thousand Cases, Jour. A. M. A., July 15, 1939.

2. Holt and McIntosh: Diseases of Infancy and Childhood. D. Appleton-Century Company, Eleventh Edition, 1940.

3. Porter and Carter: Management of the Sick Infant. C. V. Mosby Company, Fifth Edition, 1938.

4. Blumer, George: Bedside Diagnosis. W. B Saunders Company, 1928.

5. Fischer, Louis: Diseases of Infancy and Childhood. F. A. Davis Company, Eleventh Edition, 1928.

6. Griffith, J. P. Crozer: The Diseases of Infants and Children. W. B. Saunders Company, Second Edition, 1937.

7. Darrow, Daniel C.: Pediatrics. D. Appleton-Century Company.

8. Kerley, Charles Gilmore: The Practice of Pediatrics. W.B. Saunders Company, Third Edition, 1924.

At the end of the fifth round, the heavyweight staggered to his corner in a dazed and battered condition. His manager approached him and whispered in his ear. "Say, Slugger, I've got a swell idea! Next time he hits you, hit him back!"

Treatment of Burns

JOHN F. BURTON, M.D., F.A.C.S.

OKLAHOMA CITY, OKLAHOMA

Thermal injuries continue to be one of medicine's unsolved problems. Progress has been made in their management, especially in the general treatment of the individual and in definitely establishing good surgical principles in the management of the local areas, but the satisfactory therapeutic measure for all burns has not been found.

For the sake of clarity and at the same time attempting to be concise, I have divided the treatment of burns into the following divisions:

1. First aid treatment of burns.
2. Hospital treatment of recent burns.
3. Hospital treatment of old burns.
4. Treatment to promote closing of epithelial defects—skin grafting.

FIRST AID TREATMENT OF BURNS

The first consideration is an examination of the patient for shock. This must be done before any attempt is made to examine the burn. If the patient is not in shock, treatment of the burn may be instituted. If the patient is in shock, he should receive immediate treatment.

a. Treatment of Shock

The patient should be put completely at rest by placing him in a reclining position with head slightly lowered. The body should be protected by wraps to establish and maintain body heat. The pain should be relieved. No drug is better than morphine, but it must be remembered that it should be given in large doses. One-fourth to one half grain doses hypodermically can be given the average sized adult. It should be repeated when necessary. If the patient is conscious and will swallow, give fluids freely by mouth. Hot coffee, tea and clear bouillon with salt are especially useful. Should plasma be available, it should be given at once, giving 5 cc. per pound of patient's estimated body weight.

b. Treatment of the Burn

This treatment is only for those cases not manifesting shock, or those cases that have responded to appropriate shock treatment.

1. The clothes are carefully opened and if necessary, removed with the idea of determining the degree and the extent of involvement. As treatment is concerned, burns should fall into two divisions, Minor Burns and Major Burns.

2. *Minor Burns* should have thorough scrubbing of the surrounding skin and gradually include the burned areas with plain white soap and water, using plenty of water to wash away all dirt and loose debris. With sterile gloves and instruments, the blisters are opened and all loose skin cut free following with free rinsing with sterile saline solution.

After this cleansing, the treatment may be varied, depending upon the part of the body involved. Such areas as the face, hands, feet and genitals are best treated by some form of sterile oiled gauze and bandage. Recently, I have been using gauze impregnated with 5 per cent sulfathiazole ointment with good success.

Other parts of the body may be treated with 5 per cent tannic acid solution followed with 10 per cent Silver Nitrate Solution producing a quick tanned coagulation.

3. *Major Burns.* As a rule, other than removing any clothing sticking to the burn and cleansing away gross dirt, very little cleansing is recommended for these cases. They should be quickly covered with powdered sulfathiazole and sulfanilamide. Over this is laid a layer of sterile oiled gauze, several layers of plain gauze and then sheet wadding or sterile pads, wrapping the entire dressing with stockinet or elastic bandages and sending on to a hospital.

HOSPITAL TREATMENT OF RECENT BURNS

The initial procedures would be the same as those outlined under First Aid Treatment, and the same precautions as to response to shock treatment before any local treatment is attempted, holds good. In the hospital, oxygen can be used in the management of shock.

When the response to shock is satisfactory, move the patient to a warm room preferably around 80° F.

All attendants should wear caps and masks.

All clothing and dressings are removed and the patient is placed upon a bed made up with sterile sheets and over which is a canopy frame equipped with electric lights to maintain warmth. Over this frame are placed covers as necessary.

Tests are then made to guide the future general treatment before any local treatment is started.

These are complete blood counts including a hematocrit reading and as indicated general treatment can be carried out along with the local treatment.

The attendants scrub up as for a surgical operation and with proper dress and drapes, thoroughly scrub the burned areas with white soap and water, spending as much time as necessary. Gentleness and assurance to the patient will go a long way in obviating an anesthetic. In those cases where the pain is too severe, an anesthetic may be used. After the cleansing, sterile instruments are used to open all blisters and to remove all loose devitalized skin.

The burn is now ready for local treatment. This treatment will vary according to the degree of burn, to the location of the part, the materials at hand and the experiences of the attendant.

The following have been tried and found efficacious:

Face—(1) Continuous, warm, normal saline packs; (2) 5 per cent sulfathiazole ointment gauze and a pressure bandage.

Hands and feet—(1) Continuous, warm, normal saline packs; (2) 5 per cent sulfathiazole ointment gauze with pressure bandage and splints to maintain position of function.

Genitals—(1) 5 per cent sulfathiazole ointment applied after frequent warm saline irrigations.

Arms and legs—(1) 5 per cent sulfathiazole ointment gauze, plenty of padding and pressure bandages, leaving dressing alone for eight to ten days.

Rest of body—(1) 5 per cent Tannic Acid Solution followed with 10 per cent Silver Nitrate Solution.

HOSPITAL TREATMENT OF OLD BURNS

This treatment will vary according to the general condition of the patient, the time elapsed since burn was sustained, and the amount of infection present.

Those patients receiving first aid with the sulfanilamide and sulfathiazole dressing, if seen within the first twenty-four hours from the time of incidence, may receive the treatment of a fresh burn. After that period they are treated as infected burns.

The aims of this treatment are to clear infection and promote healing. To accomplish this sometimes taxes the ingenuity and perseverance of the attendant.

The general condition must be evaluated and such measures as are necessary to re-

store normal physiology, are instituted. These will include adequate diet, fortified with vitamins, administration of liver and iron, blood transfusions and internal chemotherapy.

Locally, we strive to establish normal cleanliness of the surrounding skin and open wounds as rapidly as possible. We use the following: Daily tubbing from 30 minutes to one and one-half hours, drying out for 30 minutes under cradle and light, occasionally using ultra-violet light, then applying 5 per cent sulfathiazole ointment gauze, over which are applied warm normal saline packs. Extremities are kept in position of best function and both active and passive motions are encouraged.

It is surprising how many of these will completely heal. Those cases that do not heal and those cases where the loss of skin is great must receive other treatment.

TREATMENT TO PROMOTE CLOSING OF EPITHELIAL DEFECTS—SKIN GRAFTING

Any burn case, whether received fresh or late, that has not healed within two weeks, must be evaluated and studied relative to therapeutic measures that will be of assistance.

In this evaluation, we must know if the wound is clean and as to whether infection is present; we must know if there are complicating factors interfering with the healing. These would be such conditions as abscesses, general constitutional disease as diabetes and arteriosclerosis, nerve injuries producing trophic effects, and last due to extent and location of pressure ulcers.

Naturally, abscesses would demand incision and drainage; the general diseases should be treated and, when possible, pressure areas should be relieved. The nerve injuries are slow to respond and sometimes have to await regeneration of the nerve.

In the uncomplicated case of an unhealed burn that is clean at the end of two weeks, nothing is of more value than a skin graft. It is our preference to use the intermediate thickness or "Split Skin Graft" for all areas on the body when possible. We feel that this type has the greatest chance for healing. It closes the open wound and if the area is located such as would demand another type of graft later, the latter procedure can be followed in a clean and sterile manner.

What is the age at which the greatest number of deaths occur? In the United States, as constituted today, more persons die at age seventy-one than at any other age, except in the first year of life. In 1939—the latest year for which we have data available—there were 108,-846 deaths of infants under one year of age and about 30,000 deaths of persons at age seventy-one.—Statistical Bulletin, Metropolitan Life Insurance Bulletin.

Patent Ductus Arteriosus: A Report of Two Cases*

FRANK T. JOYCE, M.D.**

CHICKASHA, OKLAHOMA

Although it is difficult to make an exact diagnosis in congenital heart disease and the treatment is very discouraging at best, considerable interest has been aroused since 1938 when Gross[1] successfully ligated a patent ductus arteriosus in a young girl. The operation remedies a defect which, if allowed to remain, may cause retarded physical development, fatal subacute bacterial endocarditis, congestive heart failure, or any combination of these complications.

Congenital heart disease is uncommonly seen and is usually regarded as a medical curiosity for which little or nothing can be done. It is my opinion that in many cases where heart murmurs are discovered in infancy and in childhood, with or without cyanosis, the physician does not attempt to locate the lesion and assumes a negative attitude regarding the treatment. This attitude was not unreasonable in the past but now it can no longer be excused until an uncomplicated patent ductus arteriosus has been excluded. Congenital heart disease consitutes a small percentage of the cases seen by the cardiologist and it is rarely seen by the general practitioner, yet, a patent ductus arteriosus is present in one of every four cases of congenital heart disease. This is somewhat misleading because a patent ductus arteriosus is present as the *only* lesion in but one of every ten cases of congenital heart disease. Abbott[2] made a detailed study of 1,000 cases of congenital heart disease and found that a patent ductus arteriosus was present alone in 92 cases and coexisting with other anomalies in 242 cases. If it can be reasonably established that a patent ductus arteriosus exists alone, then that patient has a good chance to avoid by operation the fatal outcome so frequently seen later on in life. Establishing that fact, however, can be difficult and this is illustrated in one of my cases in which the patent ductus arteriosus acted as a compensatory mechanism for a coarctation of the aorta. The coarctation was not recognized because the cardinal finding was not present, i.e., the patent ductus arteriosus

*Read before the Oklahoma State Internists Society, Chickasha, December 4, 1941.
**Doctor Joyce is now a Lieutenant in the Air Corps and is stationed at San Antonio, Texas.

acted as a safety valve, as it were, not allowing the high systolic blood pressure to exist proximal to the coarctation. The other case is interesting because the patient is markedly under-developed physically and infantilism is one of the indications for ligating a patent ductus arteriosus. In this case, however, there is considerable question as to whether the retarded development is the result of the heart lesion.

In reviewing the embryology and physiology of this defect, it is interesting to note that there is no definitely established time of closure of the ductus arteriosus. Christie[3], in a careful analysis of 558 "normal" cases, found that at the age of eight weeks 88 per cent of the ducts were closed, and at the age of one year 5.6 per cent of the ducts were still open. I have been unable to find any critical studies of this subject in normal children beyond one year of age, but it can be assumed that the remaining few must gradually close within a period of a few years since certainly this congenital defect does not exist in such a large percentage of normal adult individuals.

In considering the pathological physiology, several factors will be reviewed: Burwell[4], et al, were able to make circulation measurements in nine cases which were operated for ligation of the ducts arteriosus. In all of their cases, the ductus measured 7 mm. or more, in diameter. They found that from 45 per cent to 77 per cent of the aortic blood (8.0 to 19.5 liters of blood per minute) was shunted through the patent ductus arteriosus to the pulmonary artery. This large arterio-venous fistula causes the left ventricle to put out from two to four times more blood than the right ventricle. If this loss of blood from the peripheral circulation is great enough, it is easy to understand why many of these patients have a retarded physical development which has been stressed by Gross[5]. The overloading of the pulmonary circuit caused some degree of pulmonary congestion and dilatation of the left auricle in all of those cases when there had not yet developed any clinical signs of congestive failure. Another feature which has been brought forth by the surgical exposure of this defect is the fact that occlusion of the patent ductus arteriosus does not abolish the murmur in many cases. It had been previously thought that the typical continuous murmur with systolic accentuation was produced entirely by the flow of blood through the ductus arteriosus, and its continual nature was caused by the higher pressure existing in the aorta during diastole. That this is often not the case has been demonstrated by several surgeons who have ligated the patent ductus arteriosus. They found that a murmur existing after ligation of the duct could be abolished by compression of the pulmonary artery. In all cases where the ductus is wide enough to produce sufficient findings to make a clinical diagnosis, the pulmonary artery is of greater diameter than the aorta, sometimes it is greatly dilated. It is now believed that the murmur which exists after ligation is caused by eddy currents in the dilated pulmonary artery—and does not, as some believe, prove that another congenital lesion coexists.

The diagnosis is not so difficult to make in an uncomplicated case. Cyanosis does not exist unless there is an associated congenital defect or unless the patient is in cardiac failure. There is a very characteristic continuous (machinery) murmur which is accentuated during systole, and heard best at the second intercostal space on the left. The murmur may be transmitted to the axilla and/or to the apex. Very often there is a distinct systolic thrill over this area. With the above exceptions the other findings are similar to the signs of an aortic insufficiency or a large arterio-venous fistula. There is a high pulse pressure which is affected chiefly by a lowering of the diastolic pressure. In a normal individual, the diastolic pressure is elevated following exercise but in these cases the diastolic pressure is lowered after exercise. There is usually a variable enlargement of the left ventricle. The electrocardiogram shows no specific changes. An X-ray of the chest usually shows an enlargement of the pulmonary artery or a prominence in that area. It is frequently mentioned that the pulmonary arteries pulsate—but the classical "hilar dance" was not present in but one-third of Burwell's cases and was not present in either of my two cases.

The fate of patients with this congenital defect has been summarized by Bullock[6], Jones, and Dalley in a study of 80 cases. These cases were all over three years of age and rarely was difficulty encountered by the patient before the age of six. Twenty-three per cent died of cardiac failure and 53 per cent died of bacterial endocarditis, making a total of 86 per cent dying as a result of their congenital anomaly. Eleven per cent were

dead at the age of 14 years, 50 per cent at the age of 30 years, and 71 per cent at the age of 40 years. Two patients lived to the age of 66 years, one of whom went through eight pregnancies without trouble.

Munro[7], in 1907, suggested that these cases might be benefitted if the patent ductus arteriosus could be ligated but no attempt was made to do this until 1938 when Strieder[8] ligated the ductus in a patient who had subacute bacterial endocarditis. The patient died. In August, 1938, Gross[1] first successfully ligated an uncomplicated patent ductus arteriosus in a seven and one-half year old girl. Since then many cases have been reported in the American literature[9-5-10-4-11-12-13-14] with a total of 33 cases most of them successful but with a few sudden deaths occurring because of hemorrhage when the operation was performed on patients who had subacute bacterial endocarditis at the time. Hubbard[15] has carefully considered the indications for operation and lists the following: (1) To forestall the development of bacterial endocarditis, (2) To prevent the onset of cardiac failure (it should be kept in mind that occasionally a patent ductus arteriosus is a compensatory mechanism for a coexisting pulmonary stenosis, aortic stenosis, or coarctation of the aortic arch), (3) Infantilism or delayed physical development.

Case 1, B.E.H., age 31, was first seen on December 2, 1940, complaining of weakness and anemia of three and one-half years. This patient had always been in good health and worked hard as a farmer until June 7, 1937, when he had severe pain in the left chest. Two days following the onset, he had chills and fever and a diagnosis of malaria was made. He was treated with quinine but did not respond to the drug. The physician who saw him during this first illness stated that the patient did not have a cardiac murmur but that the spleen was palpable. The fever and chills persisted for several weeks and finally another physician discovered a murmur over the pulmonic area. A diagnosis of subacute bacterial endocarditis was made and several blood cultures were done, all but one being negative. One culture was positive for staphylococcus and on that basis he was treated for a staphylococcic endocarditis. He was given anti-staphylococcal serum but in spite of very large doses of the serum the patient continued to have a progressively developing anemia, high fever, and his spleen gradually enlarged. He had several transfusions because of the anemia. In 1939, he was started on sulfapyridine and was given huge doses (the exact doses could not be determined) without any blood level studies. Blood began to appear in the urine and gradually he developed gross hematuria. Sulfapyridine was given over a period of several months and was finally discontinued because of severe nausea.

During the course of his illness he had had some precordial distress and repeated attacks of pleurisy, but he had never had hemoptysis. He later began to have numerous petchia, especially on the legs and face. There was some soreness of the fingers but no abscesses developed. Edema of the legs and face began about eight months before I saw him and had gradually increased. Along with this, there was increasing dyspnea on exertion. The patient had not had a temperature above 100 degrees for eight months prior to the time that he came to me.

The past history is essentially negative. This patient had previously been in good health, did not know that he had ever had anything wrong with his heart, and was able to do hard manual labor without discomfort.

Physical examination: Patient was 74 inches tall, pale, the face was puffy, and his legs were edematous, the weight was 150 pounds. Examination of the head was normal except there were about five petechia in the conjunctiva of the right eye. There was no upper respiratory infection and the teeth were in good shape. Examination of the spine and neck was normal. The chest was well developed, expansion was equal, but there was some dullness in both bases. Breath sounds were normal and there were no rales. The right border of the heart by percussion was 1 cm. to the right of the sternum. The left border was at the left mid-axillary line. The rate was 100 per minute and the rhythm normal. The blood pressure was 135/80. There was a continuous murmur in the second interspace to the left of the sternum. This was transmitted upwards and towards the apex. The murmur was accentuated during systole. The murmur was what is called a "machinery" murmur. The abdomen was distended, the spleen was greatly enlarged, the lower border was beyond the midline to the right. Because of the large spleen it was impossible to determine whether ascites was present. The liver could not be palpated. The remainder of the physical examination was normal except for the previously mentioned edema of the legs and there was questionable clubbing of the fingers. An electrocardiogram was normal except for left axis deviation. The blood counts: Hemoglobin 6½ gms.; white blood cell count 5,200, normal differential; red blood cell count 3,400,-000. The urine contained 4 plus albumin, with gross hematuria, and numerous casts. The serum protein: total 6.93 gms., albumin 3.5 gms., globulin 3.4 gms. A diagnosis of patent ductus arteriosus was made complicated by an endocarditis with apparent recovery, however, right heart failure was present to explain the splenomegalia and the edema of the extremities.

The patient was put to bed and treated for the congestive heart failure which was present. Although the liver and spleen became a great deal smaller and the brawny edema of the legs disappeared, he developed signs of edema due to nephritis with puffy swelling of the face and hands. This became worse and he became comatose. Finally, 18 hours after a convulsion, he expired. Death was attributed to uremia.

AUTOPSY

The autopsy was done on January 23, 1941, two hours after death. The body was well developed and appeared to have been well nourished. There were no external markings or scars. The ears, eyes, nose and mouth appeared normal.

Lungs: There was no fluid in either pleural cavity. Numerous old dense fibrous adhesions on the lateral and basilar surfaces of both lungs held them firmly attached to the chest wall. In addition to those adhesions there were many plaque-like scars varying from 2 to 5 cm. in diameter scattered over the surfaces of both lungs. Cut sections were dry and crepitant but showed several old, healed infarcts. There were no recent infarcts. Other than this, the lungs were normal with no evidence of congestion or cavitation.

Heart: About 30 cc. of straw-colored fluid was present in the pericardial sac. There were no pericardial adhesions. The heart, arch of the aorta and the pulmonary artery were removed in toto and weighed 906 grams. There was moderate hypertrophy of the right ventricle and an enormous hypertrophy of the left ventricle (Fig. 1). There was moderate dilatation of both auricles. The valve circumferences were as follows: tricuspid 13 cm., pulmonary 9 cm., mitral 10.5 cm., and aortic 7 cm. There was no evidence of old healed, or recent valvulitis except that the mitral valve leaflets were definitely thickened at the free margin and the chorda tendinea of those leaflets appeared to be shortened.

The pulmonary artery was 8.5 cm. in circumference and was larger than the aorta which had a circumference of 7.5 cm. There was a patent ductus arteriosus which was located between the bifurcation of the pulmonary artery and the first portion of the descending aorta (Fig. 2). The ductus had a hourglass constriction at its halfway point. The funnel-like opening of the aortic end of the ductus measured 1.3 cm. The similar shaped opening of the ductus into the pul-

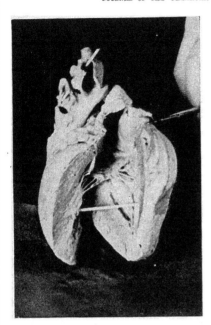

Fig. 1
Showing the enormous hypertrophy of the left ventricle.

monary artery measured 0.9 cm. The lumen of the ductus at the point of constriction was not more than 2 mm. in diameter and would admit an applicator only with difficulty. There was an area 4x3 cm. on the surface of the pulmonary artery where the intima was thickened, scarred and wrinkled. The distal margin of that area was adjacent to the opening of the ductus arteriosus. There were several firm, white warty vegetations crowded around the pulmonary artery opening of the ductus. There was a thin, translucent plaque about 4x6 mm. in the wall of the ductus proximal to the constriction (blood flowed from the aorta to the pulmonary artery). The above described lesions in the pulmonary artery and the ductus constituted the only evidence of inflamation in the heart and great vessels. The aortic valve and pulmonary valve were competent. The ascending aorta and the arch of the aorta appeared normal except for a few atheromatous plaques. However, beginning at the ductus arteriosus the diameter of the descending aorta became smaller and at a point 3 cm. distal to the ductus the circumference of the aorta was only 5 cm.

The myocardium appeared to be normal in color and consistency with no visible evidence of scarring. The left coronary artery was almost twice as large as the right, otherwise, those arteries appeared normal.

Liver: The liver weighed 3284 grams. It was reddish brown in color. On the cut surface, the liver showed the typical nutmeg appearance of passive congestion.

Spleen: The spleen weighed 1359 grams. On the surface the pulp could not be scraped with a knife. No scarred areas were seen.

Kidneys: The left kidney weighed 380 grams. The capsule stripped with ease. On cutting through the substance of the kidney it seemed to be very congested, and numerous small calculi were seen ranging from 0.5 to 2 mm. in diameter. Some of these were present in the pelvis of the kidney. On running the finger across the cut surface of the kidney in some places, it felt gritty. The kidney pelvis was very small. Numerous small hemorrhagic areas could be seen in the cortex and in the medulla. These hemorrhagic changes were more evident in the left kidney than in the right. The right kidney weighed 260 grams and was similar in

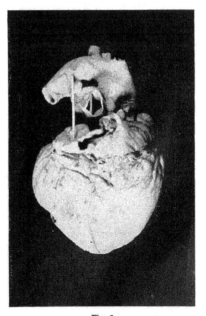

Fig. 2
The heart and vessels as seen from the right. The marked narrowing of the aorta is well shown.

appearance to the left, but no stones were found in the right kidney.

The entire gastro-intestinal tract was not removed from the body, but it appeared to be normal. The pancreas did not appear to be abnormal grossly. The bladder and prostate were not disturbed.

Brain: The brain weighed 1812 grams. There was nothing abnormal in its external appearance except that it was wet and heavy. The brain was cut 11 days after having been fixed in formaldehyde. The convolutions over the cerebral convexities were slightly larger than normal but were not flattened and the sulci were not narrowed. The blood vessels at the base of the brain appeared normal. Palpitation did not reveal any hard areas. Coronal sections were made beginning from the tips of the frontal lobes and extending backwards. At the level of the tips of the anterior horns an area of softening was found in the white matter of the left frontal lobe. This extended backwards almost to the beginning of the posterior horn. It was 7 cm. in diameter. This area was like thin paste and there was no evidence of hemorrhage into it. The blood vessels in and around the lateral ventricles of both hemispheres were congested and quite prominent. The area of softening in the left hemisphere involved the internal capsule and the basal ganglia. The ventricles were not displaced nor flattened. There was no evidence of internal hydrocephalus.

Microscopic Findings: The kidney showed some of the glomeruli to be very large and cellular. The capsules were wide. There were areas of fibrosis with lymphocytic infiltration in the cortex. In some of the tubules red blood cell casts were found. The epithelium in some of the convoluted tubules was low and degenerated. No sulfapyridine crystals were found in the tubules. The liver showed some areas of focal necrosis with round cell infiltration. There were no abscesses. The spleen showed many sinuses filled with blood cells. The lymphfollicles were large.

Final Diagnosis: Patent ductus arteriosus and coarctation of the aorta, healed subacute bacterial endarteritis, chronic passive congestion of the liver and spleen, chronic hemorrhagic nephritis, renal calculi, healed pulmonary infarction (multiple) with fibrous pleural adhesions, and encephalomalacia.

Comment: The enormous hypertrophy of the left ventricle reflects the great amount of work required by the heart to maintain an adequate peripheral circulation in the presence of a patent ductus arteriosus. There is little evidence to indicate that the endarteritis was responsible for this hypertrophy except late in the course of the disease when

the ductus became almost closed leaving the coarctation of the aorta as an etiological factor. The part played by the coarctation in causing the hypertrophy was not very great, however, because the coarctation was not severe and there was no hypertension proximal to the coarctation after the closure of the patent ductus arteriosus. It seems reasonable that the resistance to the circulation offered by the coarctation, little as it may have been, did cause a larger blood flow through the ductus than would otherwise have occurred, thus placing some additional load on the left ventricle. There is no question that a patent ductus arteriosus may be a compensatory mechanism for a coarctation of the aorta, stenosis of the pulmonary artery, or stenosis of the aorta proximal to the ductus resulting in a reverse flow of blood from the pulmonary artery to the aorta (fetal type), however, in the latter two conditions cyanosis would probably be present depending upon the severity of the stenosis. It follows that if a coexisting stenosis of the great vessels is present then ligating the ductus would throw a greater load on the heart and may hasten death.

The endarteritis being confined almost entirely to the ductus and pulmonary artery explains the numerous healed pulmonary infarcts and pleural adhesions. No emboli could reach the peripheral circulation without first passing through the pulmonary circuit. This occurs in almost all cases of this type. The vegetations are confined to the pulmonary artery. This process is just the opposite to the usual case of bacterial endocarditis where the vegetations occur primarily on the mitral valve and in the left side of heart, resulting in peripheral abscesses due to infected emboli being carried away. This man never had any lesions to suggest peripheral abscesses, even when he was having frequent pulmonary infarctions.

Although the large doses of sulfapyridine apparently cured the endarteritis, at least there was no evidence of activity for eight months prior to death and at autopsy the vegetations appeared old and healed, the kidneys suffered tremendously because of it. Though he had been acutely ill for many months before sulfapyridine was given, he had never noticed hematuria. Soon after the drug was started he had hematuria almost constantly until he died—and long after sulfapyridine was stopped. Helwig[16] has recently suggested that permanent kidney damage may result from the use of the sulfonamide drugs, and it seems in this case that the hemorrhagic nephritis was not on the basis of embolic phenomena as is usually present with bacterial endocarditis.

The patient had consented to have the

patent ductus arteriosus ligated and was anxiously awaiting some improvement in his general condition so that the operation could be more safely done. Instead of improving he died of nephritis with associated softening of the brain. At autopsy the very thin translucent wall of the ductus was discovered. This thin wall probably could not have been recognized during life and any attempt at ligation would probably have caused immediate rupture and death from hemorrhage. Several months before death he developed congestive right heart failure with enlargement of. the liver and spleen. This may have occurred regardless of whether the ductus was ligated.

In conclusion, it seems safe to say that this man's death was caused by a complication of the treatment for a bacterial endarteritis which in turn was a complication of a patent ductus arteriosus. Had the ligation been done early in life at least the contributing cause of death would have been removed. In retrospect, it seems likely that he could have lived with the coarctation of the aorta since many patients live longer than he did with more severe coarctation. Congestive hear failure may have been forestalled but, of course, it is not assumed that it would not have eventually developed.

Case 2, B.J.S., age six, was first seen on March 2, 1941, because of a temperature of 100 degrees and a history of a severe sore throat and high fever of several days duration. She made an uneventful recovery from this throat infection. On examination, it was suspected that the child had a patent ductus arteriosus. The mother states that the delivery was normal, she was breast fed, and nothing abnormal was noted at birth except that the baby was short. She weighed 8¾ pounds, and the weight gain at first was normal. When the child was about three or four months old, the mother, who is a nurse, noticed that the baby's heart was pounding.

She was seen by a pediatrician at the age of two because of her small stature, and at that time a diagnosis of congenital heart disease was made. It was thought by him that the diagnosis was a patent foramen ovale. The small stature was though to be on the basis of a thyroid deficiency, and she was given thyroid medication for a period of two years. During that two year period, there was no spectacular gain in height or weight. This child has not been ill except when she was two and one-half years old when she had pneumonia which lasted for three days. She has never had heart failure and is able to run and play without any limitations. She is of average intelligence and is doing well in school.

The physical examination at the age of

six and one-half years: Weight is 40 pounds, and the height is 39½ inches with shoes. The child is well proportioned and resembles a pituitary dwarf. Examination of the head, the eyes, the ears, nose and throat elicited no abnormal findings. The neck and spine were normal. The chest is normal in shape and expansion is equal. Both lungs are clear. The heart: The left border is at the left midclavicular line and there is no enlargement to the right. There is no cyanosis and no evidence of right heart failure. Her blood pressure is 110/40, and the pulse rate is 80, rhythm normal. There is a loud continuous murmur located in the second interspace to the left of the sternum. This is transmitted in all directions. It is a typical "machinery murmur" with accentuation during systole. There is a palpable thrill over the area where the murmur is most intense. The electrocardiogram is normal and an X-ray of the chest indicates that the heart and great vessels are normal. There is no visible pulsation of the pulmonary artery (hilar dance). The abdomen is normal. A diagnosis of a pure, uncomplicated patent ductus

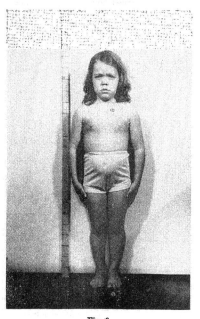

Fig. 3

Case 2, B. J. S. Now 7½ years old. Height 41 inches. The circle on the chest is where the "machinery murmur" is loudest.

arteriosus, and dwarfism, probably a pitui-tary type, was made.

Comment: There is a reasonable question whether the retarded physical development is related to the patent ductus arteriosus since her stature is similar to that type seen in pituitary dwarfism rather than the asthenic type which is usually present when a patent ductus arteriosus is the etiological factor.

The diagnosis of patent ductus arteriosus was confirmed at a well known clinic in the midwest where she was referred to have the ductus ligated. The operation, however, was not advised, the only reason given was that she should be observed for a time—now, almost a year. Regardless of the etiology of the dwarfism which in itself will not shorten her life, there remains the very likely possibility that she will develop subacute bacterial endocarditis sooner or later. In patients who do not have, or, have not had this usually fatal complication, the operative risk is not great. Every sore throat and upper respiratory infection is an obvious invitation to the development of subacute bacterial endocarditis in her present condition. An unfortunate aspect of this case is that the parents returned home firmly convinced that the operation will never have to be done.

Conclusion: The successful closure of a patent ductus arteriosus has been accomplished by ligation in a number of reported cases. This outstanding surgical contribution now affords a positive therapeutic measure for many patients with this disease who are otherwise almost certainly doomed to premature death or maldevelopment. Two cases have been presented: One to illustrate what may happen to such a patient without having the operation done, the other is presented as an unusual case of dwarfism with a patent ductus arteriosus who should have the operation done.

BIBLIOGRAPHY

1. Gross, Robert E., and Hubbard, John P.: Surgical Ligation of a Patent Ductus Arteriosus, J.A.M.A., 112: 729, 1939.
2. Abbott, Maude E.: Atlas of Congenital Cardiac Disease, American Heart Association, 1936, New York.
3. Christie, Amos: Normal Closing Time of the Foramen Ovale and the Ductus Arteriosus, Am. J. Dis. Child., 40: 323-328, 1938.
4. Burwell, C. S., Eppinger, E. C., and Gross, R. E.: Tr A. Am. Physicians, 55: 71-79, 1940.
5. Gross, R. E.: Experiences with the Surgical Treatment in Ten Cases of Patent Ductus Arteriosus, J.A.M.A., 115: 1257, 1940.
6. Bullock, Lewis T., Jones, John C., and Dolley, Frank S.: J. Pediatrics, 115: 786-801, 1939.
7. Munro, J. C.: Ligation of the Ductus Arteriosus, Ann. Surgery, 46: 335, 1907.
8. Graybiel, Ashton, Strieder, J. W., and Boyer, N. H.: An Attempt to Obliterate the Patent Ductus Arteriosus in a Patient with Subacute Bacterial Endocarditis, Am. Heart J., 15: 621, 1938.
9. Jones, John C., Dalley, Frank S., and Bullock, Lewis T.: The Diagnosis and Surgical Therapy of Patent Ductus Arteriosus, J. Thoracic Surg., 9: 413-430, 1940.
10. Touroff, Arthur S. W., and Vessell, Harry: Experiences in the Surgical Treatment of Streptococcus Viridans Endarteritis Complicating Patent Ductus Arteriosus, J. Thoracic Surg., 10: 59-83, 1940.
11. Miangiolarra, C. W., and Hull, Edgar: Successful Ligation of Patent Ductus Arteriosus, Surgery, 9: 597-602, 1941.
12. Gale, J. W., Pohle, F. J., and Romaine, Hunter: Successful Ligation of Patent Ductus Arteriosus, Wisconsin M. J., 40: 296-298, 1941.
13. Gebauer, Paul W., and Nichol, A. D.: Ligation of the Patent Ductus Arteriosus, Ohio State M. J., 37: 538-543, 1941.
14. Touroff, A. S. W., Vessell, Harry, and Chashoff, Julius: Operative Cure of Subacute Streptococcus Viridans Endarteritis Superimposed on Patent Ductus Arteriosus, J.A.M.A., 118: 890-892, 1942.
15. Hubbard, John P., Emerson, Paul W., and Green, Hyman: Indications for the Surgical Ligation of a Patent Ductus Arteriosus, New England J Med., 221: 481-485, 1939.
16. Hellwig, C. Alexander, and Reed, H. Lester: Fatal Anuria Following Sulfadiazine Therapy, J A.M A., 119. 561-563, 1942.

A Radiologist's Viewpoint In the Treatment of Some Common Diseases*

EDWARD D. GREENBERGER, M.D.**

MCALESTER, OKLAHOMA

In the past two decades, irradiation therapy of physiological and pathological diseases and dysfunctions has expanded so rapidly in every specialty of medicine, that the average physician has not been able to assimilate or get acquainted with the multiple uses of this therapy. The radiologists as a group have been backward in their endeavors to inform their colleagues in their respective communities of the uses of X-Ray and radium irradiation as a supplement or compliment to their usual therapeutic measures. Perhaps it has been the thought or discomfort of being accused of-competing with his colleagues that is responsible for this reticent attitude. The radiologist's approach in the past has therefore been "let me demonstrate the value of

*Read before the Pittsburg County Medical Society, September, 1942
**Doctor Greenberger is now in the Army and is stationed at Carlisle Barracks, Pa.

irradiation therapy in this particular case." The teaching process has therefore been necessarily slow, but these personal demonstrations have helped to place irradiation therapy on a conservative and sure footing in the community served by the radiologist.

In the following paragraphs, this radiologist expresses his viewpoint on the treatment of some of the more common diseases, as tonsillitis, sinusitis, hyperthyroidism, inflammatory lesions, benign uterine bleeding, carcinoma of the breast and womb. Each unrelated subject is presented in the style or manner that I would use in writing or talking to one of my colleagues in my community who consulted me in regard to the particular subject.

CARCINOMA OF THE BREAST

Carcinoma of the breast is either a surgical problem or essentially a radiological problem. In Group one cases, where the tumor is confined to the breast, radical mastectomy is indicated. No definite improvement in results can be expected by pre or post operative irradiation. In Group three cases, where more than two axillary glands larger than two centimeters are present, and the skin over the breast is fixed or involved by the tumor, a radical mastectomy will tend to hasten the patient's death rather than aid in recovery. Such patients should be treated by irradiation alone. In Group two cases, where only a few minute axillary glands are present and the skin is not involved, pre-operative and post-operative X-Ray irradiation will increase the number of five year survivals.

There is no place for a simple mastectomy in treatment of carcinoma of the breast, even for palliation in a foul ulcerating lesion. X-Ray irradiation will clean up such ulcerating lesions easier and better than surgery.

In Group two cases, it is advisable to have roentgen studies of the entire spine, pelvis and chest before the mastectomy in order to detect any possible metastasis.

CARCINOMA OF THE CERVIX

This is entirely a radiological problem. An amputation of the cervix can be done in the rare Group one cases, but the surgeon can't be sure that there is not already a lymphatic spread to the fornix and adnexa. The radical Wertheim hysterectomy is definitely contraindicated in the treatment of cancer of the cervix.

Radium therapy is the most valuable agent in treating all types of cancer of the cervix. It should be applied only by a physician who understands the necessity and importance of distributing the radium so as to obtain the most effective dosage in the vaginal fornices and adnexa and within the cervix and body of the uterus of the particular case treated. Radium thus properly distributed in the vagina and womb will destroy the carcinoma in the cervix and in the adjacent parametrium for about three to four centimeters. If a cure is desired in Group two and three patients where the adnexa are involved, a series of deep X-Ray treatments given over the pelvis through multiple ports must supplement the radium therapy.

TUMORS OF THE UTERUS

An endometrial biopsy should be performed on every woman with abnormal uterine bleeding a few years before, at, or beyond the menopause, and a radium tandem inserted in the womb after the curretage. A dosage of 1500-2400 mg/hrs. of radium should be given if the scrapings look benign, a dosage of about 3600 mg/hrs. if carcinoma is suspected.

If the biopsy confirms the clinical impression of a carcinoma of the fundus of the uterus, then a radical hysterectomy is performed about five to six weeks after the radium therapy. This combined treatment of radium and surgery will cure a larger number of patients with fundus cancer than when surgery is used without preliminary irradiation.

Radium therapy alone is used in treatment of fundus cancer only when the patient is considered a poor risk for hysterectomy. By distributing the radium evenly throughout the fundus by means of multiple tandems and thus administering large doses, many cures by radium therapy alone are obtained.

BENIGN UTERINE BLEEDING

(a) Due to Fibroid Uterus.

Hysterectomy is the treatment of choice in all large uterine tumors and most small tumors. Surgery definitely determines whether the tumor is uterine or ovarian, whether it is benign or malignant.

If the diagnosis of fibroid can be definitely determined and the uterus is less than four months gestation in size, external irradiation alone or combined with intra uterine radium therapy will promptly stop the bleeding and later cause a marked regression in the size of the uterus and fibroid tumor. The same therapy is used with only fair results in the large fibroid uterus and therefore used only in patients who are poor surgical risks.

(b) Due to Endocrine Dysfunction.

I do not believe that any surgeon should perform a hysterectomy on a young woman with a normal size uterus and normal adnexa because of her profuse menstrual bleeding. When the proper endocrine preparations fail, a small dose of radium applied within the womb (about 500 mg/hrs.) will stop the bleeding promptly, and in most cases will not cause any permanent damage to the ovaries.

When the abnormal bleeding is due to menopausal changes, external irradiation to the pelvis is the ideal treatment to permanently stop the uterine hemorrhage.

HYPERTHYROIDISM

Is X-Ray irradiation for hyperthyroidism preferable to thyroidectomy? Many radiologists claim that irradiation is the better treatment for hyperthyroidism except in those patients who have large tumors sufficient to cause pressure symptoms and those who are extremely toxic with B.M.R. of about 70 plus.

Many good statistical papers have ben presented by these radiologists. Their percentage of cures run about 80 to 85 per cent. Most surgeons doubt these figures, and feel that surgery should be done on all toxic thyroids.

I feel that thyroidectomy performed by an experienced surgeon is preferable to irradiation therapy, but irradiation is far superior to bungled thyroid surgery. A patient with a B.M.R. of over 35 requires strict bed rest and supervision. The surgeon is the one who can enforce such proceedures, the radiologist can not.

The hyperthyroid patient usually referred to me by my colleagues for irradiation therapy are patients (1) whose B.M.R. is less than 35, not toxic enough to require an operation, (2) recurrence of toxic symptoms following thyroidectomy, (3) patients with some systemic disease where surgery is considered inadvisable and (4) those who refuse any surgery.

NASAL SINUSITIS

In those cases of acute sinusitis where no relief from pain is obtained by the usual therapeutic measures, the application of one or two small doses of X-Ray irradiation will often produce prompt relief from the severe headaches.

Irradiation therapy is a real adjunct in the better management of those cases of sub-acute and chronic sinusitis who continue to have pain and purulent discharge in spite of proper topical nasal applications and surgical drainage of the affected sinuses. In over 60 per cent of the cases treated with X-Ray, a marked prompt clinical improvement or cure can be expected. The roentgen rays act directly on the inflamed edematous or hypertrophic mucosa.

The dose usually administered is about two-thirds of an erythema dose delivered in one to four treatments.

The results of X-Ray irradiation in the treatment of chronic sinusitis with large polypoid formation is not good. The Caldwell-Luc or similar operation is the better therapy in these cases. X-Ray irradiation is of little value in allergic sinusitis.

Irradiation therapy is the simplest and the best proceedure in the treatment of sub-acute and chronic sinusitis in children. Medical management is usually difficult and surgical drainage usually inadvisable in children. The percentage of cures in children thus treated are much higher than in adults.

TONSILLITIS

A few years ago, several popular magazines extolled the virtues of X-Ray treatment for chronic tonsillitis. The radiologists subsequently received many requests from patients who desired this non-operative form of therapy. To have accepted all these patients for such therapy would have invited just criticism from the otolaryngologist and general practitioner. I feel that the radiologist has a useful role in the management of certain cases of tonsillitis without competing with the otolaryngologist and general practitioner.

Tonsillectomy is the simplest and best proceedure in the treatment of chronic tonsillitis in children. In twenty-four hours, the child is ready to partake of its regular diet. If there is a marked or moderate enlargement of the tonsillar and cervical glands associated with the tonsillitis, X-Ray irradiation of the glands should preceed the tonsillectomy. A small single dose of X-Ray will cause a rapid decrease or a disappearance of the glands within ten days. The radiologist receives excellent cooperation from the otolaryngologist in treating such cases.

Many physicians procrastinate in performing a tonsillectomy for badly infected tonsils in children below three years of age. Otitis media is a frequent complication in such cases. A few small doses of X-Ray applied to the tonsil area in these youngsters will cause the pain, swelling, dysphagia, and the infection in the tonsil to disappear. The tonsillectomy can be done when the child is older.

In contrast to children, an adult who undergoes a tonsillectomy usually continues to have a sore throat and malaise for several days after the operation. This is especially true in the elderly individual. In this group of patients, X-Ray irradiation to the tonsils produces results comparable to tonsillectomy without the associated discomfort. The dose administered is about an erythema dose (500-600 r) to each side, applied in three to four treatments.

Irradiation therapy is preferable to tonsillectomy in all cases where the tonsillar or lymph tissue is scattered on the pillars, tongue, and adjacent pharyngeal wall. The lymphoid tissue is very responsive to the small doses of X-Ray, and the tonsil tissue in these cases disappears completely.

. Irradiation is of value in recurrent tonsillitis following tonsillectomy. X-Ray irradiation is the treatment for patients who have bleeding tendencies, and others who can not undergo a tonsillectomy.

INFLAMMATIONS

X-Ray irradiation is the most effective tool that the physician can use in the treatment of his patients with single or multiple boils and carbuncles, particularly those located on the face, back of neck, auditory canal, and axilla. If applied early, X-Ray causes resolution without suppuration. When applied to the full blown lesion, X-Ray causes the lesion to point and thus permit early drainage.

X-Ray therapy is most effective in all inflammatory lesions of the skin, in cellulitis, lymphangitis, and erysipelas, and associated infectious adenitis.

It is the ideal treatment in acute parotitis the gland either subsides or it becomes fluctuant in two or three days and thus ready for surgical drainage. The application of radium or X-Ray irradiation to an acute parotitis that follows some abdominal operation is often life saving.

NEURITIS AND NEURALGIA

Any agent that can relieve or stop completely the severe pain in many of the patients afflicted with neuritis or neuralgia is worth a good trial. X-Ray irradiation directed to the involved roots or nerves accomplishes such clinical improvement and cures in many cases, and therefore should be used before any nerve block or nerve resection is contemplated. I have had fairly good results in treating trigeminal neuralgias, peripheral facial nerve neuralgia, and herpes zoster, with X-Ray irradiation. Also, a large percentage of cases with functional pruitis of the anus or vulva are relieved or cured by irradiation.

CONCLUSION

The reason for this unorthodox type of paper is to enable me to present a summary on the management of some common and important diseases—from a radiologist's viewpoint. I purposely included three highly controversial subjects—hyperthyroidism, tonsillitis, and sinusitis. Irradiation therapy has a definite place in the treatment of these diseases. The type of cases suitable for such therapy have been briefly outlined.

I hope this paper serves as a guide to some physicians and surgeons by enabling them to evaluate the aid they can expect from irradiation therapy in their management of the diseases discussed.

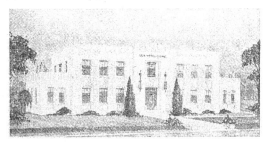

• THE PRESIDENT'S PAGE •

Office for Emergency Management
WAR MANPOWER COMMISSION
Washington, D. C.

Procurement and Assignment Service for
Physicians, Dentists, and Veterinarians .

November 30, 1942

James D. Osborn, M.D.
President, Oklahoma State Medical Association
Frederick, Oklahoma

Dear Doctor Osborn:

On behalf of the Directing Board of the Procurement and Assignment Service, I wish to express to the Oklahoma State Medical Society its sincere thanks and appreciation for the loan of Mr. Richard H. Graham to work in our Central Office. Mr. Graham did an excellent piece of work with us, and we deeply appreciate his services.

It is gratifying to learn that the State Medical Societies are cooperating in every way possible, and I want you to know that the Procurement and Assignment Service in Oklahoma is doing an excellent job.

With kind regards and many thanks, I am

Sincerely yours,

Frank H. Lahey, M.D.
Chairman, Directing Board

(President's comment: The above letter is self-explanatory, and the commendation of our Executive Secretary will not be surprising to any member of the State Medical Association. The service to the Procurement and Assignment Service of the War Manpower Commission is in line with Oklahoma's response to Procurement and Assignment, and the State Medical Association is proud to have had this opportunity to serve.)

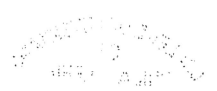

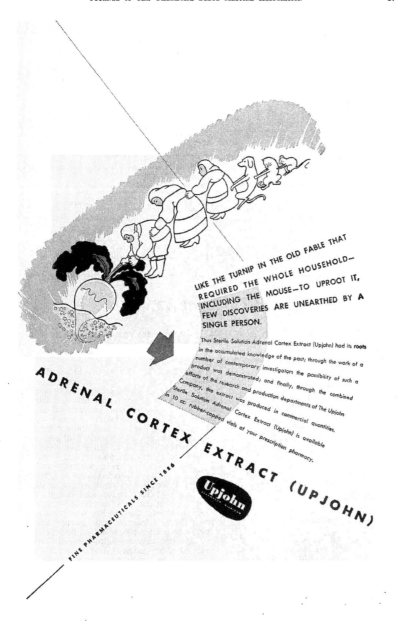

LIKE THE TURNIP IN THE OLD FABLE THAT REQUIRED THE WHOLE HOUSEHOLD— INCLUDING THE MOUSE—TO UPROOT IT, FEW DISCOVERIES ARE UNEARTHED BY A SINGLE PERSON.

Thus Sterile Solution Adrenal Cortex Extract (Upjohn) had its **roots** in the accumulated knowledge of the past; through the work of a number of contemporary investigators the possibility of such a product was demonstrated; and finally, through the combined efforts of the research and production departments of The Upjohn Company, the extract was produced in commercial quantities. Sterile Solution Adrenal Cortex Extract (Upjohn) is available in 10 cc. rubber-capped vials at your prescription pharmacy.

ADRENAL CORTEX EXTRACT (UPJOHN)

FINE PHARMACEUTICALS SINCE 1886

Upjohn

The JOURNAL Of The
OKLAHOMA STATE MEDICAL ASSOCIATION

EDITORIAL BOARD

L. J. MOORMAN, Oklahoma City, Editor-in-Chief

E. EUGENE RICE, Shawnee

NED R. SMITH, Tulsa

MR. R. H. GRAHAM, Oklahoma City, Business Manager

CONTRIBUTIONS: Articles accepted by this Journal for publication including those read at the annual meetings of the State Association are the sole property of this Journal.

The Editorial Department is not responsible for the opinions expressed in the original articles of contributors.

Manuscripts may be withdrawn by authors for publication elsewhere only upon the approval of the Editorial Board.

MANUSCRIPTS: Manuscripts should be typewritten, double-spaced, on white paper 8½ x 11 inches. The original copy, not the carbon copy, should be submitted.

Footnotes, bibliographies and legends for cuts should be typed on separate sheets in double space. Bibliography listing should follow this order: Name of author, title of article, name of periodical with volume, page and date of publication.

Manuscripts are accepted subject to the usual editorial revisions and with the understanding that they have not been published elsewhere.

NEWS: Local news of interest to the medical profession, changes of address, births, deaths and weddings will be gratefully received.

ADVERTISING: Advertising of articles, drugs or compounds unapproved by the Council on Pharmacy of the A.M.A. will not be accepted. Advertising rates will be supplied on application.

It is suggested that members of the State Association patronize our advertisers in preference to others.

SUBSCRIPTIONS: Failure to receive The Journal should call for immediate notification.

REPRINTS: Reprints of original articles will be supplied at actual cost provided request for them is attached to manuscripts or made in sufficient time before publication. Checks for reprints should be made payable to Industrial Printing Company, Oklahoma City.

Address all communications to THE JOURNAL OF THE OKLAHOMA STATE MEDICAL ASSOCIATION, 210 Plaza Court, Oklahoma City.

OFFICIAL PUBLICATION OF THE OKLAHOMA STATE MEDICAL ASSOCIATION
Copyrighted January, 1943

EDITORIALS

THE VALUE OF COD LIVER OIL AND TOMATO JUICE IN THE PREVENTION AND TREATMENT OF INTESTINAL TUBERCULOSIS COMPLICATING PULMONARY TUBERCULOSIS*

The family physician occupies a singular and important position in the treatment of pulmonary tuberculosis. It is he who treats the majority of tuberculosis patients for weeks or months before sanatorium care is available. Experience has taught us that intestinal tuberculosis frequently develops during this period. As it is the most frequent, and one of the most serious, complications of pulmonary tuberculosis, it seems worthwhile to emphasize a simple, effective means of prevention and treatment which can be employed in the humblest household.

Intestinal tuberculosis was generally regarded as a fatal complication of pulmonary tuberculosis prior to 1921. In that year, Blanchet demonstrated that ultra-violet irradiation was a valuable method of treatment, and his findings were confirmed by other workers. There were, however, certain disadvantages to the general application of this form of therapy, including the cost of the apparatus and the need for electrical installation.

Therefore, in 1926, we sought an effective method of treatment which could be used in any home or sanatorium. For reasons stated elsewhere, cod liver oil and either tomato or citrus fruit juice were administered to patients suffering from intestinal tuberculosis. These studies disclosed that the administration of the remedy, as here outlined, was more effective in the treatment of intestinal tuberculosis than ultra-violet irradiation; the patients responding more promptly and in greater numbers. This led to the routine use of the "cocktail" in treating intestinal tuberculosis at Ray Brook and many other sanatoria both in this country and abroad.

Subsequently, the remedy was tried as a prophylactic measure with gratifying results. For example, prior to its use as a prophylactic measure, approximately eleven per cent of our patients with moderately and far advanced pulmonary tuberculosis developed intestinal tuberculosis while under observation; whereas, subsequent to its routine administration, the incidence fell to one per cent, and has remained at that low level for the past fourteen years.

*This editorial was contributed by Dr. Mack McConkey of Ray Brook, New York. Dr. McConkey is an honored son of Oklahoma whose cod liver oil cocktail, now widely employed in this country and abroad, has saved much suffering and prolonged many lives.

The method of administration is simple and few patients object seriously to the remedy when it is properly given, but attention to detail is important. Three ounces of tomato, or cirtus fruit, juice are placed in a glass about half the size of an ordinary tumbler. On the surface is floated half an ounce (a large tablespoonful) of plain cod liver oil. The "cocktail" is chilled and served immediately after each meal. The patient should be told that slight gaseous eructations savoring of cod liver oil may be experienced for the first week or so of treatment, but that they will not be noticed thereafter. In certain instances, it is necessary to substitute cod liver oil in ten minim capsules for the usual half-ounce of oil for a week or so. Patients suffering with intestinal symptoms are given one quart of milk daily in addition to the "cocktail."

SILENCE AND SUNSHINE

In the year 1847, Kussmal was studying at the University of Vienna. Much of his time was spent "in the small, poorly equipped morgue" where the great pathologist, Rokitansky was making his daily contributions to our knowledge of gross pathology and building his astounding record of 30,000 autopsies.

Kussmaul left the following interesting picture of Rokitansky. If the reader permits his imaginatiton to flow between the lines of this paragraph, he will sense the motivating principles in the lives of these two great men.

"The facial features of Rokitansky bore the stamp of great kindness of heart and of dependableness. Everyone respected him. He was extraordinarily silent. In the morgue he opened his mouth only to dictate the protocol. After I had been a constant visitor at the morgue for four months, it happened one beautiful autumn morning that the scalpel rested for a short period. I took advantage of the short recess by stepping to the door in order to enjoy the fresh air. Soon after Rokitansky came and stood near me in the sunlight, which he enjoyed noticeably. Suddenly he turned toward me, greeted me pleasantly, and said: 'This is nice weather.' I was dumbfounded. Had the daughter of Jairus suddenly arisen from the dead and come to me from the morgue with a loud greeting I would not have been more surprised. I composed myself, however, and answered: 'Yes, this certainly is a nice day.' The conversation was finished. It was the first and only conversation in which I heard him take part."

OUR STATE MEDICAL ASSOCIATION

Among the institutions to which we as doctors and good citizens owe allegiance stands the State Medical Association. While the church stands for religious freedom and fosters the moral and spiritual integrity of the home, the State Medical Association represents the orthodox practice of medicine without which the physical welfare of the home would be insecure.

In this day of organization for political and economic preferment often at the expense of those who are passive or disinterested, it is time for doctors to stand by the one organization which champions their legitimate cause. The State Medical Association is not asking any favors or seeking any advantages which are not in keeping with the public weal. For its members, it merely seeks the privilege of continuing the individual practice of medicine as it has always been carried on in the United States and as it should be pursued in every free country. All doctors who are interested in their professional freedom and the physical welfare of their people should liberally support the State Medical Association.

During the war, this responsibility rests heavily upon those doctors who remain at home. Our professional way of life must be preserved. We must keep the faith with those who face the guns. Through organized effort, we must take care of the civilian needs and save a place for those members of our profession who wish to return to civil practice. We must find a solution for all our local problems and thereby relieve the Federal Government and big industry of the excuse for various government and pre-paid group services which rob the doctor of personal dignity and initiative, making him a kin to the inanimate cog in the so-called wheel of progress.

These ends can be achieved only through organized effort directed by the State Medical Association. This means keeping up membership in the State Association even though dues have been increased: also, ready response to every call for service including faithful attendance upon committees and scheduled county and state meetings.

In addition, every member, through his professional and public relationship, should strive to bring medicine into popular esteem. Only through the loyalty and integrity of its individual members can the State Medical Association attain the high position it deserves and wield the influence necessary to protect the doctor and society from the devastating influence of regimented medicine.

THE DOCTOR'S REWARD

Everywhere from the smart-set to the slums, the honest, capable doctor is welcome. Regardless of the social or economic level, he seeks only the truth and the opportunity to serve. He is never too seedy for the fastidious, never too polished for the poor.

The sun and the moon stand still when the doctor is urgently needed. His arrival is a signal for people to give way and humbly stand by because of his unobtrusive authority.

There are moments in the mansion when the doctor takes precedent over the most important social and financial events. There are crises in the slums which shatter all class distinctions and call for the best medicine can give. To come natural to people and to be sought by all classes, when trouble strikes, means more than silver and gold.

THE ALPHABET ABUSED

The innocent old alphabet never anticipated spelling "bureaucrat" and submitting to the flagrant abuse of its modest characters through the capitalized designation of government bureaucracies. The word "Bureaucrat" does not appear in Samuel Johnson's Dictionary (1799). He describes bureau as "a chest of drawers with a writing desk."

The Encyclopedia Brittanica says the term bureau "is used of certain subdivisions of the executive departments" and goes on to say "the term bureaucracy signifies the concentration of administrative power in bureaux of departments, and the undue interference of officials outside the scope of state interference."

Webster gives the following definition of bureaucracy: "a system of government by bureau heads, responsible only to administrative officers above them, having complete power over subordinates and, in official duties generally, not subject to the common law of the land." Webster says a bureaucrat is "an official confirmed in a narrow and arbitrary routine or established with great authority in his own department; a member of a bureaucracy."

Under his definition of bureau, Samuel Johnson quotes Swift as saying:

"For not the desk with silver nails,

Nor bureau of expense,

Nor standish well Japaun'd avails

To writing of good sense."

Our American application of the word bureau has not absolved it from Swift's criticism. The exercise of good sense is not a distinguishing mark of the bureaucrat. About 1805, the statesman, Fisher Ames said: "It is party that bestows emolument, power and consideration, and it is not excellency in the science that obtains the suffrages of party."

The regular medical profession, always in search of the truth, has never been guilty of embarrassing the alphabet. Science is truth, it thrives on silence and obscurity, it is eternal, it seeks no fan-flare, but is content to appear in small type in order that it may find room among the world's treasures.

The search for knowledge in the field of medical science and its practical application are incompatable with bureaucratic control and can never click with the clock on any fixed hourly basis.

It is to be hoped that medicine may escape the leveling influence of the cold impersonal, arbitrary control of bureaucracy. Voluntary service, free initiative and independent action constitute the doctor's chief ailment. Without these, medicine will become an anemic, spiritless profession incapable of sustaining its fine traditions.

The people must be permitted to judge the inequalities of medical skill and professional virtue. They must have the privilege of choice. The medical profession should not be humiliated by bureaucratic control with an alphabetical designation. Already bureaucratic blanks coming out of Washington with enigmatic books of instruction are giving the average citizen who would like to be about his country's business, an obdurate headache, which destroys his equanimity and devours his initiative.

As the honest doctor contemplates socialized medicine, with its annulling thralldom, he thinks of the free spirit of Patrick Henry with glowing admiration. He wonders if medicine should not take a stand, not so much in behalf of a great profession, but for the welfare of a free people, who in the face of government concern, must be born, must encounter the ills of the flesh and ultimately die. These are intimate, personal experiences, sacred to the individual and the home and, as a rule, shared only by trusted and privileged medical and spiritual advisors.

(Since the above editorial was written a hard-working doctor-friend has reported that, while seeking a C gasoline card, he appealed to a Washington representative of the Gasoline Rationing Bureau and received the following response: "Oh, yes, you are one of these doctors, who expect everything and give nothing." This agent of the bureaucrats, who is wholly dependent upon the taxpayers for a living, was insulting a good citizen whose service to the poor annually runs into thousands of dollars.)

"I congratulate poor young men upon being born to that ancient and honorable degree which renders it necessary that they should devote themselves to hard work."—Andrew Carnegie.

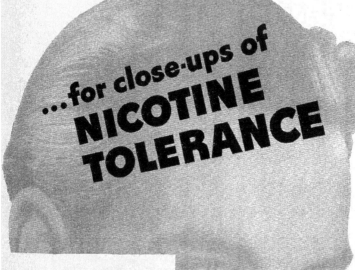

ASSOCIATION ACTIVITIES

FIRST MEMBER OF ASSOCIATION KILLED IN ACTION

Word has been received of the loss in action of Captain James C. Smith of Ardmore. Doctor Smith was associated with the Hardy Sanitarium and, while living in Ardmore, served as the Secretary of the Carter County Medical Society until entering the military service.

Doctor Smith was a graduate of the Harvard Medical School, and entered the Medical Reserve Corps as a First Lieutenant February 13, 1941. He was subsequently promoted to Captain in March of 1942. He was killed during a bombing raid on September 9 somewhere in New Guinea. His death is the first

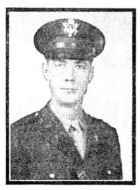

1907-1942

among members of the Association serving in the military forces, however, one other member is reported missing in action and is believed to be a prisoner of the Japanese.

FIRST DISTRICT MEETING HELD AT FORT SUPPLY

The annual meeting of the First Councilor District convened on December 3 at Fort Supply with twenty-five physicians in attendance.

Members of the Association and their wives were guests at a dinner given by Dr. John L. Day, Superintendent of the Western Oklahoma Hospital.

Guest speakers for the meeting were Dr. James Stevenson of Tulsa, President-Elect of the Oklahoma State Medical Association, and Dr. Grady F. Mathews, Oklahoma City, State Commissioner of Health.

Dr. O. E. Templin, Alva, Councilor for the First District, presided at the meeting and introduced the guests which included, in addition to the speakers, Captain Katzner and Lieutenant Baine of the U. S. Army Medical Corps.

Following the meeting, there was a business session of the Woodward County Medical Society for the purpose of electing officers. The following physicians were elected and will serve during 1943: President, Dr. C. E. Williams; Vice-President, Dr. D. W. Darwin, and Secretary-Treasurer, Dr. C. W. Tedrowe.

INSIGHT

"Skilled physicians, gifted with peculiar insight into human nature, can often estimate a personality with remarkable accuracy in a few minutes or even seconds, but in general the more a doctor knows of his patient's background the greater advantage he has in handling the case."—Doctor and Patient by Francis W. Peabody, M.D.

ANNUAL A. M. A. CONFERENCE OF SECRETARIES AND EDITORS

Each year the American Medical Association holds a conference at the headquarters of the Association in Chicago to which are invited the Secretaries of State Medical Associations and the Editors of the various State Medical Journals. The 1942 meeting was held on November 20 and 21 with an approximate attendance of two hundred including officers of the various branches of the United States Armed Forces in addition to the officials from state organizations. The program of the Conference dealt wholly with the wartime policies of American Medicine.

The Friday meeting was called to order by Dr. Roger I. Lee, Chairman of the Board of Trustees of the American Medical Association. Dr. H. H. Shoulders, Secretary of the Tennessee State Medical Association and Speaker of the House of Delegates of the A. M. A., was chosen Chairman and presided over all sessions throughout the Conference.

Colonel Fred W. Rankin, President of the American Medical Association, welcomed the guests to the meeting, and in his remarks emphasized the curtailment of large medical meetings but urged that they be replaced by smaller meetings in various sections at properly spaced intervals. He also emphasized the need for the maintenance of the present high standards of medical education regardless of the fact that medical schools are now operating on an accelerated program basis.

The Navy

Admiral Ross T. McIntire, Surgeon General of the United States Navy, explained the place of the Reserve Medical Officer in the wartime setup of the Navy Medical Corps, and further stated that the medical profession should start planning now for the post-war period since the problems arising would be those of specialization. Admiral McIntire remarked that physicians will return to civilian practice with an entirely different viewpoint; and because of their wide experience during service, they will feel they should no longer be compelled to practice only one specialty. The speaker emphasized that organized medicine should start thinking constructively now on the problem of meeting the cost of medical care at the close of the war as Government control would be undesirable.

Procurement and Assignment Service

Dr. Frank H. Lahey, Chairman of the Directing Board of the Procurement and Assignment Service, paid tribute to all those who have in any way cooperated with the work of the Committee. He explained that states having provided more than their quota for 1942 would be given credit for 1943, and that states not reaching their 1942 quota would be required to provide more in 1943. Doctor Lahey stated that, at a recent meeting of the representatives of the various branches of the service, the ratio of physicians to men was set at 6.5 physicians per 1,000 men in the navy and air force, and it was felt the army would probably accept the same figure. It was further pointed out that one physician for each 1,500 civilians was thought to be satisfactory and that recruitment would be based on the same decision. Doctor Lahey mentioned the problem of dislocating physicians and stated that Procurement and Assignment Service was attempting to work out a satisfactory solution.

Dr. Harold M. Diehl of Minneapolis, Minn., a member of the Directing Board, also appeared on the program in behalf of the Procurement and Assignment Service. In his discussion regarding dislocation, Doctor Diehl stated that a committee to investigate needs should be set up in each state. He said the Central Office would be willing to send State Chairmen lists of interns and physicians physically disqualified for military service who, in turn, might be utilized in needy areas.

The Army

Brigadier General Charles C. Hillman, a representative from the Office of the Surgeon General of the United States Army, spoke on the personnel problem of the Army and explained how the Reserve had been built up since 1918. He explained how the Army had worked with Procurement and Assignment Service in calling doctors into service thereby preventing confusion and disruption. General Hillman further observed that the War Department is working on a plan of keeping an adequate supply of students in the medical schools.

A. M. A. President-Elect

The first speaker on the Friday afternoon session was Dr. James E. Paullin of Atlanta, Ga., President-Elect of the American Medical Association. Doctor Paullin is also a member of the Directing Board of Procurement and Assignment Service. He mentioned the redistribution of physicians and stated that it was his opinion that most of the problems would be considered on a state level inasmuch as it was not possible to solve all problems in the same manner. The President-Elect informed the Conference that 218 doctors in 154 communities in 29 different states had been relocated on a voluntary basis. Doctor Paullin suggested temporary licensure as one possible solution to the problem but further pointed out that each state should be able to work out a satisfactory solution in the time of war.

Public Health Service

Thomas Parran, Surgeon General of the United States Public Health Service, explained that his agency was cooperating with state and local public health agencies. The objectives of National Public Health, according to General Parran, are to aid state departments in replacing personnel in boom areas; to strengthen and develop industrial hygiene to keep up with the changing population; to aid in the control of venereal disease; to operate the malaria control program around industrial sections; and to provide the medical staff of the Office of Civilian Defense base hospitals erected in target areas. It was General Parran's belief that redistribution could be more satisfactorily worked out on a voluntary basis rather than through legislation.

Selective Service

The medical needs of the war and the Selective Service System was discussed by Colonel Leonard G. Rowntree, Chief of the Medical Division of the Selective Service System. He stated the war had made many demands on medicine, and listed four separate branches —military medicine, public health and industrial medicine, research medicine and civil practice. Colonel Rowntree stressed the need for deferment of medical students and other allied problems to meet future needs. The speaker also discussed the problem of rehabilitation and stated that, at present, the best program in this field was being conducted by the State of New Jersey.

The Air Corps

Brigadier General David N. W. Grant of the United States Army Air Force presented the aims of the medical officers in the Air Corps, and stated that every attempt was being made to improve the physician for his return to civilian practice. Because of the far flung fields of operation, a new and very necessary development is global medicine. General Grant stated that every effort was being made by officials to see that flyers returned to their post following hospitalization in better mental as well as physican condition. All hospital staff members have been urged to associate with local medical societies.

Physicians for Civilians

Dr. Creighton Barker, Secretary of the Connecticut State Medical Society, presented the important problem of maintaining an adequate supply of physicians for the civilian population. He stated that the public looked toward medicine for medical care rather than to the Government. Doctor Barker observed that the public should be educated in order that the doctor's time and energy might better be utilized.

War Participation Committee

Dr. Walter F. Donaldson, Pittsburgh, Pa., Chairman of the War Participation Committee of the American Medical Association, discussed the desirability of every state medical association's development of such a committee to coordinate the activities of all agencies engaged in war work. Doctor Donaldson emphasized the fact that it was the duty of those who remained at home to be on the alert in order to protect and safeguard the practice of medicine in the best traditions of the "good old American way."

Annual Editors Dinner

Friday evening a dinner meeting for the Editors of the State Medical Journals was held at the Palmer House. Dr. Stanley B. Weld, Editor of the Connecticut State Medical Journal, presided and, in a brief discussion, presented a number of the problems with which an editor is confronted. Dr. Julian P. Price, Secretary and Editor of the South Carolina Medical Association, discussed the subject "Improving the Methods of Transmitting Information to Physicians." A general discussion of medical magazine problems followed by several of the editors in attendance.

Medical Service Plans

At the Saturday morning session, Mr. A. M. Simons, representing the Bureau of Medical Economics of the American Medical Association, discussed medical service plans of the Farm Security Administration. His detailed explanation presented the difference between the first plans and those now in effect. Mr. Simons stressed the need for a definite understanding of the contract coverage, and further stated that a program would never be inaugurated without the consent of the local county medical society.

The development of the Massachusetts Medical Service Plan was presented by the President, Dr. James C. McCann of Worcester. Discussions followed by representatives from California, New Jersey, Michigan, Pennsylvania and Missouri. Father A. M. Schwitalla of St. Louis, Mo., appeared before those in attendance and emphatically stated that, in his opinion, the time has come for the Board of Trustees of the American Medical Association to work out the experiences of the various medical care plans for the benefit of all State Medical Associations.

Industrial Health

Recent developments in Industrial Health activities as presented by Dr. Carl M. Peterson, Secretary of the Council on Industrial Health of the American Medical Association, was the final presentation to the Conference. The speaker stressed the need for industrial health programs and urged that county medical societies recognize the problem and cooperate with industry in order that the highest level of efficiency of the employees may be maintained.

After extending a vote of thanks to the speakers and the officials of the American Medical Association, the Conference adjourned at one o'clock Saturday.

OKLAHOMA CITY INTERNISTS TO CONDUCT ANNUAL WASHINGTON BIRTHDAY CLINICS

The Fourth Annual Meeting of the Oklahoma City Internists Association will be held at the University Hospital in Oklahoma City on Monday, February 22, 1943.

Clinics will be conducted from 10:00 A. M. until 4:00 P. M. The program to be announced later will include a luncheon and roundtable discussion of all medical problems.

All physicians of Oklahoma are invited to attend.

THE VICTORY TAX AND THE MEDICAL PROFESSION*

Prepared by the
Bureau of Legal Medicine and Legislation

The Revenue Act of 1942 imposes a victory tax on individuals amounting to 5 per cent of their victory tax net income. This tax is in addition to all other taxes imposed by the new act, applies to income received after December 31, 1942, and will continue in effect during the present war. The act provides that the victory tax shall not apply with respect to any tax year commencing after "the date of cessation of hostilities in the present war." Physicians of course will be subject to this tax to the same extent as other taxpayers.

The return that a physician must file on or before March 15, 1943, will not reflect the victory tax net income of the taxpayer nor will the victory tax be payable at that time. Since the new tax applies only to income received *after* December 31, 1942, and since the next return includes only income *prior* to January 1, 1943, assuming that the physician is on a calendar year basis for income tax purposes, physicians generally need not be concerned with the payment of the victory tax until their returns are executed, in 1944, for the tax year 1943. There are certain aspects, however, of the victory tax provisions of the new act that will impose requirements on physicians beginning with the first of the year.

Physicians Who Are Employers

If a physician on or after January 1, 1943, employs any person, subject to certain exceptions discussed later on, and pays to such a person a wage in excess of $12 a week, or $624 a year, he must withhold the 5 per cent victory tax from that wage and transmit it to the government at quarterly intervals.

What Constitutes Wages.—Affirmatively, the term "wage" means all remuneration, other than fees paid to a public official, for services performed by an employee for his employer, including the cash value of all remuneration paid in any medium other than cash.

Negatively, the term does not include remuneration paid (1) for services performed as a member of the military or naval forces of the United States, other than pensions and retired pay; (2) for agricultural labor; (3) for domestic service in a private home, local college club or local chapter of a college fraternity or sorority; (4) for casual labor not in the course of the employer's trade or business; (5) for services as an employee of a nonresident alien individual, foreign partnership or foreign corporation, if such individual, partnership or corporation is not engaged in trade or business in the United States; (6) for services as an employee of a foreign government or any wholly owned instrumentality thereof, and (7) for services performed as an employee while outside the United States, unless the major part of the services performed during the calendar year by such employee for his employer are performed within the United States. Persons who perform services in the foregoing seven categories are not exempt from the payment of the victory tax, but their employers are not required to withhold the tax from their wages.

The definition of the term "wage" therefore, is broad enough to include the remuneration paid by a physician to an assistant physician, an office nurse, a stenographer, a secretary, a receptionist and other personnel employed by the physician in connection with his practice.

Withholding Deductions.—Not all of an employee's wage is subject to the victory tax; only that in excess of $624 a year. In computing the 5 per cent victory tax to be withheld, therefore, the employer will disregard the wages paid for each payroll period in accordance with the following schedule:

Payroll period	Withholding Deduction
Weekly	$ 12
Biweekly	24
Semimonthly	26
Monthly	52
Quarterly	156
Semiannually	312
Annually	624

That is, if the payroll period for a particular employee is a week, the tax does not apply to the first $12 paid the employee; if the payroll period is a month, the first $52 escapes the victory tax, and so on. All wages paid in excess of the indicated amounts for each payroll period are subject to the tax and employers must either withhold 5 per cent of that excess or an amount in accordance with tables set forth in the act. These tables indicate optional amounts an employer may withhold instead of the actual 5 per cent of the wage. As an example, for a weekly payroll period, if the wage paid is over $12 and not over $16, 10 cents weekly may be withheld. If the wage is over $20 but not over $24, 50 cents may be withheld and so on for different wage groups for different payroll periods. The use of these tables will simplify greatly the withholding process and physicians should ascertain from the office of the collectors of internal revenue where copies of the table may be obtained.

The law provides that, if a payroll period is less than one week, the excess of the aggregate of the wages paid during each calendar week over the deduction allowed for a weekly payroll period must be used in computing the tax required to be withheld. For example, if an employee is paid on a daily basis at the rate of $5 a day, the employer will not withhold any of the wage paid for the first two days of employment in any calendar week. The wages paid for a third day in the same calendar week will be subject to withholding on $3, the excess of the aggregate of three days' wages, or $15, over the weekly deduction of $12. All subsequent wage payment during the same calendar week will be subject to withholding on the entire amount of each payment. If a payroll period is not covered specifically by the foregoing table, the deduction allowed against each payment of such wages will be the deduction allowable in case of an annual payroll period divided by 365 and multiplied by the number of days in such period, including Sundays and holidays.

In any case in which wages are paid by an employer without regard to any payroll period or other period, the deduction allowable against each payment of such wages will be the deduction allowable in the case of an annual payroll period divided by 365 days and multiplied by the number of days, including Sundays and holidays, which have elapsed since the date of the last payment of such wages by such employer during the calendar year, or the date of commencement of employment with such employer during such year or January 1 of such year, whichever is the later.

In withholding the victory tax, the employer gives no consideration at all to the marital status of the employee or to any dependents that the employee may have, or to any possible deductions to which the employee may be entitled, other than the basic deduction of $12 a week.

Transmission of Withheld Tax to Government.—The employer who has withheld the victory tax from wages paid to employees is required to transmit the withheld tax to the government on or before the last day of the month following the close of each quarter of each calendar year. The first report to be made by an employer to the government, therefore, will be due on or before April 30, 1943. Such an employer must keep such records and render under oath such statements with respect to the tax withheld and collected as may be

*Taken from the Journal of the American Medical Association, Volume 120, No. 14, December 5, 1942, Pages 1143-1145.

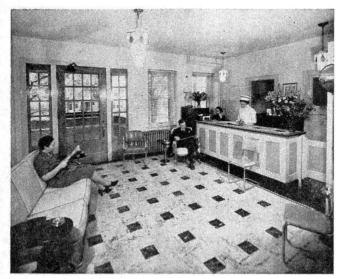

required under regulations prescribed by the Commissioner of Internal Revenue with the approval of the Secretary of the Treasury.

Receipts to Employees.—Every employer withholding the victory tax must furnish to each employee, on or before the close of the calendar year, on the day on which the last payment of wages is made, a written statement showing the period covered by the statement, the wages paid by the employer to such employee during such period, and the amount of the tax withheld and collected. Duplicate copies of such statements must be transmitted to the Commissioner of Internal Revenue along with the final report made by the employer for the calendar year.

Physicians Who Are Employees

A physician who is an employee may expect deductions to be made from his wages in accordance with the procedure outlined. The deductions will be made by the employer, subject to the exceptions previously noted, whether that employer is the federal or a state government, a county, a municipality, any agency or instrumentality thereof, a hospital, an industrial or business concern or other person or agency paying wages to a physician. While physicians generally will not be required to pay the victory tax until 1944, and then on income received during 1943, physicians who fall in the category of employees will start paying the tax periodically in 1943 as it is deducted from their wages by their employers.

At the end of the tax year 1943 the victory tax that has been withheld from the wages of a physician employee will be adjusted. This adjustment will take place when the return from 1943 is filed the early part of 1944. At that time the victory tax will be redetermined on the return then filed and credit taken from the amounts that have been withheld from wages. Since the amounts so withheld are based on 5 per cent of the *gross* income in excess of $624 a year and since the actual victory tax imposed is 5 per cent of the *victory tax net income*, that is, gross income minus specified deductions in addition to the $624, there will in many instances be an excess in the amount withheld over the tax actually due. In such cases that excess may be deducted from the income tax that will be payable. In all cases, therefore, in which employers have withheld, during 1943, periodic amounts from wages on account of the victory tax, there will be adjustments between the government and the taxpayer at the close of the tax year if such adjustments are necessary.

Postwar Credit or Refund of Victory Tax

As soon as practicable after the date of cessation of hostilities in the present war, the following amounts of victory tax paid for each taxable year beginning after December 31, 1942, will be credited against any income tax or instalment thereof then due from the taxpayer and any balance will be refunded immediately to the taxpayer:

1. In the case of a single person or married person not living with husband or wife, 25 per cent of the victory tax or $500, whichever is the lesser.

2. In the case of the head of a family, 40 per cent of the victory tax or $1,000, whichever is the lesser. In the case of a married person living with husband or wife where separate returns are filed by each spouse, 40 per cent of the victory tax or $500, whichever is the lesser. In the case of a married person living with husband or wife where a separate return is filed by one spouse and no return is filed by the other spouse, or in case of a husband and wife filing a joint return, only one such credit will be allowed and such credit may not exceed 40 per cent of the victory tax or $1,000, whichever is the lesser.

3. For each dependent, excluding as a dependent, in the case of the head of a family, one who would be excluded as a dependent for income tax purposes, 2 per cent or $100, whichever is the lesser.

If for any taxable year the status of the taxpayer, other than a taxpayer whose gross income is $3,000 or under and who uses the simplified return form, with respect to his marital relationship or with respect to his dependents, changes during the taxable year, the amount of the credit or refund of the victory tax for such taxable year will be apportioned, under rules and regulations prescribed by the Commissioner of Internal Revenue with the approval of the Secretary of the Treasury in accordance with the months to and after the change. For the purpose of such apportionment, the fractional part of a month will be disregarded unless it amounts to more than one-half a month, in which case it will be considered as a month.

The law contains provisions under which a taxpayer may, prior to the cessation of hostilities, take advantage of his postwar credit or refund. To the extent of that credit or refund, the taxpayer may reduce the victory tax by deducting amounts paid during the year as premiums on life insurance in force on September 1, 1942, certain reductions of debts and certain investments in obligations of the United States. At the end of 1943 and of each year thereafter in which the victory tax is imposed the taxpayer may, with respect to that tax, do one of two things: (1) He may pay the victory tax in full and wait until the cessation of hostilities to claim his postwar refund or credit, or (2) He may at the time the victory tax is payable reduce the amount of the tax by deducting expenditures for purposes above described in an amount equal to the postwar refund or credit to which he would be entitled after the cessation of hostilities. Assume that Dr. X, an unmarried physician with no dependents, when he executes his return on or before March 15, 1944, finds himself owing a victory tax of $100. Assume, further, that during 1943 Dr. X purchased government bonds, paid premiums on life insurance and reduced indebtedness, expending a total amount of $1,000 for such purposes. Dr. X may pay the $100 victory tax during 1944 and after the cessation of hostilities receive a refund or credit of 25 per cent of the tax, or $25, or he may reduce the victory tax payable in 1944 by claiming credit for the amount expended for the purposes stated but only to the extent of the postwar credit to which he would be entitled, that is, $25. In the one case, Dr. X pays the full victory tax of $100 and gets a refund or credit later; in the other he pays $75 and will not thereafter receive a refund or credit.

No attempt has been made to discuss in detail the intricacies of the victory tax. The object has been rather to present a broad picture with many of the technical details omitted. As previously stated, the tax does not extend to 1942 incomes and physicians generally will not have to compute the amount of the tax they must pay until the returns are filed on or before March 15, 1944. Before that time arrives, it is assumed that proper regulations will be promulgated and be given wide publicity, which will simplify the procedure for the determination of the tax.

Danger in the Cabinet

Two war factors have increased the danger of poisoning from drugs and other preparations frequently found in home medicine cabinets.

One is the thinning out of doctors, which causes people to rely on their own remedies. The other is the possibility of blackouts, which make it harder to find what you are looking for.

Shoe dyes and cleaning chemicals are sometimes taken for throat gargles, and disinfectant tablets are mistaken for aspirin.

As a result, 10 children and 20 adults die each week from accidental poisoning in American homes.

The home medicine cabinet is a time-honored institution, but figuratively speaking, it is filled with high explosive.

GASOLINE RATIONING GOES INTO EFFECT

Gasoline rationing has now been in effect in Oklahoma since December 1, and comparatively few complaints have been received concerning its administration.

The following open letter to the medical profession on gasoline and tire rationing has been released through the Journal of the American Medical Association by Mr. John R. Richards, Chief of the Gasoline Rationing Branch, Office of Price Administration, and should receive the full cooperation of the medical profession:

"In the East Coast Gasoline Rationing program, made necessary by the shortage of transportation facilities for petroleum products, the indispensability of your profession was recognized by its inclusion in the categories of persons eligible for preferred mileage, that is, necessary occupational mileage in excess of 470 miles a month. Now the Office of Price Administration has been ordered by Mr. William Jeffers to institute and administer a nationwide mileage rationing program for the express purpose of conserving our rubber-borne transportation. In framing the Regulations for the new program, your profession was one of the first to be provided for.

"If we are to carry out our double task of preventing a collapse of our military and civilian transportation, we must have the complete cooperation of those groups of persons whose driving is deemed essential to the war effort. Our immediate aim is to attain the 5,000 mile national mileage average set by the Baruch Report as the maximum possible in light of the dire rubber shortage. Our experience with the East Coast program tells us that the preferred categories use one-half of the gasoline consumed, though they constitute less than one-fourth of the total number of automobile operators. Clearly, then, the great savings of rubber on a nation-wide scale must be made in the preferred categories.

"Under the Regulations, governing the mileage rationing program, physicians are eligible for preferred mileage if their essential occupational needs exceed 470 miles a month and if the mileage is needed for regularly rendering necessary professional services. Mileage traveled daily or periodically between home or lodging and a fixed place of work is not considered preferred. Physicians who conduct their practices in offices, as many specialists do, are not eligible for preferred mileage.

"Without question or hesitation, doctors have been and will be granted all the gasoline needed to carry out their professional work. We hope that they will regard their concrete symbol of their indispensability, the C book, as a moral obligation and not as a personal privilege. From another point of view, the C book is part of a doctor's equipment; it should not be used for anything but the work of humanity.

"When nationwide gasoline rationing begins, there are certain concrete things a doctor can do to live up to the high ethical standards set for him by his own profession:

"1. At the time of first issuance of rations, he can so carefully compute his necessary mileage as to make a B book adequate for his purposes though he might easily make out a case for a C book, which might be granted to him without question by his local War Price and Rationing Board eager to provide for physicians.

"2. In the computation of his mileage, he can religiously adhere to the provision of the Regulations, which makes 150 miles of his basic ration available for occupational purposes. Moreover, he can help mightily in establishing the principles that only 90 miles of the basic ration are to be used for home uses purposes and that there is no provision whatever in any ration for 'pleasure driving.'

"3. Conversely, if he should be granted a C book, he can return to the local board, at the end of the three months period, all unused coupons accruing to him as a result of a quite natural overestimation of needs or of overgenerous 'tailoring' by his board, instead of using such coupons for nonessential purposes. The moral effect of such an act on his fellow citizens will be incalculable.

"4. He can set an example by scrupulously observing the 35 mile speed limit, except in cases of emergency, in spite of the fact that doctors could easily 'get away with it.'

"5. Should he be assigned to a hospital, clinic or institution after a ration card for calling on his private practice has been issued, he can use public means of transportation at the price of personal inconvenience.

"6. He can refrain from any kind of driving whatever which might appear to be nonessential in the eyes of the public.

"Doctors are the leaders and molders of public opinion in their communities. If the average man has any reason to believe that the professional men whom he regards with great respect are indifferent or hostile to the mileage rationing program, it will be difficult, if not impossible, to make it effective. Conversely, if doctors as a group observe the letter and spirit of the Regulations, they will be a powerful force in making this absolutely mandatory war measure serve its purpose. We know that we can rely on the support of your profession, which has demonstrated its patriotism, ability and unselfishness at every opportunity."—John R. Richards, Chief Gasoline Rationing Branch, Office of Price Administration.

Gas Saving Rackets

Physicians who own more than one car are cautioned to be on their guard when approached on propositions concerning the purchase of gasoline saving devices, such as trick spark plugs and carburetor gadgets. Investigation in this field by Better Business Bureaus all over the country have not been satisfactory. Ignition systems can best contribute to motor efficiency and economy by being left to the periodic care of reputable automobile service centers.

PHYSICIANS RECENTLY LICENSED

J. D. Osborn, M.D., Secretary-Treasurer of the Oklahoma State Board of Medical Examiners, reports that licenses to practice medicine and surgery have been granted to 22 applicants during the period from August 15 to December 14, 1942.

The following doctors of medicine were granted licenses:

Aldredge, William Max, Hobart; Black, Thomas Claiborne, Clinton; Bonham, Kenneth Warren, Enid; Dennis, James Lowden, Merced, California; Engleman, Clarence Clarke, Clinton; Fair, Ellis Edwin, Oklahoma City; Felson, Benjamin (Army), Cincinnati, Ohio; Freeman, Chas. Winfred, Rocky; Funk, Robert Edward, Tulsa; Harms, Harold H., Durham, North Carolina; Haynes, Boyd Withers, Jr., Oklahoma City; Kinnaman, Joseph Horace, Ponca City;

MacKercher, Peter A., Ponca City; McQuown, Albert Louis, Des Moines, Iowa; Montgomery, Hazel Irene, Rochester, New York; Packard, Louis Albert, McAlester; Reiff, Maxine Ruth Hoffer, Oklahoma City; Reiff, William Henry, Oklahoma City; Sprinkle, Davis Lee, McAlester; Taylor, Lloyd Wilson, San Francisco, California; Weber, Roxie Adeline, Stillwater, and Weeks, Bertram Allen (Army), Carlisle Barracks, Pennsylvania.

No Widely Accepted Explanation Yet for Seasickness

A review by W. J. McNally, M.D., and E. A. Stuart, M.D., Montreal, Canada, in the current issue of War Medicine, of experimental work on the labyrinth or inner ear in relation to seasickness and other forms of motion sickness fails to bring to light any widely accepted explanation for the cause of the condition or immunity to it. "The labyrinth has been shown by experiment to play an important, probably the most important, part in the causation of motion sickness," the two physicians explain.

NEWS FROM THE COUNTY SOCIETIES

"Rheumatic Health Disease" was the topic of discussion by Dr. Clark H. Hall of Oklahoma City before the Cherokee County Medical Society at its meeting on Monday, November 23, 1942.

The following members of the Cherokee Society have been called to duty with the armed forces: Dr. R. K. McIntosh, Jr., Dr. Harry E. Barnes, Dr. Isadore Dyer and Dr. Andrew Ritan.

The Carter County Medical Society met Tuesday, December 15, at 7:00 P. M., at the Hardy Sanitarium with 15 members in attendance. Mr. John B. Turner, candidate for State Senator, was the guest speaker.

The 1942 officers of the Society were re-elected to serve during 1943; namely, President, Dr. Walter Hardy, Ardmore; Vice-President, Dr. D. E. Cantrell, Sr., Healdton, and Secretary-Treasurer, Dr. H. A. Higgins, Ardmore.

The Society extended sympathy to Dr. Hoyle Carlock in his bereavement of the recent death of his father. Doctor Carlock is serving with the armed forces.

The next meeting of the Society will be January 12 at the Hardy Sanitarium.

Election of officers for 1943 was the order of business for the Blaine County Medical Society meeting at the Watonga Hospital on Thursday, December 10.

The officers elected are as follows: President, Dr. Virginia Olson Curtin, Watonga; Vice-President, Dr. Frank Buchanan, Canton; Secretary-Treasurer, Dr. W. F. Griffin, Watonga, and Delegate to the State Meeting, Dr. Virginia Olson Curtin.

A discussion of next year's program was also held.

Dr. L. R. Kirby of Okeene will be the speaker at the next meeting of the Society on Thursday, January 21. The dentists in Blaine County will be invited guests.

Dr. William C. Miller of Guthrie was re-elected President of the Logan County Medical Society at its meeting on December 15 at the Cimarron Valley Wesley Hospital. Ten members were in attendance. Other officers elected were Vice-President, Dr. Charles L. Rogers, Marshall; Secretary-Treasurer, Dr. J. L. LeHew, Jr., Guthrie, and State Delegate, Dr. L. A. Hahn, Guthrie.

One of the subjects of discussion by the Society was that of the Grade A Milk Ordinance. The County Health Unit was discussed and a resolution passed to endorse and continue the same.

Among the projects being worked on by the Society are discussions on timely topics by the members, motion pictures and local health problems.

The annual business meeting and election of officers of the Tulsa County Medical Society was held Monday, December 14, at 8:00 P. M., at the Mayo hotel with 55 members present.

Dr. James C. Peden, President-Elect during the past year, will assume the duties of President. Officers elected to serve with Dr. Peden are as follows: President-Elect, Dr. R. A. McGill; Vice-President, Dr. H. A. Ruprecht, and Dr. E. O. Johnson was re-elected Secretary-Treasurer. Dr. H. B. Stewart was elected as a member of the Board of Trustees to serve until 1947. Dr. L. C. Northrup was elected to replace Dr. R. C. Pigford, now in the service, as a Delegate to the State Meeting. Dr. Hugh Graham was also elected as a Delegate. The other Delegates are holdovers. Dr. J. S. Chalmers of Sand Springs is the new member on the Board of Trustees.

The inauguration of the new President will be January 11 at the Mayo hotel. A motion picture, "Peptic Ulcer," in sound and color will also be presented.

Fifteen members of the Custer County Medical Society attended the dinner meeting held Wednesday, December 9, at 7:00 P. M., at Harry's Cafe in Clinton.

The following officers were elected to lead the Society during the coming year: President, Dr. F. R. Vieregg; Vice-President, Dr. Ross Deputy, and Secretary-Treasurer, Dr. C. J. Alexander. Delegates elected to represent Custer County are Dr. McLain Rogers and Dr. Ellis Lamb with Dr. C. H. McBurney and Dr. C. Doler as respective Alternates. Censors for the Society are Dr. C. H. McBurney, Clinton; Dr. T. A. Boyd, Weatherford, and Dr. E. M. Loyd, Taloga—the latter two having been elected at the recent meeting.

It was voted by the Society to pay the dues of nine members who are now serving in the military service; namely, Drs. A. W. Paulson, L. J. Kennedy, Paul B. Lingenfelter, J. R. Hinshaw, Gordon Williams, J. Guild Wood, H. R. Cushman, William C. Tisdal and Bernard Bullock.

The Society also voted to send a donation to the National Physicians Committee.

Following this order of business, discussion was held concerning the joint meeting of Washita, Beckham and Custer Counties in view of the reduced membership because of the fact that many members are serving with the armed forces. To stimulate closer union of members while so many are away and in view of the difficulties of transportation, the appearance of local men on the program was discussed.

Dr. Clinton Gallaher, Secretary of the Pottawatomie County Medical Society, presided in the absence of the President at the regular meeting of the Society on Saturday, November 21. Dinner was served at 7:00 P. M. in the Haviland Room of the Aldridge Hotel in Shawnee to fourteen members followed by the regular business session.

Nominations for 1943 officers made at the November 7, 1942, meeting were read and no further nominations were offered. The officers are: President, Dr. A. C.

McFarling; Vice-President, Dr. Charles W. Haygood, and Dr. Clinton Gallaher was re-elected Secretary-Treasurer. Delegates are Dr. G. S. Baxter and Dr. W. M. Gallaher, and Alternates are Dr. C. C. Young and Dr. E. E. Rice.

By vote, the following committees will serve during the coming year: Executive Committee; Drs. A. C. McFarling, Charles W. Haygood and J. M. Byrum; Board of Censors: Drs. M. A. Baker, A. C. McFarling and W. M. Gallaher; Board of Trustees: Drs. A. C. McFarling, Clinton Gallaher and J. M. Byrum.

Standing Committees for the year 1943 will be appointed by the incoming President, Dr. A. C. McFarling.

Following the election of officers, Dr. C. C. Young reviewed the financial condition of the Bulletin of the Pottawatomie County Medical Society and submitted an annual statement of the auditing. It was voted by the Society to continue the maintenance of the Bulletin publication under the financial advice of the Board of Trustees and business management of Dr. C. C. Young. Dr. E. E. Rice will continue as Editor.

Dr. F. P. Newlin will continue as manager of the Radio Broadcast programs which are sponsored by the Society.

Dr. C. C. Young discussed the activities of the Infantile Paralysis Foundation and called attention to the fact that it was prepared to give aid in any case where needed.

Dr. E. E. Rice, who had charge of the scientific program, spoke on the subject "Treatment of Hyperemesis Gravidorum with Vitamin B₆ (Pyridoxin Hydrochloride)." Discussions followed by Drs. J. M. Byrum, F. P. Newlin, C. C. Young, John Carson and others.

At the December meeting of the Kay County Medical Society at Ponca City on the 17th, Dr. Philip C. Risser of Blackwell was elected President, Dr. G. H. Yeary of Newkirk, Vice-President, and Dr. J. Holland Howe of Ponca City was re-elected Secretary-Treasurer. Delegates chosen are Dr. A. S. Risser, Blackwell, and Dr. Dewey Mathews, Tonkawa, and Alternates are Dr. J. C. Wagner, Ponca City, and Dr. L. H. Becker, Blackwell.

The program for the evening consisted of a moving picture and running discussion entitled "Peptic Ulcer" sponsored by John Wyeth and Brother. The text of discussion was distributed to members of the Society.

The next meeting of the Society will be January 21 at Blackwell.

Dr. W. G. Husband of Hollis was elected President of the Harmon County Medical Society at the Tuesday, December 15, 1942, meeting of the Society.

Dr. R. H. Lynch will serve as Vice-President, and Dr. L. E. Hollis was elected Secretary-Treasurer. Doctor Husband will represent Harmon County as Delegate with Doctor Hollis as Alternate.

Dr. Carroll M. Pounders of Oklahoma City discussed "Rheumatic Fever" and Dr. Elias Margo of Oklahoma City presented a paper entitled "Functional Disorders of the Feet" at the meeting of the Woods County Medical Society on November 23 in Alva at 7:30 P. M. Twelve members were in attendance.

The two above-named physicians were examiners at the Crippled Children's Clinic held at the Legion Hut during the afternoon which was sponsored by the State Commission for Crippled Children and the Alva Rotary Club.

At the business session following the program, officers were elected: President, Dr. C. A. Traverse; Vice-President, Dr. D. B. Ensor, and Secretary-Treasurer, Dr. O. E. Templin. Doctor Ensor will serve as Delegate and Dr. W. F. LaFon as Alternate.

A resolution was passed to admit all medical officers stationed within Woods County as associate members of the County Society without dues.

The next meeting of the Society is scheduled for January 26 at Alva.

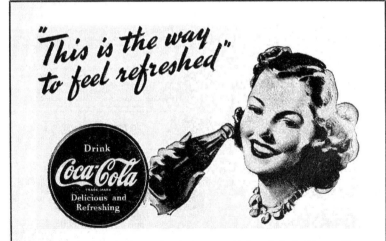

Dr. F. M. Edwards of Ringling was elected President of the Jefferson County Medical Society at the meeting on Monday, December 14, at Waurika. Elected to serve with Dr. Edwards are Dr. C. M. Maupin, Waurika, Vice-President, and Dr. L. L. Wade, Ryan, Secretary-Treasurer. Dr. W. M. Browning of Waurika was chosen Delegate.

The transfer of Dr. H. Wesley Yeats of Ringling, as a member from Bryan County, was accepted by the Jefferson County Society.

The Tri-County Society consisting of Stephens, Cotton and Jefferson Counties will meet in Waurika on Tuesday evening, February 9.

Dr. J. V. Athey read a paper entitled "Anesthetic Fatalties" and Dr. H. G. Crawford discussed "Peptic Ulcer" before the members of the Washington-Nowata County Medical Society at the meeting of the Society on Wednesday, December 9, at the Washington County Memorial Hospital in Bartlesville.

At the business session, the following officers were elected to serve for 1943: Dr. J. G. Smith, Bartlesville, President; Dr. J. P. Vansant, Dewey, Vice-President; Dr. J. V. Athey, Bartlesville, Secretary-Treasurer; Dr. K. D. Davis, Nowata, Dr. H. C. Weber, Bartlesville, and Dr. L. D. Hudson, Dewey, Delegates, and Dr. S. A. Lang, Nowata, Dr. E. E. Beechwood and Dr. Thomas Wells, both of Bartlesville, Alternates. Censors are Dr. S. P. Roberts, Nowata, and Dr. O. I. Green and Dr. B. F. Staver, both of Bartlesville.

The annual banquet of the Washington-Nowata County Society will be held January 13 at 7:30 P. M.

A film on "Syphilis" was presented at the meeting of the Stephens County Medical Society on Tuesday, November 24, at the Wade hotel in Duncan by Dr. E. A. Gillis, Director of Venereal Diseases, State Health Department, Oklahoma City. Discussion followed by Dr. F. W. Highfill, Stephens County Health officer.

Doctors representing Cotton and Jefferson County Societies were in attendance at the meeting.

Dr. John S. Lawson of Clayton was elected President and Dr. B. M. Huckabay of Antlers will serve as Secretary-Treasurer of the Pushmataha County Society for 1943, as reported by the December 15 meeting. Dr. D. W. Connally of Antlers will represent the Society as Delegate and Dr. E. S. Patterson, also of Antlers, as Alternate.

"Syphilis" was the topic of discussion selected by Dr. Paul T. Powell, Director of the County Health Department, at the meeting of the Pittsburg County Medical Society on November 20 at the Albert Pike Hospital in McAlester.

Election of officers for 1943 was the order of business of the Craig County Medical Society at its regular meeting on Tuesday, December 15, at 7:30 P. M., in Vinita. Six members and four visitors were present.

The following were chosen to serve during the coming year: President, Dr. Felix M. Adams; Vice-President, Dr. Lloyd H. McPike, and Dr. J. M. McMillan was re-elected Secretary-Treasurer. Doctor Adams will represent the County as Delegate to the Annual Meeting of the Association and Doctor McPike as Alternate. The Board of Censors is composed of Doctor McPike, Dr. W. R. Marks and Dr. P. L. Hays. Doctor McMillan, as Secretary, is in charge of the Scientific Program Committee.

Immediately following the election of officers, a film "Peptic Ulcer," sponsored by John Wyeth and Brother, was presented.

Dr. C. E. Williams of Woodward was elected President of the Woodward County Medical Society in a business session immediately following the meeting of the First

Councilor District at Fort Supply on December 3. Those chosen to serve with Doctor Williams are Dr. D. W. Darwin as Vice-President, and Dr. C. W. Tedrowe as Secretary-Treasurer.

For the duration, the Society will hold quarterly meetings in March, June, September and December. The next meeting is scheduled for March 11, at 7:00 P. M., in Woodward.

Officers elected to serve the Okmulgee County Medical Society during the coming year are as follows: President, Dr. A. R. Holmes, Henryetta; Vice-President, Dr. H. D. Boswell, Henryetta; Secretary-Treasurer, Dr. J. C. Matheney, Okmulgee; Delegate, Dr. J. G. Edwards, Okmulgee, and Alternate. Dr. G. Y. McKinney, Henryetta. Dr. S. B. Leslie, Okmulgee, was chosen as a new member on the Board of Censors to serve until 1945. Serving with him are Doctor McKinney and Dr. G. A. Kilpatrick, both of Henryetta. The Secretary with a special committee will have charge of the scientific program each month.

A short business meeting of the Payne County Medical Society was held December 1 at the Davis Funeral Home in Cushing immediately following the postgraduate lecture on Internal Medicine by Dr. L. W. Hunt. The Secretary reports that five of the meetings are being held in Stillwater and five in Cushing and that the lectures are very interesting. Regular county medical meetings will be resumed following the close of the course.

Dr. J. T. Colwick, Durant, was elected President of the Bryan County Society at a recent meeting. Other officers chosen are Dr. J. T. Wharton, Vice-President; Dr. W. K. Haynie, Secretary-Treasurer; Dr. John A. Haynie, Delegate, and Dr. A. J. Wells, Alternate. Drs. S. M. Toney of Bennington, J. T. Wharton and O. J. Colwick comprise the Board of Censors of the Society.

"Shock Therapy in Mental Disorders" was the subject chosen for discussion before the Ottawa County Medical Society at Miami on November 19, by Dr. P. L. Hays, a member of the Eastern Oklahoma Hospital staff, Vinita. Eighteen were in attendance at the meeting.

The Miami Baptist Hospital entertained the members of the Ottawa Society at a dinner meeting at 7:00 P. M., December 17. The speaker for the evening was Dr. William Kinney.

Dr. W. Floyd Keller presented a paper entitled "Intravenous Fluids" at the November 24 meeting of the Oklahoma County Medical Association.

A buffet dinner was served at 6:30 P. M. at the Oklahoma Club. Seventy-nine were in attendance.

• OBITUARIES •

Dr. James William Prowell
1873-1942

Dr. James William Prowell of Kansas, Delaware County, Oklahoma, passed away November 27. Dr. Prowell's death was caused by a Cerebral Hemorrhage which struck him as he was attempting to extricate his car from a small ditch.

Dr. Prowell came to Oklahoma in the early part of 1900, and for the last eighteen years practiced at Kansas. At the time of his death, he was County Health Officer for Delaware County. Dr. Prowell was a member of the American Legion, having served in World War I as a Lieutenant in the Medical Corps.

At the time of his death, Dr. Prowell was 69 years of age.

WOMEN'S AUXILIARY NEWS

Mrs. Frank L. Flack, our State President, urges all County Auxiliaries to endeavor to keep their organizations intact, in spite of the fact that many of their members have gone to join their husbands who are serving in the armed forces. She feels it is very important to have these Auxiliaries still organized at the close of the war, and although it may mean curtailing some of the activities, and a doubling up on the work by some of us who are left, it is our duty to keep things going at home until the others return to resume their normal lives again.

Our National President, Mrs. Frank L. Haggard, stresses that we should keep in touch with the doctor's wife whose husband is in the service, and that a note from her own Auxiliary will mean much, even if she is at home.

Mrs. S. J. Bradfield, of Tulsa, is the new Public Relations Chairman, replacing Mrs. Shade Neely, who resigned to join her husband in the service.

There have been several inquiries made about members at large of the Women's Auxiliary to the Oklahoma State Medical Association, and they may become members upon the payment of 50 cents dues to both the State and National Organizations. Any of the wives of members may send their dues to Mrs. H. Lee Farris, 2214 East 25th Place, Tulsa, Oklahoma, our State Treasurer.

Pottawatomie County

Dr. Paul Gallaher is in service in California, and Dr. Horton Hughes is in Louisiana serving his country. Dr. Alley is in service at Camp Wolters, Texas, and Mrs. Alley and the family are with him. Mrs. R. M. Anderson has charge of the Red Cross work in this community, and they have been making bandages.

Cleveland County

The following Cleveland County doctors are in the armed forces:

Dr. F. C. Buffington, is a First Lieutenant stationed at Jefferson Barracks, Mo. He and Mrs. Buffington are living in St. Louis, Mo.

Dr. Phil Haddock, First Lieutenant, is stationed at Camp Claiborne, La., and he and Mrs. Haddock are living in Alexandria, La.

Dr. James O. Hood, has been commissioned a Captain, and is stationed at Fort Devens, Mass. His family is living in Ayers, Mass.

Dr. Ben H. Cooley, Lieutenant Colonel, is stationed at Wm. Beaumont Hospital, El Paso. Mrs. Cooley and their daughters are in Norman.

Dr. Tom Beeler, Captain, is stationed in Mississippi, and Mrs. Beeler is with him.

Dr. C. R. Rayburn, Major, is stationed at Hunter Field, Ga. He and the family are living in Savannah.

Dr. R. J. Reichert, Captain, is stationed at Camp San Luis Obispo, California. Mrs. Reichert remained in Moore, Oklahoma.

Dr. Wm. A. Loy, First Lieutenant, reported August 21 to Fort Sill, and Mrs. Loy accompanied him.

Dr. M. P. Prosser, Captain, is stationed at Camp Gruber, and Mrs. Prosser plans to join him.

Dr. D. G. Willard, Lieutenant Commander, is stationed at the Naval Hospital, San Diego, California. Mrs. Willard and the family are living in San Diego.

Pontotoc County

The Pontotoc County Auxiliary has sponsored a surgical dressing institute for the Red Cross, and so far, there have been nine counties from that district represented at the meetings.

Tulsa County

The Tulsa County Auxiliary met for its regular monthly luncheon on December 3 in the home of Mrs. Fred Y. Cronk, and the hostesses were the Mesdames D. L. Garrett, Paul Grosshart, C. O. Armstrong, Hugh Graham, J. W. Rogers, and W. S. Larrabee. The members brought toys for their annual toy shower for the children in Tulsa Hospitals on Christmas, and they will be distributed by the Philanthropic Committee. The members also donated 24 new garments to the Needlework Guild.

The members of the Tulsa County Auxiliary donated 38 Christmas boxes for the orphaned soldiers stationed at Camp Gruber. These were turned in to the A. W. V. S. Headquarters for delivery to Camp Gruber. This Auxiliary has also furnished a day room at Camp Gruber, and has partially furnished several others.

Mrs. F. D. Sinclair, and sons, Franklin and Johnson, have joined Captain Sinclair at Fort Sam Houston, Texas.

We are happy to report that our State President, Mrs. Frank L. Flack, is able to be active again, and was at the December 3 meeting of the Tulsa Auxiliary. Best wishes to her for a complete recovery.

AWARDS OFFERED FOR SCIENTIFIC PAPERS

Announcements have been received in the Office of the Association that the American Urological Association and the National Society for the Prevention of Blindness are offering awards for outstanding medical papers in their respective fields.

The Urology Award will be for an essay or essays on some specific clinical or laboratory research in Urology. The amount of the prize will be based on the merits of the work presented. Competitors shall be limited to residents in urology in recognized hospitals and to urologists who have been in such specific practice for not more than five years.

Essays must be forwarded to the office of the Secretary, Dr. Thomas D. Moore, 899 Madison Avenue, Memphis, Tennessee, by March 1, 1943.

The prize offered by the National Society for the Prevention of Blindness. is in the amount of $250.00 and will be awarded to the paper judged to contribute the most to the present knowledge on the diagnosis of early glaucoma.

Papers should be in the office of the National Society, 1790 Broadway, New York City, by September 15, 1943.

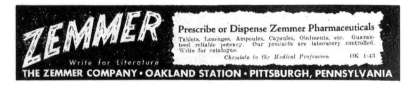

Office of Civilian Defense

I. PROGRESS REPORT OF EMERGENCY MEDICAL SERVICE.

1. The county health and housing committees have been organized in all counties.

2. Emergency Medical Service has been organized in all counties. Emergency Medical Service in some counties is very well organized, and there are other counties where a mere skeleton organization exists. County Medical Societies could aid the County Emergency Medical Chief in further perfecting the local Medical service for any eventualities from any war activities.

3. A central control system has been perfected covering all of the seventy-seven counties in the state.

4. A full-time State Nurse Deputy was appointed October 1. Nursing Councils for War Service have been set up in seventeen counties. A number of other counties are now in the process of perfecting their Nursing Councils for War Service.

5. There are now enrolled in Emergency Medical Service OCD in our state approximately eight hundred Physicians and Surgeons.

6. There are now enrolled in the Eremgency Medical Service approximately one thousand nurses.

II. HOSPITALS.

One hundred and thirty-eight hospitals have been contacted and are now working wholeheartedly with the Emergency Medical Service.

Twelve hospitals are approved for giving courses to Nurses Aides. These twelve hospitals are located in eight different counties. The National Red Cross has approved, or has in the process of being approved two additional counties. A survey of the 138 hospitals discloses that 1,825 beds are available for evacuation casualties in case of an Emergency. One base hospital has been approved by the War Department in the state, and two other base hospitals are being given some consideration. The State Emergency Medical Service has made available four Mobile Emergency Medical Hospital Units. This project was made possible by the Highway Department, State Health Department and the Emergency Medical Service. The Highway Patrol furnishes the trailer and transports same to the point of disaster where the local Emergency Medical Service will take over the manning and operation of the Unit.

III. BLOOD PLASMA.

Ninteen hospitals in the state are manufacturing blood plasma. Most of these hospitals have a limited amount of blood plasma units available to be turned over in case of an emergency to Civilian Defense. The Medical Division of the Regional Eighth Corps Area expects an inventory of the blood plasma manufactured in the State of Oklahoma, therefore, a monthly inventory is made.

IV. AMBULANCE SERVICE.

One thousand and seventeen ambulances located in various counties of the state are enrolled in the Emergency Medical Service for regular ambulance service. Arrangements have been made for emergency cars to be used for ambulance purposes in case of disaster due to the War.

V. DEFENSE FILMS.

The Defense Films shown under the auspices of the local emergency medical service continues to be in demand. The films have been shown in many parts of the state.

If your County Medical Society desires to have these films shown, have your Emergency Medical Chief make written application.

VI. IMMUNIZATION PROGRAM.

The immunization program continues in practically all parts of the state. (This immunization program is sponsored and agreed to by the State Medical Association, State Department of Health and the Emergency Medical Service).

VII. CHILD DAY CARE PROGRAM.

Proper facilities for child day care have been set up, and are in the process of being set up in five different areas.

VIII. MUTUAL AID WATER SERVICE PROGRAM.

To provide the most effective water service during an emergency, a Mutual Aid has been devised which will function under the direction of a State Water Supply Coordinator, who is also the Chief Engineer of the State Health Department in cooperation with the County Civilian Defense Committees. Under this program the state has been divided into five districts, corresponding with the five engineering districts of the Health Department. Each district will be served by the district engineer of the Health Department, and this person together with his assistants, will have access to a complete record of all trained personnel in the local communities, the location and quantity of supplies and equipment within the districts which will be available for use in any emergency involving a water system.

The following are some of the names of bulletins sent to the Emergency Medical Service over the State.

1. Municipal Sanitation Under War Conditions.

2. Emergency Mortuary Services.

3. Protection and Maintenance of Public Water Supplies Under War Conditions.

4. Volunteers in Health Medical Care and Nursing.

5. Gas Consultant.

6. Medical Field Team Equipment.

University of Oklahoma School of Medicine

The Christmas vacation for the School of Medicine will start at 5:00 P.M., December 19, 1942, and class-work will be resumed at 8:00 A.M., December 28, 1942. Final examinations will begin on January 7, and the Faculty Board will hold its annual meeting at 7:30 P.M., January 15, 1943. The enrollment for the second semester will be on January 15 and 16, and the second semester will begin at 8:00 A.M., January 18, 1943. According to the present calendar of the University, Commencement exercises will be held on May 7, 1943.

The University of Oklahoma School of Medicine was well represented at the meeting of the Oklahoma Academy of Science on December 4 and 5, at Stillwater. The following members of the faculty were included on the program:

Dr. Samuel A. Corson, who gave three illustrated lectures: "Comparative Permeability of Living Cells to Cations and Anions;" "A Quantitative Method for Microinjecting Controlled Quantities of Aqueous Solutions into Living Cells;" and "An Optical Torsion Micro-lever for Measuring Cell Permeability."

Dr. Donald B. McMullen gave an illustrated talk on "Recent Developments in the Control of Water Itch."

Dr. Mark R. Everett and Mr. Louis E. Diamond had a joint paper on "Gasometric Studies of Carbohydrate Oxidation by Hydrogen Peroxide."

Dr. Everett, Clifford F. Gastineau (Junior Student), and Miss Fay Sheppard had a joint paper on "The Catalysis of Carbohydrate Oxidation by Iron and Copper Salts."

Vitamin-rich oil, which is also suitable for varnish making, is contained in the tomato seed, according to reports from Brazil.

AMERICAN BOARD OF OBSTETRICS AND GYNECOLOGY EXAMINATIONS TO BE HELD

The next written examination and review of case histories (Part I) for all candidates will be held in various cities of the United States and Canada on Saturday, February 13, 1943, at 2:00 P.M.

Arrangements will be made so far as possible for candidates in military service to take the Part I examination (written paper and submission of case records) at their places of duty, the written examination to be proctored by the Commanding Officer (medical) or some responsible person designated by him. Material for the written examination will be sent to the proctor several weeks in advance of the examination date. Candidates for the February 13, 1943, Part I examination, who are entering military service, or who are now in Service and may be assigned to foreign duty, may submit their case records in advance of the above date, by forwarding the records to the Office of the Board Secretary. All other candidates should present their case records to the examiner at the time and place of taking the written examination.

The Office of the Surgeon General (U. S. Army) has issued instructions that men in Service, eligible for Board examinations, be encouraged to apply and that they may request orders to Detached Duty for the purpose of taking these examinations whenever possible.

All candidates will be required to take both the Part I examination, and the Part II examination (oral-clinical and pathology examination). Candidates who successfully complete the Part I examination proceed automatically to the Part II examination to be held later in the year.

The Part II examination will be held at Pittsburgh, Pennsylvania, from May 19-25, 1943. Notice of the exact time and place of the examinations will be sent all candidates well in advance of the examination date. Candidates in Military or Naval Service are requested to keep the Secretary's Office informed of any change in address.

If a candidate in service finds it impossible to proceed with the examinations of the Board, deferment without time penalty will be granted under a waiver of our published regulations applying to civilian candidates.

Applications are now being received for the 1944 examinations of the Board.

For further information and application blanks, address Dr. Paul Titus, Secretary, 1015 Highland Building, Pittsburgh (6), Pennsylvania.

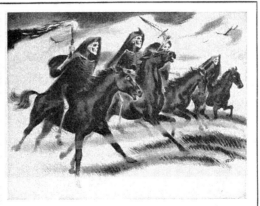

Blue Cross Reports

Enrollment in Blue Cross Hospital Service Plans has increased a hundredfold in the past few years and now protection has been extended to more than 11,000,000 workers and their dependents.

The voluntary non-profit movement for providing hospital care through the joint action of community hospitals has become and is recognized as a national influence in the provision of health service. The action of the American Hospital Association in permitting use of the seal of the Association superimposed upon a Blue Cross has been a great factor in the growth of the movement. The snowball started by a few hospitals ten years ago has become an avalanche of community action throughout the nation, or to change the metaphor, a powerful genie which serves the American people in removing the uncertainty and dread of hospital bills.

The example of Blue Cross service sponsored and guaranteed by community hospitals has led to two additional developments in the provision of hospital care; namely, the offering of hospitalization benefit policies by numerous private insurance companies, and, more important, the suggestion for a federal system of hospitalization benefits under the Social insurance provisions of the Social Security Act.

It is, perhaps, only natural that commercial insurance companies would feel justified in extending their protection to include hospitalization contracts, because the American people had been made "hospital conscious" by the Blue Cross movement. Probably some six million participants are today enrolled in commercial and industrial plans. A composite picture of all Blue Cross plans in America reveals that the operation costs for 1941 was less than 12 per cent. Since the remainder must go for payment of hospital bills or increased benefits to members, it is obvious that no serious threat exists from commercial companies that, of course, do not operate as non-profit organizations. Then, too, there is usually no conflict with a cash indemnity rebate and the Blue Cross service agreement.

A compulsory system can be avoided by the voluntary hospitals. If the hospitals of America will continue to support their Blue Cross Plans, they can avoid great inconvenience and regimentation which would develop from a system in which most of their revenue will be received through a single agency.

The present satisfactory hospital income should not obscure the actual facts or present trends in the provision of hospital care. Much of the present high occupancy and income of community hospitals is derived directly from war activity. A very large portion of hospital care is now rendered to patients employed by firms whose products are purchased by government agencies, which, in turn, are financed by local, state, and federal taxation. After the war, a momentary demand will be made for more, rather than less, government support of essential services which have been regularly supplied to members of the Armed Forces. A firmly established voluntary, non-government system of distributing hospital care for employed workers and their families will permit the government, at that time, to concentrate upon service to the unemployed, indigent, and other recipients of public assistance.

The tremendous acceptance of Blue Cross Plans has not been solely because of the rates and benefits offered, but mainly because these non-profit corporations, operating as they do, fulfill their functions in such a manner as to preserve individual self-help and freedom and the perpetuation of our voluntary health system.

A man will talk much of his experience, and make the same mistake every day.

News From The State Health Department

Health in Industry

The health of the American worker has become the topic of much writing and conversation during the past year. People in all walks of life are looking with increasing interest toward the problems of health in industry. The United States Bureau of Labor Statistics has estimated that, as of April 1, 1942, approximately nine million workers were engaged in the typical war industries. By the close of 1942, many more will be so employed. Of this number the great percentage will be made up of men in the older age groups, women, and younger workers who have been rejected from military service for physical or mental disability. The responsibility of guiding the employment of these sub-standard workers and of assisting in the reduction and prevention of accidents and illnesses rests with the physician who derives even a small part of his practice from industry, the general practitioner as well as the surgeon.

The pre-employment medical examination must be used as a means of proper placement of workers in jobs for which they are best suited and in which they will be of least danger to themselves, their fellow workmen and to the industry. In all industries, large and small, engaged in vital war production, medical examinations should be instituted without delay where they do not now exist. In order to make such activity worthwhile, it is important that the physician have a working knowledge of the actual operations within the plant and of the real or potential hazards which may exist. This information may be obtained only by visiting the plant and observing all of the operations involved.

Industrial medicine is no longer concerned only with treatment of traumatic injuries and occupational diseases. Prevention of occupational and non-occupational diseases and injuries is of paramount importance at this time. This is absolutely necessary not only because of the employment of sub-standard workers but because there is the problem of fewer available physicians should sickness and accident rates increase. New substances and processes have been introduced into industry, many of which are potentially harmful. Other substances of known toxicity which were replaced by less toxic or non-toxic substances in peace time, must now be used in industry again, due to shortage of materials and priority restrictions. There are many other reasons why medicine must devote a great part of its attention to industry at this time. Local and Governmental agencies are ready and willing to do their part for conservation of manpower.

The Oklahoma State Health Department has an active Industrial Hygiene Service which is available and capable of giving assistance to the physicians of industry. Through plant surveys and studies, and medical and engineering consultation, effective service for the health protection of workers in industrial plants is available. Requests for assistance are given prompt attention.

Classified Advertisements

MEDICAL PREPAREDNESS

Physicians To Be Dislocated

The following release has been received from the Directing Board of the Procurement and Assignment Service with the request that it be given immediate publicity:

"It is of the utmost importance that the Procurement and Assignment Service for Physicians, Dentists and Veterinarians, immediately has the name of any doctor who really is willing to be dislocated for service, either in industry or in over-populated areas, and who has not been declared essential to his present locality. This is necessary if the medical profession is to be able to meet these needs adequately and promptly. We urgently request that any physician over the age of 45 who wishes to participate in the war effort send in his name to the State Chairman for the Procurement and Assignment Service in his State."

Oklahoma physicians above the age of 45 should give careful consideration to the above request before enrolling with Dr. W. W. Rucks, 210 Plaza Court, Oklahoma City, the Procurement and Assignment Chairman for Oklahoma.

In the past, there have been far too many physicians who, in a spirit of patriotism, have offered their services in any field in which the Procurement and Assignment Service felt they could be utilized; and when they were subsequently called upon, found that circumstances in their local locality had been altered to such an extent that their original desire to serve in a dislocated capacity or non-military governmental agency could no longer be considered without creating a medical shortage in their own community.

With this new appeal from the Procurement and Assignment Service needing immediate response, it is urged that before a physician enrolls his name he first consult with his local Procurement and Assignment Service Committee as to whether he is considered available for dislocation.

While new quotas for 1943 have not been announced, there is little doubt that Oklahoma will have to supply additional physicians for the armed service during the coming year. On September 1, the 1942 quota for Oklahoma stood at 121 per cent, which will mean the 1943 quota will be reduced in proportion to the number now in the service over and above last year's quota.

The announcement from Selective Service concerning the induction of men over the age of 38 will obviously place a greater responsibility for volunteering on the physicians under that age. In all probability, the majority of the age groups up to 38 years of age will be invited to make applications for commissions; however, physicians between the ages of 38 and 45 will not be excluded from securing commissions, if they are available for service from the standpoint of medical care in their local community and can meet the qualifications of the military Medical Corps.

BOOK REVIEWS

"The chief glory of every people arises from its authors."—Dr. Samuel Johnson.

THE TOXEMIAS OF PREGNANCY. William J. Dieckmann, M.D., Professor of Obstetrics and Gynecology, the University of Chicago and Chicago Lying-in Hospital and Dispensary. C. V. Mosby Publishers, 521 Pages.

Dr. Dieckmann, in the very first chapter, outlines and discusses the present day classification of the toxemias of pregnancy with a very excellent review of the classification suggested by the American Committee on Maternal Welfare. He stresses the importance of placing all patients in one group or another with a definite diagnosis, even if it is found necessary to reclassify them later. He recognizes two big groups, namely: A. Toxemia where the disease is not peculiar to the particular pregnancy, having existed prior to the present pregnancy and B. Where the toxemia is peculiar to or dependent upon the pregnancy, stating the pre-eclampsia and eclampsia are true complications of pregnancy and occur only in pregnant women.

The incidence of the different types of toxemia are dealt with and he especially does review and discuss the incidence of eclampsia the world over.

Dr. Dieckmann does not feel that, as yet, we have any characteristic pathological lesion that could be interpreted as being specific of eclampsia. He has identified similar lesions in the livers and kidneys, at times, in non-pregnant persons where death was caused by other diseases. His review of the different causes of death in 41 patients with eclampsia is very timely. Circulatory failure was the most frequent cause of the immediate death.

Section II, dealing with normal and abnormal physiology is presented in masterly form. By reading and understanding this portion of the book one's knowledge of the normal physiology is so refreshed that the abnormal physiology is more easily understood. By taking advantage of the author's knowledge of biochemistry, his wide experience of interpreting certain laboratory and chemistry reports the obstetrician can save many dollars for his patients as Dr. Dieckmann elaborates on the laboratory procedures that are valueless as well as those that are of value.

The chapter on recording the blood pressure is well worth while. The different sounds and phases are considered. Normal blood pressures in pregnant and non-pregnant patients are discussed. Special tests that might affect the blood pressure are discussed.

No place in the present available literature could one learn so much in so few pages as he could in the two chapters on the physiology of the kidneys and liver. Dr. Dieckmann's knowledge of their physiology and his evaluation of the functional test are worth any physician's time. His assimilation of data and their evaluation represents years of work and study.

The two chapters on the relation of the endocrine glands to the toxemias are interesting but, as in endocrinology in general, lacks definite experimental evidence and background, as yet, to be supplied. The pituitary and thyroid gland seem to be associated with toxemia more than the other glands.

The section on the physiology of the development of edema in pre-eclampsia and eclampsia gives one a better understanding of why it develops and how to treat it. The signs and symptoms are described in such a way and so thoroughly elaborated upon that all who are interested in obstetrics should read and re-read these chapters. The individual discussion on the various types of toxemias are considered with well prepared case reports. Complications, prognosis and the obstetrical management of these different types are individually

considered. In the chapter on pharmacodynamics, the hypnotics, anesthetics and sedatives are discussed thoroughly and individually. Here one can find the present day opinion of these drugs as they should be used or not used in the treatment of the toxemias.

The procedures used and methods of treatment are discussed and presented in detail. One of the most important chapters of the book is Chapter XXVI where it deals with the indication for terminating pregnancy, the methods of choice and precautions to take. This is followed by chapters on the obstetrical treatment of eclampsia and the non-convulsive toxemias.

Maternal and fetal mortality, as well as morbidity, is presented in Section VI. After reading this section one will want to re-read the book, for here is published by an authority on the subject data not only of the deaths caused by the toxemias but pathological changes that take place resulting in partial or complete invalidism.

This book of Dr. Dieckmann's represents years of work and continuous study of this most important subject. All who are interested in obstetrics will be stimulated and more determined than ever before to evaluate and do something about these treacherous signs and symptoms, namely: excessive weight gain, edema, headaches, alleviation of blood pressure and albuminuria as they occur or are found in pregnant women. Let this be the book of the year for the obstetrician or the general practitioner who does obstetrics.—J. M. Parrish, Jr., M.D.

DR. COLWELL'S DAILY LOG FOR PHYSICIANS. A brief, simple, accurate financial record for the physician's desk. Colwell Publishing Company, Champaign, Illinois, 1942. Price $6.00.

Dr. Colwell's Daily Log appointments and accounts has saved many a dollar and many a headache for the busy doctor. It supplies a simple but comprehensive system of bookkeeping which enables the office secretary to accurately record the "days run" as she attends to other routine duties. The convenient arrangement of the book with outlines for every transaction encourages consecutive recording. In this way, the hazards of memory and recollection are safely negotiated.

The summary sheet appearing at the end of each calendar month keeps the secretary and the doctor informed, offers a ready comparison with previous months and with the same month in previous years, and, what is more important, it supplies ample data for the compilation of income tax reports.

For the benefit of those who are not familiar with this record book, may we add that it provides an obstetrical waiting list, narcotic records, social security, deaths and notifiable diseases.

If you are worried about your haphazard handling of the above items, you may want to consider Dr. Colwell's Daily Log.—Lewis J. Moorman, M.D.

WHEN DOCTORS ARE RATIONED. Dwight Anderson and Margaret Baylour. Pp. 255. 1, chapters. Coward-McCann, Inc., 2 West 45th Street, New York City. Price $2.00.

This volume is intended primarily to assist those millions who, because of the needs of the United States Armed Forces and the interests of the public, have temporarily, at least, lost their family physicians. One of the co-authors is Director of Public Relations, Medical Society of the State of New York, and an introduction is by Dr. Nathan B. Van Etten, who recently served with distinction as President of the American Medical Association.

It therefore follows that the subjects discussed and the advice offered has been done in an orthodox manner. All activities and institutions which are related in any way to the art of medical practice are given due consideration. These include clinics, hospitals, standardized and otherwise, drug stores, prescribing druggists, self-treatment, specialists, quacks and the irregulars.

If the prospective patient follows the advice given by the authors, the procedure usually followed in the selection of a new doctor will, to say the least, be considerably extended. A friendly neighbor or an acquaintance may, as in the past, be asked to recommend a physician, but he will also be asked whether the physician belongs to his county medical society and takes postgraduate courses. If satisfactory information is not obtained in this manner, the prospective patient is told that good public libraries usually contain medical directories which contain up-to-date information on every legally licensed doctor in the country; also, directories of the various specialists. A differentiation is made between a qualified specialist and one who, without such qualifications, has set himself up as such.

The "Bedside Manner" of a strange doctor often wins or losses a client with the first contact, and there are not a few otherwise well qualified physicians who, because of a lack of that "something," cannot win the confidence of the patient. Many of our younger doctors receive their clinical training in charity wards of general public hospitals where the necessity for a tactful approach to the patient is not given serious consideration largely because the patient does not have the privilege of making a choice. Chapter XIII of this book should serve to correct this lack of very necessary training if and when the building of a private practice is under consideration.

The authors have also lectured the prospective patient on "How to Be a Good Patient" to the end that the most satisfactory results possible may be obtained under existing circumstances.

Finally, a warning is sounded as to the future of medical practice. That an attempt will be made to continue rationing of doctors after the war is an almost forgone conclusion. Even before the war and for several years this move has been under way—largely from influences originating outside the profession.

Apropos of this warning, the volume is brought to a close with this paragraph: "One of the most important decisions which the people have to make, or have made for them, when the war is over, is whether they will have the doctor of their choice, one toward whom the feeling of confidence is most likely to flow, or a doctor rationed to them, whom they must accept whether they like him or not, or go without medical care."

A wide-spread reading of this volume by the public could not result otherwise than good in helping to continue the march of medical advance in our beloved country after the war is over.—Horace Reed, M.D.

Warn Against the Use of Sulfathiazole For Infections Within the Skull

Their findings in experimental investigations of the use of the sulfonamide drugs for intracranial infections constitute "a clear warning against the intracranial use of sulfathiazole," Cobb Pilcher, M.D., Ralph Angelucci, M.D., and William F. Meacham, M.D., Nashville, Tenn., report in the July 18 issue of The Journal of the American Medical Association.

The development of convulsions in a very high percentage of their investigations following the implantation of sulfathiazole, the three physicians say, "prompts this preliminary report, as a warning against the clinical use of this drug in this manner. . . . Sulfanilamide and sulfadiazine do not appear to have the same irritating effects on the cerebral cortex, but until microscopic studies are completed no conclusion can be drawn in this regard."

MEDICAL ABSTRACTS

"TRANSPLANTS TO THE THUMB TO RESTORE FUNC-
TION OF OPPOSITION: END RESULTS." C. E. Irwin,
M.D. Southern Medical Journal. Vol. XXXV, P. 257.
March, 1942.

Lack of opposition power in the thumb is a serious
handicap to the usefulness of the hand. The grasping
ability of the hand is decreased to the extent that its
function is hardly more than a hook, and the finer movements of the hand are lost. The various movements of
the thumb are discussed. Following an attack of infantile paralysis, many of these movements may be lost.
A basic transplant to restore the usefulness of the thumb
includes the following features:

1. The course of the transplanted tendon from the
muscle belly to the pulley must be in a straight line.

2. The pulley must be so constructed that its original
position will remain constant.

3. The pulley must be so constructed that it will
allow free gliding movement of the tendon.

4. The tendon must lie in front of or toward the
flexor side of the metacarpophalangeal joint as it passes
to its insertion in the base of the proximal phalanx.

5. The tendon is fastened directly to the bone, entering the proximal phalanx of the thumb on the border
adjacent to the web.

The details of the mechanical advantages of this transplant are described. The flexor sublimis tendon to the
fourth finger is passed through a tendinous pulley,
formed at the pisiform bone by a part of the flexor
carpi ulnaris, is extended subcutaneously, and is attached
to a tunnel in the second phalanx of the thumb. Contraindications and postoperative treatment are discussed.
The results obtained were good, twelve; fair, four; and
poor, three.—E. D. M., M.D.

"CALCIFICATION AND OSSIFICATION OF VERTE-
BRAL LIGAMENTS (SPONDYLITIS OSSIFICANS
LIGAMENTOSA); ROENTGEN STUDY OF PATHO-
GENESIS AND CLINICAL SIGNIFICANCE." Albert
Oppenheimer, M.D. Radiology, Vol. XXXVIII. P. 160.
Feb., 1942.

The pathogenesis of this condition is disputable. The
longitudinal ligaments are often calcified or ossified in
the presence of vertebral infections, such as, tuberculosis
typhoid, staphylococci osteitis, syphilis, and malta fever;
after trauma; and less commonly, around malignant
metastases. It may be present in juvenile and in senile
kyphosis.

Bone hypertrophy always follows rarefaction. When
vertebrae adjacent to a thinned disc are constantly injured mechanically, because of the loss of thickness and
elasticity of their natural buffer, traumatic rarefaction
results—a reaction corresponding to callus formation.
A triangular area between the anterior vertebral edge,
the attachment of the longitudinal ligament to the body
above this edge, and to the disc below, presents a vertebral surface devoid of ligamentary covering. It is in
this space that vertebral osteophytes form. Instead of
playing an active part in the formation of osteophytes,
the vertebral ligaments mold them and set a limit to
their growth.

The longitudinal ligaments may be calcified or ossified
in the absence of other vertebral lesions. This tends to
occur where the ligament is relaxed, as opposite a reduced
intervertebral space or on the concave side of a kyphosis
or scoliosis. Calcification and ossification of vertebral

ligaments are not typical of any disease, and should not
be confused with arthritis. In their presence, vertebral
mobility is normal, unless there is also present disease
of the apophyseal joints or vertebral bodies. Complete
spinal rigidity has been observed in Marie-Strumpell
disease, in the entire absence of calcification or ossification of ligaments. This condition does not cause pain.
It is not a pathological or a clinical entity, but a secondary reaction, often indicating the coexistence of a lesion
or the vertebral bones or joints.—E. D. M., M.D.

"THE GEOGRAPHIC PATHOLOGY OF ST. LOUIS EN-
CEPHALITIS." Albert E. Casey, M.D., Birmingham,
Alabama. Southern Medical Journal, Vol. 35, No. 10,
October, 1942.

In this report, it seems that the author has contributed
information resulting from a study of the graphic distribution of encephalitis of a distinct type which occurred
in St. Louis and St. Louis County in 1933 and 1937,
which may be exceptionally important.

It was found to be significantly distributed along the
small streams in St. Louis and St. Louis County, all
of which carried sewerage, and in areas characterized
by weeds and garbage dumps; and it was significantly
scarce in both epidemics in those areas not characterized
by weeds, open sewage and ponds. Using an adequate
control series and biometrical methods, no foci were
found along the most traveled highways in St. Louis
County, along the principal boulevards in St. Louis,
along the interstate railroads, and there was no relation
of the disease to congested housing. There was no
evidence that in 1937 the population in the heart of
the city where the disease was significantly scarce contained more immune persons than were to be found in
the areas of greatest concentration of the disease. In
fact, there was a possible significant preponderance of
immune persons in the areas of greatest concentration
(the disease occurred in the same districts in 1933).
The distribution of the disease was different from that
of measles. The possibility of a mosquito vector was
considered.

The discussion of this report was also enlightening.
Dr. Goronwy Owen Broun of St. Louis, an authority,
had the following to say:

"The status of mosquito transmission of this disease
at the present time is as follows: The distribution of
the case of St. Louis encephalitis as Dr. Casey has
pointed out, is such as you would expect from an insect-
borne disease where the insect lives along streams. That
would be in favor of the mosquito as vector.

"It would be necessary, of course, to show that
mosquitoes biting an infected animal could acquire the
virus. That has been done in the case St. Louis encephalitis, by Webster, in the case of the Anopheles
mosquito, and in our own laboratory we have shown
that the Culex pipiens, which is the most common mosquito in this neighborhood, is able to harbor the virus
after biting an infected animal.

"Thirdly, it should be possible to find infected mosquitoes in an epidemic neighborhood. That has been
done, as Dr. Smith has pointed out, with mosquitoes
captured in the state of Washington during an epidemic,
a variety of Culex, Culex tarsalis, being found spontaneously infected with virus.

"Locally here we have captured mosquitoes in the
last several years, but I would like to point out that
this was in the period between the epidemic outbreaks.

So far, in this area, we have not found any infected mosquitoes.

"There is a final point still needed to prove the possibility of mosquito transmission of St. Louis encephalitis. So far it has not been demonstrated that once a mosquito acquires the virus and bites a second animal, that the animal will become infected with encephalitis. Webster attempted to do this with infected Anopheles mosquitoes, and we have done similar experiments with infected Culex. The animals bitten by the mosquitoes did not become ill with encephalitis.

"It is, of course, known that the virus, when injected under the skin of mice does not cause encephalitis. If injected into a nerve or introduced into the nasal passage so that it comes in contact with the olfactory nerve, then the animal becomes infected. The proof of transmission by the bite of infected mosquitoes is therefore still missing in evidence needed to prove mosquito transmission.

"Recent work has shown that in the case of lymphocytic meningitis, the temperature to which the mosquito is subjected prior to biting an animal is important, and this may be a factor in the transmission of St. Louis encephalitis.

"Still another method of transmission deserves some mention, namely, entry of the virus through the gastrointestinal tract. That the intestinal tract is a possible portal of entry for the infection is shown by the observations of Harford, Sulkin and Bronfenbrenner. These investigators have shown that an adult mouse after devouring infected young, may become infected with encephalitis.

"Dr. Mezera working in our laboratory introduced the virus directly into the gastro-intestinal tract by injection after laparotomy. In only one instance among fifty did the virus so introduced into the intestine result in production of encephalitis."—H. J., M.D.

"THE INHERITANCE OF DIABETES INSIPIDUS." Harry Blotner, M.D., Associate in Medicine, Peter Bent Brigham Hospital, Boston, Mass. American Journal of the Medical Sciences, August, 1942, Vol. 204, No. 2, Pages 261-265.

"The term diabetes insipidus means a marked polyuria and polydipsia which usually ranges from at least six to ten liters a day and is relieved by pituitrin. The polyuria and polydipsia are even present during the night, when the patient is in bed."

The functional pathology attending the mal-functioning of the pituitary glands and its anatomic environs, have been known in its relation to Diabetes Insipidus for a long time. Tumors of the hypophysis and regional anatomy, fractures, infections, and many etiological factors have been attributed to its development. The most common cause is Idiopathic, where neither x-ray biochemistry or meticulous history taking has given a clue as to its onset. The experience of its being a familial disease has been studied by several continental clinicians. The most notable being Adolph Weil, 1884, when he studied four generations of a family of 91 members, headed by a man with Diabetes Insipidus and found that 24 of these had the disease. His son followed up and found in five generations of this family that there were 35 cases among 225 members. Another case studied by Chester and Spiegel with both maternal and paternal ancestry affected, had one child by one marriage, and one child by another marriage so affected.

The author has followed a case for five years in which the mother and grandmother had the disease. Since there is so little in American literature about its family proclivities that he has meticulously reported this case and reviewed the literature on this subject. Among the 70 cases of this trouble in the records of Peter Bent Brigham Hospital, this seemed to have been the only one. The author concludes, however, that when this disease is inherited it may be found rather frequently in such a family. He claims the disease may appear shortly after birth or in later life. He says there is a rather general impression that the familial Diabetes Insipidus is due to a dominant gene and transmitted through many generations of a family through maternal and paternal side to either female or male.—L. A. R.

"UNUSUALLY HIGH INSULIN REQUIREMENTS IN DIABETES MELLITUS." William I. Glass, M.D.; Clifford L. Spingarn, M.D.; and Herbert Pollack, M.D., New York. Archives of Internal Medicine, Vol. 70, No. 2, August, 1942. Pages 221-235.

No two cases of diabetes mellitus are treated alike. They vary from day to day during the course of the disease and its complications. The Dextrose-Insulin ratio is changed by so many fundamental factors. Bizarre conditions are frequently met with when enormous doses in insulin resistent cases present themselves. The author divides the insulin resistent cases into two groups: one, those connected with some complication, as diabetic ketosis, infection, endocrine disorder, and hepatic disease. Two, a large group probably called idiopathic, where clinical and post-mortem findings do not identify the etiology.

The case the author reports is one which was observed for six months, giving 85,000 units of insulin with some days reaching 2,800, 2,500, 2,700, to relieve the ketosis. The cases ultimately managed on five units a day. This case emphasizes the statement of Martin "that there is not necessarily any upper limit to the number of units of insulin that may be given."

His guide for the administration of insulin was the presence of acetone and dextrose in the urine and the general condition of the patient. The persistent acetonuria caused an effective level to be reached, only on giving 200 units hourly for ten hours. He was prepared to raise the dose to a higher level if need be. He says "this experience supports the concept of Taussig that in case of insulin insensitivity, the law of mass action of inorganic chemistry is valid with respect to the action of insulin."

He changed diets, insulin, gave intravenous phosphates, various endocrine substances, low potassium diet, desensitization, procedures to depress the activity of the anterior lobe, by roentgen ray of pituitary area. It is known that the anterior pituitary and pancreas are antogonists and that excessive antutiary secretion weakens the pancreatic hormones so x-ray therapy was centered on the silla turcica, but if results were obtained that was only three months treatment. Diabetes in dogs can be produced by long injection of anterior pituitary substances. Lipocaic, a fat free extract of pancreas is effective in maintaining depancreatized dogs alive, but it was not sure that was effective in this case, although given. It was felt by the author that there was only slight hepatic dysfunction.

A transient bacillary diarrhea was noted to upset the ketogenic anti-ketogenic balance temporarily. Tests for hepatic efficiency were done and not found abnormal, even though hepatomegaly was present, and even slight icterus at one time.

The insulin resistance gradually diminished so that after a six months period, management was carried on with only five units of insulin a day on a prescribed diet.

This case is quite educational because the outcome would have been very different had not treatment with heroic doses of insulin, under proper guidance, been instituted. This also emphasizes the fact that insulin insensibility may be only of short duration and the one in charge should be alert to the daily changes.—L. A. R.

"PITRESSIN TANNATE IN OIL IN THE TREATMENT OF DIABETES INSIPIDUS." Harry Blotner, M.D., Boston, Mass. Journal A. M. A., Vol. 119, No. 13, July 25, 1942.

The treatment of diabetes insipidus has gone through many stages of evolution since it was found to have its etiology in the base of the brain, and the harmone of the posterior pituitary body was isolated. He first used obstetrical and surgical pituitrin by hypodermic

I like S-M-A!

IN INFANT FEEDING ...IT SAVES MY TIME

● Directions on how to mix and feed S-M-A can be explained to the mother and nurse in two minutes.

● S-M-A is more easily digested by the normal infant because of the all-lactose carbohydrate and the unique S-M-A fat.

● With S-M-A nothing is left to chance. All the vitamin requirements, except ascorbic acid, together with additional iron are included in S-M-A in the proper balance, ready to feed.

● S-M-A fed infants compare favorably with breast-fed infants in growth and development.

Prescribe S-M-A!

*S-M-A, a trade mark of S.M.A. Corporation, for its brand of food especially prepared for infant feeding—derived from tuberculin-tested cow's milk, the fat of which is replaced by animal and vegetable fats, including biologically tested cod liver oil, with the addition of milk sugar and potassium chloride; altogether forming an antirachitic food. When diluted according to directions, it is essentially similar to human milk in percentages of protein, fat, carbohydrate and ash, in chemical constants of the fat and physical properties.

S. M. A. CORPORATION • 8100 McCORMICK BOULEVARD • CHICAGO, ILLINOIS

injection, and then found that by insufflating it, it had even a better effect, since some thought it was absorbed closer to the hypophysis. Then the pituitary powder was commercially available and its insufflation was effective and more economic. Insufflation was only a fair weather treatment that was not dependable when a cold or allergy prevented its absorption. Now since pituitary glandular substances has so many harmones, it was found that the posterior pituitary contained a pressor substance which is precipitated by tannic acid. This was filtered out, dried, and dissolved in peanut oil. This pressor substance, Pitressin Tannate in Oil, does not have the oxytoxic effect, nor does it produce the intestinal cramp, diarrhoea, headaches, palpitation or pallor. The effects of the water soluble or powdered form is very short, lasting only a few hours, and later may produce sore arms. The sudden absorption was the cause of the unpleasant effects, so it was found the slow absorption in peanut oil added decidedly to the efficiency and length of the therapeutic effect, as insulin combined with protamine and zinc, by its slow absorption, has added good qualities to the therapy of diabetes mellitus.

The Pitressin Tannate in Oil in one c. c. ampoules will cause a diminution in urinary output in a few hours, and the following day the amount will be diminished. The daily injection of this ampoule seems to have a cumulative effect, so that after a few days one ampoule will control the polyuria and polydipsia for as much as 48 to 60 hours in eight cases he studied. (The reviewer has noticed that emotional factors produced a lessened efficiency and required a larger dosage of this drug, as it correspondingly does in protamine zinc insulin.)

The urinary output in adequate dosage would lessen the thirst and bring down the output to the physiological amount, but would not reduce it below that point unless heroic dosages were given. The author found in the case of the brain tumor, that the polydipsia and polyurias refractory to the solution of posterior pituitary, but the use of Pitressin Tannate in Oil reduced to an intake of 3200 to 2400 c. c. The output was 1100 to 1195 c. c.

The author has given the clinical histories and charts showing the relative effects of Pitressin Tannate in Oil with no treatment on the daily output of a patient with diabetes insipidus. Various blood tests were done and one c.c. of the drug was always given. The specific gravity of the urine would raise from 1000-1010, to 1024-1036. The weight of the patient did not seem to have been affected. The author said it was interesting to note the increased saliva and improved appetite and digestion. The dryness of the mouth disappeared more definitely with Tannate than plain water soluble post-pituitary therapy. (The reviewer noticed one case of a pregnancy in diabetes insipidus was relieved of her vomiting and the bad effects of pregnancy when started on this therapy, only to return when the effect of her medicine wore off.) This treatment has certainly been a boon to those so afflicted, as they would be unable to sleep but a short time at night, or go out in society or places of amusement, because of the frequency or urination and in such large amounts. The secondary effects was the dilatation of the portions of the urinary tract. The life expectancy was not affected, as these cases frequently live to a ripe old age, going through pregnancies as otherwise normal individuals.—L. A. R.

"IRON IN NUTRITION (REQUIREMENTS FOR IRON)."
Clark W. Heath, M.D. Journal of A. M. A., October 3, 1942, Pages 366-369.

"There is no more useful field in nutritional research at the present time than the exploration of the adequacy and inadequacy of different foods and enriched foods in supplying substances necessary to the health of man."

Iron he calls a one way substance, i. e., it is not lost to the body economy by the normal kidney, bowel, or other emunctories. The iron lost to the blood by excessive absorption is stored up in the liver, kidneys, spleen, and other organs as a depository for future use if needs be.

The matter of growth, pregnancy, menstruation, lactation and other physiologic functions may call on added intake to replace the drainage from these depositories. The study of patients having hypochromic anaemia which is alleviated by iron medication shows that serious blood loss can usually be demonstrated. Even when on a very poor diet with inadequate iron and mal-absorption by a disordered gastrointestinal tract, the real cause will be found to be in blood loss. Even then when a patient has achylorhydria or gastrointestinal disturbances, interfering with adequate iron in a diet, the anaemia will respond to inorganic iron in large doses. "The child at birth has a certain amount of stored iron which is available for use. In prematurity and twin births, this may be considerably limited and these infants are later vulnerable to iron deficiency."

The amount of iron absorbed into the body is quite large. One experiment of the absorption of 6 gms. of iron, was more than is assumed to be present in the normal body. The increased storing of iron gets pathologic in haemachromatosis where over 50 gms. may be recovered from the tissues. Hence there must be a delicate mechanism which controls the normal amount of iron in the tissues. In dogs and man, iron absorbed is retained in greater amounts when needed for blood regeneration. Iron is absorbed in the upper intestine. (The reticulocyte response to large iron dosage following blood loss, is like that in primary anaemia following liver therapy.)

The need of iron varies in different ages and under different conditions. Chlorosis has disappeared because of the outdoor activities and heliotherapy of our modern girls. Iron requirements are greatest in infancy, early childhood, and puberty, being larger in females than males, and increased during pregnancy. Consequently, when physiologic needs are not supplied, iron deficiency anaemia will occur.

. Sixteen per cent of the female patients entering Boston City Hospital medical wards have iron deficiency. If stores of iron are deficient, then these stores must be replenished by dieting and iron. The synergistic effect of copper, cobolt and manganese is still subjudice, because of the proportion of these elements in the usual iron derivatives.

The problem regarding iron in enriching flour has to do with the choice of iron preparation, the ease and efficiency of mixing palatibility and availability, together with the possible detriment on other constituents. It is fairly certain that iron as a simple salt added to flour will be more available than the iron in close organic combination in original flour. "There has also been shown a relationship betwen the utilization of iron and the amounts of phosphorus and calcium in the diet." On the other hand, there is no definite indication that harm would result from the addition of small amounts of iron salts to flour.

"At the present time, it would appear that if whole grain flours were widely used and the advantages of widely chosen and adequate diet were promulgated, nutritional requirements for iron and other minerals would be adequately supplied."—L. A. R.

"EPIDEMIC KERATOCONJUNCITIVITIS (SUPERFICIAL PUNCTATE KERATITIS, KERATITIS SUBEPITHELIALIS, KERATITIS MACULOSA, KERATITIS NUMMULARIS) WITH A REVIEW OF THE LITERATURE AND A REPORT OF 125 CASES." M. J. Hogan and J. W. Crawford. American Journal of Ophthalmology, Vol. 25, Pp. 1059-1078. September, 1942.

The acute inflammatory eye disease appeared in the region of San Francisco in September, 1941, and spread rapidly among the shipworkers in a form of epidemic. It has been called by various names. The term of epidemic keratoconjunctivitis is a good descriptive term since the affection is characterized by edema of the lids and conjunctiva, followed by intense hyperemia, but with very little discharge, keratitic spots developing in from five to eight days just beneath Bowman's membrane.

The disease is now being seen in various parts of the United States. The authors have recognized and treated a good many cases, and base their present report upon 125 observations. It is not a new disease, since, in 1889, Stellwag described it as a peculiar form of keratitis. Since that time, many other ophthalmologists have studied it and observed it all over the world. Only recently a widespread epidemic has been reported in Germany and Southern Europe. In the United States the first epidemic occurred in 1938 in San Fernando, California. In 1941, Holmes recorded about 10,000 cases in an epidemic that occurred on the island of Oahu, Hawaii, from where the disease was probably imported to San Francisco.

Epidemic keratoconjunctivitis has been described in so many different pictures that it seems there are many possible variations in the disease. The conjunctival symptoms may be mild followed by severe keratitis, or they may be mild followed by a mild keratitis. The corneal signs are also subject to considerable variation; some lesions can be seen only with the slitlamp, while others are disciform in appearance.

In the epidemic observed by the present authors, the course of the disease was as follows. Acute conjunctivitis was the first symptom. The patients complained of a "sandy" sensation as if a foreign body were present. In some patients there was intense itching. Within a few hours, glassy edema of the caruncle and semilunar fold appeared and spread to the lower cul-de-sac and bulbar conjunctiva. At this stage there was a little hyperemia. Within 24 hours slight edema of the lids and skin with pseudoptosis became evident. Within from 36 to 48 hours the swollen conjunctiva became congested and red and there was some lacrimatoin. The bulbar conjunctiva was elevated somewhat at the limbus. Most characteristic at this stage was the intense hyperemia and swelling without discharge. In about three-fourths of the patients the regional lymph nodes were enlarged (preauricular, angular, submandibular, and cervical).

In the more severe forms so much edema was present that the conjunctiva was sometimes ballooned out through the palpebral fissure. In this form, severe keratitis nearly always followed. The conjunctivitis was follicular in several patients. A few of them developed bilateral conjunctivitis, either simultaneously in both eyes, or the second eye became affected four or five days later. In some instances, the conjunctivitis was accompanied by conjunctival hemorrhages. Several patients developed extensive, white, fairly thick pseudomembranes covering the palpebral conjunctiva, caruncle and fold. Other patients had transient, milky pseudomembranes on the tarsal conjunctiva of the lids, especially on that of the lower lid. The average duration of the conjunctivitis was 13 days.

Keratitis occurred in about 80 per cent of the patients. It began between the second and eighth days after the onset of the conjunctivitis. Deep lesions of the substantia propria were found in a few patients of whom a smaller number had also iritis with small creamy, round, sharply defined keratitic precipitates, an aqueous flare, and cells. The early corneal changes were tiny punctate infiltrates of the epithelial-erosion type; they healed as the conjunctivitis regressed, and could be stained with fluoresceine. On about the eighth day, typical macular infiltrates could be observed; first, a general haze was noticed; very soon dotlike opacities appeared, which soon coalesced, forming larged foci. The well-developed lesions were 0.5 to 1.5 mm. in diameter, round or oval, sometimes angular, and varied in number from 10 to 100 or more. They were located chiefly in the superficial substantia propria. Characteristic was a lack of ulceration and of vascularization of these lesions.

The corneal infiltrates outlasted the acute conjunctival symptoms by a considerable period. In most cases the lesions became faint within three months. A few patients showed, however, dense corneal maculas and diminution of visual acuity to 20/40 at the end of four months. The prognosis for ultimate vision was good in most of the cases, and even in the most severe cases 20/30 vision was usually attained at the end of three months.

It is probable that the disease is endemic in the Far East where the largest epidemics have been reported. It is believed that the disease is not highly contagious. The disease in the San Francisco epidemic spread by close contact, with direct transfer of the infectious agent. Individual susceptibility played a great part in the transfer of the disease. The organism probably survives only a short period when out of contact with the human body. Close contact, unhygienic surroundings, and a susceptible population probably played a part in the recent American edipemic. Preventive measures have so far been ineffective. It is suggested that patients contracting the disease be isolated from their fellow workers for a period of at least 15 days, or until the conjunctivitis is nearly well.

The cause of the disease is not yet determined. Herpetic virus, other viruses, bacteria, neuropathic, allergic, and nutritional causes have been mentioned. For many reasons it seems probable that the disease is caused by virus. The occupation itself seems to have no bearing on onset of the disease, as there were many instances in which housewives, druggists, dentists, bankers, and business men, as well as the industrial group, were affected. All patients were in excellent general health and in a good nutritional status.

The diagnosis can be made early from the sudden onset, early petechial hemorrhages, absence of discharge, enlargement of regional lymp nodes, absence of bacteria, and presence of lymphocytes in conjunctival smears instead of polynuclear leukocytes.

Therapy is of little avail except possibly in the early stages and in milder cases. The disease is self-limited. For mild cases iced compresses, one percent atropine drops, two percent quinine bisulfate ointment massaged into the eye, roentgen therapy and five per cent sulfonamide ointment may give some relief.—M. D. H., M.D.

"THE CHANGING CONCEPTION OF THE MANAGEMENT OF CHRONIC PROGRESSIVE DEAFNESS." F. T. Hill. The Annals of Otology, Rhinology and Laryngology, Vol. 51, Pp. 653-661. September, 1942.

Twenty-five years ago the treatment of so-called catarrhal deafness was usually some form of inflation, based on the theory of negative pressure as the etiological factor. Tonsils and adenoids were removed and certain intranasal operations performed but largely with the idea of overcoming tubal obstruction. Then came the era of focal infections and the possibility of toxic absorption causing deafness began to displace the negative pressure theory. This time was characterized by eradication of supposed infective foci, which method, though satisfactory in some cases, proved to be rather a disappointing effort. Roentgen therapy of deafness aroused some interest around 1920, soon to be followed by theories of endocrine imbalance and nutritional deficiencies as possible causes of deafness. Meanwhile the treatment for otosclerosis consisted largely of advising patients as to readjustment to future deafness.

For many years surgical efforts to circumvent obstruction to sound waves reaching the internal ear have interested otologists. In and around 1870, division of the posterior fold of the drum membrane and tenotomy of the tensor tympani were practiced by otologists. Various other operations have been suggested since then until 1910 when Barany made a fistula into the posterior semicircular canal and found that there was a slight transient improvement in hearing. Jenkins Holmgren, Sourdille, Lempert, and Campbell perfected this fistulization operation so well that now hearing improvement is more stationary, yet no one can claim that the progress of otosclerosis is completely checked.

All of these procedures have been in the nature of orthopedic otology, ignoring efforts to remove the underlying pathology. Meanwhile, but little attention was paid to research in the physiology of hearing and the pathology of deafness. Even so, we have gained now a better conception of cochlear function, and we developed the audiometer as a precise means for testing hearing.

Our present conception of treatment of chronic progressive deafness is that adequate treatment depends upon correct diagnosis. This frequently requires considerable study and observation. A comprehensive history and careful examination should give a good conception of the otological condition, its functional status and some idea of its probable etiology. When there are definite indications of tubal obstruction, we may employ the eustachian catheter, and sometimes the bougie. The treatment of deafness is the treatment of its cause, and the cause of tubal obstruction will be found usually in the sinuses or the nasopharynx. Recognition of probable factors such as lymphoid hypertrophy, sinusitis, enlarged posterior tips of inferior turbinates, nasopharyngeal cysts and tumors, or allergic manifestations should lead to more effective therapy.

We keep in mind the possibility of toxic absorption and strive to eradicate foci of infection when indicated. We consider the effect of occupation or environment, and realize the importance of good general health, and advise the correction of any nutritional or endocrine deficiency.

For the majority of the patients with established deafness, sufficient to be handicapping, correction by amplification will be preferable. Operative treatment may be suggested to those who, after critical study, meet all the requirements laid down as essential to successful fenestration. But, after all, we realize the impossibility of curing deafness, and all of our therapeutic efforts finally come down to prevention, and rehabilitation.—M. D. H., M.D.

"RIBOFLAVIN; SIGNIFICANCE OF ITS PHOTODYNAMIC ACTION AND IMPORTANCE OF ITS PROPERTIES FOR THE VISUAL ACT." M. Heiman. Archives of Ophthalmology. Vol. 28, Pp. 493-502. September, 1942.

In 1932, Warburg and Christian described the "yellow enzyme," of which riboflavin is an important part. The photodynamic action of flavin was soon recognized, and also the fact that this flavin can be found in large quantities in the retina. In 1935, Theorell stated that flavin has something to do with vision. In 1939, other observers related clinical ocular disease with visual disturbance to a deficiency of riboflavin. It was also found that administration of riboflavin can re-establish visual function in certain visual disorders characterized by dimness of vision, impaired visual acuity and photophobia.

The author experimented with riboflavin, and found that it belongs to the group of photodynamic substances. These experiments made in 1936 were later confirmed by other observers. Riboflavin is also characterized by its yellow-green fluorescence. The author believes that fluorescence and photodynamic action together are important functions, guaranteeing the proper function of the eye in reduced light. Riboflavin, by its photodynamic action, supports the visual function during weak light; it also forms a protection against strong light. The excess of light is screened off, and injury to the photosensitive cells is avoided. A dearth of riboflavin becomes noticeable clinically as photophobia.

The various clinical symptoms of ariboflavinosis are associated with different manifestations of the function of riboflavin. The dimness of vision corresponds to the photodynamic action and the fluorescence, being caused by their reduction. Since carotene is also present in the retina, it seems that both riboflavin and carotene share in these functions, but riboflavin excels carotene in importance in the visual act. Cones and riboflavin form a functional unit.—M. D. H., M.D.

"DINITROPHENOL AND ITS RELATION TO FORMATION OF CATARACT." Warren D. Horner, M.D., San Francisco. Archives of Ophthalmology, Vol. 27, No. 6, June, 1942.

This is an interesting subject about which much has been written. Since this is the most complete presentation of the subject that I have read, I am giving the author's own summary of the subject below.

1. The pharmacologic properties of four phases in the use of dinitrophenol are traced: (a) as a laboratory curiosity in 1895, (b) as a health hazard in the munitions industry (1914 to 1918), (c) as metabolic stimulant with possible clinical applications (1933), and (d) as a potent drug which was used in the treatment of obesity (1934-1935) and which exhibited certain unfortunate side reactions.

2. The majority of these reactions were trivial, a few were fatal, and a middle group, affecting the skin and the blood, were severe, but the most serious of all was the development of cataracts.

3. Cataracts occured with recommended doses of the drug and without other demonstrable reactions.

4. Cataracts developed in a total of more than 177 persons after the use of either dinitrophenol or dinitroorthocresol, an estimated incidence of 0.86 per cent. Of the patients, 98 per cent were women who averaged about 45 years of age.

5. The cataracts, all of one type, were bilateral, developed rapidly, and were accompanied with visual loss and occurred at any time up to a year after the drug had been discontinued.

6. Medical treatment was without effect, but surgical extraction proved successful, excellent visual acuity being obtained in a large percentage of cases.

7. Late secondary cataract was of frequent occurrence after extraction, as was shown by a reported incidence of 88 per cent in one series.

8. All attempts to produce experimental cataracts in laboratory animals by various and repeated doses of dinitrophenol have been successful.

9. Dinitrophenol does not alter the permeability of the lens in vivo or in vitro, nor does it increase inordinately the oxygen consumption of the lens as compared with other tissues. It does not hasten or otherwise affect the artificial production of lactose cataracts in animals.

10. The cause of cataracts following the treatment of obesity with dinitro bodies is unknown, and its relation to the ingestion of these substances is unproved. The argumentative strength of post hoc, ergo propter hoc, cannot be denied, however. This argument has been used successfully to obtain monetary damages in medicolegal actions filed by patients.

11. Since the dinitro compounds found widespread and generally enthusiastic acceptance because of the beneficial results they produced, it is regrettable that they had to be discarded because of the secondary reactions. Additional studies are therefore needed to determine whether related products may not be developed that will retain the metabolic potency with a lessened amount of untoward effects or even their complete absence. Some attempts along this line have proved at least partially successful, and others will doubtless be made. The chief deterrent to such studies is the necessity of being certain that the animal experiments can safey be used as guides to the potential clinical toxicity of the compounds elaborated.—M. D. H., M.D.

KEY TO ABSTRACTORS

E. D. M. ....Earl D. McBride, M.D.
H. J. ....Hugh Jeter, M.D.
L. A. R. ....Lea A. Riley, M.D.
M. D. H. ....Marvin D. Henley, M.D.

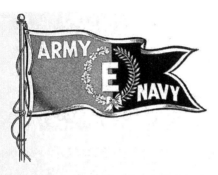

OFFICERS OF COUNTY SOCIETIES, 1943

★

COUNTY	PRESIDENT	SECRETARY	MEETING TIME
Alfalfa	H. E. Huston, Cherokee	L. T. Lancaster, Cherokee	Last Tues. each Second Month
Atoka-Coal	J. B. Clark, Coalgate	J. S. Fulton, Atoka	
Beckham		E. S. Kilpatrick, Elk City	Second Tuesday
Blaine	Virginia Olson Curtin, Watonga	W. F. Griffin, Watonga	
Bryan	J. T. Colwick, Durant	W. K. Haynie, Durant	Second Tuesday
Caddo			
Canadian	P. F. Herod, El Reno	A. L. Johnson, El Reno	Subject to call
Carter	Walter Hardy, Ardmore	H. A. Higgins, Ardmore	
Cherokee	P. H. Medearis, Tahlequah	James K. Gray, Tahlequah	First Tuesday
Choctaw			
Cleveland			Thursday nights
Comanche			
Cotton			Third Friday
Craig	F. M. Adams, Vinita	J. M. McMillan, Vinita	
Creek	H. R. Haas, Sapulpa	C. G. Oakes, Sapulpa	
Custer	F. R. Vicregg, Clinton	C. J. Alexander, Clinton	Third Thursday
Garfield	Paul B. Champlin, Enid	John R. Walker, Enid	Fourth Thursday
Garvin	T. F. Gross, Lindsay	John R. Callaway, Pauls Valley	Wednesday before Third Thursday
Grady	Walter J. Buze, Chickasha	Roy E. Emanuel, Chickasha	Third Thursday
Grant	I. V. Hardy, Medford	E. E. Lawson, Medford	
Greer			
Harmon	W. G. Husband, Hollis	L. E. Hollis, Hollis	First Wednesday
Haskell	William Carson, Keota	N. K. Williams, McCurtain	
Hughes			First Friday
Jackson	E. S. Crow, Olustee	E. W. Mabry, Altus	Last Monday
Jefferson	F. M. Edwards, Ringling	L. L. Wade, Ryan	Second Monday
Kay	Philip C. Risser, Blackwell	J. Holland Howe, Ponca City	Third Thursday
Kingfisher	C. M. Hodgson, Kingfisher	H. Violet Sturgeon, Hennessey	
Kiowa	B. H. Watkins, Hobart	J. William Finch, Hobart	
LeFlore			
Lincoln	H. B. Jenkins, Tryon	Carl H. Bailey, Stroud	First Wednesday
Logan	William C. Miller, Guthrie	J. L. LeHew, Jr., Guthrie	Last Tuesday
Marshall	O. A. Cook, Madill	Philip G. Joseph, Madill	
Mayes			
McClain			
McCurtain	A. W. Clarkson, Valliant	N. L. Barker, Broken Bow	Fourth Tuesday
McIntosh	James L. Wood, Eufaula	William A. Tolleson, Eufaula	First Thursday
Murray			Second Tuesday
Muskogee-Sequoyah-Wagoner			First and Third Monday
Noble	C. H. Cooke, Perry	J. W. Francis, Perry	
Okfuskee	L. J. Spickard, Okemah	M. L. Whitney, Okemah	Second Monday
Oklahoma	Walker Morledge, Oklahoma City	E. R. Musick, Oklahoma City	Fourth Tuesday
Okmulgee	A. R. Holmes, Henryetta	J. C. Matheney, Okmulgee	Second Monday
Osage	C. R. Weirich, Pawhuska	George K. Hemphill, Pawhuska	Second Monday
Ottawa			Third Thursday
Pawnee			
Payne	L. A. Mitchell, Stillwater	C. W. Moore, Stillwater	Third Thursday
Pittsburg	John F. Park, McAlester	William H. Kaciser, McAlester	Third Friday
Pontotoc			First Wednesday
Pottawatomie	A. C. McFarling, Shawnee	Clinton Gallaher, Shawnee	First and Third Saturday
Pushmataha	John S. Lawson, Clayton	B. M. Huckabay, Antlers	
Rogers	C. W. Beson, Claremore	C. L. Caldwell, Chelsea	First Monday
Seminole	Max Van Sandt, Wewoka	Mack L. Shanholtz, Wewoka	
Stephens			
Texas			
Tillman			
Tulsa	James C. Peden, Tulsa	E. O. Johnson, Tulsa	Second and Fourth Monday
Washington-Nowatu	J. G. Smith, Bartlesville	J. V. Athey, Bartlesville	Second Wednesday
Washita			
Woods	C. A. Traverse, Alva	O. E. Templin, Alva	Last Wednesday
Woodward	C. E. Williams, Woodward	C. W. Tedrowe, Woodward	Second Thursday

THE JOURNAL
OF THE
OKLAHOMA STATE MEDICAL ASSOCIATION

| VOLUME XXXVI | OKLAHOMA CITY, OKLAHOMA, FEBRUARY, 1943 | NUMBER 2 |

The Exigencies of Cardiovascular Origin*

GEORGE HERRMANN, M.D.

GALVESTON, TEXAS

The most dramatic exigencies of cardiovascular origin are those in which there is a momentary falling out or somewhat prolonged loss of consciousness. There are usually some premonitory symptoms as giddiness, vertigo and visual disturbance. The progression to syncope may be very rapid, and fleeting unconsciousness of only a few minutes duration. Recovery is usually rapid and complete. When the unconsciousness is persistent and prolonged, a state of more or less profound coma may intervene and last for hours.

Attacks of unconsciousness are fear-inspiring and usually of most serious moment. Not only the life of the afflicted one may be endangered, but when he is one in a responsible position, the safety of others may be threatened by his abrupt incapacitation. Therefore, studies of the conditions that produce these serious episodes are warranted. The subject is always worthy of review in order that we may be prepared to meet these emergencies any time they arise.

The cardiovascular conditions that contribute to clinical pictures of syncope and coma will be found to rank at the very top of most statistical studies of cases of unconsciousness in civilian life. In war, of course, trauma outranks all other causes of coma, yet we may still quite properly consider the medical conditions that we might encounter most frequently in general practice.

The Clinical Picture

The unfolding of the symptom complex of syncope and coma is usually quite rapid. Premonitory symptoms are few and of very short duration. Giddiness, vertigo, weakness, staggering, visual disturbances, unsteadiness, restlessness, and confused speech are usually kaleidoscopic or cinematic in their development or progression. Occasionally one notes drowsiness, yawning, nausea and vomiting and complaints of headache, loss of memory and inability to concentrate are common. Aphasia, paresthesia and paralysis may precede the loss of consciousness or the development of convulsions or coma. The rather insidiously developing status are quite as serious as are the precipitate attacks.

The adjective "cerebral" may be properly used to designate the type of syncope with which we are here concerned. Syncope itself usually indicates the cutting off of the blood flow. Certainly this is what generally occurs in these conditions. "Syncope cerebri" is commonly of cardiovascular origin and is associated with a sudden general or local deficiency of blood flow in the brain.

Observation has shown that interruptions in the cerebral blood flow or cerebral anemia for two to three seconds produces fleeting giddiness and black spots before the eyes, "blind staggers;" for three to five seconds, momentary, transient vertigo followed by a blackout; for ten to twenty seconds, a temporary syncope and general convulsions; for twenty to one hundred and twenty seconds, profound coma and increasing cyanosis appear.

This inadequate cerebral circulation may be the result of general systemic conditions or local conditions in the brain. The most common general conditions are those that result in the fall in systolic blood pressure to levels of 60 to 70 mm. Hg. Hypotension of such grades is considered critical for the maintenance of adequate cerebral blood flow in patients with normal arteries. In those with cerebral arteriosclerosis, the critical levels of blood pressure may be higher. The

*Read before the Section on General Medicine, Oklahoma State Medical Association, Tulsa, April 22, 1942.

causes for general hypotension might well be set forth first for consideration. Among these conditions it seems desirable to begin with simple, less serious and the most frequent ones and proceed to the more serious and less common causes of syncope.

Common Splanchnic Vasosympathetic Faints

The cerebral anemia in ordinary fainting is due to hypotension incident to a reduced cardiac output. The chief or primary factor consists of reflex splanchnic vasoparesis, probably active splanchnic venous dilatation, which contributes to the decreased blood flow back into the heart.

Certain types of individuals under emotional stress or strain, or following visual shock of seeing blood, or under auditory bombardment, may suddenly or slowly become nauseated, feel giddy, see black spots before the eyes and black out.

Reflex splanchnic vasopareses and the resulting cerebral anemia with simple fainting is much more common in women than in men. Reflex dilatation of the splanchnic area usually lowers the systemic blood pressure to critical levels of 80 to 60 mm. mercury systolic. In the arteriosclerotic individuals, the pressure need not fall to this level before symptoms appear. The pulse rate is increased when the blood pressure falls too low to maintain adequate cerebral circulation.

The symptoms develop in rapid succession: giddiness, vertigo, weakness, visual disturbances, unsteadiness, restlessness, confused speech, drowsiness, yawning, usually associated with nausea and a feeling of abdominal fullness, headache, disturbances of memory and inability to concentrate. As signs, the patient usually presents a deathly, ashen pallor and falls unconscious. In a typical cerebral syncopal attack, no loss of reflexes or deviation of the eyes, no frothing at the mouth, no biting of the tongue occur. In the prone position, which the patient usually assumes, the blood pressure rises and the pulse rate drops and consciousness usually returns promptly. If there is delay, reflex stimulation of cold water to the face is effective.

. Vascular re-education is the best form of prophylactic treatment. Cardiovascular neuroses as neurocirculatory asthenia or the effort syndrome may contribute to syncopal attacks.

Shock, particularly that of psychogenic or emotional origin as well as the more frequent traumatic or that due to physical conditions, usually lowers the blood pressure most conspicuously as the result of a general vasoparesis and perhaps also the loss of fluid, blood volume and unconsciousness with intervals. Superficial or skin vasoconstriction and cold clammy sweats, pallor and greyness accompany the acute vascular letdown. These most conspicuous manifestations represent the first evidences of the physiopathological disturbances and call for immediate correction.

Nitrite Poisioning or Nitrite Fainting

Nitrites, particularly amyl nitrite, nitroglycerine, sodium nitrite and more recently erythroltetranitrate and mannitol hexanitrate have been used extensively as vasodilators in patients with hypertension. Certain individuals are hypersensitive to the nitrite action and the acute vasodilatation results in a·precipitate drop in the blood pressure to critical levels. It is not at all uncommon to have the patient faint particularly if he is standing or sitting in the upright position following the taking of the drug, even when it is taken for therapeutic effects. This reaction usually occurs when the patient is not accustomed to the drug. In a patient with angina pectoris who gets panicky and takes several doses in an attempt to get immediate relief there may be accumulative effect and usually there is a marked flushing of the face, the patient complains of throbbing and weakness. The drug effect usually wears off rather promptly.

Nitrite faints also occur in individuals who are working in nitroglycerine manufacturing concerns. The number of such exposed workers has increased with the great expansion of the production of high explosives. In this work nitroglycerine is used extensively and the workers must gradually develop a tolerance to the heavily laden nitrite atmosphere of such plants. In some workers exposed to the nitroglycerine fumes, a tolerance develops to the point where the drug is almost necessary. Some workers on leaving the nitroglycerine plant may develop a cerebral angiospasm or coronary angiospasm with resulting disturbances in the cerebral as well as the coronary circulation, even to the point of causing withdrawal faints.

Disorders of the Cardiac Mechanism

Sudden derangement of the heart action only occasionally results in syncope. This is particularly true in the more benign mechanism disturbances. It occurs more frequently in rather serious disorders. Dramatic situations however may be created by any one of the paroxysmal disturbances of the heart's mechanism. The prompt recognition and proper treatment may forestall serious complications. It is quite as important to recognize the benign or innocuous conditions that cause cerebral syncope. It is highly desirable to give them the specific treatment promptly. Carotid sinus episodes may cause significant cardiac standstill and should perhaps be considered under this same heading as well as under the heading of vagus faints. Some remarks on the differentiation and usual management, the clinical characteristics and therapeutic procedures that have been found effective are warranted. For absolute differentiation, electrocardiograms taken during an attack are of the greatest importance.

Paroxysmal Atrial Tachycardia

Attacks of a rapid succession of premature heart beats, from the ectopic focus in the atria and yet outside the usual pacemaker, the sino-auricular node, in other words attacks of atrial tachycardia, are most common. The rate rises suddenly from normal to a higher level usually between 180 and 240 beats per minute. Worry, fear and uncertainty may bring on attacks in psychologically, unstable individuals. In such cases, the blood pressure may drop to the critical level and all of the symptoms of cerebral anemia may develop. It may occur particularly in elderly individuals whose cerebral vessels are sclerosed. There may be no demonstrable precipitating factor but occasionally an emotional upset or unusual physical strain or surgical operation will bring on an attack. The paroxysm usually stops spontaneously within a short time, or it may persist for hours and occasionally for days.

The differential diagnosis must take into consideration sinus tachycardia, atrial flutter, paroxysmal ventricular tachycardia and in some instances, rarely atrial fibrillation. The abrupt onset and termination, the high rate, the constancy of the rhythm which is regular and full minute counts varying not more than two points, either unaffected by increased vagus tone or in one-third of the cases completely stopped are all characteristic. Ventricular tachycardia varies usually six to eight points in minute to minute counts and is usually of much more serious moment and accompanies myocardial damage.

Treatment consists of increasing the vagus tone by carotid sinus pressure which stops the attack immediately in about one-third of the cases. Quinidine sulphate in 5 gr. doses taken every hour for not more than eight doses is perhaps as safe and successful as any form of therapy. Ipecac syrup in one to two dram doses of the fresh preparation by mouth will usually result in nausea and vomiting in fifteen to forty-five minutes and interrupt most cases of paroxysmal atrial tachycardia. In elderly individuals morphine sulphate ⅛ gr. to ¼ gr. doses is seemingly the treatment of choice. In heart failure digitalis extract 10 cc. (3.5 cat units) or digifoline or digiglucine solution in 10 cc. doses, digilanddid, 1½ to 2 mg. or lamataside are most successful, particularly in the presence of heart failure. Starr and Stroud found mecholyl, 10 to 30 mg. subcutaneously to be very effective. Key's

studies suggest that neosynephrin 5 to 10 mg. doses subcutaneously, may be a valuable vagatonic drug. St. Feher and Dressler have advised the use of a 20 per cent solution of magnesium sulphate intravenously, 5 cc. slowly and then 5 cc. more rapidly.

Paroxysmal Ventricular Tachycardia

Paroxysmal ventricular tachycardia is a rapid succession of ventricular premature contractions. It begins suddenly and usually stops suddenly. It often follows attacks of pains of an anginal nature and thus suggests the presence of myocardial damage, which may be of most serious moment. It is not nearly as common as the atrial and junctional types of tachycardia. The blood pressure usually drops lower and sometims it is difficult to determine it during a paroxysm. The differential diagnosis is similar to that of paroxysmal atrial tachycardia. The rate of the ventricular paroxysm is usually not as high as that of atrial tachycardia but usually is higher than that of sinus tachycardia and atrial flutter. It characteristically varies five to six points between minute to minute counts. In this it differs from atrial tachycardia and from flutter. The signs of myocardial infarction are usually present and sometimes evidences of left ventricular failure appear when the precipitating thrombosis occurred in the large anterior descending branch of the left coronary artery.

As treatment, the specific or sovereign remedy for this condition is quinidine sulphate. It is given by mouth in five grain doses every hour for six, seven or eight doses. It is usually effective in stopping a paroxysm after three or four doses.

Paroxysmal Atrial Flutter and Fibrillation

Paroxysmal atrial fibrillation and flutter are very rarely accompanied by syncope. Flutter however, when there is a one to one block, (instead of a usual two to one block), may decrease the filling of the heart so that the blood pressure drops to very low critical levels. One to one flutter, with the rate rising to 300 per minute, is a condition of serious moment. Such rates have been so recorded by the electrocardiographic method. It is characteristic of flutter for the regularity of two to one atrial flutter to be disturbed by carotid sinus stimulation temporarily only, and returns in spite of continued stimulation. Atrial fibrillation is characterized by absolute arrhythmia.

The patient often feels the irregular action or palpitation and exercise increases the disorder. Treatment is sometimes necessary and usually desirable even though the attacks frequently end spontaneously. Quinidine sulphate again is the drug of choice in 5 gr. doses every hour for five to eight doses will usually stop an attack and reestablish normal mechanism at the slow rate. In the presence of heart failure digitalization by the intravenous method administering 10 cc. of the digitalis extract of standard potency is first tried. Digitalization is sometimes successful in itself in turning over the mechanism to normal but usually a subsequent course of quinidine sulphate is necessary to restore sino-atrial rhythm.

Ventricular Asytole, Heart Block or .... Ventricular Fibrillation

Paroxysmal ventricular flutter or fibrillation have occasionally been recognized clinically as the cause of syncopal attacks. Ventricular fibrillation is considered the most common cause of sudden death. Ventricular fibrillation has been shown experimentally to produce a state of diastasis. There is no propulsion of the blood out of the ventricles. The diagnosis may be suggested by the sudden onset, by the absence of all heart sounds, by the presence of fibrillary movements in the pulse of the congested jugular veins. Other symptoms as cerebral anemia, shock, vertigo, syncope along with convulsions are likely to appear. The diagnosis of this condition should not be made without corroboration of electrocardiographic study.

Adams-Stokes' Syndrome with Convulsions

The classical clinical picture of ventricular asystole, that of Adams-Stokes' attacks, is quite similar to that of temporary ventricular fibrillation. The attacks may be suspected in patients who have varying grades of heart block in which complete A.-V. dissociation appears now and then and the ventricular pacemaker fails to take up the function immediately.

The second type of attack in which there is no preceding conduction disturbance but sudden complete block and at the same time low grade ventricular irritability. Development of the symptom complex is very rapid and complete, and the patient is usually given no time to complain of vertigo since syncope promptly intervenes.

Failure of the ventricular beat, even for a short period of time is a matter of serious moment. The blood column is at a standstill with the loss of the drive of ventricular activity or contraction. The moments of suspension of the heart beats are precious ones and no one can know whether or not the ventricle will develop an idioventricular pacemaker to start the beating again. Likewise when ventricular fibrillation is reason for the asystole, chances for return of concerted ventricular activity are very slight. Within two minutes after the onset, the patient is usually in coma, convulsions have developed and usually cyanosis has become intense. It is doubtful whether any patient

would survive more than four or five minutes suffering from such an attack. Patients have, however, been reported to have lived after eight minutes of suspended heart action.

Treatment

In the emergency it seems desirable to rapidly administer quick, sharp, hard blows of the fist over the precordium, in the hope that the transmitted force may stimulate the ventricle to contract and reestablish circulation. During ventricular asystole the only possibility of intravenous injection of epinephrin reaching the heart would be by possible gravitation from the jugular bulb with the patient in the upright position. Preparation of a sterile syringe with a long 2½-inch 22gauge needle containing three to five minims of adrenalin should be quickly prepared.

If there is no recognizable activity of the heart within four minutes, heroic intracardiac injection of adrenalin is warranted It is justifiable to thrust the long needle through the fourth interspace into the heart at its left border and penetrate the ventricular cavity. The needle is slowly withdrawn as the three to five minims of epinephrin are injected.

Prevention of attacks or recurrences of the same should receive careful consideration. Some clinicians use quinidine sulphate routinely in small doses after attacks of coronary thrombosis to prevent ventricular fibrillation. Patients with heart block that is changing from a partial to a complete block with episodes occuring at each change, should be digitalized. The hope is for the establishment of a complete block with a relatively high and adequate ventricular rate of about forty or above, to prevent attacks. The ventricular muscle may be kept irritable by use of ephedrine hydrochloride, ⅜ gr. three times a day or paredrine, 1/6 gr. (10 mg.) three times a day or adrenalin in oil 5 to 10 mg. doses (1:1000 solution). These are all rational procedures but are sometimes contraindicated because of subsequent rise in the blood pressure. Barium chloride, ½ to ¾ gr. (30 to 40 mg.) three times a day seemingly has been successful in keeping the ventricular muscle irritable and thus preventing episodes.

Acute Cor Pulmonale, Cardiovascular Shock With Critical Hypotension

The bombardments of the nervous system in acute massive pulmonary embolism and the pain of coronary occlusion may produce such profound peripheral circulatory collapse or forward failure as to result in syncope. This happens more often, relatively speaking, after pulmonary embolism or obstruction than after major coronary occlusion and extensive myocardial infarction, even though the pain is not so severe, and is shorter in duration. The rich sympathetic innervation of the pulmonary arterial bed probably accounts for the greater severity of pulmonary obstruction shock. The acute cor pulmonale is overactive particularly in the conus region area and rough basal friction sounds are generally heard. The pulmonary second sound is accentuated loudly. The electrocardiograms may show characteristic signs of cor pulmonale; namely, a prominent S1 in a rare case S2 and a prominent Q3, and signs of right ventricular strain. Occasionally electrocardiographic changes are quite similar to those of conorary occlusion with myocardial infarction. If the patient is unconscious there may have been a reflex spasm in various arterial beds. Myocardial infarction has been shown to occur along with pulmonary embolism in twenty to thirty per cent of the cases.

Acute cor pulmonale calls for emergency treatment. Papaverine and morphine along with heparin may be used intravenously. Papaverine in 1 gr. dose may relax the spasm about the embolus and allow it to pass on further to disintegrate. Heparin will prevent the secondary thrombosis. Oxygen by the B.L.B. mask may be beneficial by mass action. Aminophyllin may be used intravenously as a vasodilator in 7½ gr. doses diluted to 10 cc. and given slowly. The source of the emboli is usually evident and if in an accessible place, the vein should be tied off when it is possible to do so. In this country, pulmonary embolism cases are subjected to embolectomy, the Trendelenburg operation, only after the patient has expired. In order to accomplish this the patient must be placed in the operating room, ready for the operation, and vigil kept until exitus has intervened. The surgeon must be prepared to go ahead as soon as respirations cease. This may seem ultraconservative compared to the heroic attempt of pulmonary embolectomy as done in Sweden, but it is definitely more justifiable.

Major Occlusion with Extensive Myocardial Infarction

Coronary occlusion with myocardial infarction may occasionally produce such great cardiovascular shock and forward failure as to result in syncope. Excruciating pain and massive left ventricular infarction with forward failure may be combined to produce a dramatic picture. The pain is usually substernal or epigastric. The blood pressure usually falls abruptly and to critically low levels. A friction rub may appear and the electrocardiogram is usually striking with an RST elevation and beginning T wave negativity. The fluoroscopic examination may show defective movements of the in-

farcted left ventricular wall. Within a day or two leucocytosis or increased sedimentation rate may be found. Electrocardiograms characteristically show progressive changes in the RST segment and T waves.

The emergency treatment of acute coronary occlusion episodes consists in relieving the pain with morphine sulphate, ¼ gr., and atropine sulphate, 1/100 gr. This may be given intravenously and repeated once if necessary. If dyspnea is present, oxygen in 100 per cent atmosphere through a B. L. B. mask, should be administered. Oxygen will not only relieve the pain but will also combat shock. Sex hormones in 10,000 unit doses, intramuscularly twice a week for the slow vasodilating effect and its sympathetic stimulating action on the intestinal canal for the relief of distention. Aminophyllin in 7½ gr. doses intravenously diluted ten times or in 3 gr. enteric coated tablets three times a day may improve the coronary circulation by virtue of the dilating effect of the drug, which is desirable in the development of the collateral channels.

Paroxysmal cardiac pain, that is angina pectoris, rarely produces cerebral anemia primarily because it is promptly relieved by the inhalation of amyl nitrite or the taking of spirits of nitroglycerin. A sharp rise in the blood pressure usually accompanies angina pectoris. When the pain is not relieved by the nitrites and persists, myocardial infarction has occured. A sudden or continuour drop in blood pressure is the result of myocardial infarction. The critical levels of hypotension may be reached but syncope is only occasionally present.

Interference with the Outflow From the Heart

Pathological changes in the root of the aorta and in the ascending arch, obstruct or interfere with outflow from the left ventricle and thus contribute to the production of cerebral anemia and syncope. Concomitant low blood pressure will make more likely the development of cerebral symptoms. The loss of the elasticity of the aorta itself and aortitis in aneurysmal formation is barely sufficient to seriously reduce the cerebral circulation but aortic change may be a significant factor in elderly or aged people. A poorly sustained blood column due to the presence of aortic regurgitation likewise in itself rarely produces syncope unless the systolic blood pressure is low as well as the diastolic.

Aortic stenosis on the other hand is usually associated with considerable valvular calcification and calcium deposits at the root of the aorta, so much so that the designation calcerous disease has been assigned to this condition. The primary lesion is probably a rheumatic aortic valvulitis with some fusion of the cusps and subsequent gradual calcification. Ejection of blood from the left ventricle is obstructed, the systolic blood pressure is consequently low and the pulse pressure is very low. Patients with this lesion are very prone to have attacks of vertigo and syncope. It has been pointed out by Marvin that such patients, besides having the very low systolic blood pressure and low pulse pressure, also have a very sensitive carotid sinus. Sudden reflex vagatonia may therefore appear upon mechanical stimulation of the carotid sinus.

This gives the clue for the only therapeutic procedure indicated in such patients. This consists of atropinization with belladonna, atropine itself, or syntropan in regular doses two or three times a day to remove the vagus tone. The removal of the vagus effect will often prevent the recurrences of the syncopal attacks in which vagatonia has played a part.

Sudden Causes of Deficient Cerebral Blood Flow

In the third group of the exigencies of cardiovascular practice, I might well discuss disturbances in the intracranial cavity itself. Some of these are very common and some are very rare, some easy to establish, others difficult to diagnose; any one of them may be a factor of significance in a patient with syncope or coma. Most of them are of very serious moment.

Intracerebral Obstruction of the Blood Flow To the Brain

Localized cortical cerebral angiospasm is perhaps the mildest of any of these and at the same time the most difficult one to establish. Spastic segments in the retinal arteries, when present, corroborate the diagnosis. The spontaneous relief within some hours or the prompt response to papaverine or nitrites are almost diagnostic.

Cerebral arteriosclerosis is usually accompanied by extensive tortuosity the broad white streak and irregularities of the lumena of the retinal arterioles are characteristic.

Intracranial disturbances produce cerebral anemia by compression and usually result in coma which frequently terminates fatally. Subarachnoid hemorrhage is to be suspected if the slowly developing coma has been preceded by severe headache and the rigidity of the neck with or without abducens palsy can be demonstrated.

Cerebral thrombosis produces a slowly developing coma without stiffness of the neck. It occurs most often in elderly individuals with cerebral arteriosclerosis and low blood pressure. Cerebral hemorrhage is followed promptly by deep coma, paralysis and pathological reflexes usually in patients who have had hypertension. The blood pressure usually rises.

Meningitis often produces coma and usually presents Kernig's and Brudzinski signs and the etiological factor is usually demonstrable in the purulent cerebrospinal fluid. Syphilis of the meninges or central nervous blood vessels or tissues or general paralysis of the insane may be recognized by pupillary and deep reflex changes and by positive spinal fluid serology and cytology attacks of coma and convulsions are common in paresis.

Epilepsy can usually be recognized as the cause for a state of coma and convulsions by the characteristic signs as the cry, the biting of the tongue, the loss of sphincter control, the tonic and clonic spasms and the previous and familial histories. Brain tumor coma is usually accompanied by signs of increased intracranial pressure in the eye grounds and some times by localizing signs. The electroencephalogram and roentgenograms or air surrounding the brain or in the ventricles may be necessary to prove the diagnosis of tntracranial neoplasm as a cause for coma.

Summary

The cardiovascular causes of syncope and coma have been reviewed. The analysis of the circulatory exigencies, which produce cerebral anemia, has been carefully presented. The disorders of the cardiac mechanism which give rise to syncope have been stressed, because they are so much more amenable to treatment. The common emergency therapeutic methods have been discussed.

Injuries to the Heart

Injury to the heart and adjoining structures caused by blows to the chest or to distant parts of the body is often overlooked because of the prevailing idea that the chest wall and the cushion effect of the lungs prevent such injury, Louis H. Sigler, M.D., Brooklyn, declares in The Journal of the American Medical Association for July 11. He emphasizes the importance of bearing in mind that such injury to the heart may occur in any bodily injury and that such patients should be given frequent heart examinations.

The types of blow or impact that may result in heart injury in man, he says, include (1) direct blow to the chest, especially if applied to the region over the heart or stomach; (2) compression of the chest between two solid objects; (3) sudden extreme increase in the pressure within the abdomen by external violence; (4) lifting of an extremely heavy object or other severe strain thrown on the body.

"It must be stressed that it is not the latent force but the velocity of travel of the force when it strikes the body which produces the injury," Dr. Sigler declares.

The presence of disease of the arteries of the heart in advanced age is a sensitizing factor for the production of heart disturbances, if not actual damage, by comparatively little force.

Tuberculous Tracheobronchitis

RICHARD M. BURKE, M.D., F.A.C.P.

OKLAHOMA CITY, OKLAHOMA

For the past few years tracheobronchial tuberculosis has been a much discussed subject among phthisiologists. It provides an example of another one of the re-discoveries of medicine. Over one hundred years ago it was described, and its not infrequent occurrence noted on the basis of autopsy studies. In the intervening years, this complication of pulmonary tuberculosis was lost sight of from a clinical standpoint. As time went on it was commonly thought that this condition was rare, and of little clinical importance. This situation was changed about fifteen years ago. With the widespread and successful use of collapse therapy, greater clinical interest was aroused in the patient and his symptoms. Investigators began to trace the source of wheezing in the tuberculous. Autopsies were done on some of these patients, and stenosis found. Papers were published telling about tuberculosis of the bronchi simulating asthma. More interest was shown in "blocked cavities." Their relationship to bronchial diseases was demonstrated. Then came the much wider use of diagnostic bronchoscopy in pulmonary tuberculosis. It was soon learned that the procedure carried very little risk provided one showed respect for active laryngeal tuberculosis. By 1935, clinicians were beginning to be very much on the alert for this complication, and by 1940, it reached a point where bronchoscopy was being advocated routinely for virtually all sanatorium patients. Others a little less enthusiastic were urging its routine use prior to thoracoplasty. (A by-product of the wide use of the bronchoscope has been bronchospirometry, a procedure which enables one to measure separately the vital capacity of each lung.) There is yet much to be learned about bronchial ulcers as evidenced, for example, by the conflicting statements regarding its incidence, its pathology, and its treatment.

The number of bronchoscopies done at the Western Oklahoma Tuberculosis Sanatorium has been increasing during the past four years. Our present series is still small. In this preliminary report we should like to review briefly the subject and give a few of the impressions gained thus far.

INCIDENCE

In a series of 120 bronchoscopies done on tuberculous patients, 105 individuals were examined, of whom nine per cent showed tracheobronchial tuberculosis. The majority of these examinations were done to discover the cause and source of unexplained positive sputum, rather than because the patient had frank symptoms suggestive of ulcer. Most of the patients showed the typical ulcerogranulomatous changes, while three presented a localized, intense area of inflammation just distal to the tracheobronchial juncture. This latter group, we felt, were precursors of the granulomatous lesions which follow. The simple diffuse reddening secondary to bronchitis was not included. In the literature one finds the incidence varying from three per cent, as reported from autopsy studies by Flance and Wheeler[1], to 60 per cent, as reported by Conklin[2], from bronchoscopic studies. Hawkins[3], reports an incidence of 25 per cent among 516 selected patients, and Warren[4], 13.3 per cent in a series of prethoracoplasty bronchoscopies.

Females predominate (74 per cent in our series). A rather common experience is to find ulceration on the left side in a young woman with moderately advanced pulmonary tuberculosis. This preponderance of ulcers in the female has brought forth many hypotheses, but as yet no satisfactory explanation has been advanced.

PATHOLOGY

A common route of infection, according to pathologists, is by direct extension. Auerbach[3], states that these lesions extend beneath the bronchial mucosa from the original parenchymal focus. Eventually they may reach the large bronchi. The typical lesion is located in the submucosa, and is an inflammatory tuberculous infiltrate. As it progresses, it erodes through the mucosa, forming an ulcer. This ulcer is soon transformed to a granuloma through proliferation of the tuberculous infiltrate which goes on to occlude completely the lumen. As the healing occurs, there is a replacement of the granuloma by fibrous tissue. In the healing process, the lumina of the larger bronchi are reopened. In the smaller air passages, the lumen remains closed and the original infectious focus is closed off from the rest of the bronchial tree. According to the teaching of Myerson[6], tracheobronchial tuberculosis will heal spontaneously in the majority of cases. For this reason he feels that cautery and local therapy are contraindicated as this interferes with nature's way of healing, and it may spread the infection. Furthermore, the ulcer is too widespread, and cautery only reaches its presenting edge. We are not so optimistic as Myerson as to spontaneous healing of these ulcers, but we do feel that topical applications have little to offer.

Implantation or contact is said to lead to ulceration. It is commonly taught that positive sputum can implant infection at distant points such as the larynx and bowel. This appears to occur at the point of greatest stasis, such as the posterior commissure of the larynx or the ileocecal region of the bowel. In persons who have an unsatisfactory collapse maintained for a period of months, stasis in the bronchial tree on the affected side is apt to result. This is because the ventilatory power of the lung is impaired and sputum, as a result, is not properly expelled. This theory attempts to explain the ulcers sometimes seen in such cases. Hematogenous seeding in the tracheobronchial tree, with resultant ulcers, may occur. These are usually shallow and multiple.

SYMPTOMS AND INDICATIONS FOR BRONCHOSCOPY

The only means of determining the presence of ulcer is by bronchoscopy. The common indications for such an examination are:

1. Unexplained positive sputum, 2. Wheezing or noisy respirations and 3. Unexplained atelectasis.

Unexplained positive sputum: This is the most common indication for bronchoscopy. Quite often a patient has a pulmonary lesion which appears to be well controlled by collapse therapy, yet the sputum continues to be positive. Such a patient should always be bronchoscoped, particularly before any supplementary collapse measures are done in an attempt to render the sputum negative. Again we may have a patient with a minimal lesion, or even with no pulmonary disease evident on X-ray, who will continue to raise tubercle bacilli the origin of which could be ulcer.

Wheezing or noisy respirations: When the airways are narrowed by bronchial disease, wheezing develops. This wheezing is unilateral, and persists after coughing. Besides this, a number of other symptoms may be present, such as difficulty in raising the sputum which is mucoid and thick. These patients find it difficult to take a deep breath. Often they will tell you when they are or are not breathing with the affected lung. There is dyspnoea out of proportion to the amount of pulmonary involvement. Cyanosis is not common. On physical examination, rhonchi often are heard. Listening with the stethoscope before the open mouth is an aid in detecting the wheezing. When stenosis is marked and of long standing, the diagnosis is readily made by X-ray.

Unexplained atelectasis: This is always an indication for bronchoscopy. Sometimes soon after initiating a pneumothorax, and giving a few refills, one suddenly finds a lobe or all lobes atelectatic. This may mean that bronchial disease with narrowing is present. As a result of collapsing the lung, this narrow airway then completely closes. It further means that an unnecessary pneumothorax has been started which will be hard to re-expand. This can best be further explained by citing a case where such an error was made.

A white female, age 25, entered the sanatorium on May 19, 1940, with a haziness in the extreme left apex, and some scattered infiltration at the level of the second rib. The sputum was positive for tubercle bacilli. A preliminary rest period of six weeks was tried. Sputum continued to be positive. Chest X-ray showed no change. Pneumothorax was then instituted and a good collapse obtained, except for a few apical adhesions. The sputum was still positive, so closed pneumonolysis was done following which the entire lung became atelectatic. And still positive sputum was present, so bronchoscopy was finally done on March 1, 1941. An ulcerogranuloma was found almost closing the left main bronchial opening. An aspirator was introduced through the narrowed opening and secretions removed. Bronchoscopy was done six weeks later, and topical application of ten per cent silver nitrate was made. In the meantime, pleural fluid developed which has persisted for the past eighteen months. Periodic aspiration has been done. The lower half of the lung has partially re-expanded, but the remainder appears atelectatic. A recent bronchoscopy showed there remains a concentric swelling, practically occluding the bronchus, and with little adjacent surface ulceration. This patient had a slight wheeze at the time of admission which was overlooked. Also the density in the apex was probably an atelectasis of a lobule as a result of a branch bronchus occlusion. If bronchoscopy had been done first, the patient would not have been subjected to collapse therapy and its attendant complications.

In children, we occasionally see atelectasis of the lower lobes secondary to enlarged tracheobronchial glands obtruding on the lumina.

Sometimes the question of which side the positive sputum is coming from arises. Here, bronchoscopy may be an aid if we happen to see purulent sputum at the time of the examination on one side or the other. If from both sides, noting the amount from each side is helpful. Smears may be taken. In the presence of unexplained hemoptysis we have a helpful ally in the bronchoscope. The examination can be done while the patient is hemorrhaging. We recently did so, and found from which side the bleeding was coming. The patient suffered no ill effects.

At present, we do not routinely bronchoscope prior to thoracoplasty. Tracheobronchial tuberculosis in itself is not a contraindication to thoracoplasty unless stenosis exists which would interfere with collapse and drainage. This is not common and can ordinarily be suspected by the symptoms and X-ray appearance after which bronchoscopy can then be performed.

TREATMENT

Considerable controversy exists regarding the proper handling of these patients. There is disagreement both as to the use of local therapy to the ulcer, and in the use of collapse therapy in the presence of ulcer.

Many believe like Myerson[5], that topical application such as silver nitrate serve little or no purpose as far as aiding in healing the lesions. (Recently we have been experimentally using Promin*, a sulfa drug, which offers some promise of being of value for such lesions.[7-8]) Others[2], feel that local treatment is of distinct value in aiding healing, particularly for isolated ulcers. Electrocoagulation seems to be in disfavor at present, one objection being the danger of stenosis following its use. Cauterization may be helpful in relieving obstruction, where exuberant granulation is present. Where there is a diffuse swelling closing the bronchus, I have found nothing of value. Davenport[9], feels that irradiation is of help in such instances. Where the ulcers have healed leaving a fibrotic stenosis, dilatation and aspiration are often employed. This offers no permanent relief, and it is in such instances that lobectomy or pneumonectomy is being advocated.

When and when not to use collapse therapy in the presence of ulcer is a vexing problem. In treating pulmonary tuberculosis, we know that we must control the source of infection,

and convert the sputum from positive to negative. In a great many cases this can be done by collapse therapy, particularly artificial pneumothorax. Where ulceration happens to be present in the main bronchi, however, we are faced with the choice of one of two evils. If we do not collapse, the disease is very apt to progress and the patient die. If we do collapse the lung, we often produce an atelectasis. This is frequently complicated by an effusion, and a lung which may remain collapsed a long time. Moreover, we do not influence by collapse measures the positive sputum coming from the bronchus. My feeling is that when encountering an early infiltration with persistently positive sputum, one should be careful to rule out bronchial tuberculosis. A small patch of atelectasis in the apex should make one suspicious. The symptoms and findings as given above should be kept in mind. Shortness of breath out of proportion to the extent of the lesion visualized is suggestive. Where advanced pulmonary tuberculosis is present collapse therapy is the lesser of the two evils.

SUMMARY

An incidence of nine per cent tracheobronchial tuberculosis was encountered in performing 120 bronchoscopies at the Western Oklahoma Tuberculosis Santorium. Bronchoscopy has become an essential diagnostic aid in the management of pulmonary tuberculosis. The presence of tracheobronchial tuberculosis should always be kept in mind in the presence of wheezing, unexplained positive sputum, and unexplained atelectasis. Local treatment by cautery is largely of mechanical value to relieve obstruction. One should be aware that inducing pneumothorax in the presence of bronchial tuberculosis may sometimes lead to harmful complications.

BIBLIOGRAPHY

1. Flance and Wheeler: Post-mortem Incidence of Tuberculous Tracheobronchitis, Am. Rev. Tuberc. 39: 633, 1939.
2. Conklin, William S.: Tuberculous Tracheobronchitis, Diseases of Chest. 8: 178, June, 1942.
3. Hawkins, Lawrence: Tuberculous Tracheobronchitis, Am Rev. Tuberc. 39: 46, 1939.
4. Warren, W., Hamond, A. E., Tuttle, W. M: Diagnosis and Treatment of Tuberculous Tracheobronchitis, Am. Rev. Tuberc. 37: 315, 1938.
5. Myerson, M. C.: Tuberculosis of the Trachea and Bronchus, Jour. A.M.A. 116: 1611, 1941
6. Myerson, M. C.: The Limitations of Bronchoscopy in the Treatment of Tracheobronchial Tuberculosis, Ann. Otol. Rhin & Laryng. 47: 722, Sept, 1938.
7. Barach, Alvan L., Melomut, Norman, Soroka, Max: Inhalation of Nebulized Promin in Experimental Tuberculosis, Am. Rev. Tuberc. 46: 269, Sept., 1942.
8. Zucker, Gary, Pinner, Max, Hyman, Harold Thomas: Chemothrapy of Tuberculosis, Am. Rev. Tuberc. 46: 277, Sept., 1942.
9. Davenport, L. F.: Tuberculous Tracheobronchitis, Am. J. Roentgenol. 45: 494, April, 1941.

The successes of the tuberculosis campaign are measured by the thousands who have lived their allotted span in spite of tuberculosis, and the failure in the thousands who are ill and incapacitated because of this serious disease.—Editorial, *Bulletin Canadian Tuber. Assn.*, March, 1942.

---

*Promin supplied us through the courtesy of Dr. E. A. Sharp, Parke, Davis & Company.

The Irritable Bowel*

TURNER BYNUM, M.D.

CHICKASHA, OKLAHOMA

Colonic disturbances of systemic origin are difficult to describe, for they lack definite manifestations and the resulting conditions indicate abnormal colonic irritability. Obviously, this irritability of a hollow tube, which contains longitudinal and circular muscles and which is lined with mucous membrane and covered by peritoneum and innervated by two sets of delicately balanced nerves, is indicated by a variety of responses.

It is easy to understand, then, why so many names have been suggested for the syndrome. Thus, there are the terms "irritable colon" and "unstable colon," simple colitis, spastic colitis, mucous colitis, catarrhal colitis, mucomembranous colitis, mucous colopathy, myxomembranous colitis, myxorrhea membranacea, myxoneurosis intestinalis, fermentative colitis, toxic colitis, sore colon, and other similar designations that attempt to describe a syndrome of varied symptoms. All indicate colonic manifestations of systemic origin, but none adequately direct attention to the basic trouble.

ETIOLOGY

The condition has been designated as an enteropathy afflicting nervous patients. The etiology may be divided into those factors arising from the outside and those from the inside of the colon. The term "irritable colon" suggests at once that the intestinal disorder is only part of a general disorder, and leads one to investigate not only the colonic difficulty but the basic trouble, there is a derangement of functional behavior not only in the large intestine, but also in other parts of the gastro-intestinal tract as well. The symptoms do not seem to be associated with actual inflammation of any part of the colon, there do appear however in many patients, after a prolonged period of time actual changes in the bowel wall, with thickening and loss of haustral markings in the sigmoid and frequently even the descending colon.

FACTORS AFFECTING THE BOWEL FROM THE OUTSIDE

Our present-day life, with its hustle and

*Read before the Southwest Oklahoma Medical Society, Clinton, September 16, 1942.

bustle, its tremendous competition in wage earning, and its every urge for speed, often interferes with proper care of intestinal functions. There results, therefore, a "nervous indigestion" in which the colon plays no small part. After a morning rush to the office, there often follows an all-day rush in a highly competitive business. A person does not have time to stop for evacuation of the bowels. The farmer's activities are of a different type, but he too must rush, and even the common laborer is at times beset with the hurries of life which are too much for him. But no one is more troubled than the lady of society whose life consists of one round of competitive entertaining and of irregular eating and drinking. For such women then, come a variety of abdominal discomforts and to them, as Axel Munthe in his story of San Michele has pointed out, the term "colitis" has only too commonly been used as a placebo, to sooth their anxious minds.

Basically, the sensitive colon may be inherited, for it is common to see members of several generations of one family suffer similarly. Once a woman shows marked signs of disturbance she is likely to suffer with it at intervals for the rest of her days. Neurogenic trends almost invaribly are present. Nervous tension, anxiety, worry, the presence of crowds, introspection, insomnia, unhappiness, family difficulties and dissipation in one form or another have been given as causes which precipitated the abdominal complaints. The symptoms usually make their appearance early in life, but they may be precipitated by any nervous strain, at any time of life.

It becomes apparent then, that many types of colonic stimulation disturb colonic function, and when the delicately balanced nerve control of this hollow viscus is recalled, there should be small wonder at the variety of symptoms produced. It follows also that disturbances of other parts of the body, be they from organic disease or from functional over-stimulation, may have direct, immediate, and at times prolonged, effects on the large intestine.

In a broad sense, it may be said to result in a combination of "drive" (vagus or parasympathetic) and "brake" (the sympathetic system). When the two are in proper balance, normal peristalsis proceeds quietly and painlessly, and we are completely unconscious of any digestive activity. If, however, the "drive" is too great, we can have overactive peristalsis with diarrheal tendency, or paradoxically, such spasticity and overcontraction of the colon that no propulsion occurs, and "spastic constipation" results. If the "brake" is overactive, it may result in atonic constipation.

It has been thought that abnormal positions and unusual mobility of portions of the large intestine have been the basis of many of the symptoms discussed under this heading. However, anyone who has done many Fluoroscopic and X-ray examinations of the gastro-intestinal tract using opaque media on both well and ailing patients has demonstrated how rarely diagnoses of enteroptosis, gastroptosis, or coloptosis are justified. Positions of viscera vary with individuals, and their natural physical build and nervous make-up usually determine the position of their internal organs.

It follows then, that abdominal complaints are not the result of abnormal mobility of the ceacum or of ptosis of the colon, but rather that such complaints and abnormal positions of the organs are the result of a person's particular build and heredity.

FACTORS AFFECTING THE BOWEL FROM THE INSIDE

Naturally the inside factors are mainly food, but must include laxatives and other locally acting medicaments. Food is taken into the stomach, a mixture of liquid and solid. By addition of the gastric juice, with its chemical and enzymatic effects, the food becomes liquid before leaving the stomach. Thus it has been prepared for assimilation in its passage through the small intestine. The actual assimilation takes place through the involved and complicated mechanism of propulsive and segmentative peristalsis, which exposes the food to the villous absorptive surface of the small intestine. Finally, still as a liquid, the residue is poured into the cecum and right colon. It is now devoid of any further food values, and is ready to be eliminated from the body, the "chaff" after the "wheat" has been separated.

Colonic function from now on is a combination of dehydration and expulsion. In the ascending colon and a portion of the transverse colon, absorption of water slowly takes place until the mass is partly dehydrated. Then this mass is moved rather

quickly in "rushes" to the descending colon and sigmoid, where gradually and slowly again dehydration continues until a formed compact fecal mass results. When this mass reaches sufficient bulk to "trip the trigger" of peristaltic action, the sigmoid passes the stool into the rectum, and it is extruded by rectal contraction and anal relaxation. Normally the stool is soft enough to pass easily but firm enough to retain its cylindrical shape, and is compact enough to sink in water. It has been variously described as "cigar-shaped"—or of the consistency of butter at room temperature.

It is at once evident from these facts that if the propulsion of the fecal material through the colon is too swift, insufficient time for dehydration is allowed and the stool will be loose or liquid. On the contrary, if the propulsion is too slow, too much dehydration will occur and a hard ball-like stool will result. It also follows that if the stool is of normal consistency, the bowel is moving at the right rate, whether it be once a day—several times a day—or once in two or three days. It is not the frequency of bowel movement which determines normality, but rather the consistency of the stool actually passed.

The inside factor which stimulates the colon to act is the presence of bulk or residue in the right colon. In general, the rule holds that the greater the bulk, the greater the activity. The normal individual eating a mixed diet has sufficient residue from his vegetables and fruits to cause just enough peristaltic action to push this residue forward at the right rate so that a normal stool results.

TIME TABLE OF DIGESTION

An explanation of the "time table" of the passage of food from stomach to anus helps many patients to understand their physiology and to overcome their fears of "improper elimination." Food eaten yesterday as three meals, breakfast, lunch and dinner, was passed through stomach and small intestine during yesterday and last night, and its residue is being poured into the right colon this morning. During today and tonight the colon will move this residue, at first slowly, to the ascending colon and hepatic flexure—then, later, by "rushes" into the left colon and sigmoid. Here it will be gathered together as a mass and will be passed as tomorrow's movement.

The colon is never normally empty. One day's stool is at the rectum while the next day's stool is in the cecum and ascending colon. If a cathartic is taken tonight on retiring, it hastens the whole process in the small intestine—strikes the colon early tomorrow morning—causes the colon to act faster than normal, and when the bowel movement does occur, it is the combination of tomorrow's stool with the next day's stool. The patient is gratified by the large and "satisfactory results," little realizing that it is really two days' movement. If, on the next day, the bowel does not move because it has not had time to "catch up," our patient is likely to resort to another cathartic because he is "constipated." Many patients thus start the pernicious habit of daily cathartics.

DIAGNOSIS

The most important step in the diagnosis of irritable colon is careful taking of the history. One must often listen to an elaborate and painfully long recitation of complaints. All symptoms of a hypersensitive nervous system with particular reference to the abdomen, are possible. At times pain is severe, and occurs with extreme suddeness, and only careful observation will distinguish it from that of intrinsic organic disease. Irritable colon at times has been confused with stone in the gall bladder, renal colic, appendicitis, girdle pains of tabes dorsalis, peptic ulcer, or even angina pectoris. More commonly, however, there is annoying and persistent distress which is frequently temporarily or at least partially relieved by anything which decreases intra-abdominal pressure such as belching, passage of flatus, having a bowel evacuation, or micturition. However, the taking of alkalies does not give relief unless this is followed by belching, and the taking of food usually gives rise to increased distress, these patients frequently abstaining from food for fear of inducing pain. Abdominal soreness is frequently present and is most commonly centered over the sigmoid but may be located anywhere over the course of the colon. Constipation is the usual finding, however the patient may have regular bowel movements, diarrhea, or there may be periods of constipation alternating with mild diarrhea. As a result of an inadequate diet and many other causes, a patient of this type may go without a movement of the bowel for several days; then he will take a laxative and this may be followed by passage of many loose stools. He then wonders why no movement occurs for several days and will repeat this procedure. A vicious cycle of this type, once established, is difficult to interrupt. Many of these patients will pass visible mucus with the stool, or frequently separate from it; this is a most distressing symptom to many of these people, to most of them the thought never having occurred that the mucus might have a function. The associated systemic complaints have included headaches, vertigo, coarse tremors of the hand, breathless

awakening at night, chewing of fingernails, fainting at work, nausea, rapid talking and sensations of weariness and weakness. Dyspepsia, hyperacidity, pylorospasm, bradycardia, tachycardia, and cardiac arrythmia are commonly seen.

Even when patients realize that the intestinal upsets seem to be the result of nervous tension, it is still difficult for them to understand that there is not some basic derangement of the bowel. In all such cases, the value of following a definite program of objective investigation cannot be over emphasized. The patient is anxious, much disturbed about his condition, perhaps has received many opinions concerning his trouble, and various kinds of treatment. Here it is very important to have the patient leave the physician's office feeling that "that was the most thorough examination he ever had," an attitude which goes far toward directing proper treatment.

The physical examination may not reveal very striking abnormalities. The facies may be anxious, the heart and lungs may be entirely negative, but frequently the colon, and particularly the descending colon, will appear rope-like at intervals. Careful digital examination of the rectum may reveal minor disturbances such as cryptitis, papillitis, poor sphincter control, or large rectocele, all having a bearing on the ease of emptying the rectum. Gross and microscopic examination of the stools should be carried out before any interference with intestinal habits has taken place; that is, the patient should pass a stool for inspection without the aid of aperients or enemas. The presence of mucus is characteristically the outstanding abnormality. For microscopic examination and the finding of unusual bacteria or parasites, a liquid stool, obtained after administration of a small dose of salts is most satisfactory.

Finally, other laboratory tests and instruments of diagnosis can be brought into play. Roentgenologic examination of the thorax is advisable to be sure incipient tuberculosis does not exist. Complete studies of the blood and urinalysis, should be performed. In many cases analysis of the gastric content is indicated. Proctoscopic examination always should be done. It will reveal an essentially normal mucous membrane, somewhat congested with adherent patches of mucous. Roentgenologic examination of the colon after barium enema, in turn followed by thorough emptying of the colon usually should be the final step of the examination.

TREATMENT
Bland Diet

With the physiological background of spastic colon in mind, it is evident that in its treatment whatever food or medication enters the digestive tube should be of a non-irritating and soothing type. The bland or "smooth" diet is used at the beginning of treatment. Eggs, meats, fish, fowl, shellfish, soups, milk, buttermilk, cheese, "white" cereals (rice, farina, cream of wheat), white breads, white crackers, macaroni or spaghetti, sponge cake, angel food, custards, puddings (such as rice, tapioca, or corn starch), gelatins, potatoes, bananas, avocado pear, fruit juices, tea, coffee, and cocoa—these form the basis of the diet on which the patient starts.

No coarse breads, no vegetables either cooked or raw, and none of the fruits either cooked or raw are allowed because of their cellulose. Syrup, fudge sauces, heavy frostings on cakes, and candies, are avoided because of their tendency to increase fermentation. Nuts, spices, condiments and pickles also are offenders. However, it makes little difference in this group of cases whether foods are fried, broiled, or baked. Allowing properly fried foods often removes one of the bugaboos that the patient has, and widens his choice of foods to advantage.

Bulk Producers

With the bland diet as given, the residue in the colon is at a minimum and some means must be found to stimulate colonic peristalsis. Cathartic drugs, such as cascara, phenolphthalein, senna, magnesia and salines, must be strictly avoided since they irritate the mucous membrane of the colon much more than would the foods that have been omitted from the diet. But the various bulk producers may be used safely because they act in a physiological way, and are non-irritating to the membrane. They have the common property of absorbing water in the stomach to form gelatin-like masses which mix with the food in the passage through the small intestine. They are not absorbed, however, but are discharged into the right colon to form the bulk which is needed to initiate peristaltic activity. As they pass through the colon their physiochemical composition allows them to retain their moisture and give the stool a soft, easily molded consistency. They act—not as a drug—but by mechanical means and therefore do not "wear out" in their effect. They can be used indefinitely without leading to congestion or injury of the colonic lining. Patients taking bulk producers should be cautioned to take adequate quantities of fluids simultaneously, that is, eight to ten glasses a day.

Examples of bulk producers are agar-agar, in finely powdered form, in flakes, or in cereal-like form; derivatives of psyllium seeds, such as Metamucil, Konsyl and Mucilose; Kabaya preparations, such as Kaba, Siblin and Mucara. The usual dosage of these various products is two to three heaping teaspoonfuls a day. If the entire amount is taken in one dose, a feeling of some fullness may follow, hence it is best to give two or three smaller doses spaced through the day. Patients vary in the amount needed to secure bowel action, and large doses may be used without fear. Mineral oil has been widely used as a means of combating the hard scybalous stools and when used in small doses is of great help. However, it should not be depended upon alone to get bowel action, as it interferes somewhat with food assimilation and with absorption of some of the fat-soluble vitamins.

Additions to Diet-Drugs

The patient is kept on this regimen of diet plus bulk producer with fluids for a variable period depending on the improvement. Many patients have to remain on the bland diet more or less indefinitely, and in that case vitamins must be given separately to prevent deficiencies. As the gas, abdominal pain and local discomforts subside, additions are gradually made to the diet. First, coarse breads and cereals, then the milder cooked vegetables and cooked fruits, later raw vegetables (salads) and finally raw fruits are used to build up the diet. We aim to have the broadest diet that the patient can tolerate. If, for instance, an addition of vegetables is made too soon and increased discomfort results, we step back to the blander level for a week—or a month—more, and then try the addition again. The constant aim is to have the colon act with just that speed that results in the formed, normal stool. If the stools are loose and frequent, we reduce the amount of bulk producer, or the amount of roughage in the diet.

Drugs are used for their effect inside the bowel and include calcium carbonate, kaolin, colloid alumina, and preparations such as Kaomagna— bismuth subnitrate. Rectal instillations of olive oil or mineral oil are of help if hemorrhoids or fissures are a complication. Enemas should be used to give temporary help for constipation. For these, normal saline is preferable to soapsuds, and small amounts—one to two pints—are less irritating than large amounts. Colonic irrigations except as an occasional temporary measure are to be avoided.

Treatment of the Nervous Element

Considering now the influences that affect the colon from the outside, we must treat the nervous elements of the patient's problem. Sympathetic discussion of his emotional situation is of extreme help. Allowing a patient to pour out his worries, his hurt feelings, or his resentments will give him relief and comfort. At times, it will be possible to give actual help in adjustment of some of his difficulties. Reassurance as to the unimportance of various phases of his illness, explanation of his symptoms, so that fear as to what they might mean will be allayed, and simple elucidation of the physiological background for the diet and medication will gain his confidence and assure enthusiastic cooperation. Adjustment to his routine of work so that more time is given to relaxation or hobbies is a part of re-educating the patient to meet his responsibilities without apprehension. The establishment of a habit time for going to stool is of extreme importance. Attention must be given to sleep habits, and sedation should be used if necessary. Above all, allaying of fear, and reassurance, are the fundamentals in helping these people to a more normal attitude toward life.

Specifically, certain "digestive" fears are commonly met with in these patients. One is the fear of being poisoned by retained feces, the fear that if daily evacuation does not occur, dire ill health will result. This may be combated by explaining that the normal colon is lined by a membrane which is protective and absorbs practically nothing but water—and which acts as a barrier between the products of fermentation and putrefaction, inside the colon, and the blood stream outside. By explaining further that the whole object of our treatment is to restore the colon wall to a normal state by soothing diet and medication, we get from our patient a more complete cooperation.

The patient must be reassured that, although during the first few days or weeks of his treatment he may have many distressing symptoms of gas, abdominal pressure, even pain, and the bowels will not move regularly, this stage is a preliminary through which he must go to reach the more comfortable stages later. In following these cases from week to week, it is common to have a patient report, at the end of the first week that the bowel moved daily and very satisfactorily. At the next report, a week later, however, discouragement has developed because the bowel has moved irregularly or only with some such help as with an enema. The fear enters the patient's mind that the

diet, or the bulk producer has "worn out." The explanation should be made that the colon during the first week was still so irritable and "touchy" from the previous cathartics or rough diet that it reacted to the amount of bulk producer used. By the second week it had recovered enough so that its irritability was lessened, and more bulk was needed to cause evacuation. A simple increase in the amount of bulk producer, or addition of some of the rougher foods is usually all that is needed to correct this phase.

Another common fear is that the bowels are not moving enough—that the stools are not large enough considering the meals eaten. The answer is that these patients have been having loose watery stools, either from cathartics or rough diet, and are expecting too much, now that the stool is compact and free of fluid.

The drugs that are helpful in the nervous control of these cases are: (1) sedatives such as phenobarbital, bromides, or even codeine; (2) antispasmodics, such as tincture of belladonna, atropine, trasentin, syntropan, novatropin, calcium gluconate, and opium derivatives such as paregoric. Other measures are heat to the abdomen, by hot water bag, by electric pad, or by diathermy.

The outlook for improvement in spastic colon, if it is treated patiently and persistently, is definitely good. The course will be irregular—some weeks better, some not so well, but he should be told that weeks rather than days should be his measure of improvement. Each case is of course a different problem, with varying emphasis put on various symptoms. But with a proper understanding by both physician and patient of the physiology of the digestive tube, and by stressing the neurological aspects of the condition, careful treatment will lead to gratifying success.

"A good home or school uses a minimum of compulsion and a maximum of persuasion, and a church has no compulsion at all at its disposal, only persuasion to rely upon. . . . yet age after age, while empires rise and fall, these three go on—homes, schools, churches—the major builders of all the real goodness that mankind has."—Harry Emerson Fosdick.

Diagnosis and Treatment of Gall Bladder Disease

D. D. PAULUS, M.D.

OKLAHOMA CITY, OKLAHOMA

The diagnosis of acute cholecystitis in the absence of any history of a previous attack is often very difficult. Pain is the most constant feature present. It is a constant dull, heavy feeling in the upper abdomen, more especially in the epigastrium and under the right rib margin. The pain may be so severe as to require hypodermics for several days. Associated with this pain there is more or less constant nausea and generally vomiting.

The abdomen is distended with gas and the lack of bowel action may simulate acute bowel obstruction. Fever, malaise, weakness, prostration, generally accompany the condition. Abdominal rigidity, at first more or less generalized, may lead to confusion with acute appendicitis or ruptured peptic ulcer, or other acute surgical abdominal conditions. An acute retrocecal appendicitis, where the tip of the appendix lies under the edge of the lower border of the liver, may simulate acute cholecystitis very closely, especially in the first twenty-four to thirty-six hours. Later, however, in an acute gall bladder condition the tenderness and rigidity become more or less localized in the upper right quadrant. Another condition which may lead to confusion is an attack of coronary thrombosis, especially in those cases where the pain is localized under the lower end of the sternum and in the epigastric region.

The gall bladder usually is distended and when the rigidity begins to disappear one may be able to palpate a tender, pear-shaped mass.

Some jaundice may be present at times but it is not pronounced unless the condition is complicated by common duct obstruction of some sort. The use of the Lyon tube for diagnostic purposes may naturally aid in the diagnosis but is generally not practical because of the profound nausea and vomiting that is present. Similarly, the use of the X-ray—either through dye by the oral route or intravenously—is not practical or may be contraindicated because of possible associated acute hepatitis and cholangitis.

If the acute condition does not subside within a few days, then watch out for some complication. If the process is an acute fulminating one from the beginning, an acute empyema or a phlegmonous gall bladder is to be kept in mind.

In discussing the symptoms and diagnosis of chronic gall bladder disease, three subdivisions may be made since the treatment followed will depend to a great extent upon the subdivision into which any case might fall. These three subdivisions are: (1) Gall bladder disease dyspepsia without colic or stones. (2) Gall bladder disease with recurrent colic but no stones. (3) Gall bladder disease with stones.

The symptoms of gall bladder dyspepsia without colic are a prolonged feeling of fullness in the epigastrium or so-called "bloat" after meals, more especially after a full meal. Belching of gas, sour, bitter or burning eructations. An uneasiness or unrest through the abdomen, only partially relieved by taking an enema. There are no severe colicky pains through the abdomen in this group, but these may be some mild colicky pains more especially through the lower abdomen, due to spasm of the intestine.

Associated with the above symptoms, intolerance to some foods is common, such as fats, fried foods, cabbage, onions, beans and pork. Constipation is frequently present but by no manner of means the rule.

All of the above symptoms, while present in gall bladder disease, are also found in the so-called "colitis" cases. Gastro-enterologists prefer to call this condition "the irritable colon" since no real inflammation exists in the colon and persistent diarrhea is absent. The typical neurogenic irritable colon syndrome consists of a history of irregular bowel habits, frequent use of cathartics and the presence of mucus in the stool in many instances. Abdominal pain and tenderness is present and is variable in degree and shifting in character. Such patients are constantly aware of their intestinal activities and have been aptly called "bowel conscious." They show the same intolerance to certain foods as the gall bladder disease dyspepsia cases. On the other hand, the irritable colon cases usually show a good response to treatment with a bland diet, antispasmodics and bland bulk-forming drugs. Another condition which may be confused with dyspepsia of gall bladder disease is the aerophagia of the nervous individual. The alert clinician should, however, readily recognize these cases.

To differentiate the latter from gall bladder dyspepsia and the neurogenic irritable colon syndrome frequently becomes a difficult problem. Unfortunately the laboratory and X-ray will not help us a great deal until the gall bladder disease has progressed to the second subdivision or the gall bladder dyspepsia with colic. Surgery in the first subdivision is disappointing.

In the gall bladder disease with colic, we may be able to obtain a history of recurrent attacks which materially aids in arriving at a more definite conclusion. The attacks of recurrent colic come on gradually, last a variable period of time, even for several days, and the colic may be due to reflex pylorospasm or the so-called biliary stasis due to spasm of the sphincter at the ampulla of Vater. Associated localized pain, tenderness and rigidity are the rule. The pain and rigidity disappear, leaving localized tenderness for several days or longer. The patient may be free from dyspeptic or other symptoms. During the attack slight fever, generally nausea and sometimes vomiting are present.

Uncomplicated gall bladder disease with stones cannot be differentiated clinically from cases of colic alone. A very abrupt onset of pain, requiring several hypodermics of morphine for immediate relief, is certainly indicative of stones. When complications such as associated common duct stone occur the accompanying jaundice in most cases will further support the diagnosis.

Diagnostic methods in gall bladder disease consist of a careful, painstaking history and thorough physical examination in addition to laboratory data and cholecystography. The use of the diagnostic duodenal drainage tube has not been very helpful in our experience and has been practically discontinued.

It is admitted, however, that when used, the demonstration of cholesterol and calcium bilirubinate crystals in combination should make the diagnosis of stones fairly accurate.

Cholecystography is accepted as an exceedingly reliable aid in the diagnosis of gall bladder disease. It is not only a test for the functional integrity of the gall bladder but if the viscus fills with the opaque bile organic changes are often directly demonstrable. It should be stated, however, that it is a method that requires punctilious observance of technical details and experienced judgment in interpreting the finished cholecystogram.

It is not necessary here to go into the technical details of the method of using the dye nor the technique used by the roentgenologist to obtain the proper cholecystograms. Suffice it to say that the method we employ is the double dye technique. The patient eats an ordinary meal at noon and takes a dose of the dye in grape juice after the meal is finished. For his dinner or supper in the evening, he gets a fat free diet and takes a second dose of the dye. Early the next morning he takes an ordinary soapsuds enema and omits his breakfast. He presents himself for the first picture at 8:00 A.M. A second picture is made at 10:00 A.M., and then he is given a fatty meal or a glassful of milk and cream, "half and half," and the final picture is made two or two and one-half hours later.

In a patient of average weight or below average weight, the normal cholecystogram series will show that the gall bladder shadow is of normal density throughout; that it is smooth in contour; and that a comparison of the first and second pictures shows a change in size and position of the gall bladder. Generally, the concentration of the dye is greatest in the second or 10:00 o'clock film. After the fatty meal the gall bladder should be at least partially or almost completely empty. Too much emphasis has been placed on this last question of the ability of the gall bladder to empty itself. We now know that the gall bladder may not empty itself even within twenty-four hours, due to constant re-absorption from the intestinal tract.

If the gall bladder fails to fill with the opaque bile or dye, then the gall bladder should be considered pathologic, provided, of course, that all sources of error have been eliminated; namely, that the patient has followed directions properly, that he has not vomited within thirty minutes after taking the dye, and that gas in the colon is not obscuring the gall bladder shadow. If gas partially obliterates the gall bladder in the 8:00 o'clock film he is given pitressin and the film repeated in thirty or forty minutes. We have never seen any ill results from the use of pitressin, but it should be used with caution in the marked hypertensive individuals or old and debilitated patients.

If the shadow of the opaque bile filled gall bladder is only very faint and the outline hardly discernible, but is of normal size and is smooth in contour, then we should ascertain whether the patient is considerably overweight or obese. Frequently in this type of patient the shadow may lie high up under the liver.

If the last film shows this shadow to be materially reduced in size due to partially or almost complete emptying, we still may have a fairly good functioning gall bladder. Should, however, the shadows in all three films be the same size and density then the shadow is probably due to the gall bladder outline itself without any dye in it. Such a case suggests a distinct non-functioning gall bladder, but it should be rechecked at a later date without using the dye, to make sure that the interpretation is correct. Such cases are not common, however. It is also to be remembered that functional abnormalities of the gall bladder are often temporary. The gall bladder that fails to fill with opaque bile or dye today may show a comparatively good functioning gall bladder a month later.

Should the shadow of the opaque, bile-filled gall bladder show considerable mottling and an uneven or irregular contour, it may be due to pericholecystic diseases, either from intrinsic or extrinsic causes. All such cases should have an X-ray of the stomach and duodenum to further clarify the condition, if possible.

All of this may sound somewhat confusing but briefly stated it may be said that if no shadow of the gall bladder can be seen, or if it is visible but faint, experience has proved that with few exceptions the cause is chronic cholecystitis, with or without stones.

When gall stones are present and the dye fails to depict a gall bladder shadow, as is often the case, stones nevertheless may often be demonstrated as dense or transradiant spots. In a very large number of cases, gall stone shadows though present will not be visible. In those cases where the stones are present and the gall bladder fills with the opaque bile or dye, it will not be difficult to determine the presence of the stones. The calcium stones will cast dense shadow spots, and the cholesterol stones will be seen as transradiant areas. When looking for stones the last film, when the gall bladder is partially empty, is the one to examine most carefully since they are much easier to depict than in the first two films. The complication of stones in the common duct, associated stones in the gall bladder, or common duct stones after a previous cholecystectomy, will not be covered in this paper.

In conclusion, we may say that symptoms of gall bladder disease are extremely variable in a very large proportion of cases and that the diagnosis depends on a careful history and examination, supplemented by cholecystography which lends valuable aid.

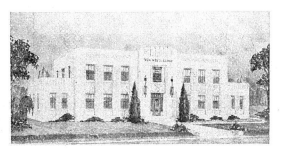

• *THE PRESIDENT'S PAGE* •

The Nineteenth Session of the Oklahoma Legislature is now in session, and a new Chief Executive has been inaugurated into office.

Robert S. "Bob" Kerr, as Governor, has already conclusively proved that he is close to the needs of the people in the matter of public health and medical care by virtue of the statements made in his address to the Legislature.

Bob Kerr has taken a stand concerning the University of Oklahoma School of Medicine that has been needed since statehood—adequate appropriations. Adequate appropriations must be secured from the Legislature or the school should be discontinued.

While it should not be the sole responsibility of the medical profession, and particularly Oklahoma City physicians, to be apprehensive about the future of the School, nevertheless, it cannot be denied that our obligation as a profession is to protect the health and welfare of the people and certainly a fight for the school and its teaching hospitals falls in this category.

Governor Kerr is sincere in his efforts, and he is entitled to the unqualified support of every physician.

Sincerely yours,

James D Osborn

President.

For timely and effective control of Scarlet Fever...

Treatment . . .

SCARLET FEVER STREPTOCOCCUS ANTITOXIN
GLOBULIN *Lederle* MODIFIED

Prevention . . .

SCARLET FEVER STREPTOCOCCUS TOXIN
Lederle

TODAY ANTITOXIN THERAPY may be administered with comparative safety —for both mild and severe scarlet fever. The advanced process of serum refinement by Parfentjev of Lederle Research Laboratories has greatly reduced the incidence of serum sickness[1]. This Globulin-Modified antitoxin usually brings about a sharp drop in temperature and prompt disappearance of symptoms[2,3]. Early administration is advised to thwart the development of complications[4].

In infected, susceptible persons, "Scarlet Fever Streptococcus Antitoxin *Lederle*" may be injected for prophylaxis, and a passive immunity is produced, lasting about two weeks. However, this temporary measure must be followed one week later by active immunization for lasting protection.

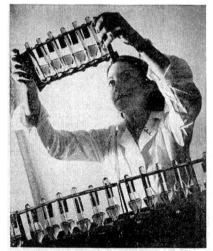

Sterility Test

"Scarlet Fever Toxin *Lederle*," for active immunization, is a highly potent and carefully standardized preparation. Complete immunization can be achieved only if a full course of undivided doses is given. By such a method 90-95% of individuals may be rendered Dick-negative, the majority remaining so for as long as 12 years[4].

Some recommend that every child be given a Dick test on entrance to school or an institution, and that a record be kept of the result[5]. Dick-testing and immunization of susceptible individuals is indicated[6] in emergencies such as threat of an epidemic. It is a timely procedure for the large numbers of children who are being moved, in many parts of the country, into over-crowded war-plant areas.

[1]KOHS, F. G.: Am. J. Dis. Child. 64:93 (July), 1942; 64:145 (Aug.) 1942.
[2]TOP, F.H., and YOUNG, D.C.: J.A.M.A. 117:2056 (Dec. 13) 1941.
[3]PALMER, L.: Kentucky M. J. 40:254 (July) 1942.
[4]MELNICK, T.: Arch. Pediat. 59:90 (Feb.) 1942.
[5]HOYNE, A. L.: Illinois M. J. 81:12 (Jan.) 1942.
[6]THOMPSON, C. G.: Connecticut M. J. 5:736 (Oct.) 1941.

PACKAGES:

Scarlet Fever Streptococcus Toxin *Lederle*
  1 complete immunization: 5 vials of 650, 2,500, 10,000, 50,000 and 100,000-120,000 S. T. D.
  10 complete immunizations: 5—10 cc. vials.
  Dose No. 5 for supplementary immunization: 1—1 cc. vial containing 100,000-120,000 S. T. D.
Scarlet Fever Streptococcus Antitoxin (Globulin Modified) *Lederle*
  5,000 U. S. P. H. S. units (150,000 original neutralizing units) for prophylaxis and 9,000 U. S. P. H. S. units (450,000 original neutralizing units) for therapeutic use.
Scarlet Fever Streptococcus Toxin for Dick Test *Lederle*
  5 Dick Tests in 1—2.0 cc. ampul.
  50 Dick Tests in 1—10.0 cc. vial.

The JOURNAL Of The
OKLAHOMA STATE MEDICAL ASSOCIATION

EDITORIAL BOARD
L. J. MOORMAN, Oklahoma City, Editor-in-Chief

E. EUGENE RICE, Shawnee NED R. SMITH, Tulsa

MR. R. H. GRAHAM, Oklahoma City, Business Manager

CONTRIBUTIONS: Articles accepted by this Journal for publication including those read at the annual meetings of the State Association are the sole property of this Journal.

The Editorial Department is not responsible for the opinions expressed in the original articles of contributors.

Manuscripts may be withdrawn by authors for publication elsewhere only upon the approval of the Editorial Board.

MANUSCRIPTS: Manuscripts should be typewritten, double-spaced, on white paper 8½ x 11 inches. The original copy, not the carbon copy, should be submitted.

Footnotes, bibliographies and legends for cuts should be typed on separate sheets in double space. Bibliography listing should follow this order: Name of author, title of article, name of periodical with volume, page and date of publication.

Manuscripts are accepted subject to the usual editorial revisions and with the understanding that they have not been published elsewhere.

NEWS: Local news of interest to the medical profession, changes of address, births, deaths and weddings will be gratefully received.

ADVERTISING: Advertising of articles, drugs or compounds unapproved by the Council on Pharmacy of the A.M.A. will not be accepted. Advertising rates will be supplied on application.

It is suggested that members of the State Association patronize our advertisers in preference to others.

SUBSCRIPTIONS: Failure to receive The Journal should call for immediate notification.

REPRINTS: Reprints of original articles will be supplied at actual cost provided request for them is attached to manuscripts or made in sufficient time before publication. Checks for reprints should be made payable to Industrial Printing Company, Oklahoma City.

Address all communications to THE JOURNAL OF THE OKLAHOMA STATE MEDICAL ASSOCIATION, 210 Plaza Court, Oklahoma City.

OFFICIAL PUBLICATION OF THE OKLAHOMA STATE MEDICAL ASSOCIATION
Copyrighted February, 1943

EDITORIALS

THE NATIONAL PHYSICIANS COMMITTEE AND AMERICAN MEDICINE

The angel of professional security first stirred the waters of ideal medical service at the bedside of the humble, the poor and the obscure wherever they were found. Luke Field's brush caught the spirit of this service when he painted the well-known picture entitled "The Doctor." In this striking portrayal, the kindly face, contemplating the fate of a sick child, is supposed to be that of Dr. James Clark (later Sir James), who rendered valuable voluntary medical service to the immortal John Keats as he lay dying of tuberculosis in the Piazza di Spagne in Rome. It was this good doctor who steered the lonely Keats through the shadow of the night and saw him silently removed "from the contagion of the world's slow stain."

The chief slogan of the National Physicians Committee is the "doctor and patient relationship." The members of this Committee and the doctors they represent should remember that to make this an effective slogan, it must first be a living reality in the American home, ranging from the widow's hovel to the plutocrat's palace. It is well for the Committee to keep this in mind.

OPPORTUNITY IS KNOCKING AT YOUR DOOR

Every doctor in the State should be interested in the forthcoming Institute on Wartime Industrial Health to be held in Tulsa on March 18 and in Oklahoma City March 19.

Your attention is called to the program which appears in this issue of the Journal. It promises interesting and constructive discussions with authoritative speakers. These two educational assemblies should be largely attended by the members of the State Medical Association.

In the past, Oklahoma doctors have been concerned primarily with the diseases caused by infections and those resulting from degenerative and metabolic conditions. But suddenly war has placed big industry upon our doorstep, and we must welcome and nurture it. In addition to our accustomed medical knowledge, we must learn much about industrial hazards, their potential evils and their prevention. Also, we must learn how to interpret symptomatology and pathology in the light of noxious gases, dust, fumes, solvents, metals and many other occupational hazards.

Today the average doctor is not prepared

to meet the challenge of industrial medicine which has been so rudely thrust upon him. There is so much that is new and so much not taught in medical schools that it becomes necessary to supplement medical education with additional knowledge such as this Institute provides.

When occasion arises, it is the doctor's duty to recognize industrial hazards and to recommend proper preventive measures. It is equally encumbent upon him to understand and to teach industrial hygiene in order that workers and their families may have adequate protection against the handicaps of occupational diseases. For the duration, this is particularly important in that it should help prevent absenteeism in war industries.

"We must beat the iron while it is hot; but we may polish it at leisure." (Dryden).

The industrial health forge is hot, the iron is ready for the hammer, the dates are — Tulsa, March 18; Oklahoma City, March 19.

THE INJUSTICE OF JUSTICE

When the Supreme Court of the United States upheld the conviction of the American Medical Association for its opposition to a questionable type of medical service, Themis, the Goddess of Justice, opened her eyes in astonishment. "This Daughter of the Heavens," representing the personification of "that divine law of right which ought to control all human affairs," lost her Olympian poise and longed for the days of the "venerable deities," when with eyes blindfolded, it was relatively safe to let her sword rest in its sheath — and to hold her scales for the accurate balance of justice which was duly meted out.

Leaving justice out of the question, how can the administration reconcile its ambition for better medical service with this obstructive attitude toward the best medical service in the history of the world?

If Themis had not deserted the Delphic oracle, we might learn the answer.

TOXIC EFFECTS OF SULFONAMIDE THERAPY

Before any one of the sulfonamides is prescribed, the possible immediate and remote toxic effects should be considered. Naturally editorial comment cannot be comprehensive, but it can serve as a reminder and a warning.

After more than six years' experience with the sulfonamides, we are warranted in the statement that all doctors should be familiar with the established indications of these drugs and keenly aware of the toxic reactions.

Available figures[1] indicate that the total important toxic reactions for the preparations most commonly employed are as follows: Sulfathiazole 18.6 per cent, Sulfapyridine 15.9 per cent, Sulfanilamide 11.9 per cent and Sulfadiazine 6.5 per cent.

Some of the most significant of these reactions are reported as follows:

DRUG FEVER—highest in sulfathiazole —6 per cent, and lowest in sulfadiazine— 1.6 per cent.

SKIN REACTIONS—highest in sulfathiazole—5.2 per cent, and lowest in sulfadiazine—1.3 per cent.

Acute HEMALYTIC ANEMIA—highest in sulfanilamide—2 per cent, next highest in sulfapyridine—1.1 per cent, and very rare in sulfathiazole and sulfadiazine.

LEUKOPENIA—highest in sulfapyridine —2.1 per cent, approximately the same in sulfanilamide and relatively low in sulfathiazole and sulfadiazine—1.5 per cent.

HEMATURIA—highest in sulfathiazole— 4.7 per cent, approximately the same in sulfapyridine—4.6 per cent, sulfadiazine—1.7 per cent, sulfanilamide very rare.

OLIGURIA or ANURIA—highest in sulfapyridine—2.2 per cent, sulfathiazole—1.1 per cent, very rare in sulfadiazine and sulfanilamide.

HEPATITIS—rare in all, the highest in sulfanilamide—0.6 per cent.

Common among the minor immediate toxic effects are nausea, vomiting, dizziness, lack of coordination with psychic and motor imbalance. These are most common with sulfanilamide and sulfapyridine and occasionally true psychoses have been observed.

The question of permanent and remote untoward effects are not yet fully comprehended. Apparently, we may safely presume that there will be no residual tissue damage or remote ill-effects in cases receiving sulfonamide therapy without obvious immediate toxic reactions. With almost equal assurance, we may say that when acute toxic reactions occur sensitivity will follow, giving rise to recurring reactions in case the same drug is subsequently administered, the reactions occurring more promptly and with greater severity.

Perrin H. Long has called attention to the danger of gradual sensitization of our population and the resulting attenuation of the great boon which chemotherapy has conferred upon suffering humanity. This possibility should be accepted as a warning against promiscuous sulfonamide therapy without specific indications. It is doubtful if these powerful preparations should ever be given in mild, acute, respiratory infections, with the vague hope of preventing more serious secondary infections. But when specific indications arise and the race between infection and resistance is definitely on, therapy should be heroic. Such a therapeutic policy demands careful attention to all safeguards including daily observation of the patient with acute awareness of the danger of toxic reactions and prompt withdrawal of the drug upon the first indication of such reactions.

We have discussed only the more severe and the most common minor toxic reactions. It is to be hoped that this brief discussion will lead to a more careful consideration of the dangers inherent in these life-saving therapeutic agents.

BIBLIOGRAPHY

1. Long, Perrin H.: The Connecticut State Medical Journal, VII: 6-10, January, 1943.

MULTI-VITAMIN MANIA

The medical profession is ever learning more about vitamins, but doctors cannot keep up with radio criers and magazine writers. Having learned much about vitamin deficiencies and having established definite indications for vitamin therapy in many conditions, it seems advisable for the medical profession to carefully consider the limitations of vitamin therapy. It is particularly important for the family physician to know something of vitamin therapy and its limitations because his patrons are annually spending millions for vitamin pills without his advice, and many of those who are too loyal to dose themselves without his approval make bold to suggest that they may need vitamins because they are constantly assailed by misguided publicity and over-enthusiastic salesmen.

At this season of the year, vitamins are squandered with the false belief that they will "keep off" colds. Every doctor should read "Vitamins for the Prevention of Colds" in the December 19, 1942, issue of the Journal of the American Medical Association.

The authors report a controlled study among students at the University of Minnesota. One group of students received capsules of multiple vitamins (hepicebrin), and a corresponding group received placebo capsules.

Similar groups received large doses of vitamin C and placebo tablets.

After reporting in detail, the authors make the following significant statement:

"An examination of table 2 does not reveal any evidence that the multiple vitamins reduced the severity of the colds. In fact, complications were more frequent among the students who got the vitamin supplements than among the control group. Furthermore, the average duration of each cold was the same for all three groups.

"This controlled study yields no indication that either large doses of vitamin C alone or large doses of vitamins A, B1, B2, C and D and nicotinic acid have any important effect on the number or severity of infections of the upper respiratory tract when administered to young adults who presumably are already on a reasonably adequate diet."

In an editorial on "Early Vitamin B Disorders" appearing in the New York State Journal of Medicine, we find the following statement: "Efforts to increase the productive capacity of individuals on an adequate diet by administration of additional vitamins have failed both in industrial and military circles. Large, continued doses of thiamine are not without risk, contrary to the general impression that a water-soluble vitamin which is freely eliminated can be given in huge doses. Reports are beginning to appear about thiamine toxicity and even fatality. The symptoms induced by doses of 10 to 50 mg. for a period of two to three weeks were nervousness, insomnia, hyper-irritability, palpitation (signs simulating hyperthyroidism), and eventually collapse, syncope, and signs of circulatory shock."

It is unfortunate that doctors must spend valuable time in an effort to correct false impressions created through premature and unwarranted claims with reference to vitamin therapy, but this duty now stands prominently among their professional obligations. The above duty is emphasized by the fact that approximately four-fifths of the vitamins consumed in the United States are purchased over the counter without a doctor's prescription, and that the individual and collective (the latter through industry) lay consumption is based upon the popular belief that vitamins administered to well-nourished people will prevent colds and increase physical capacity.

The Menninger Sanitarium

For the Diagnosis and Treatment
of Nervous and Mental Illness.

The Southard School

For the Education and Psychiatric
Treatment of Children of Average
and Superior Intelligence.

Boarding Home Facilities.

Topeka, Kansas

ASSOCIATION ACTIVITIES

COMMITTEE ON ANNUAL SESSION SELECTS DATES FOR 1943 MEETING

President James D. Osborn has announced that the Committee on Annual Session has selected May 11 and 12 for the 1943 Meeting to be held in Oklahoma City.

The meeting for this year is being reduced to a two-day session, and no attempt will be made to secure technical exhibitors.

Dr. Ben H. Nicholson, Chairman, and members of the Scientific Work Committee, are working on the scientific program which will be adapted to the war effort as it pertains to the health of the public.

Every indication points to an exceptionally interesting meeting with a distinct flavor of military officialdom being present to participate.

Any member desiring to present a scientific paper should immediately contact Dr. Nicholson, 301 Northwest 12th Street, Oklahoma City.

AMERICAN COLLEGE OF SURGEONS APPROVES FORTY OKLAHOMA HOSPITALS

The American College of Surgeons, through its chairman Dr. Irvin Abell, has announced the approval of 2,989 hospitals for 1943. This number represents an increase over 1941 of 116.

Oklahoma hospitals approved are as follows:

Valley View hospital, Ada; Hardy sanitarium, Ardmore; Washington County Memorial hospital, Bartlesville; Claremore hospital, Claremore; Clinton Indian hospital, Western Oklahoma Charity hospital, Western Oklahoma Tuberculosis sanatorium, Clinton; Cheyenne and Arapaho Indian hospital, Concho; Masonic hospital, Cushing.

Federal Reformatory hospital, El Reno; Enid General hospital, St. Mary's Enid Springs hospital, Enid; Kiowa Indian hospital, Lawton; Albert Pike hospital, St. Mary's hospital, McAlester; Oklahoma Baptist hospital, Veterans Administration hospital, Muskogee; Central Oklahoma State hospital, Ellison infirmary, Norman.

Bone and Joint hospital-McBride clinic, Crippled Children's hospital, Oklahoma City General hospital, St. Anthony's hospital, University of Oklahoma Crippled Children's hospital and State University hospital, Wesley hospital, Oklahoma City; Ponca hospital, Pawnee; American hospital, Picher; Ponca City hospital, Ponca City.

A. C. H. hospital, Shawnee Indian sanatorium, Shawnee Municipal hospital, Shawnee; Soldiers Tubercular sanatorium, Sulphur; Western Oklahoma hospital, Supply; William W. Hastings Indian hospital, Tahlequah; Eastern Okahoma State Tuberculosis sanatorium, Talihina sanatorium and hospital, Talihina; Hillcrest Memorial hospital, St. John's hospital, Tulsa.

The development of war industry areas in Oklahoma together with the continued growth of the Blue Cross Plan sponsored by the Oklahoma State Medical and Hospital Associations have materially increased hospital admissions and enabled many hospitals to expand and improve their services and make needed improvements.

Oklahoma hospitals approved by the American College of Surgeons are to be complimented for their continued adherence to the high standards necessary for recognition, especially in view of the difficulties with which they are confronted due to war priorities and depleted hospital staffs.

ASSOCIATION TO HOLD WARTIME INDUSTRIAL HEALTH INSTITUTE

An Institute on Wartime Industrial Health has been announced by Dr. Henry H. Turner, Chairman of the Postgraduate Medical Teaching Committee, and Dr. Henry C. Weber, Chairman of the Industrial and Traumatic Surgery Committee of the Association, to be held in Tulsa, Thursday, March 18, and Oklahoma City, Friday, March 19.

The Institute is being sponsored in cooperation with the Oklahoma State Health Department, and will bring outstanding industrial health authorities to Oklahoma for the two-day session. Out-of-state guests who will be present are J. J. Bloomfield, Bethesda, Md.; Carl Peterson, M.D., Chicago, Ill.; Clarence D. Selby, M.D., Detroit, Mich.; W. A. Sawyer, M.D., Rochester, N. Y.; J. Albert Key, M.D., St. Louis, Mo.; A. G. Hewitt, Chicago, Ill., and Louis Schwartz, M.D., Bethesda, Md.

The meetings will be afternoon and evening sessions beginning at 2:00 P.M. and 8:00 P.M. There will be an informal dinner at 6:30. The meetings will be held at the Biltmore Hotel in Oklahoma City and the Mayo Hotel in Tulsa.

The following is the program of the Institute as announced by Dr. Turner and Dr. Weber:

INSTITUTE ON WARTIME INDUSTRIAL HEALTH

Program

2:00 P.M.—The Puposes and Objectives of the Program on Industrial Health of the Oklahoma State Medical Association.

H. C. Weber, M.D., Chairman, Committee on Industrial and Traumatic Surgery, Bartlesville, Okla.

2:10 P.M.—Technical Assistance of the Oklahoma State Health Department Available to Industry.
Grady F. Mathews, M.D., Commissioner.

V. C. Myers, M.D., Industrial Hygiene Physician.

Carl Warkentin and R. B. Ady, Industrial Hygiene Engineers.

Eugene A. Gillis, M.D., Director, Venereal Disease Control Division.
Demonstration of Equipment.

2:40 P.M.—Industrial Hygiene in War Production.
J. J. Bloomfield, U. S. Public Health Service, Bethesda, Md.

3:00 P.M.—General Relation of Medicine to Industry.
Carl Peterson, M.D., Executive Secretary, Council on Industrial Health, American Medical Association, Chicago, Ill.

3:20 P.M.—Pre-employment Examination and Placement.
Clarence D. Selby, M.D., Medical Director, General Motors Corporation, Detroit, Mich.

3:50 P.M.—Conservation of Industry's Manpower.
W. A. Sawyer, M.D., Medical Director, Eastman Kodak Company, Rochester, N. Y.

4:15 P.M.—Medical Legal Phase and Evaluation of Disability.
J. Albert Key, M.D., Orthopedic Surgeon, St. Louis, Mo.
Clinics and presentation of cases for evaluation.
Vancil K. Greer, Chairman, Oklahoma State Industrial Commission, Oklahoma

City, Okla. Earl D. McBride, M.D., Oklahoma City, Okla. J. S. Chalmers, M.D., Sand Springs, Okla.

Discussion by Dr. Key.

5:15 P.M.—Discussion of Papers.

6:30 P.M.—Informal Dinner.

8:00 P.M.—Management Looks at Industrial Health.

A. G. Hewitt, General Superintendent, The Visking Company, Chicago, Ill.

8:30 P.M.—Occupational Diseases and Their Control. (Illustrated).

Louis Schwartz, M.D., Medical Director, U. S. Public Health Service, Bethesda, Md.

9:00 P.M.—General Discussion.

Motion Picture: ''Save a Day''—U. S. Public Health Service.

The Postgraduate Medical Teaching Committee is composed of the following physicians: Dr. Henry H. Turner, Chairman, Oklahoma City; Dr. H. C. Weber, Bartlesville, and Dr. M. J. Searle, Tulsa. Members of the Industrial and Traumatic Surgery Committee are Dr. H. C. Weber, Chairman, Bartlesville; Dr. O. S. Somerville, Bartlesville, and Dr. J. S. Chalmers, Sand Springs.

The increase in war industries in states which before the war were not considered industrialized has made the problem of industrial health one of major importance. Oklahoma physicians should avail themselves of the Institute and the opportunity it affords for postgraduate study.

LEGISLATURE CONVENES

The Nineteenth Legislature which convened January 4, under the leadership of the newly-elected Chief Executive Robert S. ''Bob'' Kerr, has the earmarks of being of the disposition to assume its obligations for wartime economy in the face of necessary large Federal expenditures.

Every indication points to one of the shortest sessions in the history of the state which, if accomplished, will please the ''home folks'' and be a credit to the legislators themselves.

Committee organization in both the Senate and the House of Representatives was announced on the opening day of the session with additional committee membership assignments being made as the occasion demanded.

Senate Committee on Public Health

The Committee on Committees in the Senate in announcing committee assignments nominated Senator Clint Braden, attorney, of Wilburton, as Chairman for Public Health and Sanitation and Louis H. Ritzhaupt, Guthrie, as Vice-Chairman. Dr. Ritzhaupt, who has always been a leader of the Senate and instrumental in fostering progressive and protective health measures, met with the Senate when it convened and was excused from serving as he is now with the military forces, presently serving at State Medical Officer for Selective Service. No additional members of this Senate committee have been announced.

House of Representatives Committees on Practice of Medicine and Public Health and Sanitation

Speaker of the House, Representative Harold Freeman, Pauls Valley, has announced the following membership for the Committee on Practice of Medicine and Public Health and Sanitation: Practice of Medicine—Chairman, Orange W. Starr, Drumright; Vice-Chairman, Elbert ''Pete'' Weaver, Stillwater; Andy Banks, McAlester; Walter Billingsley, Wewoka; D. C. Cantrell, Stigler; T. N. Crow, Hollis; George E. Davison, Arnett; B. B. Kerr, Oklahoma City; John T. Levergood, Shawnee; J. D. McCarty, Oklahoma City; D. M. Madrano, Tulsa; Kirksey Nix, Eufaula; Arthur Reed, Poteau; Amos Stovall, Anadarko; Claude Thompson, Antlers, and Paul Washington, Oklahoma City.

Public Health and Sanitation—Chairman, Raymond H. Lucas, Spiro; Vice-Chairman, Bayless Irby, Boswell; Andy Banks, McAlester; Walter Billingsley, Wewoka; Raymond Board, Boise City; D. C. Cantrell, Stigler; W. R. Dunn, Arapaho; Russell Farmer, Pauls Valley; Carl Frix, Sallisaw; Joe Harshbarger, Tulsa; Con Long, Seminole; J. D. McCarty, Oklahoma City; W. B. McDonald, Hobart; C. L. Mills, Wellston; Arthur Reed, Poteau; Orange W. Starr, Drumright; Earnest W. Tate, Ardmore; Elbert R. Weaver, Stillwater; Charles A. Whitford, Nowata; Purman Wilson, Purcell, and Henry W. Worthington, Mangum.

Dr. Starr, Chairman of the Practice of Medicine Committee, is serving his first term as a Representative from Creek County. His interest in legislation to protect the health of the public is making him an exceptionally valuable member of the House. Pete Weaver, who is Secretary of the Oklahoma State Pharmaceutical Association, is a veteran member of the Legislature as well as the Practice of Medicine Committee. Representative Weaver's interest in public health is a credit not only to himself but to his allied profession.

Raymond Lucas, Spiro, Chairman of the Public Health and Sanitation Committee, is serving his second term as Chairman. His cooperation in the consideration of public health legislation submitted by interested organizations is sound and constructive. Under the leadership of these members of the House of Representatives, Oklahoma may expect sound and judicious health legislation. Members of the profession are urged to counsel with their Representatives and Senators on public health legislation.

Legislation Introduced Affecting Public Health

Thus far in the Session, the health legislation introduced has dealt mainly with problems related to the war effort. Representative Paul Washington, Oklahoma City, has introduced three measures in the House dealing with prostitution and venereal disease. These measures are House Bills Nos. 37, 38 and 39, and have been reported out of the Committee with the recommendation ''Do Pass.''

In the Senate, Senator Ferman Phillips, Atoka, has introduced a measure to establish a county claims board for the purpose of considering medical and hospital expenses and making an appropriation of $500,000.00 for the payment of such claims .

Senator Robert Burns, Oklahoma City, is the author of a bill to recognize Naturopathy as a healing art and creating a Board of Examiners. This measure was introduced in the House at the last session, but failed to receive Committee approval.

Medical School Appropriations

The Medical School for the first time in many years appears to be in a position to receive an appropriation commensurate with its needs. Governor Kerr and the Chairmen of the Appropriations Committees in both the House and Senate, Representative Creekmore Wallace, Oklahoma City, and Senator Charles B. Duffy, Ponca City, have expressed a favorable attitude.

Public Policy Committees of the county societies will be kept advised of the progress of legislation in the field of health in order that the profession may be at all times advised.

Chickasha Physicians Honored

Three Chickasha physicians have recently been notified of their election to the College of Surgeons or the College of Physicians. Dr. H. M. McClure has been elected a fellow in the American College of Surgeons, Dr. W. Turner Bynum a fellow in the American College of Physicians, and Lieutenant T. Frank Joyce has been granted associate membership in the American College of Physicians. All are members of the staff of the Chickasha hospital, however, Lieutenant Joyce is presently attached to the medical corps of the army air force.

WHEN YOU SEND THEM

send

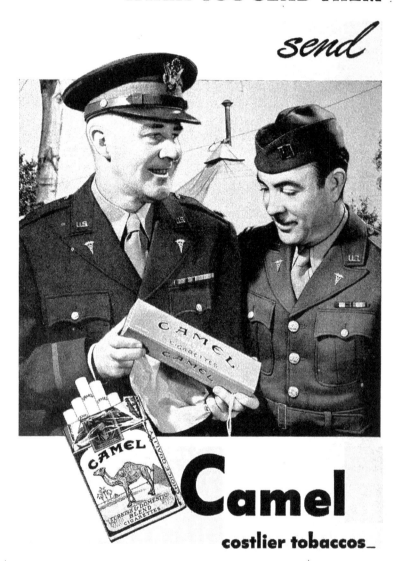

Camel
costlier tobaccos_

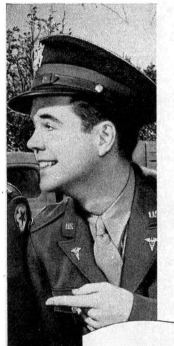

CHANGES IN 1942 REVENUE ACT

Oklahoma physicians should immediately consider the new provisions of the 1942 Revenue Act, as it pertains to their March 15 returns. The highlights of the Act, herewith presented, are only a part of the Act that might effect their returns.

It is suggested that, should a physician desire additional information, he consult an accountant or members of the staff of the Office of the Collector of Internal Revenue.

Normal Tax On Individuals:

Previously was four per cent. Has now been increased to six per cent on net income less personal exemption, credit for dependents, exempt United States interest and earned income credit.

Surtax On Individuals:

Based on surtax net income (which is net income less personal exemption and credit for dependents) the surtax is drastically increased in every bracket, starting with 13 per cent surtax net income not over $2,000 and ranging upward from that figure.

Personal Exemption and Credit for Dependents:

Personal exemptions are reduced to $1,200 for a married person or the head of a family, and $500 for a single person. The credit for dependents is reduced from $400 to $350.

Gross Income:

Excluded from gross income are amounts received as a pension, annuity, or similar allowance for personal injuries or sickness resulting from active service in the armed forces of any country.

Excluded from the landlord's gross income is the value of improvements made by the tenant, except when these improvements represent rentals.

Detailed rules are provided for allocating estate and trust income.

Deductions:

Non-Business—Amendments allow a deduction of ordinary or necessary expenses paid or incurred for the production or collection of income or for the management, conservation or maintenance of property held for the production of income (i.e., bank or agent serving to buy, sell, invest and collect income) whether or not such expenses are paid or incurred in carrying on a trade or business, and also allows a deduction for exhaustion, wear and tear of property held by the taxpayer for the production of income, whether or not the property in question is used in the trade or business of the taxpayer, including a reasonable allowance for obsolescence. The new provisions are effective for all tax years beginning after December 31, 1938.

Medical and Dental Expenses—A new provision allows a deduction for expenses paid during the taxable year for medical, dental, etc., expenses (*including accident and health insurance, and hospitalization insurance*) which *are in excess of five per cent of the individual's net income*. In the case of husband and wife, the expenses are not deductible unless they exceed five per cent of the aggregate net income of both. The maximum allowable deduction on a joint return or the return of a head of a family is $2,500, and in the case of all other individuals the limit is $1,250. (The term "medical care" is broadly defined to include amounts paid for the diagnosis, cure, mitigation, treatment, or prevention of diseases or for the purpose of affecting any structure or function of the body, including amounts paid for accident or health insurance.) Where a husband and wife both have income, and one of them incurs excessive medical expenses, it is advisable for them to file separate returns.

Interest on Indebtedness Incurred to Carry Life Insurance—Deduction is denied for any amount, whether in the form of interest or any other form, which is paid or accrued on an indebtedness incurred or continued to purchase a single premium life insurance or endowment contract. If substantially all the premiums on a life insurance or endowment contract are paid within a period of four years from the date of purchase of the contract, it is regarded as a single premium contract.

Bad Debt Deduction—Deduction for bad debts has been changed as follows: (1) Retroactive and applicable to all taxable years beginning after December 31, 1938, a bad debt is now deductible only in the year it actually became worthless; (2) The extension from three to seven years is provided for the period in which claims for refund on debts which became entirely worthless in the tax year may be made, and this amendment is retroactive to overpayments for the taxable years beginning after December 31, 1938. (NOTE: Professional services rendered for which cash compensation is not received, or services rendered for which no income was previously reported, do NOT constitute bad debts for the doctor, in filing his returns.)

Miscellaneous Provisions:

Among the miscellaneous new provisions is one which stipulates that individual returns do not have to be sworn to before a notary public, as the taxpayer will be liable for the penalties for perjury if he willfully signs a return which he knows to be false in any material respect; one that the basis of property acquired by gift shall be the same whether the gift is a direct gift or one in trust; and one that returns filed before the due date for the purpose of the limitation period on refunds and credits.

MEDICAL ADVISORY COMMITTEE REPORT*

C. R. ROUNTREE, M.D.**

OKLAHOMA CITY, OKLAHOMA

Since its organization fourteen months ago, 1,647 cases have been submitted to the Medical Advisory Committee for review as to the physical or mental incapacity of the patient. Of these, 1,263 were new cases, and 384 were receiving assistance but were presented to the committee by the Department of Public Welfare for further consideration. In 1,159 cases, the committee found that the medical report of the local physician was adequate and the findings regarding the degree of incapacity were sound. Eight hundred and fifty-four of these cases were eligible for assistance, and 305 applications were recommended for denial or cancellation on the basis of the doctor's findings.

The committee was of the opinion, in 240 cases, that further consideration should be given by the Department as to eligibility for assistance. The County had planned to give assistance to 232 of these cases, and eight cases were considered ineligible.

Forty-nine cases were sumbitted prior to County action. Of these 49 cases, the committee considered that three showed physical incapacity and that 46 were not sufficiently incapacitated to warrant an award of assistance.

Thirty-six cases were closed during this period for reasons other than listed above; such as, death, moved out of State, etc.

At present, 163 cases are pending consideration by the Medical Advisory Committee.

In reviewing these cases, the committee has recognized that rehabilitation is a major objective which should be given consideration by both the Department of Public Welfare and the committee. We have, therefore, submitted to the Department suggestions which, if followed, will be helpful in rehabilitating selected patients to such an extent that they may become wholly or partially self-supporting.

A study of 206 cases, in which it appeared that rehabilitation of the patient might be possible, has been made. The type of rehabilitation recommended falls in the following groups:

---

*Read before the Third Annual Secretaries Conference of the Oklahoma State Medical Association, October 25, 1942, Oklahoma City.
**Chairman of Medical Advisory Committee to the Public Welfare Department.

Treatment	66
Operation	58
Institutionalization	29
Dental care	7
Service	2
Vocational Rehabilitation	21

Those cases in which more than one recommendation

Operation and treatment	9
Service and dental care	1
Vocational Rehabilitation and operation	1
Treatment and dental care	5
Operation and dental care	2
Institutionalization and dental care	1
Vocational Rehabilitation and treatment	1
Vocational Rehabilitation and dental care	1
Treatment and service	2

The Department has contacted these patients explaining the recommendations made by the committee, and is working with the patient in making plans for following the recommendations. The Department has a record of contacts to 158 of these patients, 140 have indicated their willingness to accept treatment, and 18 were unwilling to accept treatment or had been advised by other doctors not to accept treatment. Of the 140 willing to accept treatment, plans for recommended treatment were initiated by the Department of Public Welfare for approximately 80 percent in less than three months after the recommendation was made, and in approximately five percent of the cases more time was needed to perfect a plan of treatment. No report is yet available for those cases in which recommendations have been made in recent months. Of the 18 unwilling to accept the recommendation of the committee, 14 were afraid for the present to follow the treatment suggested and four were advised against operation by their own physician.

The following classification shows the status of treatment for the 140 patients indicating their willingness to accept treatment and for which reports are available:

Patients following recommendation

Treatment completed	10
Receiving treatment	45
Awaiting treatment	41
Institutionalized	8
Awaiting bed in institution	6
Receiving Vocational Rehabilitation	3
Application made for Vocational Rehabilitation	9

Patients not following recommendation

Moved out of State	5
Obtained employment	3
Made other plans for self	4
Transportation to hospital not available	2
Rejected by Vocational Rehabilitation	1
Admission to Tuberculosis Hospital refused because of age (50)	1
Hospital refused to operate because of age (63)	1
Physically unable to report for treatment	1

Almost one-half of these cases indicating willingness to accept suggested treatment are awaiting treatment because of insufficient facilities.

The Department, at the present time, is able to meet only 60 percent of the basic needs of food, clothing and shelter for aid to dependent children clients. No medical fees can be included in the grants, and depending on free service is not only unsatisfactory but is also an imposition on the medical profession.

The committee will continue to study this problem and attempt to find a satisfactory solution wherein the physician and hospital will receive an adequate stipend for their services.

In July of 1942, the Public Welfare Commission authorized the Department of Public Welfare to pay stipulated fees to physicians making physical or mental examinations for persons applying for aid to dependent children. The schedule of fees recommended by the Medical Advisory Committee and approved by the Commission is $3.00 for an initial examination and $2.00 for a re-examination by the same physician. The first examination made by a physician is always considered an initial examination. The fee for an examination made on a re-application is the same as an initial examination even though made by the same physician. Laboratory fees will be paid only when they have been specifically requested by the Medical Advisory Committee. The amount to be allowed for laboratory work will be specified at the time the request for the work is made on the same basis (insofar as possible) as fees paid the United States Veterans' Bureau. In no instance will a fee be paid for a physical or mental examination unless the examination has been authorized by the County Welfare Department. The patient has the privilege of designating the physician whom he desires to make the examination. The County Department will see that the physician receives the proper form authorizing the examination.

Should there be a question concerning the degree of incapacity as shown by this examination, the Medical Advisory Committee will request the County Department to send the patient to a designated physician for another examination. The schedule of fees paid to the physician designated by the Medical Advisory Committee will be on the same basis as above.

These fees apply only to office examinations. Should a home examination be necessary, the amount of the fee will be determined by previous agreement between the County Director and the physician, before the examination is made.

The committee has spent considerable time in studying and revising the physical examination form in use at the present time. We believe each question must be answered and each item filled out completely before the examination is acceptable and can be put in line for payment of the stipulated fee. We earnestly solicit the cooperation of every examining physician in this regard. Thus far, about 75 claims for examination fees have been filed with the Department of Public Welfare. A little over one-half of these have been paid, and the others will be paid as soon as possible. The committee regrets that the law requiring all claims to be notarized or sworn to before a public official before the State Auditor can pay them is inflexible. This matter was thoroughly discussed with the State Auditor and the Attorney General's office, and we find no way to get around it. While this may seem to work a hardship on those physicians away from county-seat towns, please remember that the representative of the Public Welfare Department in your district is more than glad to assist in any way possible.

In conclusion, let me say the committee feels some progress has been made, some policies have been established and some good has been accomplished. The Aid to Dependent Children rolls seem to be decreasing. From 12 to 15 percent fewer applicants are being certified now than before the committee was appointed. We all realize that there is much that remains to be done. What we have accomplished is due, in a large part, to the splendid spirit and cooperation of the physicians who make up the Oklahoma State Medical Association, its officers, and the officers of the various County Societies.

The immediate future of this committee hangs in the balance. Gasoline rationing and transportation difficulties make it almost impossible for us to hold monthly meetings much longer. We realize, however, that the war effort comes first above all else, and with this in mind we shall mold our program accordingly.

Captain W. W. Rucks, Jr., To Washington

Word has been received that Captain Bill Rucks, Oklahoma City, who is attached to the 53rd Evacuation Hospital Unit, has been ordered to Washington, D. C., for a two-months course in tropical medicine. Captain Rucks will return to his Unit upon completion of the course.

PHYSICIANS PART IN STUDENT NURSES RECRUITMENT

To care for the sick in the Army and in the Civilian population, we must have more nurses. From May 31, 1942, to January 1, 1943, the National quota was 55,000. This is an increase of 20,000 over the pre-war period. Next year we must have 65,000.

The goal for Oklahoma, this school year, is 468. We have admitted 420 students or 90 per cent of our goal. With the classes starting in February, we hope to admit the other forty-eight.

In the Nation we have only filled 68 per cent of our quota. This means 19,000 girls must enter schools of nursing before June. Can't we help in this National Emergency?

The family doctor can direct girls into nursing. The mother often needs more information and assurance than the girl. The British Nurses slogan, "Nursing, War Work With A Future," should appeal to the mother who is thinking of her daughter's future. Federal Aid, which pays all expenses except spending money, may appeal to some. This is limited to hospitals of one hundred beds. Write to Student Nurses, P. O. Box 88, New York City, for a list of schools having this aid.

Girls, who want a college degree, may get it in nursing. This requires four or five years, but is often a good plan for the girl of seventeen who wants both college and nursing, and has the money for it.

Schools of Nursing takes girls between eighteen and thirty-five. Some schools will take a married girl if her husband is in the Army, and some permit the student to live at home while taking her training. If a woman has had college work, she may get credit for it in her nurses school. Usually nine months credit is given for a degree and six months for two years work. Write Student Nurse, P. O. Box 88, New York City, for any information.

Nurses are needed now and will be needed all over the world after peace. Nursing is a satisfying profession and one that has a place for the girl who likes to do bedside care, the one who likes to teach or the one who likes to be an administrator. The fact that it is a woman's profession opens up opportunities for leadership not found in many professions, and the service to others, one is able to do every day makes it a satisfactory one.

Nurses now may find employment in the hospital, the Doctor's office, industry, public health, or schools. Civil Service has interesting work in its Indian Hospitals and Veterans hospitals. The United States Public Health Service employs nurses for both hospital and public health work.

The Army and Navy need 40,000 new nurses this year. Eleven nurses have been sent recently to South and Central America to stimulate and assist in the organization of public health nursing, where requests for these services are made by the Government. Here at home every county needs nurses in hospitals, office, industry, and public health. It is really an interesting profession with varied opportunities for service.

WARNING

The following communication has been received from the local United States Secret Service office of the Treasury Department and is submitted for your information.

Precautions Payees of Government Checks Should Observe—for removing causes for delayed payments from improper addresses and from forgery:

1. If your name and address are not fully and correctly recorded with the agency issuing your checks, notify them at once of your full and correct name and address. All change in your mailing address should be immediately reported, in writing, to both the agency issuing your checks and to your postmaster.

2. Have your name upon your mail box. Arrange for the closest watch possible to be kept over your mail box. If possible, work out some system with your mail carriers so that you will know when he delivers your checks. Remove your checks from your mail box at once.

3. Safeguard your checks very carefully after receipt. If possible, cash your checks on the day received. Endorse your checks only at the time you cash them. If you need assistance, trust only dependable persons to aid you.

Precautions Persons Cashing Government Checks Should Observe—for preventing financial losses from forgery of endorsement and fraudulent negotiation:

1. *Know your endorsers. Beware of strangers. Require identification.* Before cashing a Government check, ask yourself this questions: "*If this check is returned, can I find the person who gave it to me?*"

2. Do not honor any card or paper for identification for check cashing purposes unless the same may be rightfully possessed and will establish identification of the holder as the payee of the check presented. Identifications attempted through other persons should receive most careful scrutiny.

3. Require checks to be endorsed in your presence. Take all other precautions needed, as by noting upon the back of checks the presenter's address and physical description, the description of the identification offered and, an impression of the presenter's thumb-print. Place your initials upon checks when received.

Crimes Committed in Violation of the Laws for the Protection of Government Checks are Felonies Punishable by Imprisonment up to Ten Years in a Federal Penitentiary. The use of proper caution serves to prevent these crimes, while failure to use reasonable and proper caution acts as an encouragement and attaches liability from affording opportunities which assist to make the commission of these crimes possible.—John E. Osborn, Agent in Charge, U. S. Secret Service.

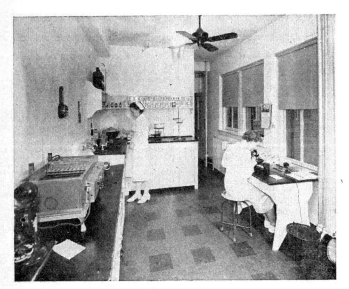

NEWS FROM THE COUNTY SOCIETIES

At a recent meeting of the Atoka-Coal County Medical Society, Dr. J. B. Clark of Coalgate was elected President; Dr. T. H. Briggs of Atoka, Vice-President, and Dr. J. S. Fulton of Atoka was re-elected Secretary-Treasurer. Dr. H. C. Huntley of Atoka and Dr. R. C. Henry of Coalgate were elected Delegates, and Doctor Briggs and Doctor Clark respective Alternates.

Election of officers for the Oklahoma County Medical Association and the Oklahoma City Clinical Society was the order of business at the December 15, 1942, meeting of the Oklahoma County Medical Association at the Oklahoma Club. One hundred members were in attendance.
The following will serve the County Association during the coming year: President, Dr. Walker Morledge; Vice-President, Dr. W. E. Eastland, and Secretary-Treasurer, Dr. Elmer R. Musick. The Board of Directors of the Association is composed of the following: Doctor Eastland, Dr. W. F. Keller, Dr. F. M. Lingenfelter, Doctor Morledge, Doctor Musick, Dr. C. R. Rountree, Dr. Gregory E. Stanbro, Dr. W. K. West and Dr. Oscar R. White. Dr. Carroll M. Pounders, Dr. L. J. Starry and Dr. Lea A. Riely comprise the Board of Censors.
Inauguration of 1943 officers was held at a Dinner-Dance, January 23, given at the Biltmore Hotel.

"Newer Treatment of Compound Fractures and Fractures of the Neck of the Femur" was the topic discussed by Dr. Earl McBride of Oklahoma City at a joint meeting of the Okfuskee and Okmulgee County Medical Societies at Henryetta on December 14.
Following the program, the Societies met separately and elected officers for 1943.

Dr. H. B. Jenkins of Tryon was recently elected President of the Lincoln County Medical Society to serve during 1943. Those elected to serve with him are Dr. E. F. Hurlbut, Meeker, Vice-President, and Dr. Carl H. Bailey, Stroud, Secretary-Treasurer. Dr. U. E. Nickell of Davenport was elected Delegate and Dr. Ned Burleson of Prague, Alternate. The Scientific Program Committee is composed of Dr. Jno. S. Rollins, Prague, and Doctor Burleson.

Nine members of the Garvin County Medical Society met at the Chamber of Commerce in Pauls Valley at 7:30 P.M., Wednesday, December 16, 1942. The paying of 1943 dues and election of officers for the ensuing year was the order of business.
Those elected to serve were President, Dr. T. F. Gross, Lindsay; Vice-President, Dr. A. H. Shi, Stratford, and Dr. John R. Callaway, Pauls Valley, was re-elected Secretary-Treasurer. Dr. Galvin L. Johnson, Pauls Valley, will serve as Delegate and Dr. Morton E. Robberson, Wynnewood, Alternate.
The next meeting of the Society is scheduled for January 20 at the Chamber of Commerce.

Dr. Paul B. Champlin of Enid was elected President of the Garfield County Medical Society to serve for the coming year at a recent meeting of the Society. Dr. Bruce R. Hinson was elected Vice-President, and Dr. John R. Walker was re-elected Secretary-Treasurer. Delegates are Dr. V. R. Hamble, Enid, and Dr. D. S. Harris, Drummond.
The Board of Censors of the Society is composed of Doctors George S. Wilson, V. R. Hamble and D. D. Roberts, all of Enid. President Champlin has assumed the responsibility of securing scientific programs.

Members of the medical staff of the United States Southwest Reformatory at El Reno were hosts to the members of the Canadian County Medical Society and guests at a tour of inspection of the reformatory including the hospital and clinic on December 16, 1942. Dinner was served following the tour at 6:30 P.M.
Dr. Eugene A. Gillis of the State Health Department presented the sound film "Syphilis" following the dinner.
Guests of the medical staff of the reformatory, in addition to the physicians from Canadian County, included physicians from Oklahoma City, Chickasha, Minco, Fort Reno and Concho.

Dr. H. R. Haas of Sapulpa has been elected President of the Creek County Medical Society to serve during the coming year. To serve with him, Dr. J. E. Hollis of Bristow was elected Vice-President, and Dr. C. G. Oakes of Sapulpa has assumed the duties of Secretary-Treasurer.
Delegates to the Annual Meeting are Dr. C. R. McDonald of Mannford and Dr. J. B. Lampton of Sapulpa, and Alternates are Dr. Frank Sisler and Dr. O. C. Coppedge, both of Bristow.

Dr. P. M. McNeil of Oklahoma City was guest speaker at the Tri-County (Grady-Caddo-Stephens) Medical Society meeting in Chickasha, Thursday, December 17, 1942, when 35 members were in attendance. "The Treatment of Pneumonia" and "Present Concepts in Treatment of Migraine" were the subjects discussed by Doctor McNeil. "Two Cases for Diagnosis" was discussed by Dr. Turner Bynum of Chickasha.
The papers and cases were discussed by staff members of the Borden General Hospital.
Following the above program, the three Societies met separately and elected 1943 officers for their respective County Societies.
The next meeting of the Society will be January 14 in Chickasha, and Dr. Robert H. Akin and Dr. O. Alton Watson, both of Oklahoma City, will be guest speakers. Special guests will be the medical staff of the Borden General Hospital.

At a recent meeting of the McCurtain County Medical Society, Dr. A. W. Clarkson of Valliant was elected

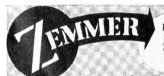

President; Dr. W. H. McBrayer, Haworth, Vice-President, and Dr. N. L. Barker, Broken Bow, Secretary-Treasurer. Dr. R. D. Williams, Idabel, and Dr. J. T. Moreland, also of Idabel, were elected Delegate and Alternate. The Scientific Program Committee is composed of Doctors Clarkson and Barker.

Fifteen members of the Osage County Medical Society met at the Duncan hotel in Pawhuska Wednesday, January 6, at which time Dr. L. W. Hunt presented the tenth lecture of the postgraduate course in Internal Medicine. Following Dr. Hunt's lecture, a sound and motion-picture film in technicolor, "Peptic Ulcer," was presented and discussed.

The following officers were elected to lead the Society during the coming year: President, Dr. C. R. Weirich, Pawhuska; Vice-President, Dr. B. F. Sullivan, Barnsdall, and Secretary-Treasurer, Dr. George K. Hemphill, Pawhuska. The Delegate and Alternate to the State Meeting are Dr. G. I. Walker, Hominy, and Dr. Roscoe Walker, Pawhuska. The Board of Censors is composed of Dr. B. E. Dozier of Shidler, Dr. G. I. Walker and Dr. Roscoe Walker. The officers of the Society serve as the Scientific Program Committee.

Dr. Nelse F. Ockerblad of Kansas City, Mo., will discuss "Urology for the General Practitioner" at a joint meeting of the Washington-Nowata, Kay, Pawnee and Osage County Medical Societies in Pawhuska on February 8.

Dr. L. A. Mitchell of Stillwater was elected President of the Payne County Medical Society at a recent meeting. Dr. P. M. Richarson of Cushing will serve as Vice-President, and Dr. C. W. Moore, also of Stillwater, was re-elected Secretary-Treasurer. Dr. John W. Martin of Cushing will serve as Delegate to the State Meeting. The Board of Censors of the Society is composed of Dr. R. E. Waggoner, Stillwater, Dr. R. E. Leatherock, Cushing, and Dr. F. Keith Oehlschlager, Yale.

Election of officers for 1943 was the order of business for the Cherokee County Medical Society at the meeting of the Society at the Hastings Hospital in Tahlequah on Friday, January 8. Six members were present at the meeting. The following officers were elected: Dr. P. H. Medcaris, President; Dr. J. S. Allison, Vice-President, and Dr. James K. Gray, Secretary-Treasurer.

The subject of discussion for the evening pertained to the present medical problems of Cherokee County .

Dr. James L. Wood of Eufaula will serve as President of the McIntosh County Medical Society during 1943. Dr. F. R. First, Eufaula, was elected Vice-President, and Dr. William A. Tolleson, Eufaula, was re-elected Secretary-Treasurer. Doctor Tolleson will represent the Society as Delegate to the State Meeting and Dr. D. E. Little, Eufaula, will serve as Alternate. The Scientific Program Committee is composed of the officers of the Society.

"Injection Treatment of Hemorrhoids" was the subject selected for presentation by Dr. W. C. Vernon of Okmulgee at the joint meeting of the Okfuskee and Okmulgee County Medical Societies at the meeting in Henryetta on January 11. Twenty members were in attendance.

The establishment of a blood bank was discussed at the business meeting following the program.

Twenty-one were present at the dinner and regular meeting of the Jackson County Medical Society on January 11 at Altus. The following were elected officers to serve during 1943: Dr. E. S. Crow, Olustee, President; Dr. R. Z. Taylor, Blair, Vice-President, and Dr. Earl W. Mabry, Altus, Secretary-Treasurer. Delegate and Alternate are Doctor Crow and Dr. John R. Reid, Altus, respectively. The Board of Censors are Dr. C. G. Spears and Dr. L. H. McConnell, both of Altus, and Dr. Thomas M. Berry of El Dorado. The Scientific Program Committee is composed of Captain Hartwick of the Altus Airport and Doctor Mabry.

Following the election of officers, the general discussion for the evening was led by Doctor Crow followed by Captain Hartwick of the Airport and Dr. M. E. Woolridge of Altus representing the dentists.

During the business session, the medical officers from the Airport were elected Honorary members of the Society and will meet with them throughout the year. Regular monthly meetings will be held in Altus the last Monday of each month and special call meetings will be scheduled at the Altus Air Field.

The next meeting of the Society will be February 22 in the Gosselin Building. The speaker for the evening will be one of the members of the medical staff from the Air Field.

Dr. E. A. Abernethy, one of the members of the Jackson County Medical Society, was injured in a car accident on December 17 and is still confined to his home.

Dr. W. M. Kinney of Joplin, Mo., was guest speaker at the meeting of the Ottawa County Medical Society on December 17, 1942, at which time he discussed "Common Sense in Treating Heart Disease."

Eighteen members of the Society attended the turkey dinner given by the Miami Baptist Hospital preceding the program.

Fifty guests and members of the Washington-Nowata County Medical Society were present to attend the annual inaugural banquet of the officers of the Society in the home of Mrs. Forerst S. Etter on Wednesday, January 13, at 7:30 P.M., in Bartlesville.

The Tri-County Society (Washington-Nowata, Osage and Kay) will meet in Pawhuska on February 8, in Ponca City in March and at Bartlesville in April.

The regular meeting of the Garvin County Medical Society, scheduled for January 20, was postponed inasmuch as the physicians of the County are presently attending a postgraduate course given as a 10-week lecture course by Dr. L. W. Hunt.

Ten members and several guests attended the meeting of the Kay County Medical Society held in Blackwell on January 21.

The regular program included discussions by Dr. A. S. Nuckols of Ponca City, Dr. T. F. Renfro of Blilings and Dr. I. D. Walker of Tonkawa on ambulant treatment in hypertension. A moving picture on Vitamin B2 was presented by a representative of Eli Lilly and Company.

Dr. Joseph Kinnamon, Blackwell, Director of the Kay County Health Unit, was a guest, and the following committee of the Society were appointed to meet with him from time to time: Dr. A. S. Risser, Chairman, Dr. C. W. Arrendell, Dr. I. D. Walker and Dr. G. H. Yeary.

WOMEN'S AUXILIARY NEWS

Mrs. Luther H. Kice, Chairman of the Legislative Committee of the National Auxiliary to the American Medical Association, recommends that the Woman's Auxiliaries carefully consider pending and proposed legislation on health, both state and federal, and that we make ourselves and our Auxiliaries part of the great American law-making system by having an understanding of what that system is, and by taking an intelligent part in its formation.

At the State Convention, held in Tulsa in April, 1942, the Women's Auxiliary to the Oklahoma State Medical Association approved a recommendation that the Auxiliary go on record as favoring legislation concerning compulsory immunization for smallpox and diphtheria for all school children. The Auxiliary was invited to have a representative at the Oklahoma Congress of Parents and Teachers Association, which was held on Tuesday, January 19, 1943, at the Skirvin Hotel in Oklahoma City, inasmuch as legislation for immunization was being studied by that group. The American Association of University Women approved this measure at their 1942 State Convention, and it has long been a project of the Parent-Teachers groups.

Mrs. Maxey Cooper, President-elect, Mrs. George Garrison, Legislation Chairman, and Mrs. S. J. Bradfield, Public Relations Chairman, represented the State Auxiliary at this Congress. If our Advisory Council approves the legislation, our State Legislation Chairman will notify all County Presidents, so that the proposed bill may be studied thoroughly by each County group.

The National Public Relations Chairman, Mrs. Frank P. Dwyer, in suggesting points for procedure in public relations, mentions as one point "Interest in Pan American Medical Unity." Inasmuch as this can contribute vitally to our post-war world unity, each organization should keep this subject in mind in preparing programs for next year.

Our State Tray Chairman, Mrs. F. Redding Hood, and her children are now in New Orleans with Dr. Hood, who is in service there.

Mrs. Maxey Cooper, the State Hygeia Chariman, has been very active, and has sent material out to all of the County Hyeia Chairmen.

Mrs. S. J. Bradfield, State Public Relations Chairman, has requested mid-year reports and plans for the balance of the year from the various Public Relations Chairmen. Tulsa County's Mid-year Report follows:

Philanthropic Committee: Thirty-five toys for Christmas toy shower to children in Tulsa Hospitals. Thirty dollars contribution to Library Fund of Tulsa County Medical Society.

Hygeia Committee: Sixty-one six-month's subscriptions donated by the Auxiliary to the Public Schools. Twelve one-year subscriptions secured.

Legislative Committee: Cooperating with State P.T.A. on a program of compulsory immunization.

War Aid Committee: Of 126 members, a survey conducted by the Red Cross showed the following: Twenty-three are registered nurses, of which four are teaching Home Nursing. One interviews personnel for Nurses' Aide Course, with two members enrolled in this course. One teaches Home Nursing and one teaches Child Care to the Girl Scouts. Mrs. Bradfield is chairman and Mrs. Ruprecht a member of a board of five appointed by the Mayor to investigate and approve boarding homes for children. Mrs. Russell and Mrs. Mishler are volunteer investigators for this board, and all are working through the Office of Civilian Defense. Mrs. I. H. Nelson heads Nutrition for the Red Cross.

Mrs. Ruprecht is a First Aid Instructor, and Mrs. Spottswood was a chairman at the Office of Civilian Defense.

Dr. Mabel Hart is City School Physician, and is extremely active in health activities of the city .

Two members are in canteen work, 26 are registered in OCD work, 19 have completed first-aid courses, five have completed staff assistant courses, 13 have completed Home Nursing courses, 13 have completed Nutrition, 11 members knit, 21 sew, and 15 prepare surgical dressings. Many members have been active in volunteering services in sugar rationing, telephone squads, etc.

Program and Health Education Committee: Camp Gruber Day Room Project: A total of $71.00 in cash and a considerable amount of furniture were contributed, resulting in the complete furnishing of two day rooms, including curtains and two pianos.

Public Relations Committee: This committee, with Mrs. S. J. Bradfield as chairman, has established a shelf of medical pamphlets at the County Courthouse for the purpose of obtaining a wider distribution of authentic medical material. These pamphlets, recommended by the State Health Department, relate to communicable diseases, nutrition, posture, tuberculosis, syphilis, child care, immunization, cancer, etc. In five weeks time, it has been necessary to replace these pamphlets four times, which indicates that this information is supplying a large demand from the general public for health education. A file of copies of these leaflets is in the Executive Office of the Tulsa County Medical Society.

Tulsa County

The Tulsa County Auxiliary is presenting its Annual Health Forum on Tuesday, February 2, 1943, at 1:30 P.M., in the Club-room of the Y.W.C.A.

The speakers for this forum and their subjects are as follows:

Mrs. Rebecca Nelson, Coordinator of Family Life Education in Tulsa Schools, "Our Concern Every Child."

Mr. Verser Hicks, Chairman Health Division of Tulsa Council of Social Agencies, "Community Cooperation in a Local Health Program."

Mrs. Rodney Nowakowski, Physical Director of Tulsa Y.W.C.A., "A War Time Program for Physical Fitness."

Mrs. I. H. Nelson, Director of Red Cross Nutrition, "Nutrition Today."

Dr. Mabel Hart, Legislation Chairman of Tulsa County Medical Auxiliary, "Immunization Facts."

Miss Velma Neely, R.N., Secretary of the Tulsa Public Health Association, "Tuberculosis and Your Community."

The Parent-Teachers Associations are cooperating as they did last year in inviting their members and their Health Chairmen to attend this forum. Mrs. W. A. Walker, of the Medical Auxiliary, and Mrs. Lawson Wood, P.T.A. Council Chairman, will handle the registration.

In appreciation of their kindnesses during 1942, the Tulsa County Medical Society at the meeting of December 14 unanimously approved a resolution of thanks to the Auxiliary.

The Auxiliary to the Tulsa County Medical Society entertained its members with a guest tea and book review on January 5, 1943, in the home of Mrs. Frank L. Flack. Mrs. James L. Stevenson reviewed "A Time to be Born" by Dawn Powell. The members of the Social Committee acted as hostesses for this tea in serving about 80 members and guests.

News From The State Health Department

TRACHOMA CONTROL REPORT

Trachoma is an endemic, communicable disease in certain sections of our State, and is second to none in the cause of blindness, being responsible for twenty-five per cent of the Blind Pensions in Oklahoma, and costing the tax payers of the State approximately $120,000 per year.

The fact that trachoma is a communicable disease made it the responsibility of the health department to take steps to attempt to reduce the prevalence. A plan was evolved to provide the necessary funds and personnel to carry on the work. The funds were made available and the personnel employed, which consisted of a consulting ophthalmologist, a clinical director, a public health nurse, a clerk, and a medical social worker. Since trachoma is confined largely to the low-income groups and in most instances to those of poor hygienic surroundings, the work has been confined to those counties of the State where the above conditions prevail to a greater extent than in other sections.

The work was begun on July 30, 1941, and carried forward until sixteen counties in the eastern and southern part of the State had been included. From July 30, 1941, to December 31, 1942, ninety-one clinics were held. 8,591 patients were examined, and 1,262 positive cases were found which were given treatment. Treatment consisted of Sulfanilamide, 1/5 grain per pound of body weight, each twenty-four hours for ten days; also, saturated solution of Sulfanilamide dropped in the eyes from four to six times daily; or, finely-powdered Sulfanilamide in the lower cul-de-sac twice daily.

An effort was made to be very conservative. In the evaluation of results, therefore, all patients were classified into five groups: (1) those showing no improvement, (2) slight improvement, (3) moderate improvement, (4) marked improvement, and (5) arrested or apparently cured. Caution was used with the term "cured."

According to the above classification, in the 1,262 positive cases, there were 72 cases showing no improvement, 60 cases showing slight improvement, 285 cases showing moderate improvement, 420 cases showing marked improvement, and 81 cases arrested or apparently cured.

Two hundred and eighty cases did not return for a second check-up; in 15 cases, no treatment was recommended; three cases were referred to the Indian Bureau; and 46 cases were admitted at final clinics during December and have not had an opportunity to return.

A great number of other eye diseases were found, and the patient advised the proper procedure for his individual care; advising him to consult physicians in his locality specially prepared for such work. In this program, only trachoma and its sequelae were treated.

Surgery was offered to all patients suffering from entropion, or trichiasis, when they were not able to pay for this service. Eighty operations were performed, with very satisfactory results. A large number of refractive errors were referred for correction.

From this limited experience, it is evident that there are great possibilities in this particular field; and with the entire medical profession lending full cooperation in controlling this insidious disease, there is no reason why it should not become as rare as diphtheria or typhoid fever.

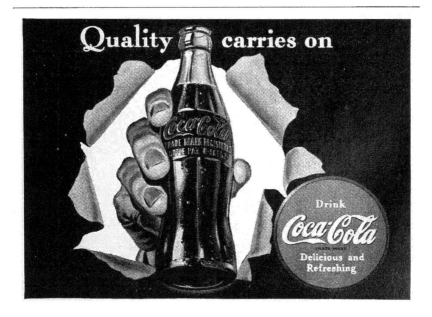

Blue Cross Reports

The Oklahoma Blue Cross Plan was host to a regional meeting of Blue Cross Plans of the Southwestern States, held in Tulsa, January 15th and 16th. N. D. Helland, Executive Director, expressed appreciation that Oklahoma had been selected for the first of a series of meetings to be held by our neighboring approved plans. Directors and representatives of ten plans from nine states were in attendance.

A principal reason for this meeting was a request for opinions from a national committee, regarding a proposed national surgical plan to supplement non-profit hospital service. The plan would, if put into operation, provide surgical benefits on a cash indemnity basis and would be designed to also serve in firms operating nationally.

Many Directors supported the idea, because they felt that service organizations guaranteed by the medical profession, would take too long to get in operation to be of any material aid in forestalling social federal regulation. The belief that prompt action is necessary was general among those attending the conference. Due to the fact that details have as yet, not been incorporated in the proposal, it was impossible to come to a definite conclusion, but the plan was approved in principle by the majority of those in attendance.

Mr. Morris J. Norby, Research Director of the Hospital Service Plan Commission and Ray J. McCarthy, Executive Director of Group Hospital Service of St. Louis, were principal speakers at a special dinner, at which time the proposed surgical plan was discussed at length. Special guests for the occasion were members of the medical profession. Trustees of Group Hospital Service in Oklahoma and Civic and Industrial leaders. All of the guests took part in the open forum conducted on the subject.

Mr. Helland deserved and received many expressions of appreciation for the splendid program that he had arranged for the two-day meeting. Contrary to customary procedure, the executive for the plan, for the greater part of the meetings, took a back seat and listened to the representatives conduct meetings and bring up for discussion various subjects on which they wanted information. Pertinent subjects such as ''reciprocity between plans'' and ''need for uniformity'' were given particular study. ,Individual expressions for those in attendance gave the Oklahoma Plan and Mr. Helland in particular, credit for arranging the most informative meeting that they had been privileged to attend. The time for the next meeting of this nature has not been determined, but it will be held in Dallas the latter part of this year.

Blue Cross Plans participating in the meeting were: ''Associated Hospital Service, Inc.'' Sioux City, Iowa, ''Associated Hospial Service in Nebraska,'' ''Colorado Hospital Service Association,'' ''Group Hospital Service in Kansas City, Missouri,'' ''Group Hospital Service in St. Louis, Missouri,'' ''Group Hospital Service in Texas,'' ''Hospital Service Association of Louisiana,'' ''Hospital Service Incorporated of Iowa,'' ''Kansas Hospital Association, Inc.,'' and ''Group Hospital Service of Oklahoma.''

Lieutenant Johnny A. Blue, formerly of Guymon, reports that he has recently been transferred from the National Naval Medical Center, Bethesda, Md., to the Bainbridge Naval Training Station, Bainbridge, Md.

Dr. Jack F. Parsons is now a Lieutenant in the Air Corps and is presently stationed at Station Hospital, Brooks Field, San Antonio, Texas. Prior to entering the service, Lieutenant Parsons practiced at Cherokee.

• OBITUARIES •

Dr. John C. Duncan
1871-1942

Dr. John Calvin Duncan, 71, pioneer Oklahoma physician, passed away November 25, 1942, at the Shattuck Hospital following a brief illness.

Doctor Duncan was born at Bradyville, Tenn., April 21, 1871, and in his early childhood moved with his parents to Hiawassee, Ark. He was united in marriage to Nora Ellen Bates of Gravette, Ark., December 25, 1895.

He received his pre-medic education at Pea Ridge Normal College, and in 1898 graduated from the Memphis Hospital Medical College.

Doctor Duncan first practiced in southeastern Oklahoma in Indian Territory prior to his removing to Forgan in Beaver County in 1915, where he has since continued to practice medicine. Doctor Duncan took an active part in county and state medical activities and was an Honorary Member of the Oklahoma State Medical Association.

He was a member of the Christian Church and the Masonic Lodge.

Surviving besides his wife of the home address, he leaves to mourn his passing three sons, Dr. Dean H. Duncan of Shreveport, La.; John Duncan of Lubbock, Texas, and Robert Duncan of Oklahoma City, in addition to four grandchildren and a host of friends.

Dr. W. D. Dawson
1869-1942

Dr. William D. Dawson, who was born at Reid Creek, Ark., May, 1869, passed away on October 17, 1942, in Henryetta, Okla., where he had practiced medicine for the past 24 years. In May of 1942 he had celebrated his 50 years in the practice of medicine.

Doctor Dawson practiced medicine in Arkansas for a number of years following his graduation from the Eclectic Medical College, St. Louis, Mo., after which time he removed to Mangum, Okla., where he practiced several years prior to his attending and graduation from the Baylor University College of Medicine, Dallas, Texas.

In 1918, Doctor Dawson established his residence in Henryetta where he continued in active practice until the time of his passing.

Survivors include his wife of the home address and one son, Leslie Dawson of Oklahoma City.

Dr. W. C. Sanderson
1875-1942

Dr. W. C. Sanderson, a pioneer physician of Henryetta and Okmulgee County, passed away October 15, 1942, at a local hospital following a prolonged illness.

Doctor Sanderson was born near Richmond, Mo., in 1875, and following his graduation from the University Medical College of Kansas City, Mo., in 1903, came to Henryetta where he continued the practice of medicine until the onset of his last illness.

Doctor Sanderson was interested in the progress of the town in which he lived and at one time served as mayor of Henryetta. He also served on the school board.

The weather was never too bad nor the nights too cold or bad that Doctor Sanderson did not go when called upon to render service to mankind, and his going will be sorely missed by his many friends and family.

Major Cole D. Pittman of Tulsa is now stationed with the Headquarters, First Mapping Group, Bolling Field, D. C. Prior to his transfer, Major Pittman was stationed at Chanute Field, Ill.

MEDICAL PREPAREDNESS

New Procurement and Assignment Classification For Physicians in 1943

Announcement has been received from the Directing Board of the Procurement and Assignment Service that a new survey of the medical manpower remaining in civilian life must be made.

The new survey will more closely correlate Procurement and Assignment classifications with those being given by Selective Service.

Dr. W. W. Rucks, Chairman of the Oklahoma Procurement and Assignment Committee, is making preparations for the calling of Councilor District meetings of County Chairmen for a discussion of the new survey.

Every physician is urged to give his complete cooperation to his County Chairman and the State Committee in the completing of his individual classification.

For the purpose of this nation-wide report, each physician will be classified in one of the following categories.

Class I. Available.

A. Potentially qualified for service, i.e., has not been rejected by Army.

1. Unmarried or married but not maintaining a home with wife and/or children.

2. Married and maintaining a bona fide home with wife and/or children.

a. Married with no children.

b. Married with 1 child.

c. Married with 2 children.

d. Married with 3 or more chidlren.

B. Not eligible, on account of age, physical disability, or other reason, for service with the armed forces, but considered available for civilian medical services associated with the war effort.

Class II. Essential for limited duration or until a replacement can be secured.

A. For community medical care.

B. For medical teaching or war research.

C. For hospital service.

D. For public health.

E. For industry.

Class III. Essential for unlimited duration.

A. For community medical care.

B. For medical teaching or war research.

C. For hospital service.

D. For public health.

E. For industry.

Class IV. Physicians not available for either military or emergency civilian services because of:

A. Physical disability or age.

B. Ethical and professional shortcomings.

C. Retirement or engagement in work not directly or indirectly connected with the field of medicine.

Class I.—Physicians considered available during the war for service other than in their present situations.

Class 1A.—Male physician under 45 years of age presumably physically qualified for service, with sub-classes 1 and 2 indicating the order of call in conformity with Selective Service laws and regualtions. For example, a physician, considered available, who is under 45 years of age and maintaining a home with wife and 2 children would be classified as 1A—2c.

Class 1B—Male physicians under 45 years of age who have been rejected for military duty but who are able to carry on civilian work; males over 45 who might be willing to relocate; females; and aliens.

Class II—Physicians for whom it is assumed that satisfactory substitutes may be obtained and those who may be released as a result of changes in their personal situations or in conditions affecting the institutions employing them.

Class III—Essential physicians for whom, according to present conditions, the chances are small of finding a satisfactory replacement.

Class IV—Physicians who cannot be expected to contribute to medical service.

Class IVA—Physicians with marked physical disabilities, including old age ,which make them incapable of practicing their profession.

Class IVB—Physicians who, because of unethical conduct or professional incompetence, are not acceptable for service in the community or elsewhere.

Class IVC—Physicians who are retired from activities connected with medical care and those who have been engaged in occupations unrelated to medicine for so long that their return to medical work is not feasible.

HOW SURGEON HELPED SAVE HOSPITAL

How a British surgeon helped save a hospital that had been bombed is described in The Journal of the American Medical Association for October 24 by the regular London correspondent of The Journal who reports that:

"High explosive and incendiary bombs fell on a hospital, setting it on fire. The house surgeon, Dr. Philip Baxter, wearing a dressing gown over his pajamas, climbed a fall pipe to the blazing roof. Then he used the girdle of his dressing gown as a rope to hoist up buckets of water, which were tied on by helpers below. He got the blaze under control. In leaping from the roof to a lower one he injured an ankle but went to the operating theater to attend the victims of the raid. When there a message came that an elderly woman was trapped under wreckage in another part of the town and that medical help was urgently needed. He went and had to crawl down a tunnel in the debris to administer morphine. He waited until she was extricated and sent to the hospital. He then hobbled back but was in great pain. While on his way a policeman lent his bicycle. Cycling was no less painful but was quicker. On arrival he returned to the operating theater and continued his work. Only after he had been on duty for several hours did his own injury receive attention. . . .''

BOOK REVIEWS

"The chief glory of every people arises from its authors."—Dr. Samuel Johnson.

MENTAL ILLNESS: A GUIDE FOR THE FAMILY. By Edith M. Stern with the collaboration of Samuel W. Hamilton, M.D., 1942, New York, The Commonwealth Fund. Pp. 121. Price $1.00.

This little volume is distinctly worthwhile and should find a large place on the working desks of mental hospital superintendents, administrative officers and social workers. It could also be read with great profit by physicians other than those immediately concerned with the care and treatment of mental cases, because it is a well-known fact that most mental cases are seen first by the family practitioner. It would probably fall to his lot to be in a position to recommend the use of this book by those for whom it is primarily intended much more often than the consulting psychiatrist.

The author gives convincing evidence of a close working knowledge of the problem that the mental case represents to the distressed family, and, in turn ,the problem that the family represents to the psychiatrist and institution where the patient is being cared for. She has covered in a most simple and convincing way, to any open-minded person, practically all of the questions that the psychiatrist is called upon to discuss and answer in the course of his work from day to day. Only one statement is clinically questionable. Certainly not every psychiatrist will agree "that most forms of mental illness follow such definite patterns, are so well recognized and classified, that he can diagnose them and foretell their course as accurately as your family physician can inform you about measles, tonsillitis or pneumonia." After a reasonable time it is probably true that diagnosis can be firmly establisheed, but if there is one thing that is relatively unpredictable it is the course of mental illness.

The book thoroughly meets the principal deficiency among otherwise well-informed and intelligent people as to the place that mental illness should occupy in our thinking. The old "bugaboos" as to the causes of mental illness and the embarrassment that it engenders, with a resulting attempt on the part of the family to cover up and thus deprive the patient of appropriate management, are most thoroughly aired and disposed of. Taken as a whole, it is a most commendable little volume, and should bring a lot of comfort to a lot of people who need to have it recommended to their perusal. —Ned R. Smith, M.D.

"NEURO-ANATOMY." Fred A. Mettler, Professor of Anatomy, University of Georgia School of Medicine, Augusta, Ga. Now associated with College of Physicians and Surgeons Columbia University, New York. The C. V. Mosby Company, St. Louis, Mo., 1942. Price $7.50.

This book, prepared as a test for medical students beginning in Neuro-Anatomy, is likewise an excellent reference for general practitioners and those of us interested in Neurology and its allied fields. It fulfills the student's need in covering the subject completely and at the same time leaving out the dispensable material lessening the confusion so often brought about by the inclusion of more controversial points. The organization being progressive carries the student along a logical sequence of facts about the gross aspects of the nervous system. This first section is followed by a second dealing with microscopic studies of the various structures and pathways.

The author is to be particularly commended for his

attention to the matter of terminology. When new terms are used they have been previously defined and properly identified with their B.N.A. equivalent.

The text has an excellent bibliography and to quote the author "will serve as a springboard into the more detailed knowledge and bibliography of particular topics." One has but to review the list of references briefly to realize that, based on many articles by contemporary neurologists, neuro-surgeons and neuro-physiologists this text has a particularly close realtionship to the practical application of its principles. He has also referred freely to the older related works which have stood the test of time.

The illustrations are plentiful. In all, 337 are used, 30 of which are in color. Close correlation of these to the text is evident. Excellent dissections by the author served as original material for the illustrations. A standard plan of reduction and enlarbement makes this material of greater value to the student in establishing his own concept of neuro-anatomy.

The subject index is conveniently arranged and a complete author's index adds materially to the value of the book as a reference volume.

The type is well chosen and the plan of the printing adds to the readability of the text.

I have recommended this work to our students without reservation and am very pleased to have this material close at hand for frequent reference.—Harry Wilkins, M.D.

"YEAR BOOK OF GENERAL MEDICINE, 1942." By Dick, Amberson, Minot and Castle, Stroud and Eusterman. The Year Book Publishers, 304 S. Dearborn St. Chicago.

The busy physician either in general practice or limiting his work to internal medicine will find that the Year Book provides one of the best means of keeping abreast of current developments in the field of internal medicine.

The five sections, Infectious Diseases, Diseases of the Chest, Diseases of the Blood and Blood Forming Organs and Diseases of the Kidney, Diseases of the Heart and Blood Vessels and Diseases of the Digestive System and of Metabolism are edited by outstanding specialists.

Some of the most important contributions to the literature are concisely summarized with occasional pertinent comments by the editors. Proper emphasis is given to articles dealing with diagnosis and treatment. Enough summaries of investigative articles are included such as the work on Penicillin to acquaint one with possible future therapeutic agents.

The section on infectious diseases is especially valuable and includes a summary of a number of articles by army and navy officials. Attention is focused upon some of the diseases rarely found in this country which may be more common incident to the war and air transportation. It also includes under 'Chemotherapy' Circular letter No. 17 issued February, 1942, by the Office of the Surgeon General of the United States Army. This very well summarizes the use of the various sulfonamides in different types of infection.

The twenty questions on the jacket providing a ten-minute quiz are well selected. The editors might expand these to cover each section separately. It would aid in practical crystallization of opinion concerning the newer diagnostic and therapeutic advances.—Bert F. Keltz, M.D.

"AFTER EFFECTS OF BRAIN INJURIES IN WAR." Kurt Goldstein, M.D., Clinical Professor of Neurology, Tufts Medical School, Boston, Mass. Grune and Stratton, Inc., 443 Fourth Avenue, New York. Price $4.00. 244 Pp.

It is particularly apropos that a work of this type be completed and available to the profession when we are entering a phase of medical care of war casualties. Dr. Goldstein has presented findings related to patients with skull and brain injuries caused by gunshot wounds, based on a large series of cases observed during and following the first World War. The information on which these findings were based was gathered during the systematic study of about 2,000 cases over a long period. Many cases were observed and studied for as long as ten years.

He points out that immediately after the injury the primary concern is for the condition of the wound and the patient's general condition. After the wound has healed externally, defects produced by impairment of function of the brain assume major importance but not to the neglect of the wound, as complications may arise even after a period of weeks or months. He calls attention to the improved methods of immediate post injury management, present transportation facilities and sulfanilamide therapy, permitting evacuation of casualties to hospitals remote from the field of battle. This permits organization of hospitals specializing in the care of the brain-injured soldiers, where the nursing problem can be more successfully solved.

The material presented in this treatise has been especially well organized with chapters covering "General Symptoms," "Neurological Symptoms," "Mental Symptoms," and "Origin of Symptoms."

Separate discussions are given of the "Psychological Laboratory examinations and Neurological and Physical Therapy" and "Social Adjustments." This final chapter deals with practical problems, such as, the Choice of a future vocation, evaluation of usefulness for military service and civilian life, the question of compensation and the problem of social care.

This small readable volume will undoubtedly provoke a more profound consideration of the things which may be accomplished in the followup treatment of the head injury cases. If so, it will have fulfilled its mission.

The illustrations are few but pertinent.

An excellent bibliography has been prepared.

The publishers have contributed to the value of the book by the excellent printing and satisfactory binding.

I should like to recommend the volume for those engaged in civilian practice as well as for those engaged in industrial and war work.—Harry Wilkins, M.D.

University of Oklahoma School of Medicine

The faculty of the School of Medicine had its annual mid-year meeting on Friday, January 15. Mr. Joseph A. Brandt, President of the University of Oklahoma, was present and discussed some of the medical school problems with the faculty. Dean Tom Lowry also attended this meeting.

Classwork for the second semester started at 8:00 A.M., Monday, January 18.

The first lecture of a series given under the direction of the Post Graduate Committee of the State Medical Association, with Dr. L. W. Hunt as lecturer, was held on Friday evening, January 15, in the Auditorium of the School of Medicine.

Dr. Joseph B. Goldsmith, Associate Professor of Histology and Embryology, left on January 16 for active duty as First Lieutenant, Sanitary Corps, Army of the United States.

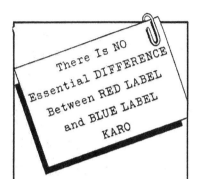
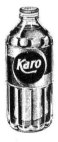

MEDICAL ABSTRACTS

"DIET AND BRIGHTS DISEASE." Soma Weiss. Connecticut State Medical Journal, V: 499-501, July, 1941.

Early Stages of Acute Glomerulonephritis and Interstitial Nephritis with Oliguria. This he evaluates from the consideration of the structural, physiological and chemical deviations from the normal.

Oliguria is common in both intra and extra glomerular conditions interferring with filtration and to tubular obstruction interferring with filtrate flow, extra cellular factors, such as low blood sodium and hypoproteinaemia are less responsible. Osmosis of fluid and chloride to the tissues fail to reach the kidneys. Low osmotic blood pressure in hypoproteinaemia causes sodium retention in the tissues.

The amount of fluid and salt therefore depends on the plasma. Thus the acids, alkaline and bases of the food are fundamental factors in its physio-chemical changes. He still emphasizes the Karrell milk diet for 3-5 days with additions then of fruit juices and lactose.

After this the increasing of fluid above the 1500 cc lost in the lungs and skin. Where water is retained in the tissues as salt solution, a fairly large amount of water will aggravate the edema less if sodium salts are not available. He emphasizes that although proteins have never proven to have harmed the kidneys, they should be restricted temporarily only. Carbohydrate diet with vitamins should be given. Salt restriction to less than 2 gms. should be continued. Potassium salts may be added to the foods to flavour, but it is questionable whether they help the edema. An acid ash diet may be helpful and later 80-120 gms. of proteid may be given in the more chronic stage.

We dealt with only part of this article, but it would be well to peruse it in its entirety since it comes from such a master clinician.—L.A.R., M.D.

"COLLES'S FRACTURE." William Darrach. The New England Journal of Medicine, CCXXVI, 594, April 9, 1942.

The author describes the anatomy, pathology, symptoms, signs, and treatment of Colles's fracture. He prefers, in the treatment, the use of the ''sugar-tong''—single plaster splint—which he generally replaces seven to ten days later, after the subsidence of the swelling, with a circular plaster gauntlet from the mid-palm to the upper forearm. The sugar-tong splint is applied so as to allow free motion of the interphalangeal and metacarpophalangeal joints, and finger movement is encouraged.

When the plane of fracture is oblique, or when there is comminution of the dorsal surface, there is a strong tendency, because of the muscle pull, for the dorsal shift and tilt to recur. This can be partially overcome if the splint is applied with the wrist in strong flexion and moderate adduction.

If the comminution is so extensive that no form of splint alone prevents collapse and shortening, he advises using double Kirschner wire and plaster, one wire through the bases of the second, third, and fourth metacarpals and the other higher in the forearm in the upper ulna, just distal to the coronoid. Reduction is obtained by traction on the wires, and a cast is applied incorporating the two wires. These are left in place for from five to seven weeks.

He describes the late disabilities and their treatment, but these do not differ from those described elsewhere, and their treatment is also similar to present accepted methods.—E.D.M., M.D.

"NUPERCAIN SPINAL ANESTHESIA FOR ABDOMINO-PERINEAL RESECTION OF THE RECTUM: A NEW TECHNIC." F. A. H. Wilkinson. M.D., D.A., Montreal, Canada. In the Journal of Anesthesiology, July, 1942, Volume 3, Number 4, Page 437-443.

Anesthesia for the operation of abdomino-perineal resection of the rectum must provide adequate relaxation for abdominal work and an anesthetic that will not wear out before perineal work is done.

Procaine will not last long enough for the average operator. Pontocaine will last for about two hours, however, this may not be long enough to complete the abdominal-perineal work. Nupercaine by using both combined heavy and light solution has proved most satisfactory. This technic was suggested by Dr. M. D. Nosworthy at St. Thomas Hospital, London, and has been modified by Doctor Wilkinson.

The technic for the combined heavy and light nupercaine spinal anesthesia, the maximum dosage of the light 1:1500 calculated by allowing 1 cc. of this solution for each inch of back length, as measured from the seventh cervical vertebra to the interiliac line with the back in full flexion, up to a maximum of 20 cc. The average adult back measured by this method, varies from 16-22 inches in length, however the author has found for abdominal work that about 15 cc. of this dose is needed, unless the person has extremely long back. The difference in back length necessitates a different time for the light nupercaine to rise.

Both the heavy and light nupercaine is warmed when injected, the interspace used is usually the third lumbar. Since nupercaine is precipitated out in the presence of alkali, care must be taken that the glassware and needles are rinsed with slightly acidified sterile water.

The patient is in the sitting position for the puncture. First, 1.5 cc. of 1:200 nupercaine (in six per cent Glucose) is injected slowly, this immediately settles down into lower spinal canal and attacks the sacral and lumbar roots. At the end of two minutes the concentrated nupercaine solution has settled down and the syringe is disconnected and replaced with a syringe containing 15-20 cc. of warmed light nupercaine (1:1500), this injected slowly so as not to swirl the dependent solution of heavy nupercaine. The time at beginning of injection is noted and the light solution is allowed to rise from forty-five to sixty seconds from the commencement of the injection, depending upon the height of anesthesia desired and the length of back. At the conclusion of the specified period, the patient is lowered backward and placed in a slight Trendelenburg position (ten degrees) and is maintained in this position in order to prevent the upward spread of the light nupercaine. A marked Trendelenburg position is contraindicated, as the heavy 1:200 nupercaine solution might spread too high above the sacral and lumbar roots where it is most needed, but a slight lowering of the head allows an adequate spread of the heavy solution. The nerves are adequately taken care of by the original sitting position. After twenty to thirty minutes from the time of injection the patient may be placed in the steepest position, as the drug has been fixed by this time.

The longest unsupplemented anesthestic was four hours and fifty minutes. The average duration of Dr. Wilkinson's surgery was two hours and eight minutes, but usually the anesthesia lasts longer than three hours. The only drug that will outlast the operation is nupercaine. The principle underlying this technic is the injection of sufficient of the heavy nupercaine to insure a long lasting perineal anesthesia, followed by only enough light nupercaine for the duration of the abdominal part. It is desirable so that when the patient is turned on his side, he is able to use intercostals muscles, hence they have better respiration, this will also aid to maintain blood pressure.

Shock arising while patient is on operating table can be successfully treated with intravenous saline, blood or plasma transfusion. The patient frequently shows a marked fall in blood pressure when his position is changed, but the use of ephedrine grain ¾ or neosynephrine ½ cc. subcutaneously about ten minutes before the turning of patient, should prevent this drop.

There were no deaths in the 33 patients in which this technique was used. Four patients had postanesthetic headache but all responded to the pituitrin ½ cc. or caffeine sodio-benzoate grains 7½. There were no other neurological complications. Two patients developed pulmonary infarction postoperatively, but in only one case could the anesthetic have played a part.

The average dose was 1.5 cc. of 1:200 nupercaine and 15 cc. of 1:1500 nupercaine. The average length of back was 19 inches and the average time allowed for light nupercaine to rise was fifty to fifty-five seconds. All cases were given ephedrine hydrochloride grains 1½, this was given five minutes before operation, this helps to maintain blood pressure. The usual premedication was morphine grain ¼ and hyoscine grain 1/150, thirty minutes before surgery and repeated once during the operation if there was no evidence of shock. Intravenous infusion of normal saline was started at beginning of surgery and this was kept running slowly. If blood pressure dropped, the rate was increased. Toward the end of the operation, saline was replaced by blood or plasma.—G. C. H., M.D.

"VALUE OF FATTY ACID DERIVATIVES IN TREATMENT OF CHRONIC OBSTRUCTIVE RHINITIS." E. A. Thacker. Archives of Otolaryngology. Chicago. Vol. 36. Pp. 336-353. September, 1942.

Treatment of the chronic obstructive forms of rhinitis has been unsatisfactory in many cases. Chronic obstructive rhinitis includes five types: 1. obstruction due to anatomic abnormalities; 2. obstruction due to specific diseases; 3. allergic rhinitis; 4. obstruction in which the mucosa does not shrink well with astringents and which does not belong to type 1, 2 or 3; 5. obstruction in which the mucosa shrinks well with astringents.

Chronic nasal obstruction may be caused by anatomical abnormalities of the septum or the bony framework of the turbinates or of such tumors as hypertrophied adenoid tissue, polyps, papillomas or malignant growths. The correction of such conditions requires appropriate treatment by surgical means or with radium or roentgen rays. In obstruction due to specific disease such as tuberculosis or syphilis, the treatment should be focused on the primary disease, with local therapy. Patients with true allergic rhinitis should be treated by desensitization or removal of the allergene if possible.

Sclerosing therapy has been recommended for the treatment of chronic obstructive rhinitis. The author found that it is type 5 of obstructive rhinitis which responds especially well to submucosal injections of sclerosing fluids. These sclerosing fluids are fatty acid derivatives, and they include sodium morrhuate, sylnasol, and monoethanolamine oleate.

The indications for treatment with these sclerosing agents are: 1. intermittent nasal obstruction of long duration, especially when it is associated with changes in temperature and humidity; 2. chronic nasal obstruction from engorged turbinates which have failed to respond to the usual therapeutic measures after one or two months' trial; 3. postnasal dripping, chronic pharyngitis, headache and neuralgic pains in the head and neck, in which intumescence of the turbinates exists and is causing pressure on the lateral nasal wall or on the septum; 4. chronic sinusitis in which there remain after treatment symptoms of nasal congestion due to engorged turbinates; 5. good shrinkage of the turbinates with astringents; this factor is important.

Conditions which contraindicate such therapy are: 1. chronic systemic disease, such as arteriosclerosis, hypertensive or other types of advanced cardiac disease, nephritis, and specific diseases; 2. anatomic defects of the nasal passages; 3. hyperplastic rhinitis; 4. definite allergy; 5. acute infections of the nose, throat and paranasal sinuses.

The technic of administration of these sclerosing agents is as follows. Two tampons saturated with an anesthetic are placed around the turbinate. A long No. 22 needle and a tuberculin syringe are excellent for injection into the inferior turbinate. A long gold needle is advantageous for injection into the middle turbinate. Only a small amount of the sclerosing agent should be administered in the first injection or if several weeks have elapsed since an injection has been made. The usual dose of 0.25 to 0.5 cc. of the fatty acid solution is drawn into the syringe. The tampons are removed. The anterior portion of the mucosa is pierced, and the needle is inserted toward the posterior end of the turbinate. The sclerosing solution is liberated as the needle is gradually withdrawn. A pledget of cotton placed within the nose will readily control bleeding from the needle puncture. The cotton is removed in five minutes, and a tampon saturated with an astringent is placed around the turbinate for ten minutes. The patient is advised to use a one percent solution of ephedrine sulfate or 0.5 percent solution of neo-synephrin hydrochloride every two hours for five days. Injection into one side of the nose only is made at a sitting. After one week the other side may be treated. Two or three weeks should elapse before another injection is made into the same tissue.

Excellent clinical results were produced with these fatty acid derivatives. As long as one year to 18 months has elapsed since the patients completed treatment with sodium morrhuate and sylnasol, and nasal obstruction has not recurred. The associated complaints of sphenopalatine neuralgia, headache, postnasal dripping, and in a few patients anosmia, hoarseness and coughing, have been either completely relieved or definitely decreased.

This method of treatment is beneficial as an adjunct in the treatment of patients with obstinate, refractory chronic sinusitis in whom the engorged turbinates prevent drainage and aeration of the sinuses.

Submucosal injection of the fatty acid solutions is preferable to most of the other forms of therapy because it is easily carried out and requires no expensive equipment and no ulcerations or adhesions and, as shown by microscopic examination, no deleterious effect or damage to the mucous membrane follows the treatment. The appearance of the tissue tends to return to that of normal nasal mucosa.—M. D. H., M.D.

"A STANDARDIZED TECHNIQUE FOR SEDIMENTATION RATE." By J. W. Cutler, M.D., Philadelphia, Pennsylvania. The Journal of Laboratory and Clinical Medicine. Volume 26, Number 3, December, 1940.

This report should be one of considerable importance. No single laboratory procedure needs classification more than doees this sedimentation rate. The author, who is one of the original investigators in the field, has described a method which is simple and the underlining principles of which seem almost universally acceptable. One principle is emphasized and that is that the maximum sedimentation rate in terms of five minute periods of the first thirty minutes is considered to be the most important. The equipment used is very simple and the procedure in no way difficult. It is a modification of the author's own original method. Results are easy to interpret, no correction is necessary for anemia and the method embodies principle applicable to all types of tubes.—H. J., M.D.

"A SEQUEL OF KNEE LIGAMENT STRAIN: PELLE-GRINI-STIEDA'S DISEASE (METACONDYLAR TRAUMATIC OSTEOMA)." W. R. HAMSA, Nebr. State Med. Jour., XXVII: 62, Feb., 1942.

The characteristic feature of this condition is the presence of an area of new bone or calcific change in the region of the medial femoral condyle, presumably the femoral end of the medial collateral ligament. The condition develops following direct or indirect trauma, and is most common in active adults. The earliest symptoms are those of synovitis — pain and swelling — followed by some improvement but not complete recovery. Limitation of motion may occur gradually and become progressive. Tenderness is localized over the medial aspect of the medial femoral condyle. Gradual enlargement of this condyle, either bony or calcific, may or may not be the cause of the disability. Joint relaxation and injury to semilunar cartilage may contribute greatly to the disability. The process seems similar to myositis ossificans.

Treatment consists of (1) immobilization in a splint or cast to remove all stimuli which may increase bone formation; and (2) deep heat, preferably diathermy, to facilitate absorption. Surgical removal is seldom necessary as the enlargement is rarely sufficient to give rise to a mechanical disorder.

The rapidity with which an area of increased density within the area of ligament attachment may appear on roentgenograms following injury is not appreciated, and for this reason alone this case report is justified.

A plasterer, thirty-nine years old complained of pain and disability of left knee following a fall which turned the left leg into marked valgus and produced severe pain. On attempting to walk he felt a snap in the knee which became freely movable but developed moderate swelling. Five days following injury, the roentgenogram showed no bone change; but eighteen days following injury, it showed calcification above and medial to the medial femoral condyle, and was interpreted as an old injury. Three months after the injury, a tender palpable hard mass appeared over the medial femoral condyle, and the roentgenogram showed the fairly smooth outline of the calcifying area proximal to the medial condyle of the femur. This case illustrates one of the earliest appearances on record.

Surgical removal in the majority of reported cases has been followed by recurrence of the bony mass. Surgery would seem to be indicated only after improvement by conservative means has ceased and after the bony mass has shown definite condensation and smooth outline.—E.D.M., M.D.

"SEMEN AND SEMINAL STAINS." A review of methods used in medico-legal investigations. By O. J. Pollack, M.D., Taunton, Massachusetts. Archives of Pathology, Volume 35, Number 1, January, 1943.

This is a subject of particular interest to those interested in the question of sterility of the male and also more particularly to those concerned with medicolegal investigations. Macroscopic and microscopic details are discussed at considerable length. Interesting data is given concerning azoospermia and aspermia. Technic of examination of the fresh fluids and details of chemical, histological and biological tests are given. Normal findings are itemized and compared with abnormal and last, but not least, 344 references are given in the bibliography. The general summary is as follows:

A wide variety of laboratory tests may be employed successfully for the identification of material of seminal origin. The choice of methods depends on the nature and the condition of the material and on the specific purpose of the investigation.

The various physical, chemical and immunologic tests applicable to the examination of seminal material have been reviewed, and their respective spheres of usefulness have been described.

Microscopic examination of suspect material for the identification of spermatozoa is the most generally useful procedure because it is least likely to be interfered with by extraneous influences. Frequently the success of such an examination depends on the utilization of special procedures by which cellular structures may be freed from the environment. Of equal and in some respects of greater specificity are the various serologic tests. Unfortunately, certain of the immune properties of seminal material deteriorate rapidly and may be destroyed by the chemical qualities of the environments in which stains are likely to be found.

The many macrochemical and microchemical tests that have been recommended through the years are of limited usefulness even under optimal conditions, and they should be employed only with full appreciation of their limitations.—H. J., M.D.

"OSTEOMA OF THE EXTERNAL AUDITORY CANAL." Joseph G. Druss and Jacob L. Maybaum. Archives of Otolaryngology, Vol. 36, No. 4, Pages 499-509. October, 1942.

The bony tumors of the external auditory canal are the most often observed by the otologist among all the bony tumors of the temporal bone. The vast majority of these tumors of the bony canal are small exostoses situated close to the tympanic membrane; they occur either as single or as multiple growths. They are not infrequently symmetric and bilateral. Large solitary bony growths occluding the external canal are relatively rare.

There seems to be a diversity of opinion with regard to the origin of bony tumors of the external canal. The preponderance of evidence favors the view that they arise as fibrous tissue tumors from the periosteum lining the os tympanum and mastoid bone. Having inherent osteogenic potentialities, these fibromas undergo a form of bony metaplasia and eventually assume the character of osseous tumors. There is no unanimity of opinion with regard to the part played in the formation of these tumors by previous inflammations of the middle ear or by mechanical irritation to the canal wall.

The small exostoses are usually situated in the bony canal close to the tympanic membrane. The large osteomas are found to arise in most instances at the margin of the isthmus of the bony and cartilaginous canal wall, in close proximity to the tympanosquamous suture, and only on rare occasions from other sites in the canal.

The large solitary osteoma of the external canal is slow growing and usually has existed for years before the patient becomes aware of its presence. It may be accidentally discovered by the patient in cleansing his ear. Or, it may cause symptoms of impairment of hearing, tinnitus, and pain in the ear. There is usually also interference with the egress of cerumen and exfoliated epidermis. In only relatively few of the cases reported was there an association of suppurative otitis media. Eczema and erysipelas of the ear are not infrequent complications. It is difficult to gage the size of the tumor from the appearance of its exposed portion. When the tumor is removed, its size may be found to vary considerably from that which was anticipated.

The authors had opportunity to study three cases of osteoma of the external auditory canal. One patient had a large osteoma which completely filled the external canal. There was an associated chronic discharge from the middle ear. The osteoma was attached to the bony canal wall by a wide bony base. At operation a large cholesteatoma was discovered in the antrum and middle ear. A radical mastoidectomy was done and the osteoma easily removed.

In the second case, the patient has experienced aural symptoms for a period of only seven weeks. The tumor, however, must have been growing for several years. The tumor was so large that the posterior bony wall of the auditory canal had to be taken down. The tumor was attached to its neighborhood by means of a soft tissue pedicle. The third base was similar to the second as to the size and comparatively asymptomatic growth of the tumor.

Until recently there has been considerable reluctance in advising surgical treatment for an osteoma of the external auditory canal. The growth itself is no indication for surgical intervention unless there are annoying or dangerous symptoms such as impairment of hearing, pain, constant sensation of fullness in the ear, tinnitus, occasional vertigo, and recurrences of external otitis because of attempts at manipulation on the part of the patient. Associated with suppuration of the middle ear, an osteoma of the canal may give rise to serious consequences. Interference with effective drainage from the middle ear and inability to observe the clinical course of the suppuration may be responsible for a menacing otitic complication.

Reluctance to interfere surgically in these cases has been due in part to the fact that certain untoward results may follow careless or inexpert removal of the growths. Whether the postauricular or the endaural approach is decided on, it must be understood that a minimum of trauma is a sine qua non to a successful result. The endaural route appears to be a better approach, for the reasons that this incision entails less trauma; it affords a far better view of the growth, and in the absence of the use of packing after the first dressing subsequent care causes little or no discomfort.

The results after operation are most gratifying; the hearing improves appreciably, and the annoying symptoms of which the patient had complained are entirely relieved. Bony growths of the external canal seldom, if ever, recur after thorough removal.

The ease with which a tumor can be removed depends on its size, its proximity to the drum membrane and the width of the pedicle. At times it can be removed without difficulty through the external canal, in a manner similar to the procedure used in the case of a nonimpacted foreign body.—M. D. H., M.D.

"OCULOGLANDULAR TULAREMIA." Edward Francis. Archives of Ophthalmology. Vol. 28, No. 4, Pages 711-741. October, 1942.

The author presents clinical and bacteriological data derived from 78 proved cases of oculoglandular tularemia observed in the United States and from 18 in foreign countries.

Ophthalmologists were the first to recognize cases of ocular tularemia in human beings. D. T. Vail, Sr., of the United States, was the first who called attention to this type of ocular infection in 1914. Wild rabbits caused the disease in 56 of the American cases, through contact with a contaminated hand, and in two cases by blood which spurted into the eye. Tick tissue mashed between the fingers was conveyed to the eye by fingers in ten cases. A fly mashed by the fingers was the cause in one case. Ground hog blood or bile entered the eye in two cases. A tree squirrel was dressed in one case. A dog scratch caused the disease in one case.

There were more male than female patients. Twenty-seven were farmers, or members of their families. Conjunctivitis of animal or insect origin and unilateral enlargement of the lymph nodes which drain the infected eye constitute the dominant local picture. This condition is accompanied by the general constitutional symptoms of fever and debility, which are a part of all forms of tularemia.

The incubation periods averaged three days, the longest being 14 days and the shortest one day. The right eye was affected in 31 cases, the left eye in 36 cases and both eyes in seven cases.

Unilateral enlargement of the preauricular lymph nodes occurred in 55 cases, of the submandibular gland in 46 cases, of the parotid in 21 cases and of the cervical nodes in 41 cases. Bilateral enlargement of the lymph nodes occurred in seven cases of bilateral conjunctivitis. Occasionally, suppuration of the lymph nodes was also seen. Small ulcers were reported on

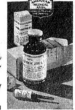

enlarged tonsils once and on the posterior pharyngeal wall once.

Several patients showed ulcers on the fingers which conveys the rabbit infection. In addition, some of the patients had enlarged axillary glands and epitrochlear glands. Dacryocystitis occurred in five cases. One lacrimal sac required incision a year after onset. The conjunctival secretion was purulent in five cases. Ulcers were located on the tarsal conjunctiva in 43 cases and on the bulbar conjunctiva in eight cases. Corneal ulcers appeared in six cases. Corneal perforation, prolapse of the iris and scarring caused greatly impaired vision in one case.

Atrophy of the optic nerve was unilateral in one case, and bilateral in another, causing complete blindness in both eyes. Enucleation was necessary in one case on account of the ulcer, ruptured globe and panophthalmitis. Death occurred in seven of the 78 cases, a mortality of 9.0 per cent, in comparison with a mortality of 6.9 per cent in 15,525 cases of tularemia of all types in the United States.

The diagnosis was confirmed by agglutination alone in 70 of the cases; by isolation of a culture from inoculated guinea pigs in three additional cases, and by direct culture of Bacterium tularense from the conjunctiva in two cases. Attempts to identify the organism from smears of the conjunctival secretion are useless.

A similarity of symptoms is noted between the American and the foreign cases, but an outstanding difference is the greater virulence of the American strains, as shown by a shorter incubation period and by the presence of corneal ulcers, corneal scarring, perforation of the cornea, impaired vision, etc. The mortality of tularemia in foreign countries is about 0.1 per cent. Cases have been reported from Alaska, Japan, Russia, Norway, Canada, Sweden, Austria, Czechoslovakia, Italy, Central Germany, and Turkey.

Pascheff, of Sofia, Bulgaria, described a conjunctival disease that he called conjunctivitis necroticans infectiosa. The clinical characteristics of Pascheff's disease resemble those found in oculoglandular tularemia.

Another disease closely resembling ocular tularemia is the pseudotuberculosis of rodents, the bacterium of which has been accused of causing human conjunctival infection of the oculoglandular tularemia type. Later, such cases have been identified with tularemia itself.

Another conjunctival inflammation which often hides the true nature of oculoglandular tularemia is Parinaud's conjunctivitis. Yet, the two diseases are not identical.
—M. D. H., M.D.

"SOME CAUSES FOR FAILURE IN FRONTAL SINUS SURGERY." Robert Lincoln Goodale. The Annals of Otology, Rhinology and Laryngology. Vol. 51, No. 3. Pages 648-652. September, 1942.

The author gives a short review of frontal sinus operations which were done at the Massachusetts Eye and Ear Infirmary during the period from 1933 to 1942. During this time there were 190 cases in which external operation on the frontal sinuses were performed. He reports on 182 cases. The indications for operation were: infection, 123; mucocele, 18; acute osteomyelitis, 33; osteoma, two; meningioma, one; cholesteatoma, one; unclassified cyst, one; fracture, one; primary carcinoma, two.

In the group of infections there were 38 recurrences requiring operation. In cases of mucocele, there were 18 recurrences. In the group of infections it was found at reoperation that certain pathological or anatomical conditions were frequently present such as scar tissue, remnants of the frontal sinus floor, and ethmoid extensions. In many of the recurrences more than one condition was present. The procedure of reoperation was to remove these conditions.

The frequency with which these conditions were found at reoperation emphasizes the need for fully understanding the important points involved in an external

operation on the frontal sinus. Unless all pockets in the frontoethmoid region are eliminated by removal of bony partitions and small shelves of bone which form ledges in the floor of the sinus, reinfection will recur sooner or later in these areas. Scar tissue will have a greater opportunity to form barriers within the sinus and conditions will appear necessitating a surgical revision.

In any type of operation (obliterative or for drainage) consideration must be given to a complete removal of the frontal sinus floor and the ethmoid cells.—M. D. H., M.D.

"LARYNGOTRACHEOBRONCHITIS IN CHILDREN; CLASSIFICATION AND DIFFERENTIAL DIAGNOSIS." T. Roy Gittins. Archives of Otolaryngology. Vol. 36, No. 4. Pages 491-498. October, 1942.

In recent years many articles have appeared in the literature of otolaryngology concerning infectious laryngotracheobronchitis. The author distinguishes four types of the disease. These are:

(1) Infectious types caused by (a) nonspecific bacteria such as streptococci, staphylococci, influenza bacillus, and pneumococcus; (b) specific bacteria such as diphtheria bacteria;

(2) Traumatic types caused by foreign bodies, or particles of solid matter in mucus, or drops of liquids;

(3) Allergic types such as those caused by angioneurotic edema or asthma; and

(4) Spasmodic types.

The diphtheria type of laryngotracheobronchitis is uncommon at present; however, cases still appear, and it is possible that the condition may be treated as nondiphtheritic if a proper differential diagnosis is not made. For such doubtful cases it is the best practice to give antitoxin early and in large doses until a definite diagnosis has been made. No harm results from giving antitoxin, and the possible foreign protein reaction is probably helpful, even in cases of non-diphtheritic infections.

Among cases of traumatic laryngotracheobronchitis there are some in which history and physical findings, often including roentgenographic and laboratory evidence suggest the presence of a foreign body in the respiratory tract, although no demonstrable foreign body other than collections of mucus is found on bronchoscopy; this mucus at times forms in sticky plugs in the bronchi, which are as obstructive as any foreign body. The author observed thirteen such cases during the past few years. In each instance there was a thoroughly definite history of sudden onset of choking, followed by varying degrees of stridor, cough, wheezing and cyanosis, in a child with no evident previous respiratory symptoms. Popcorn, peanuts, coffee beans, field corn and watermelon seeds are some of the materials which were found in the mouths of these children when the symptoms of respiratory disturbance developed. It is possible that milk, medicine, nasal oils or chemicals may enter the respiratory tract of infants and young children and set up a clinical picture which is usually associated with the presence of a demonstrable foreign body.

In all such cases there was some degree of dyspnea wheezing respiration, cough and cyanosis. The children usually had high fever and a leukocyte count up to 39,000.

Bronchoscopy, of course, reveals no demonstrable foreign body. In each case mucus, sometimes in sticky masses or plugs, was removed by suction through the bronchoscope from the trachea or from one or both bronchi. Complete recovery occurred in all thirteen cases without sequelae. Tracheotomy was necessary only in one case. The recognition and differentiation of the traumatic from the infectious type of laryngotracheobronchitis is very important because most of the traumatic cases will be cured by proper bronchial drainage, while in the infectious type, which has a much higher mortality rate, trachetotomy is more often necessary.

The allergic type of laryngotracheobronchitis is characterized by rapid noisy respiration which suddenly develops. There may be restlessness dyspnea refusal of food, fever and moderate cyanosis, and an expiratory wheeze.

The asthmatic type of laryngotracheobronchitis is not very frequent in young children, but eventually it may occur even in young infants. Such cases are best treated with small doses of epinephrine, highly humidified air and increase in the fluid intake.

The spasmodic type of laryngotracheobronchitis is better known as spasmodic croup or sometimes pseudocroup. It is characterized by suddenly developing traumatic and fearful dyspnea which is usually of short duration and not commonly dangerous to life. Most of the patients who suffer with this condition are not seen by the laryngologist. The symptoms are usually produced by spasm of the vocal cords, in an otherwise healthy larynx. Yet in some instances they may be produced by either a trauma or an infection of the bronchial tree, in which cases the spasmodic attack persists during the daylight hours, while spasms of a healthy larynx usually occur at night.

There has been much confusion between the more severe and milder forms of laryngotracheobronchitis and, therefore, the statistics of recovery are false and misleading. Infectious laryngotracheobronchitis is a very serious disease with mortality rate up to 50 per cent.
—M. D. H., M.D.

KEY TO ABSTRACTORS

E. D. M. ....Earl D. McBride, M.D.
H. J. ....Hugh Jeter, M.D.
L. A. R. ....Lea A. Riely, M.D.
M. D. H. ....Marvin D. Henley, M.D.
G. C. H. ....Grace C. Hassler

"ESSAY ON MAN"

The hart was the first pump ever invented. It never stops beeting as long as we're lucky. It pumps the blud through vanes and arteries, depending on weather its coming or going. If you axsidently cut one of your blud vessels and know a lot about fizzeology you can tell rite away weather its a vane or a artery, thus sattisfying your curiosity even if it don't make you feel any less nerviss.

If you are not quite sure how you feel, all a doctor has to do is lissen to your hart to help you find out. If he tried to lissen on your rite side hes proberly not a good doctor.

We are born with two lungs and if we have any less its impossible. They help us to breethe all day and at nite they breethe for us. If it wasent for the lungs the air wouldent have any place to go and our whole sistern would be full of drafts.

The stummick receeves all your food but it proberly dont injoy it as much as you do. No matter how polite and well educated you are your stummick also rimes with jelly.

Between your neck and your legs you are known as your trunk, proberly because allmost all of the rest of you is packed there.

The neck seperates our head from our shoulders and helps us to look sideways in a hurry. It is one of the last things we learn to wash of our own free will.

The legs are what distinguish short people from tall ones, so even if we are all born equal, later on in life we are more equal sitting down than standing.

People proberly resemble each other more on the inside than what they do on the outside, being why we use the outside to recognize each other by, specially from our necks up.

OFFICERS OF COUNTY SOCIETIES, 1943

COUNTY	PRESIDENT	SECRETARY	MEETING TIME
Alfalfa	H. E. Huston, Cherokee	L. T. Lancaster, Cherokee	Last Tues. each Second Month
Atoka-Coal	J. B. Clark, Coalgate	J. S. Fulton, Atoka	
Beckham	H. K. Speed, Sayre	E. S. Kilpatrick, Elk City	Second Tuesday
Blaine	Virginia Olson Curtin, Watonga	W. F. Griffin, Watonga	
Bryan	J. T. Colwick, Durant	W. K. Haynie, Durant	Second Tuesday
Caddo		C. B. Sullivan, Carnegie	
Canadian	P. F. Herod, El Reno	A. L. Johnson, El Reno	Subject to call
Carter	Walter Hardy, Ardmore	H. A. Higgins, Ardmore	
Cherokee	P. H. Medearis, Tahlequah	James K. Gray, Tahlequah	First Tuesday
Choctaw	C. H. Hale, Boswell	E. A. Johnson, Hugo	
Cleveland	J. A. Rieger, Norman	Curtis Berry, Norman	Thursday nights
Comanche	George S. Barber, Lawton	W. F. Lewis, Lawton	
Cotton			Third Friday
Craig	F. M. Adams, Vinita	J. M. McMillan, Vinita	
Creek	H. R. Haas, Sapulpa	C. G. Oakes, Sapulpa	
Custer	F. R. Vieregg, Clinton	C. J. Alexander, Clinton	Third Thursday
Garfield	Paul B. Champlin, Enid	John R. Walker, Enid	Fourth Thursday
Garvin	T. F. Gross, Lindsay	John R. Callaway, Pauls Valley	Wednesday before Third Thursday
Grady	Walter J. Baze, Chickasha	Roy E. Emanuel, Chickasha	Third Thursday
Grant	I. V. Hardy, Medford	E. E. Lawson, Medford	
Greer			
Harmon	W. G. Husband, Hollis	L. E. Hollis, Hollis	First Wednesday
Haskell	William Carson, Keota	N. K. Williams, McCurtain	
Hughes	Wm. L. Taylor, Holdenville	Imogene Mayfield, Holdenville	First Friday
Jackson	E. S. Crow, Olustee	E. W. Mabry, Altus	Last Monday
Jefferson	F. M. Edwards, Ringling	L. L. Wade, Ryan	Second Monday
Kay	Philip C. Risser, Blackwell	J. Holland Howe, Ponca City	Third Thursday
Kingfisher	C. M. Hodgson, Kingfisher	H. Violet Sturgeon, Hennessey	
Kiowa	B. H. Watkins, Hobart	J. William Finch, Hobart	
LeFlore	Neeson Rolle, Poteau	Rush L. Wright, Poteau	
Lincoln	H. B. Jenkins, Tryon	Carl H. Bailey, Stroud	First Wednesday
Logan	William C. Miller, Guthrie	J. L. LeHew, Jr., Guthrie	Last Tuesday
Marshall	O. A. Cook, Madill	Philip G. Joseph, Madill	
Mayes	Ralph V. Smith, Pryor	Paul B. Cameron, Pryor	
McClain			
McCurtain	A. W. Clarkson, Valliant	N. L. Barker, Broken Bow	Fourth Tuesday
McIntosh	James L. Wood, Eufaula	William A. Tolleson, Eufaula	First Thursday
Murray			Second Tuesday
Muskogee-Sequoyah-Wagoner	H. A. Scott, Muskogee	D. Evelyn Miller, Muskogee	First and Third Monday
Noble	C. H. Cooke, Perry	J. W. Francis, Perry	
Okfuskee	L. J. Spickard, Okemah	M. L. Whitney, Okemah	Second Monday
Oklahoma	Walker Morledge, Oklahoma City	E. R. Musick, Oklahoma City	Fourth Tuesday
Okmulgee	A. R. Holmes, Henryetta	J. C. Matheney, Okmulgee	Second Monday
Osage	C. R. Weirich, Pawhuska	George K. Hemphill, Pawhuska	Second Monday
Ottawa	W. B. Sanger, Picher	Matt A. Connell, Picher	Third Thursday
Pawnee			
Payne	L. A. Mitchell, Stillwater	C. W. Moore, Stillwater	Third Thursday
Pittsburg	John F. Park, McAlester	William H. Kaeiser, McAlester	Third Friday
Pontotoc	O. H. Miller, Ada	R. H. Mayes, Ada	First Wednesday
Pottawatomie	A. C. McFarling, Shawnee	Clinton Gallaher, Shawnee	First and Third Saturday
Pushmataha	John S. Lawson, Clayton	B. M. Huckabay, Antlers	
Rogers	C. W. Beson, Claremore	C. L. Caldwell, Chelsea	First Monday
Seminole	Max Van Sandt, Wewoka	Mack I. Shanholtz, Wewoka	
Stephens	W. K. Walker, Marlow	Wallis S. Ivy, Duncan	
Texas	R. G. Obermiller, Texhoma	Morris Smith, Guymon	
Tillman		O. G. Bacon, Frederick	
Tulsa	James C. Peden, Tulsa	E. O. Johnson, Tulsa	Second and Fourth Monday
Washington-Nowata	J. G. Smith, Bartlesville	J. V. Athey, Bartlesville	Second Wednesday
Washita	A. S. Neal, Cordell	James F. McMurry, Sentinel	
Woods	C. A. Traverse, Alva	O. E. Templin, Alva	Last Wednesday
Woodward	C. E. Williams, Woodward	C. W. Tedrowe, Woodward	Second Thursday

THE JOURNAL
OF THE
OKLAHOMA STATE MEDICAL ASSOCIATION

| VOLUME XXXVI | OKLAHOMA CITY, OKLAHOMA, MARCH, 1943 | NUMBER 3 |

Aviation Medicine*

LT. COL. W. M. SCOTT, M.C.

FLIGHT SURGEON, WILL ROGERS FIELD

OKLAHOMA CITY, OKLAHOMA

At the present period of the world's history, the attention of all nations is being more and more acutely directed to the air. The success up to the present time of the Axis powers, especially in their early campaigns, hinges largely on sudden and overwhelming air action, and the air force has continued to be a potent factor not only in their military effort but that of the United Nations as well. We are all more or less familiar with the rapid advances that have been made in actual flying methods and aircraft construction. We may not, however, be so familiar with the progress which has been made in the world of Aviation Medicine, the developments of which and advance in which have contributed in no small measure to the advance which aviation itself has made.

As early as 1783 we find a physician, one Dr. John Jeffries of Boston, flying from Dover to Calais in a hydrogen filled balloon, he being thus the first physician known to fly. His interests, however, were in aviation and not particularly in medicine, therefore, he cannot be called actually the originator of Aviation Medicine. This honor must be reserved for Paul Bert, a brilliant French physiologist, who as early as 1875 was interested in the effects caused by changes of altitude and made a study of a report submitted to him by one of his students, a meterologist by the name of Tissandier. In a balloon assension, which Tissandier made with two companions, the balloon ascended to 28,820 feet, then descended with Tissandier alone of the three alive. From information gathered on this flight and further study, Bert published his famous work "La Pression Barometrique," having to do, as can be de-

duced from the subject, with the effect of high altitude to the human organism. This might be called the first really comprehensive work on Aviation Medicine, and hence for Paul Bert the honor of being acclaimed the father of Aviation Medicine and the first Flight Surgeon.

During the days of World War I it was found that Germany, with the thoroughness common to that people, was studying the problems of Aviation Medicine as early as 1910. France and England were not long in following suit, and by the end of 1917 all of the Allies and Germany had medical units which were integral parts of the air service, among which medical personnel were many of their leading surgeons and scientists.

The United States, in February, 1912, published a type of examination to be conducted for flying personnel, and in 1917 Col. Lister and Col. I. H. Jones made up an entirely new physical examination form for flying which was called the Form 609. By October of 1918 American medical units in France had already contributed largely to knowledge of Aviation Medicine and removal of some of the causes of aviation accidents known at that time. In January of 1918 a medical research laboratory was established at Minneola, Long Island, and in May of 1920 a section of this medical research laboratory had been established for the specific purpose of training Flight Surgeons and in that same year was moved to Mitchell Field, Long Island. In 1921 it was recognized as a special service school, and in 1922 it was designated as the School of Aviation Medicine. In 1926 the school was moved from Mitchell Field to Brooks Field, Texas, and in October of

*Read before the Oklahoma County Medical Association, Oklahoma City, September 22, 1942.

1931 the school was moved to Randolph Field, Texas, where it is now located.

The Flight Surgeon is a sort of combination of general practitioner, specialist in Ear, Nose and Throat and in cardiology and neuropsychiatry; somewhat of a father confessor to those in need; business manager and research scientist. This may seem like a large order, and it undoubtedly is if the various duties are conscientiously carried out. We believe it to be safe to state that one of the most important of the phases of research in Aviation Medicine has been concerned with the study of altitude and its varying effects on the human organism. Extensive research work has been carried on in this as in other fields at the research laboratory at Wright Field, Dayton, Ohio, under the able direction of Major Harry G. Armstrong of the Army Flight Surgeons Corps. Intimately connected with this subject has been the effects of lack of oxygen at high altitude, with its various manifestations appearing, and treatment to correct the condition. Individuals, of course, vary in their resistance to anoxia and anoxemia, as in other clinical conditions, but much has been learned concerning the maximum rates of safe ascent and the minimum levels of altitude at which the flying personnel should begin to inhale oxygen from containers carried in the ship and the length of time, even with oxygen available, during which flying personnel may safely remain and function as combat units while performing their missions at these different altitudes.

In connection with altitude effects also has been studied the formation of nitrogen bubbles, particularly those in the spinal column which it has been found occur at high altitudes and results from a release of nitrogen contained in the tissues, this release being due to decreased barometric pressure at the higher altitudes. Recognition of the early symptoms of the onset of anoxia and anoxemia and the nitrogen problem condition just mentioned somewhat resemble the submarine diver's bends, and the prevention and treatment of these conditions have been not only the concern of Major Armstrong at Wright Field but of all Flight Surgeons on duty with Army Air Force units everywhere.

Descent also is of importance in its effect, especially on the middle ear, and maximum rates of descent have been studied and worked out as a result of investigations of the various Flight Surgeons during the years.

Acceleration and its role in aviation as it affects the human organism has proved an interesting field for the Flight Surgeon, and this also in connection with the laws of gravity, changes of direction and various other factors involving sudden changes of direction at high speeds causing "black-outs," with resultant undesirable effects in some instances. Reasons for the occurrence of this condition have been studied and found, and methods to prevent its occurrence and combat its effects have been a source of interesting study to both the pilot and the Flight Surgeon. Under the heading of research can be mentioned also the factor of comfort. As is well known to all physicians, the patient who is comfortable is a much better patient and more likely to respond favorably to therapy than is the patient who is uncomfortable. This applies equally well to military personnel on aviation missions, and the result has been that considerable thought has been given and effort expended along the lines of making cockpits more comfortable as regards the type of seats used, type and location of controls and instrument panels, adjustable lengths and heights of seats and control pedals for leg length, installation of various types of heaters, designing and testing different types of suits for the wear and comfort of the flyers to protect against the extreme cold of high altitudes, and last but by no means least, intensive study to develop a comfortable and at the same time efficient oxygen mask. Vents and appliances have even been installed in aircraft for the answering of physiological needs of the personnel in the aircraft with its natural and attendant promotion of the bodily welfare and comfort. It might appear to the casual observer that with attention to the foregoing details the Flight Surgeon's life would be indeed a busy one; however, his problems do not end here for also of intense concern to the Flight Surgeon is the detection and elimination of poisonous gases in and around the airplane. It is not uncommon for the Flight Surgeon to be called on to test for the presence of carbonmonoxide in the cockpits of ships or to examine flying personnel to determine as to whether or not they are suffering from either acute or chronic carbonmonoxide poisoning. As can easily be understood, a condition of that sort allowed to persist could readily terminate in fatal results.

There also are present the possibilities connected with the use of lead, arsenic, benzine and other toxic agents used in the dope shops, paint shops and other necessary activities connected with the construction, care and maintenance of the airplane. So it can be seen that the life of the Flight Surgeon is a busy one—but the end is not yet. On any one day the Flight Surgeon may be called on to transport ill or injured patients by air from one area to another, as we have frequently been called to do, and in many instances the Flight Surgeon has no definite knowledge of the type of case he is to handle until he actually sees his patient. Therefore, we must go on our mission pretty well equipped to handle almost anything from a compound fracture of the tibia to a cerebral concussion case.

Flight Surgeons have at various times aided in local disasters such as floods, tornadoes, etc., and by their knowledge of meeting emergencies in Army life, have been able to aid when disaster has struck at our civil components, dropping food and drugs from Army airplanes to those so stricken and in isolated areas.

Of course, the conduction of the physical examinations of applicants for flying plays a large part in the activity of the Flight Surgeon in his every-day work. It is to properly evaluate the conditions found on these examinations that we attend the School of Aviation Medicine and there receive the specialized training particularly, as mentioned before, in cardiology, Eye, Ear, Nose and Throat and neuropsychiatry. The importance of a small defect, apparently negligible in degree, might not appear great to the average physician. For ground troops this could apply, but a physical defect which would be permissible in an armored car or armored truck traveling at 40 miles an hour could easily spell disaster in a pursuit ship or bomber traveling 300. Emotional and neuropsychic instability are likewise undesirable in flying personnel, and the Flight Surgeon on duty is trained to guard against the acceptance of individuals with this defect and the prevention of its development in those already accepted. In this connection comes consideration of a very important phase of the Flight Surgeon's work—one of the most important of all; that is, observation of his pilots and other flying personnel for appearance of fatigue, occupational neuroses and other types of conditions incident to their occupation. Flying is a fatiguing occupation. There are those who may doubt that this is true, but to those who have for years been associated with flying in its various phases, it is known to be so and as each individual varies in his ability to withstand hardship, so each pilot varies in his ability to withstand fatigue. Therefore, close and accurate observation of our pilots and flying personnel is mandatory.

In the neuropsychic field also comes the role referred to previously as that of father confessor. We are all, as professional men, aware of how insistently from the subconscious field is intruded into the realm of the conscious, problems which are of deep concern to us at the moment. No difficulty should be encountered to envision the result if a pilot making a vertical turn or a steep banking turn at 200 miles an hour allows his field of thought to become occupied with the note that he has due at the bank rather than with the operation of his airplane. The Flight Surgeon is ready and willing at all times to listen to the problems of the flying personnel and to advise with them concerning the solution of same, regardless of whether it be the aforementioned note at the bank, illness of the pilot's mother-in-law, of a family squabble arising from the fact that Mary Jane paid too much for her new red dress. Seriously, though, the ability to understand the problems and to kindly and understandingly advise on them constitutes one of the greatest justifications for the flying personnel's trust and confidence in their Flight Surgeons. They know that when they come to us with these things, they will find one who will lend a sympathetic ear and follow it up with helpful advice and, if necessary, with action. How many times we have in the past quietly talked with some young officer and advised him to moderate his visits to the Club bar, or understandingly advised on the solution of family problems, the solution of which took a load from his shoulders and left his mind free for the observation of his instruments and the handling of his airplane when coming in for a landing at 100 miles an hour.

The pilot may, of course, give indications that he has been flying too much and many of these youngsters, being filled with the pride of youth, may hesitate to frankly tell the Surgeon that they are tired and need a rest. It is up to the Flight Surgeon to observe these things, detect them sometimes without being told, and to take action to insure periods of rest and relaxation which will bring this young man back to his normal high plane of physical and mental activity.

Along this same line comes the care of the family of the flying personnel, for in addition to all the duties mentioned previously, the care of their families and the competent advice of their medical officers removes this hazard from the mind and everyday working world of the flying crews.

This, in very brief form, is a picture of the life and activity of the Flight Surgeon —the doctor who flies. Out on the hangar line a bomber stands, and responsible for that airplane and its flying conditions is the Crew Chief of that ship. He is usually a noncommissioned officer of some years of service, and it is his responseibility that that ship is either ready to fly or that all repair measures are being undertaken to make it so at the earliest opportunity possible. The Flight Surgeon is the Crew Chief of the men who fly. They fly 'em — we keep 'em flying.

The opinions reflected in this article are personal ones and do not necessarily constitute an indorsement of same by the War Department.

Industrial Dermatoses

EVERETT S. LAIN, M.D.

OKLAHOMA CITY

According to recent United States Public Health reports, industrial skin eruptions now constitute more than 65 per cent of all industrial injuries. Nearly 30,000 cases of occupational injuries were reported last year to the various state industrial commissions. Doubtless thousands of others occur which are adjusted without being reported. In addition to the discomfort and suffering of the worker, the economic loss to our nation runs into millions of dollars.

The advent of phenol-formaldehyde, cellulose nitrate and acetate and casein groups of resinoid products under the general term of plastics, together with other valuable synthetic products which are rapidly springing from chemical research laboratories, has resulted in a marked increase of skin eruptions.

The manufacture of multiple machines of industry, their finish with protective paints, varnishes and anti-rust coatings are handled by many individuals who have previously been unaccustomed to such work. Grinding and shaving of machine bearings and fittings require a constant flow of so-called cutting oils of a special chemical composition. The systematic and periodic cleaning and refinishing of these machines call for another type of complex chemicals known as solvents. No cutting oils or solvents for cleaning machinery have yet been compounded which are absolutely harmless to all classes of workers.

It is of interest to note that not only have laborers and technicians in industrial plants suffered serious skin eruptions during this period of advancing chemical science, but also domestics, housewives and others who use or come in contact with water softeners, powdered or chipped soaps and laundry bleaching products.

Textile manufacturing plants which supply us with ready-made clothing in their attempt to outstrip competition have resorted to chemistry for various new products with which to treat their goods in order to improve the weight, luster or wearing qualities, only to discover that under certain body conditions of heat or moisture the wearer may absorb a sufficient amount of these chemicals

to suffer an acute and sometimes violent dermatitis. It should be remembered that clothing eruptions are not confined to fashionably dressed women. During the past two or three years many cases of violent dermatitis, requiring hospitalization, have occurred on the hips and genitals of men who have worn new and chemically treated shorts .

Since the beginning of our war program with its hunreds of new building projects, installation of machinery with subsequent manufacturing of munitions and chemicals for combat service, there has been an alarming rise in the frequency and variety of occupational eruptions and new hazards. Therefore industrial injuries have become of major importance both to the state and federal departments of public health.

We are living in an age of rapid progress of industry with its multiplying numbers of synthetic products and manufacturing of machine arsenals, airplanes, ammunition and chemical gases. These changing conditions have found the average busy practitioner of medicine unacquainted with their complex chemical formulas and the possible contacts of individuals. Hence, he may fail to recognize on first sight the various types of eruptions which afflict a certain percentage of industrial workers.

Only recently a strike was called in a large shipbuilding yard on the Pacific Coast by the electricians' union engaged in splicing and welding of heavily insulated electric wires because so many employees had developed acne-like pustules and furunculosis. The United States Department of Public Health dispatched Col. Schwartz to the scene, and after a few days' study he proved the cause to be due to a new synthetic resinous gum used in coverings of most electric wires now on the market.

The Fifth Annual Congress of Industrial Health which met in Chicago on January 11, 1943, devoted all of three days and nights to a discussion of industrial injuries in general. On the same date there was begun in Northwestern University Medical School a two weeks' lecture and training course or

Industrial Dermatoses conducted by Col. Louis Schwartz and Major S. M. Peck, United States Public Health Service. Their chief emphasis of this training school consisted of lectures on methods of differential diagnosis and preventive measures. This course also included several days spent in visiting industrial plants around Chicago where clinic cases and possible hazards were pointed out. About thirty-five dermatologists and several full-time industrial physicians were in attendance.

The safety personnel of many industrial plants has long recognized industrial hazards, and many buildings have been constructed with adequate light, ventilation, shower baths, etc. Also, rigid rules have been instituted such as frequent change of clothing, protective gloves, sleeves and gowns made of impervious fabrics which must be worn while at work. Others have attempted to solve this problem by employing only those who appear to have a texture of skin which seems to possess natural or acquired immunity.

Col. Schwartz, after long and wide experience in this field, has recently announced a more optimistic and economical policy of handling sensitive individuals. Namely, it has been learned that after a period of careful and gradual exposure together with the use of protective bland creams, harmless varnishes and clothing, a large percentage of workers eventually become desensitized and can continue their former work without any discomfort whatsoever.

Chemical laboratories have already placed on the market bland protective creams and skin varnishes which are being used with a fair degree of success.

Amidst a rapidly progressive scientific age of advancing industry the Utopia of preventive medicine may never be fully realized. However, it is encouraging to know that both our national and state departments of public health, in spite of occasional political handicaps, are sincerely and laboriously striving toward the ideal of adequate protection of health for all our citizens.

TREATMENT

A careful and complete history of each case will many times reveal the probable cause or produce an enlightening lead for a further investigation of causative factors, including possible afterworking hours contacts instead of industrial.

The distillation and refining of oils and their multiple products usually require strong acids, alkalis, chlorides or metallic salts, etc. The change now taking place in manufacturing from natural to synthetic rubber products calls for a special insight into new and somewhat complex chemical formulas of solvents, anti-oxidants, accelorators and plasticizers.

A good rule of treatment to remember in most cases of external dermatitis may be summarized as follows: First, acute, moist or weeping, edematous eruptions suggest mild, cooling, astringent, drying, germicidal wet packs and lotions. Second, a dry, subacute or chronic skin condition usually demands slow acting, stimulating, reducing chemical agents incorporated in soothing oils, common ointment or one of the late products of a water soluble ointment base.

Ultraviolet light or x-radiation when cautiously and not too frequently administered in suberythema doses may stimulate cellular metabolism and hasten resolution in certain acute and in many cases of chronic industrial dermatoses.

IMPORTANCE OF GENERAL PRACTITIONER

The general practitioner is again taking his rightful place in the practice of medicine—and with a background of study and training that justifies the highest confidence in his ability, John Joseph Nutt, M.D., New York, declares in Hygeia, The Health Magazine for November, asserting that ''if specialists would accept no patients except those referred by family physicians it would benefit the patient, the family physician and the specialist.

''The patient would, of necessity, have a physician who would be friend and adviser in all things pertaining to health. The prevention of illness has become a large part of the practice of medicine, and surely this is work for the family physician, who knows his patient from top to toe. He also should be the judge of the good or evil of treatments, drugs, foods, exercise and climates. . . . No matter where he lives, the most recent advances in science are available to the family doctor through medical journals, circulating medical libraries and medical societies. By consulting him in small matters his patients may often avoid serious consequences. . . . The specialist would not be called on to treat conditions which the family physician can treat exactly as well; he would be consulted only for those conditions which come within his special field. The final result would be the thinning-out of the ranks of the specialists—only the really fit surviving—and the return of the family physician to his own. . . .''

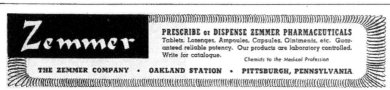

Five Year Report of University of Oklahoma Student Health Service*

W. A. FOWLER, M.D., DIRECTOR.
NORMAN, OKLAHOMA

I have the honor to present herewith the report of the Student Health Service during the five years of my incumbency as your director of student health from September 1, 1937, to September 1, 1942.

At the invitation of President Bizzell I met with the Board of Regents before the final decision as to my selection and acceptance as director of student health. There seemed to be a wholehearted agreement that our Student Health Service should be dynamic and constructive and on a par with the excellence of results in other phases of this university life; and that we should strive to equal or surpass other universities of equal rank in meeting the responsibilities and realizing the benefits of student health work. This report should give some idea as to how well we have met this challenge.

ENTRANCE EXAMINATIONS AND FOLLOW-UP. One of the first problems was the organization and improvement of entrance examinations and follow-up procedures. This required the organization and direction of a staff of more than 60 doctors, nurses, technicians, and other helpers during entrance examinations. Our entrance examination is now quite comprehensive and thorough and includes examination for visual acuity, audiometer testing, urinalysis, Wassermann, tuberculosis and undulant fever testing, in addition to the routine examination of the eyes, ears, nose, throat, heart, abdomen, reflexes, bones, muscles, etc. Our follow-up procedures have been improved and are of great value to student health, but because of an inadequate staff much is yet to be desired in this respect.

BUSINESS ECONOMIES. The obligation to avoid waste and to use wisely the funds of the department was fully realized. The business of the department was carefully reviewed with Miss Fleming. The policy of buying from wholesalers and producers where possible and after competitive price quotations rather than from the corner store

*Presented to the President of the University, members of the Board of Regents and members of Coordinating Board on September 1, 1942.

was established. These details are now handled so well by Miss Fleming that I am almost entirely relieved of this burden.

STAFF SCHEDULES AND STAFF UNIFICATION. Careful arrangement of staff schedules has increased the efficiency of the service, has saved the students valuable time, and has eliminated much deserved criticism of the service. Locating all doctors' offices in close proximity in the south end of the infirmary and the establishment of a central record office in charge of a record librarian greatly increased the efficiency of the service. It has encouraged more frequent consultations and better understanding between members of the staff and has made possible improvements and uniformity in our records. It has eliminated criticism by giving dispensary patients a choice of physicians from the entire staff regardless of sex. It has made the service an integrated, unified whole instead of divided elements.

STAFF ADDITIONS. The financial help and economies referred to elsewhere made possible the employment of an additional physician, a director's secretary, and one additional infirmary nurse the first year. Because of the illness of Miss Willie Fanning, R.N., who had been superintendent of the infirmary for many years, the selection of a new superintendent was necessary. Miss Katherine Fleming, R.N., who had been assistant superintendent of nurses at Crippled Childrens' Hospital, Oklahoma City, for eight years, was secured for this vacancy. Her able administration has been a large factor in the maintenance of the high quality of service in the infirmary and her good business management has been a substantial contribution to our ability to carry forward our program within the limitations of the budget. Later we added a full time, registered, laboratory technician; a full time, record librarian; and a dispensary nurse during the winter session. On the resignation of Dr. Elizabeth Dorsey, September, 1939, we were able to secure the servics of Dr. F. T. Gastineau, who had had special training in dieaseses of the eye, ear, nose, and throat, and who for 16 years was a member of the staff of the state hospital for nervous and mental diseases at Vinita, Oklahoma. We are indeed fortunate to have the services of a psychiatrist of such wide experience and a specialist in diseases of the eyes, ears, nose, and throat.

During the last two years Dr. Paul C. Colonna, Chief Orthopedic Surgeon at Crippled Childrens Hospital, Oklahoma City, has been coming to Norman twice a month for consultation in orthopedic conditions at no expense to the service except his traveling expenses. During the past three years our chest x-ray films hav been interpreted by Dr. L. J. Moorman, well-known chest specialist of Oklahoma City. · This has added much to the value of our x-ray service.

Since it does not seem possible to arrange for sabbatical leave for members of the staff to keep abreast with medical progress, one member of the staff is given three months leave with pay each summer for postgraduate study. Dr. Atkins spent the summer of 1940 in orthopedic surgery at Crippled Childrens' Hospital, Oklahoma City; Dr. Fowler the summer of 1941 in internal medicine and student health at the University of Minnesota; and Dr. Schmidt the summer of 1942 in diseases of the heart at Harvard University. The wisdom of this policy is obvious. These administrative changes and additions to our staff made possible the remarkable increase in volume as well as the quality of our work.

NEW EQUIPMENT. Our x-ray equipment five years ago was quite inadequate, and our films were pronounced by experts as worthless for early diagnosis of tuberculosis and as of limited value for other types of work. With the approval of the comptroller's office, the president, and the Board of Regents, we bought better x-ray equipment at a cost of $2,750.00; and we have employed a part time, registered, x-ray technician so that our x-rays compare favorably with the best. Other items of new equipment are a Leitz microscope so important in differential diagnosis; a photometer necessary for blood chemistry as in determining blood sugar and sulfonamide compound levels; a telebinocular instrument for better vision testing; drums and other containers for sterile goods; examining tables, treatment chairs, cuspidors; an orthopedic carriage, a food warmer, a laboratory incubator, floor coverings, and two surgical beds. These have added to the quality of service. On the other hand, we are still deficient in equipment necessary to give our students the full benefits of modern scientific medicine. Much of our equipment is old, and we are without funds for replacement when this becomes necessary. Our mattress-

es are old and worn and are not up to the quality to which the average well student is accustomed.

STAFF TEACHING. It is generally accepted as desirable that courses pertaining to health be taught by instructors with the broad knowledge of physicians. Teaching also provides a very desirable intellectual stimulus to the physicians and tends to bind them more closely to the university as a whole. I have therefore encouraged the assignment of staff members to limited teaching duties. All the members of the medical staff are engaged in some curricular teaching. The most important teaching function is inherent in the operation of the service itself. By demonstration of correct health procedures it is meeting a basic principle of modern pedagogy.

FINANCIAL SUPPORT. For the maintenance of the highest quality of service, good administration and a competent and conscientious staff are indispensible, but alone are not sufficient. Our equipment should be in line with the highest standards of modern, scientific medicine. Our staff should be sufficient to assure every patient unhurried, careful, and reasonably prompt attention. Only in this way will we be able to approach the fineness of the family doctor and patient relationship. The terms of employment should be worthy of the value and dignity of the work so as to attract and hold the highest type of personnel. The doctors should have more time to search for disease in its earliest and most curable stages, opportunity to read the best medical literature, and time to analyze and report results of work being done, and thus stimulate staff interest and perhaps add to the sum of medical knowledge. We should not be so overworked as to lose inclination to participate normally in university life.

In the face of difficulties, which I fully appreciate, Dr. Schmidt's salary was transferred to another budget in recognition of the curricular teaching of the staff members and the teaching value of the service itself. Two years ago the student health fee was increased from $3.00 to $3.50 per semester. These measures are largely responsible for the progress which we have been able to make. That the problem of inadequate financial support has not been fully met has been due to the difficult circumstances under which the university has been operating rather than to the fault of any individual.

We have problems of financial support, however, for which I hope we will be able to find a solution. Our student health fees are too low. For instance, our near neighbors to the north, The University of Kansas and Kansas State College, which are fairly representative, each has a student health fee of $5.00 per semester whereas our fee is $3.50, and their incidental charges are comparable to ours. Incidental charges, such as for chest x-rays, are frequently a source of dissatisfaction and limit the services for which they are made. This is often in the very class of patients financially handicapped, who because of overwork and other conditions are most likely to need them. The results may not only affect the health of the student involved but may endanger the health of other students, as in chest x-rays for tuberculosis case finding. A more satisfactory policy seems to be to have a somewhat larger general student health fee and fewer, if any, incidental charges.

As a general rule the state provides the buildings, building upkeep, and equipment. Here, however, these items so far have been paid from the student health funds. The infirmary at the Oklahoma A. & M. College, copied after our plan but with more private rooms, was provided by a state appropriation. So far we have been unable to get the state to assume our bonds. They amount to nearly $10,000.00 per year, which is the equivalent of deducting about $1.00 of the student health fee.

The unfavorable factors suggested above should not be permitted to continue to operate if possible to avoid it. A student health fee of $4.50 or $5.00 with retention of incidental charges as of the present, or a fee of $6.00 with the elimination of most incidental charges, would afford considerable relief. If in addition to this the state could be induced to assume the infirmary bonds, we should be on a financial parity with some of the best student health services.

VOLUME OF WORK. It has been our purpose to emphasize quality and not merely volume of work. To a large degree the volume of work would seem to reflect the friendliness and confidence of the students. The enclosed table shows the increase in the average annual volume of work compared with the previous year.

APPROVAL BY C. S. AND A. M. A. In ethical procedure and professional quality of work we have met the high standards of the American Medical Association and the American College of Surgeons. We have recently received the official certificate of approval of the American College of Surgeons. Except a few services operated in connection with university hospitals, there are only three other health services among the universities having this recognition. We are proud of this distinction.

I want to express my appreciation of the fine and helpful support given to this work by President Bizzell, President Brandt, and the members of the Board of Regents and the Coordinating Board; and of the loyal cooperation of members of the staff during my incumbency as director of student health. I promise my continued best efforts to maintain the highest possible degree of efficiency in this important phase of university life.

PART II

GENERAL OBSERVATIONS AND CASE ILLUSTRATIONS. It might be well to ask why have a student health service. Student bodies are coming to constitute population groups of considerable size; the subgroups representing more intimate associations are increasingly large; and students are usually nonresident, quite young, and living away from home for the first time. Health hazards are inherent in such conditions and inevitably become a concern of parents, students, and university authorities. Outbreaks of commun-

TABLE

	1937-38	1938-39	1939-40	1940-41	1941-42	Five Yr. Avg.	1936-37
Physical examinations	4459	4132	4294	4745	5449	4615.8	2945
Dispensary services	22671	30233	27779	29171	32957	28565.2	16128
X-rays	428	549	803	859	997	728.2	146
Physiotherapy treatments	1392	341	216	1344	99	678.4	868
Laboratory examinations	3422	7462	7831	7817	6875	6681.4	1864
No. hospital admissions	1105	1368	1239	1326	1223	1252.2	1040
Total days hospitalization	3066	4156	4083	3833	4001	3827.8	3045
Daily hospital average	9.8	13.0	13.0	12.1	12.6	12.2	9.8
Major operations	17	37	36	30	33	30.6	22
Minor operations (in hospital)	50	67	63	60	36	55.2	29
Deaths in infirmary	2	1	2	0	1	1.2	2

icable disease among student bodies, deaths from heart disease, tuberculosis, and similar conditions among athletes and others, and the analysis of rejections of draftees during the first world war brought forcibly to the realization of university authorities that student health is not merely a matter of chest and biceps measurements but of basic physical soundness and physical and mental functional efficiency. Student health then began to be made a concern of leaders of the highest administrative and medical ability. The results were highly satisfactory to students, to their parents, and to university authorities with the result that the growth of organized student health services has been a remarkable characteristic of higher education. For instance, at the University of Michigan the office clinical visits per thousand students enrolled in the winter session increased from 4.041 in 1925-26 to 11,613 in 1933-34; the expense rates per thousand students for the same periods increased from $6,539.00 to $14,103.00. Their present student health fee is $7.50 per semester, and the university furnishes the building, building upkeep, and equipment.

To know that the health of students will be safeguarded by a service administered by the university and providing the highest quality of medical and hospital care is reassuring to parents, and in some cases may be the determining factor in the selection of a university. To the university authorities a good student health service will satisfy the humane impulse to safeguard the students' health. Aside from this, the university has a considerable investment in each students' education. It is good business and wise administration to safeguard this investment by whatever may avoid preventable deaths and promote physical and mental efficiency.

The distribution of medical cost among the members of the student group is sound ethically and economically. The medical profession is concerned that such procedures be maintained upon the highest ethical level. This means simply that there should be no exploitation of the patient or profession and nothing which in the long run would result in a deterioration in the quality of medical service. It is our earnest concern to maintain these ideals. We have maintained cordial relations with the medical profession.

PHYSICAL EXAMINATIONS AND FOLLOW UP. General physical examinations are given to all entering freshmen who are under 21 years of age and are required to take military science or physical education, to members of athletic teams, and to individual students upon the evidence of special need for such examination. The potential value of this examination is universally recognized by auth-

orities. Its value depends entirely upon the quality of the examination. A slipshod examination is of little if any value to the student and may actually do harm by giving a false sense of security. Its educational value is definitely less than nothing. The purposes of the general physical examination are to assure that the student will be assigned to university sponsored activities that will be helpful rather than harmful; to discover defects, the correction of which will improve his scholastic efficiency and social adjustment; to discover communicable conditions which might endanger the health of other students; to furnish an available health inventory in connection with the students' subsequent medical care, and advice to deans, counselors, and others in determining the student's work load; and finally to reassure students who are basically sound.

A follow up study of all entrance examinations by a member of the staff is desirable. This would include a recheck or more complete investigation of all abnormalities noted and an explanation to the student of the significance of the examination in his case. Incidentally, an important feeling of friendliness and confidence would be promoted. We were able to review most of our entrance examination records and follow up a considerable number. This is a very fruitful field of student health work, as is illustrated by the following case:

M26467 DLR. At entrance examination 9-15-39 this young man, six feet tall, weighing 179 pounds, would certainly not have suggested to the casual examiner anything but perfect health. He gave a history of having had hay fever and malaria, and of being subject to colds. His temperature was 99.4, pulse 116, and he had a tumor of his right breast. The history and physical examination were otherwise quite normal. He was asked to return for recheck of his pulse and examination of his sinuses. His resting pulse on recheck was 105; the thyroid gland was slightly enlarged; transillumination revealed cloudiness of sinus regions. A basal metabolism test and x-ray of sinuses were ordered. His basal metabolism was minus 18, indicating thyroid deficiency; and x-ray revealed "maxillary sinus somewhat cloudy, showing some trabeculation, right maxillary showing more trabeculation than left." He was referred to a private endocrinologist who confirmed the diagnosis of hypothyroidism. The right maxillary sinus was irrigated. The culture from sinus washings was negative. He was treated with small doses of thyroid substance, which he has continued to take. He states that his grades have been better and that he definitely experiences more zest and joy in living than ever before. This student's thyroid deficiency was evidently such as to perceptibly slow down his physical and mental processes. Certainly no casual examination would have afforded him benefit.

CONTROL OF COMMUNICABLE DISEASES. Examination of food handlers, instruction to dish washers and food servers, and articles in the Oklahoma Daily are measures routinely used for prevention of communicable diseases. When a contagious disease occurs more active measures are indicated and undoubtedly frequently prevent epidemics. The following case illustrates the procedure used:

M33934 JLP. The patient was seen in the outpatient department 10-2-41 with a temperature of 101.4, pulse 102, and physical symptoms and signs indicative of an upper respiratory infection. He was referred to the infirmary. The following morning a fine rash was noticeable. He was immediately isolated, and throat smear and culture were taken. The culture revealed streptococci, and the patient developed typical signs of scarlet fever. All known contacts were notified, throat cultures taken, and prophylactic nose and throat sprays were used. Each morning before going to class each contact visited the dispensary to have his temperature and pulse taken, throat examined and sprayed, and skin examined for rash. Anyone found with elevated temperature, redness of throat, or rash indicative of possible scarlet fever was sent to the infirmary for isolation. Others attended classes regularly. No additional case occurred. We rather frequently have cases of contagious disease develop in the students. To our knowledge no additional cases have occurred during the past five years with the exceptions of a mild.epidemic of German measles and a moderate epidemic of mumps.

According to statistics from services where there are very adequate tuberculosis case findinig programs, about 0.5 per cent of university students have some degree of tuberculosis. The following case illustrates the problem:

M34602 GP. A Latin American university student, age 23, had not had the entrance physical examination since he was not required to take military science, being past 21 years of age. He came to the outpatient department 1-26-42 complaining of "run down" feeling for two months during which time he had lost 10 pounds of weight, of pain in the right side of chest, and inability to sleep well. A tuberculin test was made, and he was given an appointment for physical examination two days later. Physical findings were strongly suggestive of active tuberculosis although the x-ray report was negative. He was referred to the infirmary for further observation and study including daily examinations of sputum for tubercle bacilli.

The first two specimens were negative. Examination of aspirated contents of the stomach and of sputum on the third day revealed tubercle bacilli in both. He was referred to a chest specialist for confirmation of diagnosis and treatment. Sanatorium treatment was instituted, and his condition promptly improved with a complete arrest of the condition after a few months. He has already resumed his university education.

His intimate contacts were examined for tuberculosis. One of these was found to have active tuberculosis for which he is taking treatment at the Saranac Lake Sanatorium, New York, which reports very favorable progress, and a complete arrest is expected within a few months. No other active cases were found, but the contacts that return to the university will be re-examined this winter. The contact referred to as being treated in New York gave a history of previous attacks of pleurisy. These were probably tubercular, and it is entirely possible that he was the source of infection for case 34,602.

The compartively early discovery of thiƚs case might have saved this student's life and the lives of some of his associates. The x-ray is perhaps the most dependable single procedure in the diagnosis of early tuberculosis. It will be noted, however, that it was negative in this case. This illustrates the importance of thorough and complete examination rather than dependence upon a single method or a single examination of sputum. This case also illustrates the importance of careful examination of all entering students. Such an examination might have revealed tuberculosis in its earlier stage when interruption of his education might not have been necessary and the health of other students not endangered.

The following two cases illustrate the effect which physical defects may have upon scholastic ability and social adjustments and the importance of careful and scientific search for their detection.

M20013 EW. This student had no general physical examination because not eligible for military science. He came to the Student Health Service 7-22-39 complaining of progressive weakness for 15 months, vague gastro-intestinal symptoms, and irritability. The analysis of gastric contents was negative; smear for malaria negative; urine negative. A blood count showed pronounced anemia. Stool examination revealed blood and hookworm ova, for which he was given appropriate treatment with very satisfactory results. Had this student been given a slipshod examination and symptomatic treatment, his scholastic efficiency in the university and his later usefulness to society would have remained greatly impaired.

M22822 CRMc. This boy entered the university in September, 1937, when entrance examination was essentially negative. He was a brilliant student and in 1940 was a junior Phi Beta Kappa. During the second semester of his junior year he noticed a general "run down" feeling, and during his senior year his work deteriorated to the point where it appeared he would not be able to graduate. He was referred to the Student Health Service by Dean Meacham for a recheck of his physical symptoms. He was distressed not only because of his physical symptoms but because of the deterioration of his scholastic work, which he felt might be due to beginning mental disease. A careful recheck revealed defective vision, which was corrected with proper glasses. In addition he was found to have a maxillary sinusitis of long standing. The sinus was lavaged and culture revealed a mixed staphlococcic and streptococcic infection. Surgical drainage was deemed advisable, and he was referred to a specialist for operation. Recovery was uneventful. He gained 15 pounds of weight within a few weeks and resumed the former quality of his scholastic work.

The cases reported above are illustrative only. Reports of similar cases could be multiplied many times. In a student body of the number at our university medical problems with great potentialities for good or for ill are continually present. Their determination depends upon the quality of the medical service available. A high quality of service for students obviously ill is important but should not be enough to satisfy us unless opportunity is afforded to extend benefits in the highest possible proportion of even obscure conditions that may endanger the students' lives, happiness, or efficiency. Only such a service is worthy of a great university and of the medical profession.

SUMMARY

To THE PRESIDENT OF THE UNIVERSITY OF OKLAHOMA:

MEMORANDUM OF CONVERSATION OF JANUARY 12, 1943

RE: FINANCIAL SUPPORT OF THE STUDENT HEALTH SERVICE

The difficulties under which the Student Health Service, University of Oklahoma, is operating may be listed briefly as follows:

First, inadequate student health fees. Our fees of $3.50 per semester are not in line with those of other universities undertaking to maintain a good health service. This will generally range from $4.50 to $12.50 per semester. (University of Minnesota $4.50 with higher incidental fees; University of Kansas and Kansas State College of Agriculture and Applied Science $5.00; University of California $6.00; Princeton University and University of Michigan $7.50; University of Missouri and Carleton College $12.50.)

Second, the infirmary bonds are paid out of the student health fund. I know of no other university which places this burden on the student health fund. The amount of these bonds is equal, approximately to $1.00 per semester of the student health fee. This leaves us an operating fee of approximately only $2.50 per semester.

Third, we have less support from other sources than most universities. Fo rexample, Cornell University has a student health fee of $5.00, and the University more than matches that amount from university funds. The University of Wisconsin pays all salaries. At the University of Minnesota the athletic department pays $300.00 per year on the salary of the orthopedic surgeon, $445.00 entrance examinations, and three-fourths of the salary of the athletic physician; and the Athletic Association for Women pays $445.00 for entrance examinations. While there might be discussion as to whether or not such support is proper, it would seem obvious that if it is lacking, our fees ought to be correspondingly larger, if we are to realize financial parity with the student health services of these universities.

Fourth, our incidental charges for special services are among the lowest .

As a solution we should have financial support equivalent to a student health fee of at least $6.50 per semester. This should enable us to make salary adjustments, which in my opinion are absolutely necessary if serious disruption of our staff is to be avoided. It would relieve the almost certain considerable deficit on the present basis during the war emergency and would permit the accumulation of such funds as to remove the constant threat of deficit and enable us to purchase needed equipment which should be available at a bargain after the war is over. It should also be possible to improve the quality of the service and make it more satisfactory to students by removing most of the incidental charges, a source of frequent misunderstanding and friction.

If this program meets with the approval of the president, the Board of Regents, and the Regents for Higher Education, may I suggest the following:

First, that at their next meetings the Board of Regents and the State Regents for Higher Education pass a resolution recommending that legislation be enacted permitting incidental fees of an amount to make possible a student health fee of $6.50 per semester.

Second, that friends of the university be asked to endeavor to get such legislation at the present session.

I realize, of course, you and the Boards of Regents may not agree that the plan suggested is wise or possible at this time and that you may have a wiser solution than I have suggested. I am offering the suggestions because I am thoroughly convinced that the present basis of support necessitates an unreasonable work load and stress if there is the aspiration and the conscientious desire to approach the standards of student health service that have been well establish-

ed. It also leaves no hope of continued, orderly progress and indeed makes it unlikely that we can even maintain our present standards within the physical and administrative limitations of the present staff. The program offered is a sincere effort on my part to find a solution for a condition which makes necessary for your director to choose between frustration in spite of overwork on one hand or unimaginative complacency on the other. Very frankly I am unwilling to be compelled to make this choice.

Very truly yours,

W. A. Fowler, M.D., F.A.C.S.
Director of Student Health Service.

Management of Peptic Ulcer

ARTHUR W. WHITE, M.D., F.A.C.P.

OKLAHOMA CITY, OKLAHOMA

As one scans the literature, of the past number of years, pertaining to Peptic Ulcer he is impressed by the vast number of symposia in which noted surgeons and serious minded physicians have battled for their methods of diagnosis or special plan of therapy, each leaving the field after these Homeric conflicts more convinced of his one special plan and the weakness of others. This is not difficult to understand as diagnosis or treatment without an understanding of the basic factors, and without certainty as to the characteristic symptoms must be unsatisfactory, Hence, any diagnostic plan and certainly any therapeusis, must be predicated on a study of etiology and a knowledge of the normal physiological action, both motor and secretory, of the organs involved.

The views as to the contributing causes are myriad; a disturbance of the circulation, as a weakening of a vessel, an embolus, or a thrombus, to a disturbance of the nervous system, either general or special, and Criles's contention of primary imbalance of the endocrine glands or by reason of the influence of a particular gland, supra-renal or thyroid. Eppinger, several years ago, called attention

to an instability of the vagus and sympathetic systems as an underlying cause. Disturbances in the motor sphere, peculiarities in the form of the stomach, ptosis, congenital malformation, anatomic abnormalities affecting the stomach or duodenum. Toxaemias as in hyperthyroidism or tuberculosis, in some way affecting the secretory action of the stomach, and focal infections have been advanced as causative factors.

It has long been accepted by the unbiased student that the corrosive or irritating action of the hydrochloric acid is the immediate cause as well as the continuing cause of ulcer. Wagenstein[1], a few months ago reported producing all of the ulcer types in dogs by the continuous use of Histidine, refuting the statement frequently made that hydrochloric acid has no bearing on the ulcer question and re-enforcing the preposition first advocated by Sippy, and the premise on which most successful treatment has been carried out for several years. Recently it has been emphasized, notable in the teachings of Lehey, that "Pylorospasm is the most prominent factor," but there is such an interdependency between the pylorus and the glandular function of the stomach that this is very likely, in most cases, at least, another form of expression.

To one who has had an opportunity to observe the action of the pylorus in its relation to the hydrochloric acid content, in any great number of instances, it is obvious that while, there are extragastric influences on the pyloric action and antral muscles, the neutralization of the hydrochloric acid sooner or later brings about a complete relaxation of the pylorus in at least 80 per cent of cases. Having a like influence on the normal as well as the ulcer affected stomach.

In the normal stomach, the ratio between the ingredients of the gastic juice is constant, while in the ulcer type of patient there is always an imbalance, except possibly at those times at which the patient is entering the quiescent stage following a spring or fall exacerbation of symptoms, i.e., after the subsidence of symptoms. The hydrochloric acid being out of the normal ratio and showing either a relative or absolute increase, or both. Further, the normal period of digestion is approximately five hours, at the end of which time, in the normal stomach there is found practically no free hydrochloric acid. In the ulcer type, however, there is frequently found an amount of hydrochloric acid equal to or greater than that found in the same case at the height of digestion, i.e., one hour after a carbohydrate meal. In other words there is a definite tendency to a continuing secretion of digestive juice during the twenty-four hours and not limited to the normal digestive period, a condition found often before a defect can be demonstrated, this to my mind is the crucial factor. Hypersecretion, especially noted in the latter part of the day or during the night, while not so constant, is also an important consideration.

Therefore, our attitude toward this problem might be expressed in algebraic form: —X + A + B = Peptic Ulcer. X, representing the unknown underlying cause which, so far as present day knowledge goes, may be any one or all of the vast number of conditions previously mentioned. A, indicating the corrosive action of the hydrochloric acid on the gastric mucosa and on the motor action of the pylorus. B, indicating the lowered resistance of the gastric, duodenal, or jejunal mucus membranes at some point. This latter is susceptible to a very satisfactory explanation from a study of the position and distribution of the blood vessels in relation to position of the stomach and duodenum, as well as the emptying ability of the duodenum, a discussion of which does not belong in this paper.

The symptoms from this type of trouble should be obvious, however, it is a notable fact that often there are not characteristic symptoms. We are reminded of the great number of healed ulcers found at autopsies, there having been no symptoms during life to make one think of ulcer; of the number of cases i nwhich the first evidence was hemorrhage or perforation; again, of the number of cases which present more or less classical symptoms when no ulcer could be demonstrated at the operating table. So that a careful correlation of all of the possible evidences obtainable is necessary to arrive at a dependable conclusion upon which to base an accurate form of management.

Pain, the most outstanding symptom, when present, may be one of two types and the analysis of this symptom is of most importance. Chemical distress, often referred to as ulcer pain is undoubtedly what the above term implies and is associated with the chemical state of the stomach, despite the recurring statements in literature to the contrary, that varying amounts of hydrochloric acid have been introduced into the stomach without producing distress whether in the normal or ulcerated stomach. This type of pain occurs at a time distant from the ingestion of a meal. The threshold being determined by the height of hydrochloric acid secretion, although the presence of an ulcer seems to lower that threshold. A different type of pain, appearing during or immediately after a meal, is of mechanical origin and does not occur except in an advanced state of destruction of the mucosa.

Palmer and Heinz[2] in most conclusive studies of the manner in which pain arises, the site of origin, and to the nature of the stimulus, found, "That ulcer pain arises from the site of the lesion and is not dependent on the pylorospasm, gastrospasm, or intragastric pressure, but on the presence of a stimulus acting on the pain producing mechanism in the region of the ulcer — and that the increased irritability depends on the continued action of acid gastric juice; conversely, desensatization may be produced by continued neutralization of the hydrochloric acid. The action of the stimulus may be mechanical due to the peristaltic action, or chemical due to the highly acid chyme, but in either case the action of the stimulus is probably exerted directly on the nerves rendered hyperirritable through the destructive action of the acid gastric juice."

Referring again to the algebraic equation, the elimination of the A, necessitates the protection of the lining of the stomach and duodenum constantly and consistently from the corrosive and irritating action of the hydrochloric acid.

The plan most effective is that laid down by Dr. Sippy many years ago, that of frequent feedings of bland food with the intervening doses of alkali of sufficient strength to neutralize the hydrochloric acid for a definite period. This is the most successful plan as yet suggested for the control of the acid. The stomach contents must be examined at frequent intervals to determine for a certainty that proper correction is maintained. Lavage late at night is often necessary to take care of the hypersecretion.

The B in the equation is best taken care of by keeping the patient as nearly as possible in the prone or supine position, by reason of the anatomic arrangement of the blood vessels, the circulation is definitely favored by this position.

All peptic ulcers are found on or near the lesser curvature of the stomach, the pylorus, or the duodenum. The blood supply in this region arises from vessels well outside the lesser curvature, the superior and inferior gastric arteries, the branches taking on a folded or cork-screw appearance in the walls of the stomach so that the upright position brings about more or less interference with the blood supply of the affected area by changing the position of the somach. Again, interference, which may be due to pressure or position, with the emptying of the duodenum plays a definite part in bringing about a disturbance of the gastric secretions, in addition to an increased exposure of the duodenum to the corrosive action of its contents. It has been impressed upon me that a determination of the position of the duodenum is an important factor, this can only be done by the use of the fluoroscope.

The X-ray is of great value as one of the procedures in obtaining information as to the condition of the stomach following the plan developed particularly by Akerlund and Berg[a], i.e., the mucosal relief technique. The fluoroscope is of special value, as muscular action is not registered in films and the duodenum is rarely seen on a film. Further, the defect in an ulcer may not be so situated as to be exposed to the film when taken in the ordinary position.

X, the unknown quantity, may sometimes be determined by careful observation and examination of the patient. In any event, anything discovered that could in any way affect the general health of the patient should be eradicated, whether it be of a pathological nature, or whether it be functional, or a matter of external influence, if a permanent result is to be expected. Hence, the basis for developing the management of these cases is plain.

The help of surgery is required in prob-

ably, not to exceed, 20 per cent of all cases and then because of complications as: persistent hemorrhage, perforation, or fixed obstruction, either because of scar tissue or because of thickening of the pyloric ring which occasionally occurs in cases of long standing with marked pylorospasm.

The choice of operation should be determined by the condition present. But whatever surgical proceedure is instituted and for whatever complication, the underlying principal must be remembered and faithfully prosecuted, that of neutralization or absorption of the hydrochloric acid continually. It is the experience of the writer that the average of two years of observation and control is necessary to insure against return of the ulcer or the production of a new one, although all demonstrable evidence of a defect may disappear in a few weeks, as the habit of secreting an excessive amount of hydrochloric acid, which is so well established in these cases, is difficult to overcome and may again exert its damaging influence. Occasional fluoroscopic examination is most helpful in determining the size, type and character of the peristalsis, as well as the action of the pylorus, and of course, the determination of defects which, as already stated, can be done more dependably with the fluoroscope than from films.

Anything like satisfactory results for sufferers from this type of trouble depends upon the interpretation and care of the case as an individual problem. There is nothing in the armament of the physician that can as yet be considered a specific in the treatment of Peptic Ulcer, although recently several so-called specifics have been placed on the market none of which, from the evidence at hand, presents any basic claim for favorable expectation and from clinical observation on a somewhat limited number of cases, none of these have proved anything but a disappointment.

There is no specific cure for ulcer. Medicine does not cure, food does not cure, surgery does not cure. It must be given an opportunity to heal by taking care of the thing which hinders the healing; i.e., by any method which consistently protects the lining membrane of the stomach from the corrosive action of the hydrochloric acid. This probably will be true until such time as we are able to completely eliminate the basic cause, as yet unknown.

BIBLIOGRAPHY

Palmer, W. L.: The Stomach and Military Service, Jour. A. M. A, Vol 119. No. 15, 1155-1159, August 8, 1942.

Palmer, W. L.: Archives of Internal Medicine, 53-269, February, 1934.

Wangensten, Owen H.: The Mayo's Clinic, Reported at College of Physicians Meeting, February, 1942.

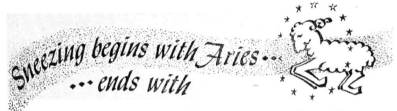

Sneezing begins with Aries...
...ends with

POLLEN ANTIGENS
Lederle

FOR COUNTLESS CENTURIES the sign of Aries (the ram) has ushered in the season of growing plants—warning of the inevitable pollen season in the months to follow.

No satisfactory cure for Hay Fever has yet been discovered, but it can often be prevented or alleviated by Pollen Antigen immunization in advance of the season.

"Pollen Antigens *Lederle*" are glycerinated extracts possessing adequate stability, prepared and standardized with great care in our laboratories. Their use during recent years, in all sections of the United States has given satisfactory relief in many thousands of cases.

Lederle literature on the various pollen antigens of the United States may help you solve some of your troublesome cases.

Specify Lederle

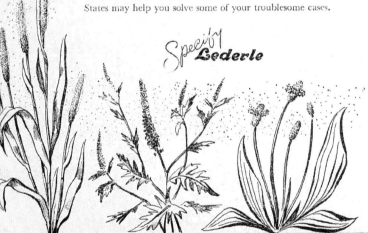

• *THE PRESIDENT'S PAGE* •

At the Annual Congress on Medical Education and Licensure held in Chicago, February 15 and 16, an outstanding program was presented. Through the cooperation of the Council on Medical Education and Hospitals of the American Medical Association and The Federation of State Medical Boards, this meeting has constantly grown in stature and importance until it has reached a place of prominence rivaled by no other like meeting. Physicians and hospital owners and administrators receive great benefit from the knowledge and experience gained by the exchange of ideas and the approaches being made to the problems of medical education and licensure.

The practice of medicine and its effect upon the health of the nation is fully dependent upon the leadership developed in meetings such as these. Leadership thus developed must be conservative; it must withstand the panzer attacks of theorists who would promulgate untried procedures and schemes for the educating and licensing of physicians.

In the present emergency certain changes must be made to meet certain demands, but to accomplish this end there must be no disposition on the part of those in authority to create physicians who are not qualified to accept the responsibilities of the physician either in civil or military life. American health has been brought to its present high plane mainly by reason of the safeguards that have been developed in the field of the healing arts with reference to the standards of medical education and licensure. To sacrifice this attainment would be folly.

Medicine today has assumed the responsibility of protecting the health of the public, and it will achieve its goal if unhampered by governmental interference and with aggressive leadership from within its own ranks. Now is the time for the American Medical Association to act. It must be ready to assume the leadership in medical economics as well as scientific medicine.

May I urge every delegate to the Annual Meeting of the Oklahoma State Medical Association House of Delegates to be giving careful and earnest thought to the medical problems of the day. Let those thoughts not only cover scientific medicine, but the field of economics. In this day and age one is as important as the other.

Sincerely yours,

James D. Osborn

President.

The JOURNAL Of The
OKLAHOMA STATE MEDICAL ASSOCIATION

EDITORIAL BOARD

L. J. MOORMAN, Oklahoma City, Editor-in-Chief

E. EUGENE RICE, Shawnee   NED R. SMITH, Tulsa

MR. R. H. GRAHAM, Oklahoma City, Business Manager

CONTRIBUTIONS: Articles accepted by this Journal for publication including those read at the annual meetings of the State Association are the sole property of this Journal.

The Editorial Department is not responsible for the opinions expressed in the original articles of contributors.

Manuscripts may be withdrawn by authors for publication elsewhere only upon the approval of the Editorial Board.

MANUSCRIPTS: Manuscripts should be typewritten, double-spaced, on white paper 8½ x 11 inches. The original copy, not the carbon copy, should be submitted.

Footnotes, bibliographies and legends for cuts should be typed on separate sheets in double space. Bibliography listing should follow this order: Name of author, title of article, name of periodical with volume, page and date of publication.

Manuscripts are accepted subject to the usual editorial revisions and with the understanding that they have not been published elsewhere.

NEWS: Local news of interest to the medical profession, changes of address, births, deaths and weddings will be gratefully received.

ADVERTISING: Advertising of articles, drugs or compounds unapproved by the Council on Pharmacy of the A.M.A. will not be accepted. Advertising rates will be supplied on application.

It is suggested that members of the State Association patronize our advertisers in preference to others.

SUBSCRIPTIONS: Failure to receive The Journal should call for immediate notification.

REPRINTS: Reprints of original articles will be supplied at actual cost provided request for them is attached to manuscripts or made in sufficient time before publication. Checks for reprints should be made payable to Industrial Printing Company, Oklahoma City.

Address all communications to THE JOURNAL OF THE OKLAHOMA STATE MEDICAL ASSOCIATION, 210 Plaza Court, Oklahoma City.

OFFICIAL PUBLICATION OF THE OKLAHOMA STATE MEDICAL ASSOCIATION
Copyrighted March, 1943

EDITORIALS

MEDICAL-RED CROSS RELATIONSHIPS

A letter has been received from Albert McCown, M.D., Medical and Health Service Director, American Red Cross, Washington, D. C., announcing the appointment of Dr. G. Foard McGinnes as Director of the Medical and Health Service of the Midwestern Area with Headquarters in St. Louis.

The officers of county medical societies are urged to make note of this appointment and the availability of Dr. McGinnes for co-operation in Medical-Red Cross relationships. Dr. McGinnes comes to this post with a rich store of experience in the field of public health, and can be counted on for a broad and sympathetic response to all medical and health service problems.

This announcement should help renew our interest in the Red Cross with its world-wide resources, its individual and composit energies and activities devoted to the promotion of health, the prevention of disease and the welfare of mankind. In this world crisis when want and destruction, death and disease encircle the globe, it is well for doctors to remember that the primary purpose of the Red Cross is to take care of the wounded and the sick.

THE STATE MEETING

The members of the State Medical Association are urged to mark their calendar for the Annual State Meeting scheduled for May 11 and 12.

The program will be streamlined to meet the home front demands, and to prepare the doctor in civilian practice for military emergencies. When doctors are expected to do more with less, they must be succored with scientific assemblies. Considering the influence of civilian medicine on community health and the maintenance of manpower, no military school of indoctrination could be more important than the State Medical Association Meeting in time of war.

At home we must keep 'em well so the boys abroad can give 'em hell.

THE UNIVERSITY OF OKLAHOMA STUDENT HEALTH SERVICE

On September 1, 1942, Dr. W. A. Fowler, Director of the Student Health Service and Professor of Hygiene and Public Health at the University of Oklahoma, made a five year report of the activities of this service. It is regrettable that this report cannot be placed in the hands of every citizen in the State of Oklahoma. One of the most important features of this report is the unobstrusive revelation of the laudable spirit which has animated this service.

Because the report is of such vital interest to the medical profession, it is being reproduced in this issue of the Journal. With the aid of the student health service the family physician can follow the children of his patrons through this critical period of their development. With this in view, it is highly important that the scientific character of this service should inspire professional confidence, and warrant the family physician's approval. The parents of students realize the need of adequate guidance and health protection for their sons and daughters when they are launched upon their first independent adventure in the art of living. When the psychological moment arises, the family physician's assurances may quiet many parental misgivings.

As indicated in this report, the student health service should be psychosomatic. It should deal wisely with both the psychological and the physical. In other words, it should recognize the unity of body and mind, and impartially exhibit both the art and the science of medicine. If university students, representing the best of our citizenry, could have four years exposure to such a health service, they would be better fitted for the age old battle of life, and the position of the medical profession would be correspondingly elevated.

Considering the financial and physical handicaps under which the present staff has labored, it is remarkable that so much has been accomplished. Yet it is quite obvious that the service has not reached the high standard it should attain because of inadequate financial support. It is equally obvious that both the quality and the quantity of service now available must deteriorate unless adequate support is provided.

Legal opinion indicates that increased financial support can be negotiated only through the recommendation of the Board of Regents of Higher Education and legislative enactment. A letter addressed to the Board of Regents of Higher Education, State Capitol, should help initiate a plan for the necessary legislation. Every doctor in the state is urged to write such a letter and to communicate with his State Representative, stressing the importance of providing adequate salaries, equipment and maintenance for this service. When the average legislator is called upon to consider the overhead per capita investment in university education, he should readily realize that it is good business to protect this investment through the provision of good health and the consequent lowering of morbidity and mortality.

ALIEN PHYSICIANS

Attorney General Biddle announced on January 16, 1943, that the naturalization of alien physicians would be expedited because of the shortage of civilian doctors throughout the United States. Biddle stated that he had instructed the immigration service to hold hearings in advance of their regular order on the calendar in the cases of practicing alien physicians or aliens who would be qualified to practice if they were citizens.

The State of Oklahoma requires full citizenship before a license to practice medicine will be granted. All other states with the exception of seven, namely, Arizona, California, Florida, Indiana, Oregon, Tennessee and the District of Columbia, require citizenship or at least the granting of first papers as a pre-requisite for practice (fourteen states require only the filing of first papers).

Oklahoma is fortunate in this respect in being situated in the Middle West where alien physicians have never been a problem, but because of the depletion of the ranks of the physicians by the armed forces and the attitude of the administration, this state will soon be faced with a serious problem in this respect.

Alien physicians coming from the various medical schools in Europe with their varying premedical and medical requirements will create a serious problem with the various state boards unable to verify their qualifications due to the lack of availability of the records of the schools of graduation and internships of these physicians.

There are at present over 42,000 physicians in the armed forces of the United States, and the requirements for 1943 are said to be an additional 12,000. This number will represent about 75 per cent of the younger practicing physicians of the country. The physicians who have remained to care for the civilian population have the additional burden of caring for the work of teir absent colleagues, which they gladly and willingly have assumed.

The physicians in the armed forces have given up their private practices, left their homes, their families, their economic security, so that this war may be won as quickly as possible. Few other professions or trades have made such sacrifices as the physician, with his ten to fifteen years of specialized training, the difficulty in establishing his practice, and his attempt to secure his own social security without government subsidy.

It is the duty of the physicians who remain at home to secure and maintain the same excellent standards of private practice so the men serving their country will be able to return to their patients and practices in the same location with a minimum of adjustment and not find their places in the community filled by alien physicians.

It is felt that the best way to maintain the practice of these men is to render the best possible medical care to the people who are dependent upon the physicians remaining, and not by flooding the country with a group of alien, probably poorly qualified, physicians.

Every physician remaining is more than willing to do an even greater amount of work, spend more hours in practice and in the clinics, forego the usual vacations, and resume general practice at the expense of his specialty if necessary, to assure these men that there will be something worth while to which they can return.

The move to flood the country with alien physicians, who are definitely not needed at this time, should be opposed in every way by the profession.—E.E.R., M.D.

OCCUPATIONAL DERMATITIS

In this issue of the Journal there is a timely article on "Industrial Dermatoses." In connection with this subject, attention is called to the following statement by Warren F. Draper,* Assistant to the Surgeon General:

"Recently we conducted a two-week course in occupational dermatitis, which was attended by twenty-two leading physicians from every part of the country. The formal lectures were followed by visits to various war plants. We believe that when these doctors return home, they will be better equipped —not only to help themselves, but also to pass along some of the experience they have gained. Since more time is lost from work because of occupational dermatitis than because of any other occupational disease, we are certain that our course is a big step in the right direction."

*An address given before the Round Table on Health in Industry, Associated Industries of Massachusetts, Boston, October 29, 1942.

War Production Board Order Affects Vitamin Capsules

To conserve vitamin A supplies during wartime, W.P.B. order L-40 limits the content of capsules to 5,000 vitamin A units.

In compliance with this order, capsules of Mead's Oleum Percomorphum 50 per cent With Viosterol now contain 83 mg. of oil, equivalent to 5,000 vitamin A units and 700 vitamin D units per capsule.

The new size capsule is now supplied in boxes containing 48 and 192 capsules — about twice the number of capsules without increase in price.

THE LIBRARY OF THE TULSA COUNTY MEDICAL SOCIETY

VENETA R. BARLOW, LIBRARIAN

TULSA, OKLAHOMA

The Tulsa County Medical Society believes that the successful doctor of medicine must read; he must continually supplement his knowledge with the knowledge of others who are now and who have been in years past interested in his subject. The Society believes that this need of the modern physician can best be met by a library to which all members contribute; that a group of doctors can build a greater repository of scientific knowledge than can one doctor alone.

For study and discussion a few farsighted physicians in 1932 organized the Journal Club and subscribed to a handful of periodicals, which was really the beginning of the Tulsa County Medical Library. Through persistent personal effort, they sustained during dark days and lean years their growing orphan.

It was, indeed, an orphan, suffering all the pains of young institutions, until 1941, when Dr. J. C. Brogden, the incoming President of the Medical Society, made the improvement of the Library and its facilities the principal project of the year ahead. Subsequently, in August of the same year it was accredited by the Medical Library Association. Since then it has expanded in size to more than 3,000 volumes, and is receiving the support of a constantly increasing endowment fund.

Not all of these volumes have come by slow accumulation, for among them are the gifts of three notable private libraries; namely, the valuable books of Dr. Paul R. Brown, donated by Dr. Paul R. Brown, III, in memory of his distinguished father; the Library of Dr. Gary Garabedian, considered by many the finest library pertaining to pediatrics in Tulsa, donated by Mrs. Garabedian as a memorial to her late husband; and the Library of Dr. Gregory S. Wall, donated by Dr. Wall after his retirement from practice. The last comprises hundreds of books on surgery.

The 3,000 volumes are classified in sections pertaining to internal medicine, obstetrics, gynecology, dermatology, neurology, psychiatry, radiology, pediatrics, ophthalmology, otolaryngology, urology and surgery. A new section on medical history, biography and autobiography is developing rapidly. Of importance also, are the bound volumes of sixty current journals each of which has been bound into one, two or three volumes a year, as the case may be. The Journal of the American Medical Association is complete from the year 1911 to date, and the Annals of Surgery from 1907 to date.

Of interest to the antiquarian is the collection of old books published before 1850. Among these are "The Practice of Physic" by William Cullen, M.D., published in 1792 by Parry Hall, Philadelphia; "The New Domestic Medicine or a Treatise on the Prevention and Cure of Diseases" by William Buchan, M.D., published in 1809 by Thomas Kelly, London, England; "Medical Inquiries and Observations" by Benjamin Rush, M.D., pubilshed at Philadelphia in 1818; "Treatment of Children" by William DeWees, M.D., published at Philadelphia in 1829; "The Principles and Practice of Obstetrics, Medicine and Surgery, in Reference to the Process of Parturition" by Francis H. Ramsbotham, M.D., published in 1849 by Lea and Blanchard at Philadelphia.

The Library seeks to serve the profession in every way possible. It observes regular hours, from nine until five, Monday through Friday, and from nine until one o'clock on Saturday, with evening and Sunday privileges, if circumstances warrant; it assembles bibliographies at the request of a member of the profession; it loans books and periodicals for a period of ten days with extension privileges upon request under certain conditions; it loans current issues of periodicals for over night or for a week end; it secures any book or periodical, either domestic or foreign, on loan from any other Medical Library within a few days time, without cost to the borrower, other than express or postage; it has the privilege of Micro-film service from the Army Medical Library, when volumes are too bulky for shipping; it maintains a file of duplicate material, which last year supplied 365 pieces of medical literature to 56 other libraries, including one each in China, Puerto Rico and Canada; it publishes in the Bulletin of the Tulsa County Medical Society, an informative page, pertaining to gifts, reviews and announcements regarding the Library; it aids in the preparation of any scientific paper, at the request of a physician.

The facilities of the Library are available not only to more than 200 regular members of the medical profession in the Tulsa area, but to the Medical Divisions connected with the various Military Service units in, and near Tulsa. Also to laymen having proper credentials, attorneys, club women, teachers and pre-medic students.

The Library, which occupies the long west side of the 12th floor of the Medical and Dental Arts Building in Tulsa, has an atmosphere of quiet charm which is conducive to thought and study. Much of this charm is due largely to Dr. H. B. Stewart, who as

President, guided the Society through the year 1942, and to the Auxiliary to the Tulsa County Medical Society, who have made the Library pleasant as well as useful. Easy chairs, growing plants and cheerful windows enhance the appearance of the two long rooms.

The Tulsa County Medical Library is one of an increasing number of medical libraries in the United States, which are maintained by county medical societies. It is the only public medical library in the State of Oklahoma other than the one connected with the Medical School at the State University. A pioneer of sturdy growth, it has set for itself and seeks to maintain, a high standard of service to Tulsa County and to the State.

A DOCTOR'S PLEA IN WARTIME

The doctor's life, in times like these,
Is not exactly one of ease.

For, on the home front, each M.D.
Is busier than any bee!

He's shouldering the burden for
The other docs, who've gone to war.

This leaves your doctor precious little
Time to sit around and whittle.

And indicates the reason why
You ought to help the poor old guy.

HOW?

1. By keeping yourselves in the best of condition
   Thus avoiding the ills that demand a physician.
2. By phoning him promptly when illness gives warning,
   But - unless very serious—waiting till morning.
3. By cheerfully taking whatever appointment
   He makes for prescribing his pills or his ointment.
4. By calling on him where he works or resides
   Instead of insisting he rush to your sides.
   (Of course, he'll come 'round when there's need for his service
   But spare him the trip when you're nothing but nervous.)
5. And, last but not least, you can help in this crisis
   By carefully following Doctor's advices.

If these commandments you'll adhere to
A doctor's heart you will be dear to!

1943 MEETINGS CANCELLED

Notice has been issued of the cancellation of two annual meetings due to the war conditions. The American Urological Association June meeting scheduled for St. Louis has been cancelled, and also the American College of Chest Physicians meeting which was scheduled to be held jointly with the annual session of the American Medical Association in San Francisco.

ASSOCIATION ACTIVITIES

FIFTY-FIRST ANNUAL MEETING MAY 11, 12—OKLAHOMA CITY

As announced in the February issue of the Journal, the Annual Meeting of the Association will be held in Oklahoma City at the Skirvin Hotel on May 11 and 12.

The Scientific Work Committee is preparing a full two day program, using Oklahoma and Army and Navy physicians as speakers. The program is being planned to coincide with the present war needs as related to medical and health problems.

Section meetings will be held during both days, and four formal papers will be presented. An innovation will be round-table discussions during the noon hour for the purpose of discussing the section papers presented in the morning.

The Council will meet Monday afternoon, and the House of Delegates Monday evening and Tuesday and Wednesday mornings. On Tuesday evening the Army and Navy will present a scientific program, which will be preceded by a buffet dinner; and on Wednesday evening will be the President's inaugural dinner-dance.

The complete program of the meeting will be carried in the April Journal.

DR. J. D. OSBORN NOMINATED FOR PLACE ON NATIONAL BOARD OF MEDICAL EXAMINERS

Dr. J. D. Osborn, Frederick, President of the Association and Secretary of the Oklahoma State Board of Medical Examiners, was one of three physicians to be nominated by the Federation of State Medical Boards at its annual meeting in Chicago on February 16, for membership on the National Board of Medical Examiners.

That Dr. Osborn should be accorded this honor will come as no surprise to the medical profession of this state who have seen his efficient work as secretary of the Oklahoma Board of Examiners during the past nine years.

Governor E. W. Marland first appointed Dr. Osborn to the Board of Examiners, and he has served continuously since that time. While his many friends may believe that his first insight to the problems of medical licensure came with his appointment to the Board the record will prove otherwise. His father and his brother, Bryce E. Osborn of Cleburne, Texas, both served as secretaries of the Texas State Board of Examiners, and it was through this early association that he first came in contact with medical licensure problems.

Should Dr. Osborn be elected by the National Board of Medical Examiners to membership, it will be the first time an Oklahoma physician has been so honored.

ECONOMICS COMMITTEE MEETS WITH FARM SECURITY ADMINISTRATION OFFICIALS

The Economics Committee of the Association held a meeting on February 28 with officials of the Farm Security Administration and the Oklahoma Hospital Association for the purpose of discussing medical and hospital care for the recipients of F.S.A. assistance.

In attendance at the meeting, in addition to representatives of the Medical and Hospital Associations and the F.S.A., were Mr. N. D. Helland, Director of Blue Cross for Oklahoma, and Mr. Virgil Bishop and Mr. Glenn Gabbard of the same organization.

The Committee was advised by the representatives of F.S.A. that about 20,000 families in Oklahoma are receiving assistance, and that about the same number were on the rolls in 1941-42. In Oklahoma 29 counties, in cooperation with county medical societies, are operating some kind of medical plan with a variance of success.

Following a general and comprehensive discussion of the problem of medical and hospital care, it was agreed that the F.S.A. representatives should consult further with the Blue Cross Plan of Oklahoma in an attempt to use its facilities to give hospital care to the F.S.A. clients, and if such a plan were successful, additional study would be given to the medical phase of the program.

INSTITUTE ON WARTIME INDUSTRIAL HEALTH HELD IN TULSA MARCH 18, OKLAHOMA CITY MARCH 19

Approximately 400 physicians and industrial plant managers attended the Institute on Wartime Industrial Health held in Tulsa and Oklahoma City on March 18 and 19.

The Institute, sponsored by the Postgraduate and the Industrial and Traumatic Committees of the Association in cooperation with the State Health Department, brought the following outstanding medical authorities to Oklahoma for the two day session: J. J. Bloomfield, Sanitary Engineer, U. S. Public Health Service, Bethesda, Maryland; Carl Peterson, M.D., Executive Secretary, Council on Industrial Health, American Medical Association, Chicago; Adolph Kammer, M.D., Medical Director, Inland Steel Company, Hammond, Indiana; Clarence D. Selby, M.D., Medical Director, General Motors Corporation, Detroit, Michigan; A. G. Hewitt, General Superintendent, The Visking Company, Chicago; Louis Schwartz, M.D., Medical Director U. S. Public Health Service, Bethesda, Maryland.

That the Institutes were of such outstanding success clearly points out the sincere and intelligent approach being made by both the medical profession and industry to a common problem; namely, absenteeism due to illness and injury which could be prevented or kept to a minimum through cooperation and scientific planning.

Oklahoma physicians and industrial representatives participating in the program included: H. C. Weber, M.D., Bartlesville; G. F. Mathews, M.D., Commissioner, State Health Department, Oklahoma City; V. C. Myers, M.D., Industrial Hygiene Physician, State Health Department, Oklahoma City; E. C. Warkentin, Industrial Venereal Disease Control Division, State Health Department, Oklahoma City; Eugene A. Gillis, M.D., Director Venereal Disease Control Division, State Health Department, Oklahoma City; Frank P. Bertram, D.D.S., Dental Service, State Health Department, Oklahoma City; E. J. O'Connor, Executive Vice President, Associated Industries of Oklahoma, Oklahoma City; Paul Pugh, Commissioner, Oklahoma State Industrial Commission, Oklahoma City; Earl D. McBride, M.D., Oklahoma City; J. S. Chalmers, M.D., Sand Springs, Oklahoma; J. C. Peden, M.D., Tulsa; Barton T. Sibole, Executive Vice President Stanolind Pipe Line Company, Tulsa; Henry H. Turner, M.D., Oklahoma City; R. A. Hefner, Mayor of Oklahoma City.

The doctor* oughta
know about this...

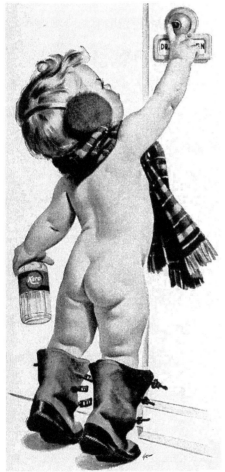

WITH an empty Karo bottle, the baby has a right to complain. And perhaps, Doctor, so have you. We admit that occasionally grocers do not have Karo syrup.

The situation is this: The great demand for Karo by the armed forces and a huge increase in domestic needs so tax our capacity that we are not always able to keep all grocers supplied.

We cannot step up quantity any further without letting down on quality and this we will *never* do.

If any patient complains that she is unable to obtain Karo for her babies, please tell her to write us direct, giving us the name and address of her grocer and we will promptly take steps to provide this grocer with Karo.

CORN PRODUCTS REFINING COMPANY
17 Battery Place, New York, N. Y.

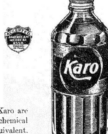

* INCIDENTALLY, Doctor, Red Label Karo and Blue Label Karo are interchangeable in standard feeding formulas. Their chemical composition is practically identical; their caloric values are equivalent. So if your patients cannot get the flavor you prescribe, please suggest that either Blue or Red Label may be used.

A. M. A. HOUSE OF DELEGATES MEETS JUNE 7

The House of Delegates of the American Medical Association will meet in Chicago, June 7. The meeting will take the place of the ninety-fourth annual session originally scheduled for San Francisco.

Cancellation of the annual session is the third in A.M.A. history, the other two being in 1861 and 1862 during the Civil War.

ASSOCIATE MEMBERSHIPS TO BE ACTED UPON AT ANNUAL MEETING

At the 1942 Annual Session the By-Laws of the Association were amended to provide for associate membership.

Under this amendment three applications have been received in the office of the Association for presentation to the House of Delegates. The Pottawatomie County Medical Society has proposed for associate membership Dr. David W. Gillick of Shawnee, and the Council of the Association will offer the name of Dr. Louis A. Turley of the University of Oklahoma School of Medicine. The Muskogee-Sequoyah-Wagoner County Medical Society will submit the name of Dr. S. G. Mollica of Muskogee.

WESTERN CHARITY HOSPITAL SUPERINTENDENT APPOINTED

Dr. James O. Asher, formerly Resident Physician at Wesley hospital in Oklahoma City, has been appointed by the State Board of Affairs as Superintendent of the Western Oklahoma Charity hospital at Clinton. Dr. Asher has moved his residence to Clinton, and has assumed his duties there.

DR. EUGENE A. GILLIS TO TEXAS

Dr. Grady F. Mathews, Commissioner of Health, has announced that Dr. Eugene A. Gillis, who for the last four years has been Venereal Disease Officer for the State Health Department on loan from the United States Public Health Service, has been transferred to the State of Texas. Dr. Gillis will report to Austin, Texas, on April 1.

During Dr. Gillis' stay in Oklahoma he has appeared before the majority of the county medical societies in the interest of venereal disease control, and his contribution in his specialized field has been exceptionally meritorius.

Dr. John Cowan, who at the present time is health officer for Sioux City, Iowa, will succeed Dr. Gillis.

POTTAWATOMIE COUNTY SOCIETY ANALYZES MEMBERSHIP

An interesting breakdown of the physicians of Pottawatomie County as related to membership of the County Medical Society has been received in the office of the Association. It is suggested that perhaps if other county societies would follow a like procedure, they might be able to increase their membership by knowing who to interest in society affairs.

The breakdown as reported by Dr. Clinton Gallaher, secretary of the society, is as follows:

1. Regular active membership in the Pottawatomie County Medical Society: Out of town—8, Shawnee residents—18.

2. Members in the armed forces: Regular—2, Associate—1.

3. Associate members—1.

4. Honorary members—2.

5. Other classifications (transfers have been requested, dues unpaid because of sickness, etc.)—6.

6. Other medical doctors in the county not members of the Society—4.

SCHEDULES FOR TWENTY WAR SESSIONS ANNOUNCED BY AMERICAN COLLEGE OF SURGEONS

New developments in military and civilian medical and hospital service will be brought to members of the medical profession at large, and hospital representatives, through a series of twenty War Sessions, beginning March 1, to be held throughout the United States under the sponsorship of the American College of Surgeons with the cooperation of other medical organizations and of the Federal medical services.

Each War Session will consist of an all-day program, lasting from 9:00 o'clock A.M. to 10:00 P.M., including luncheon and dinner conferences. Nationally known representatives of the United States Army, the United States Navy, the United States Office of Civilian Defense, the United States Procurement and Assignment Service, and the United States Public Health Service, will address the meetings and will lead discussions, in addition to participation by prominent leaders in civilian medical practice and hospital service.

Topics to be discussed relating to military medicine will include care of the ill and injured in combat zones and after evacuation. The newer types of injuries encountered in this war, such as crush and blast injuries, will be especially considered, together with prevention and treatment of infections, and treatment of burns, shock, and injuries of specific parts of the body. Anesthesia, plastic surgery, and the psychoneuroses of war, will be some of the other topics. Problems of civilian medical care in wartime which will be discussed will include the responsibilities of individual doctors and hospitals; personnel problems of hospitals; organization of emergency medical services; maintaining adequate supplies, furnishings, and equipment; maintenance of high standards of medical and nursing education, and of hospital service in general; hospital public relations; and administrative adjustments in professional staffs of hospitals. The opening meeting of each session will be devoted to discussion of "Medical and Surgical Aspects of Chemical Warfare," led by a representative of the United States Office of Civilian Defense, and the closing meeting will be a panel discussion on problems in wartime civilian medical practice. Some of the topics for consideration at this meeting will be endemic and epidemic diseases, including tropical diseases; medical services in industry; medical and surgical practice; and supplementary postgraduate education for medical officers and civilian doctors.

The session scheduled for Oklahoma and vicinity will be held in Kansas City, Missouri, at the President Hotel on Thursday, April 1.

AMERICAN PUBLIC HEALTH ASSOCIATION CONFERENCE ANNOUNCED

The Executive Board of the American Public Health Association announces that the Association will sponsor a three-day Wartime Public Health Conference in New York City, October 12, 13 and 14. The 72nd Annual Business Meeting of the Association will be held in connection with it.

The Conference program will be devoted exclusively to wartime emergency problems as they affect public health and the public health profession.

BOARD OF OPHTHALMOLOGY EXAMINATIONS ANNOUNCED

Announcement has been made that the 1943 examinations of the American Board of Ophthalmology will be held in New York City on June 4 and 5, and in Chicago on October 8 and 9. Candidates will be required to appear for examination on two successive days. Formal application blanks may be secured from Dr. John Green, Secretary, 6830 Waterman Avenue, St. Louis, Missouri.

NINETEENTH LEGISLATURE WORKING TO CLOSE

The nineteenth session of the legislature is tentatively scheduled to complete its work by the first week in April. If this can be accomplished, it will be one of the shortest sessions on record.

In the field of health legislation the session has been exceptionally free from bills that would tend to act in a detrimental manner to public health. House Bill 222 introduced at the request of the State Board of Medical Examiners, and having the support of the Public Policy Committee of the Association, has passed the House, and from all indications will receive successful consideration in the Senate. This bill, which would authorize the Board of Examiners to review its own actions with reference to suspension and revocation of physician's license, should receive the support of the entire profession.

The venereal disease control measures, House Bills 37, 38 and 39, which have had a stormy time in the House, have had a variance of success. House Bill 39, which gives a broader definition to prostitution, has become law; while House Bills 37 and 38 have been rewritten and combined into one measure, which is now known as House Bill 37. In redrafting the bill, the conference committee deleted that part of the bill which would have given public health officials the right to quarantine any person having a venereal disease.

The Parent-Teachers Association sponsored immunization bill (House Bill 175), which would make it unlawful for all persons attending public schools to do so unless immunized against smallpox and diphtheria, was amended in committee to exclude those persons having religious beliefs in conflict with the provisions of the bill. The measure is now on third reading and final passage in the House, with a splendid chance of becoming law. Physicians should give their individual attention to this measure and consult their Representative and Senator on this important piece of health legislation.

Senate Bill 98, which would give the physician the right to take a viable baby from a dead mother who had met accidental death, though performed without the consent of those in whom the law has recognized as having a legal right of possession of the body of the deceased, has passed the Senate and is now before the House for action.

Senate Bill 56, the only measure so far introduced in the legislature that has been deemed by the Public Policy Committee to be not in the best interests of the public, it still in the Senate Committee on Public Welfare and Sanitation. Since the measure would establish and recognize the practice of Naturopathy in Oklahoma, there is a possibility that public hearings will be held in the near future to discuss the necessity of such an act. No doubt your representative in the legislature would appreciate the advice of the profession on this bill.

There is no doubt that the committees of the legislature considering health legislation in this session have been more keenly aware of the problems involved than any other like committees in recent years.

Medical School and Hospital Appropriations

Appropriations for the Medical School and its teaching hospitals together with all eleemosynary institutions have had sympathetic consideration from not only the legislature, but also Governor Kerr. The Governor, while attempting to keep appropriations at a minimum, has felt keenly the needs of the medical school and the hospitals of the state. While at the time of going to press the Appropriations Committee had not made its final recommendations, there is every reason to believe there will be substantial increases in the budget of these institutions.

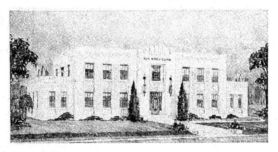

NEWS FROM THE COUNTY SOCIETIES

The Muskogee, Sequoyah, Wagner County Medical Society met February 1, at 8:00 P.M., at the Oklahoma Baptist Hospital in Muskogee with 16 members in attendance. Dr. Lawrence McAlister presented a paper on "Cancer of the Cornea," and Dr. H. T. Ballantine discussed "An Interesting Case Report."

The next meeting will be a buffet dinner on March 1, at 7:00 P.M. in the Officers' Club at the Sever's Hotel in Muskogee. Dr. James D. Osborn, President, and Dr. James Stevenson, President-Elect of the Oklahoma State Medical Association, have been invited as special guests.

A motion picture on "Syphilis" sponsored by the State Health Department was presented by Dr. E. A. Gillis, and Dick Graham, Executive Secretary of the State Medical Association, spoke on "War Manpower" at the meeting of the Woods County Medical Society at Alva on January 26. The program was preceeded by a dinner. Guests present included Dr. G. F. Mathews, State Commissioner of Health, and Dr. John L. Day, Superintendent of the Western Oklahoma Hospital at Supply.

A special film sponsored by John Wyeth and Brother will be presented and discussed at the next meeting in Alva on March 30, at 7:30 P.M. Other guests and speakers will also be present.

Dr. L. E. Silverthorn presented a paper on "The Indications For the Use of Blood Plasma" at the meeting of the Payne County Medical Society held at Stillwater on February 15. General discussion followed on the actual technique of making a blood plasma bank.

The next meeting will be in Cushing on March 18, when Dr. C. W. Moore will report on County Health Department activities. Dr. R. E. Waggoner will also discuss the Farm Security Program.

The Tri-County Medical Society composed of Jefferson, Stephens and Cotton Counties met for a chicken dinner and program at Dawson Hall in Waurika on February 9.

The program was opened by an address by Senator Charles Storms, Editor of the Waurika News. Dr. W. E. Crump of Wichita Falls, Texas, then presented a paper on "Diagnosis of Pelvic Conditions," which was followed by discussion. A paper, followed by discussion, on "Some Urological Conditions Found in General Practice" was given by Dr. J. R. Reagan, also of Wichita Falls.

The 1943 officers of the Pontotoc County Medical Society were installed by Dr. Clinton Gallaher of Shawnee at a meeting of that Society on February 13. The officers installed were: Dr. O. H. Miller, President; Dr. W. H. Lane, Vice-President; Dr. R. H. Mayes, Secretary-Treasurer.

Dr. G. S. Baxter of Shawnee was the invited guest speaker, and had prepared a paper on "Thoracoplasty in Tuberculosis," but was unable to be present because of illness. Dr. Clinton Gallaher, however, read the paper for Dr. Baxter. Dr. P. V. Annadown of Sulphur discussed the subject of "Artificial Pneumothorax."

Forty-five members were present at the meeting of the Osage County Medical Society in Pawhuska on February 8.

The guest speaker for the evening was Dr. Nelse F. Oekerblad of Kansas City, Missouri, whose topic was "Urology for the General Practitioner." His talk was followed by round-table discussion.

The next meeting of the Society will be in Pawhuska on March 8.

"Injuries to the Eyes" was the subject selected for presentation by Dr. Donald V. Crane of Tulsa for the meeting of the Ottawa County Medical Society at the Baptist Hospital in Miami on January 21.

A regular business meeting followed the program, and refreshments were served by the Miami Baptist Hospital.

The inaugural dinner-dance for the new president and officers of the Oklahoma County Medical Society was held at the Biltmore Hotel on January 23 in Oklahoma City.

Dr. R. Q. Goodwin, retiring president, reviewed the accomplishments of his administration, giving credit to his officers and board members. The incoming president, Dr. Walker Morledge, introduced his officers and new board members, and expressed his gratitude for the honor bestowed upon him by electing him to the presidency of the organization.

The speaker of the evening was Mr. L. Clark Schilder, Warden of the Federal Reformatory at El Reno.

The Garvin County Medical Society met on February 15 in Pauls Valley with 15 members in attendance. The program was devoted to the post-graduate lecture on Internal Medicine by Dr. L. W. Hunt.

At a meeting of the Craig County Medical Society on February 16 at Vinita, a resolution was passed lauding the life of Dr. Louis Bagby who passed away on February 15.

The current project of the Okmulgee-Okfuskee Medical Society is the establishment of a blood plasma bank to serve those two counties. At a dinner meeting of the Society held in Henryetta at the Georgian Hotel on February 8, the entire program was devoted to that subject.

A sound picture, "Blood Plasma Bank," was presented by Mr. Frank G. Couper of the Frank G. Couper Surgical Supplies, Inc., of Tulsa. Dr. A. Ray Wiley, Tulsa, spoke on the subject of "Shock and Certain Other Conditions in Which Blood Palsma is Used."

A motion picture in color, "Peptic Ulcer," was shown at the dinner meeting of the Garfield County Medical Society at the Youngblood Hotel in Enid on February 25. The guest speaker for the evening was Dr. Wendell Long, Oklahoma City, whose subject was "Ovarian Dysfunction."

The next scheduled meeting for the Society will be at the Youngblood Hotel in Enid on March 25, at 6:45 P.M.

Lieutenant R. L. Alexander, formerly of Okmulgee, has recently been transferred from the Induction Center, Oklahoma City, to Company C, 50th Medical Battalion, Camp Maxey, Texas.

Lieutenant Joe H. Coley, M.C., U.S.N.R., of Oklahoma City reports his present address as U.S.M.C. Unit No. 1025, care Postmaster, San Francisco, Calif.

WOMEN'S AUXILIARY NEWS

The Women's Auxiliary to the Oklahoma State Medical Association will hold its annual convention on May 11and 12 in Oklahoma City, during the convention of the Oklahoma State Medical Association. A complete program of the convention will be carried in the next issue of the Journal. Mrs. Henry H. Turner of Oklahoma City is our Convention Chairman.

Oklahoma County

The Oklahoma County Medical Auxiliary met at 10 o'clock on January 27 in the Venetian Room of the Y.W.C.A., and sewed on layettes, which were placed at the disposal of the city hospitals for mothers who need them. Hostesses for the day were Mrs. Carroll M. Pounders, Mrs. R. L. Murdock, Mrs. R. H. Akin, and Mrs. Hugh Galbraith. The meeting closed at 12:30 o'clock, with 35 present. Mrs. Floyd Keller presided.

The special project of this Auxiliary for this year, in addition to the sewing, is the meeting of the troop trains on the third Friday of each month and serving the boys gum, candy and cigarettes. Of 32 members interviewed, it was found they have averaged over one hundred hours each in war service. This includes first aid, nutrition, home nursing, canteen, red cross surgical dressing, knitting and sewing, C.D.V.O., Motor Corps, troop transit, and U. S. O. Mrs. R. O. Early tops the list with 800 hours, and she is still going strong.

Pottawatomie County

The Pottawatomie County Medical Auxiliary met on January 27, 1943, with seven members present. An election of officers was held, and the following new officers were elected: Mrs. C. C. Young, President; Mrs. John Carson, Vice-President; Mrs. Chas. Haygood, Secretary-Treasurer; Mrs. J. W. Byrum, Historian. This Auxiliary has been actively supporting the Nursery School and has placed Hygeia in all of the city schools.

LeFlore County

We regret that the Le Flore County Medical Auxiliary has been forced to disband for the duration of the war. Inasmuch as several of the members are obliged to drive a number of miles to the meetings, and due to the gasoline rationing and tire shortage, it is impossible for this Auxiliary to continue at this time.

Tulsa County

Lieutenant Commander S. Charlton Shepard is now in service with the United States Navy at Memphis, Tennessee. Mrs. Shepard and their daughter, Charlotte, have accompanied him.

Captain F. D. Sinclair has been transferred from Fort Sam Houston, Texas, to Memphis, Tennessee, where he is in charge of the new Obstetrical Division of the Kennedy General Hospital. Mrs. Sinclair and their two sons are now making their home with him in Memphis.

Mrs. Charles H. Eads and her children, Mary Carolyn and Charles Henry, Jr., have left for Riverside, California, where they will join Captain Eads, who is stationed at March Field.

We report with regret the death of Mrs. Fred W. Insull, the mother of Mrs. Gifford H. Henry, a member of the Tulsa County Medical Auxiliary.

The December issue of the Bulletin of the Woman's Auxiliary to the American Medical Association carried a poem from the West Virginia Club Woman, which we feel worthy of repetition here.

"Which Am I"

Are you an active member, the kind that would be missed?
Or are you just contented that your name is on the list?
Do you attend the meetings, and mingle with the flock,
Or do you stay at home and criticize and knock?
Do you take an active part and help the work along?
Or are you satisfied to be the kind that "just belong?"
Do you ever go to visit a member who is sick,
Or leave the work to just a few and talk about the clique?
So come to the meeting often and help with a hand and heart—
Don't just be a member, but take an active part.

New Red Cross Home Nursing Textbook Published

A new textbook on Red Cross Home Nursing, written in a simple, popular style, yet bearing the stamp of approval of the authorities in the fields of nursing, medicine and public health, has recently been published, according to Miss Mary Beard, Director of the American Red Cross Nursing Service. Prior to its publication, two million copies were ordered by the Red Cross for the use of homemakers, both old and young, masculine and feminine, in Red Cross home nursing classes throughout the country.

The new textbook will replace one which, though revised upon occasion, was written originally in 1913 by Jane A. Delano and Isabel McIsaac. The new textbook has been entirely prepared and brought up to date by Miss Lona Trott, R.N., B.S., Assistant Director of Health Education, Red Cross Nursing Service.

Bound in the familiar gray cover with red trimming, the publication is divided into four sections: "Health and Happiness in Home Life"; "How the Community Protects the Health of Home and Family"; "How to Take Care of Mother and Baby"; and "What to Do When Sickness Invades the Home." The book is priced at 60 cents and is illustrated with about 100 pictures and drawings, many of them helpful in teaching home-nursing procedures. It may be procured from any Red Cross chapter.

Dr. Frank M. King is presently stationed at the Station Hospital, Camp Gruber, Okla., having recently been transferred from Station Hospital, Fort Sill. Prior to entering the service, Dr. King was Director of Woodward and Harper County Health Units.

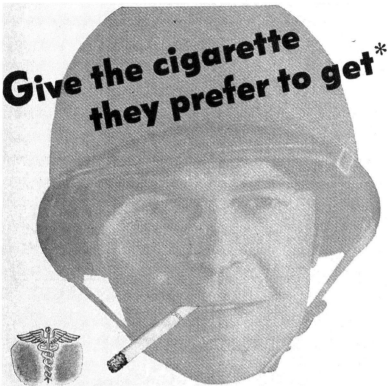

Give the cigarette they prefer to get*

IT'S EASY to understand why cigarettes are the preferred gift in the armed services. But did you know that among them the best-liked brand* of cigarette is Camel? Camel is the popular choice of millions and millions of smokers for its finer flavor and superior mildness.

Send Camels, the service man's favorite, to those friends or relatives who are fighting our battles —fighting them efficiently and unselfishly. Your thoughtfulness will be appreciated.

Tobacco stores feature Camels by the carton. See or telephone your dealer today.

Remember, you can *still* send Camels to Army personnel in the U. S., and to men in the Navy, Marines, or Coast Guard *wherever they are*. The Post Office rule against mailing packages applies only to those sent to the overseas Army.

* With men in the Army, the Navy, the Marine Corps, and the Coast Guard, the favorite cigarette is Camel. (Based on actual sales records in Post Exchanges and Canteens.)

Camel
costlier tobaccos

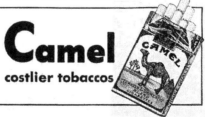

MEDICAL PREPAREDNESS

New Procurement and Assignment Survey to be Made

As announced in the February Journal, the Procurement and Assignment Service has requested a complete new survey be taken of the medical manpower of the nation for the purpose of determining the number of physicians available for both military service and dislocation in the field of civilian practice.

For the purpose of the survey the blank below will be utilized. During the month of March this blank will be mailed to every physician in the state, and it is the patriotic duty of every physician to immediately complete and return the questionnaire to the Procurement and Assignment Service, 210 Plaza Court, Oklahoma City.

Name.................... (Last) (First) (Middle)	Office street address........................ Home street address........................
Address.................... (City) (County)	
SEX: Female .... Male	RACE: White .... Negro .... Specify other	CITIZENSHIP: Citizen .... Alien	Country of birth .... Year of birth ....

MARITAL STATUS:

Single ....

Married, living with spouse ....

Married, living apart from spouse ....

Widowed, divorced, or legally separated ....

DEPENDENCY STATUS:

No dependents ....

Collateral dependents (ones other than spouse or child)

Spouse ....One child....................

2 children....................3 or more children....................

METHOD OF PRACTICE:

Individual ....Partnership ....

Group ....Intern ....

Resident ....Retired ....

Not in practice ....Other (specify) ....

APPOINTMENTS: (Official health agency, hospital, etc., specify)

TYPE OF WORK:	Full time	Part time
General practice		
Special practice		
Industrial practice		
Teaching		
Research		
Other (specify)		

SPECIALIZATION: (Name field of specialty or special interest if any) ....

MILITARY STATUS:	Date
Commissioned in Army	
Commissioned in Navy	
Rejected by Army	
Rejected by Navy	
Other (specify)	

Reference may be made to the Medical Preparedness page of the February Journal for an explanation of the method by which classification will be given the individual physician from the information given on the questionnaire.

Army's Recruiting Program Will Require 6,900 Physicians

Outline Of Procedure Reveals None Will Be
Commissioned Until Found Available By
Procurement And Assignment Service

The 1943 recruiting program of the Surgeon General of the Army calls for the commissioning of 6,900 physicians and approximately 3,000 hospital interns and residents, it is reported in The Journal of the American Medical Association for March 13 in an outline of the new procedure of processing physicians, dentists and veterinarians for the Army. The program also calls for the commissioning of 4,800 dentist sand 900 veterinarians.

Physicians will be procured from the following twenty states and the District of Columbia: California, Colorado, Connecticut, Illinois, Iowa, Maryland, Massachusetts, Minnesota, Missouri, Nebraska, Nevada, New Hampshire, New Jersey, New York, Ohio, Oregon, Pennsylvania, Rhode Island, Vermont and Wisconsin.

The following states have already contributed more physicians to the armed forces than the sum of their 1942 and 1943 quotas and will not be called on to furnish any more physicians, except interns and residents and except special cases for specific position vacancies, during 1943: Alabama, Arizona, Delaware, Georgia, Idaho, Kentucky, Louisiana, Mississippi, New Mexico, North Carolina, South Carolina, Tennessee, Texas, West Virginia and Wyoming.

It is stated that at present there will be no procurement of physicians, except interns and residents and in special cases for specific position vacancies, in those states not listed above. There will be no procurement of dentists, except special cases for specific position vacancies, in the following sixteen states: Alabama, Arizona, Arkansas, Delaware, Florida, Georgia, Kentucky, Louisiana, Mississippi, New Mexico, North Carolina, Oklahoma, South Carolina, Tennessee, Texas and Virginia.

At the present time there are no restrictions on the recruiting of veterinarians.

In the instructions issued by the Army it is pointed out that the Surgeon General has discontinued all medical officer recruiting boards and that under the new procurement program no physician, dentist or veterinarian will be commissioned in the armed forces of the United States until he has been declared "available" by the Procurement and Assignment Service of the War Manpower Commission.

In each state the Procurement and Assignment Service has set up three state chairmen: medical, dental and veterinary. Each of these prepares a monthly quota list of physicians, dentists and veterinarians who are apparently suitable and who are available, for commissioning in the Army of the United States. This list is submitted to the central office of the Procurement and Assignment Service which sends a communication inviting such individuals to apply for service with the armed forces. On the reply card enclosed with the invitation the individual states his preference for the Army, Navy or Medical Department of the Air Forces. These reply cards are sent by the potential applicants to the state chairmen of the Procurement and Assignment Service who in turn submit lists of such potential applicants to the Officer Procurement Service of the Army.

On receipts of such lists the officer procurement district office contacts the potential applicant and arranges for an interview regarding a commission.

Applicants will be requested by the officer procurement district office to complete all papers and take all steps required of them within fourteen days of the date of such request. If this is not complied with, a report thereon will be transmitted by the officer procurement district office to the state chairman of the Procurement and Assignment Service.

The decision as to the grade and appointment to be recommended for each candidate rests with the Surgeon General, not with the Officer Procurement Service.

DOCTORS ASKED TO HELP IN SURVEY TO LOCATE ALL GRADUATE NURSES

The physicians of the nation are being urged to cooperate in a survey being made to locate all graduate registered nurses in the country, The Journal of the American Medical Association points out in its March 13 issue. The Journal says:

"The National Nursing Council for War Service, which represents the voluntary, professional nursing organizations in the total war program, urges every physician in the country to lend his help and support to the current nationwide effort to locate all graduate registered nurses. A second national inventory of nurses, a follow-up on the inventory of 1941, was begun in January 1943. To date (February 25) responses from nearly 50 per cent of the nurses in the country have been reported. To help bring in responses from the remaining 50 per cent, physicians are asked to:

"1. Encourage the nurses who may be associated with them, especially the nurses in their employ, to respond without delay to the postcard questionnaires sent to them by the special state agent of the United States Public Health Service in January of this year.

"2. Urge nurses they may know who have not received questionnaires (many physicians' wives who are nurses have failed to receive them) to request cards from the special agent in their states. If they do not know the agents' address, the National Nursing Council for War Service, 1790 Broadway, New York, will forward their requests.

"Information provided by the inventory will furnish the basis of operation for the nursing supply and distribution unit now being formed in the War Manpower Commission. The purpose of the unit, as the name implies, is to determine the availability of nurses for local, state and national emergencies and to aid in the equitable distribution of nurses, so that the nursing needs of the armed forces and of civilians will be adequately met. This distribution will be on a voluntary, not a compulsory, basis. The inventory is being conducted by the United States Public Health Service and has the approval of the National Nursing Council for War Service, the War Manpower Commission and the Health and Medical Committee, Office of Defense Health and Welfare Services, Federal Security Agency."

University of Oklahoma School of Medicine

Dr. H. W. Brown, Dean, School of Public Health, University of North Carolina, Chapel Hill, North Carolina, and Professor of Public Health, Duke University, gave two lectures in the auditorium of the School of Medicine Building on Tuesday, March 16.

The expenses and honarium for these lectures are being furnished from a grant from the John and Mary R. Markle Foundation, and the arrangements are being made by the Vice Chairman of the Division of Medical Sciences, National Research Council.

Dr. Herbert B. Shields, Class of 1937, Major, M. C., has been decorated with the Silver Star for bravery during an attack on a Field Hospital in New Guinea.

In a recent communication from Colonel Rex Bolend, who is in command of the 21st Evacuation Hospital, he gives a detailed summary of the activities of this Unit.

The personnel of the Unit now consists of 46 officers, 42 nurses, and 326 enlisted men. Most of the officers are members of the faculty and staff of the School of Medicine and the University Hospitals, and the nurses have been recruited from the State of Oklahoma.

Dr. H. A. Shoemaker, Assistant Dean, attended the Annual Congress on Medical Education and Licensure of the American Medical Association, on February 15th and 16th, at the Palmer House in Chicago. He also attended a special meeting of the Executive Council of the Association of American Medical Colleges and representatives of the various schools of medicine.

• OBITUARIES •

Dr. Louis Bagby
1875-1943

The Craig County Medical Society met on February 16, 1943, and voted the following resolution in honor of our departed brother:

BE IT RESOLVED, That the death of our friend and brother, Dr. Louis Bagby, is a great loss to our Craig County Medical Society.

He came to Vinita in 1900 when he established a medical practice. He was a charter member of the Craig County Medical Society and a staunch supporter of the Society.

He has been a friend and advisor to all doctors of medicine, and his great success has been through his kindliness and pleasing personality.

We regret his loss very much, but he leaves with us a memory of a man who gave his life to reaching the pinnacle of success as a Christian gentleman, a scholarly physician and a friend to his fellow man.

Craig County Medical Society.

Dr. Jesse S. Little
1877-1943

Dr. Jesse S. Little passed away at his home in Minco on January 18. Dr. Little had practiced medicine in Minco for 30 years, and was one of the pioneer physicians of the county.

He was born at Fayetteville, Tennessee, and received his education at Fayetteville Institute, University of Tennessee Medical School, Kansas City Medical School and Fort Worth Medical School. He was given his M.D. degree in 1903, and began his practice in Minco during the same year.

Dr. Little is survived by his widow; his mother, Mrs. F. H. Little, Minco; two brothers, J. L. Little of Custer City and Dr. Aaron Little of Minco; and a sister, Mrs. Ellen Scott of Skellytown, Texas.

Dr. F. E. Rosenberger
1874-1943

Dr. F. E. Rosenberger was born in Greenview, Illinois, July 12, 1874. He was recently stricken with coronary thrombosis and died in the Polyclinic Hospital on February 8, 1943. Dr. Rosenberger was graduated from the Beaumont Medical College, St. Louis, Missouri, in 1901. Dr. Rosenberger has practiced medicine in Oklahoma since 1904. He was a member of the Oklahoma County and State Medical Associations, American Medical Association, Oklahoma County Sanity Board, Knights of Pythias and Masonic Lodges, and an elder in the Maywood Presbyterian Church.

Dr. Rosenberger is survived by his wife, Eliza Charlotte Rosenberger who lives at the family home, 3137 N. W. 22nd Street, Oklahoma City.

Dr. Rosenberger had a host of friends among the doctors and citizens of Oklahoma who mourn his passing.

Dr. F. A. DeMand
1892-1943

Dr. Francis Asbury DeMand was born in Kansas City in 1892, and died February 11, 1943. He came to Oklahoma City in 1914 when his father, Dr. John DeMand, a Methodist minister, accepted a pastorate here. In 1917 he was graduated from the University of Oklahoma Medical School and in the same year married Miss Ruth Newell, daughter of Judge Wm. Newell of Norman, Oklahoma.

Dr. DeMand served as a First Lieutenant in the Medical Corps during World War I, and spent 13 months in France in a base hospital.

He was a member of the Oklahoma County Medical Association, Oklahoma State Medical Association, American Medical Association, and of Phi Beta Pi, medical fraternity. He was a member of the University Sooner quartet while in school, and Phi Beta Pi male quartet.

Dr. DeMand will be remembered by his friends for his fine sense of humor, his winning smile and his willingness to sing whenever asked. He is survived by his wife and one son William Newell DeMand, a junior at Classen High School, one brother and four sisters.

Dr. W. M. Browning
1869-1943

Dr. W. M. Browning, pioneer physician of Jefferson County, passed away at the Medical Arts Hospital in Dallas, Texas, February 5. Dr. Browning had been in failing health for a number of years, but had kept up his office practice until about three weeks prior to his death.

Dr. Browning was born at Lewisburg, Kentucky in 1869. He was educated at Bethel College, Russelville, Kentucky, and received his medical education at Hospital College, Memphis, Tennessee, and at the Hospital College in Louisville, Kentucky.

He first began practice at Terral, Indian Territory, in 1897. Two years later he moved to Kemp, Texas, where he owned and operated a drug store and practiced medicine. In 1902 he moved to Hastings, Oklahoma, to practice medicine and in 1916 he located in Waurika where he has since practiced his profession.

He is survived by his widow; one daughter, Mrs. W. E. Peebles of Frederick; two brothers, Lem Browning, Merkle, Texas, and Merritt Browning, Perrytown, Texas; and one sister, Mrs. Duncan Briggs of Merkle, Texas.

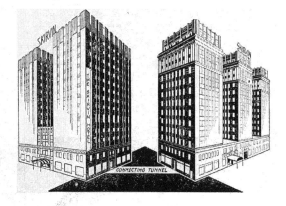

Office of Civilian Defense

PLASMA FOR CIVILIAN DEFENSE

The Medical Division of the Office of Civilian Defense and the United States Public Health Service report the current status of the blood plasma program which was initiated in the early spring.

The report indicates that 130 hospitals have now received grants-in-aid, and are preparing reserves of plasma to total at least 63,130 units. In addition to this reserve, 27,500 units of frozen plasma have been obtained through the Army and Navy from blood collected by the American Red Cross. This supply has been distributed. The Medical Division has also procured 37,500 units of dried plasma from blood collected by the American Red Cross, and this supply is in process of distribution. The total reserve, which is largely concentrated in the 300 mile coastal target areas, will be 126,630 units for treatment of casualties resulting from enemy action. In addition, 1,250 units are in Puerto Rico, and 250 in Alaska.

In addition to these sources of plasma, the Red Cross is distributing to target areas 5,000 units which will be available to the Office of Civilian Defense for treatment of civilian casualties resulting from enemy action. Many hospitals, which have not received grants under the OCD — U. S. Public Health Service program, are also preparing palsma reserves which total approximately 50,000 units.

The plasma required for the treatment of war-related injuries may be obtained by any community through its Chief of Emergency Medical Service. To meet such emergencies, plasma may be transferred: 1. Within a State by the State Chief of Emergency Medical Service,

2. Within a Region by the Regional Medical Officer, 3. From one Region to another by the Medical Division, U. S. Office of Civilian Defense.

Nineteen hospitals in Oklahoma are manufacturing blood plasma. Most of these hospitals have amounts of blood plasma that are available for Civilian Defense. The names and addresses of the hospital are as follows:

St. Mary's Hospital, 502 East Oklahoma, Enid; University Hospital Foundation, Enid; Chickasha Hospital and Clinic, Chickasha; Cottage Hospital, Chickasha; Ponca City Hospital, Ponca City; Oklahoma Baptist Hospital, Muskogee; St. Anthony Hospital, 601 W. 9th, Oklahoma City; University Hospital, 801 N. E. 13th, Oklahoma City; Wesley Hospital, 300 N. W. 12th, Oklahoma City; Osage County Infirmary, Pawhuska; Pawhuska City Hospital, 1800 Lynn Avenue, Pawhuska; American Hospital, Picher; Picher Hospital, Picher; Valley View Hospital, Ada; Claremore Indian Hospital, Claremore; Hillcrest Memorial Hospital, Tulsa; St. John's Hospital, Tulsa; Florence Hospital, Cordell; Memorial Hospital, 1504 Fourth St., Woodward.

In addition to the manufacturing of blood plasma in the nineteen hospitals of Oklahoma, U. S. Civilian Defense has stored within this state 500 units, 250 units stored with Dr. G. F. Mathews, State Chief of Emergency Medical Service, at Oklahoma City, and 250 cc's stored at Tulsa with Dr. D. L. Garrett.

Classified Advertisements

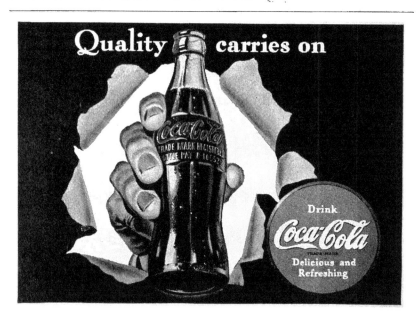

Blue Cross Reports

Mr. N. D. Helland, Executive Director of Group Hospital Service, attended the annual mid-winter conference of Blue Cross Plans in Chicago, February 8th, 9th and 10th.

Among the many distinguished speakers for the conference were Mr. James Hamilton, President of the American Hospital Association; R. H. Bishop, Jr., M.D., Chairman of the Approval Committee of the Hospital Service Plan Commission and Lewis H. Pink, President of Associated Hospital Service of New York City.

The central thought of the meeting this year, according to Mr .Helland, could be divided into three phases, namely: 1. The need for a national surgical plan. 2. The growing demand for national uniformity among the Blue Cross Plans. 3. The need for and methods of obtaining increased membership.

Due to the activities of commercial insurance companies in the field of hospital care placing emphasis on certain indemnities for surgical care, considerable discussion took place on the possibility of a non-profit surgical plan on a strictly cash basis. Blue Cross directors, generally speaking, were in accord in the belief that there is a definite need for such a plan to supplement the hospitalization program, which would be essentially the same in principle as those now being offered. A committee has been appointed to draft the details of such a plan, to be submitted to the 77 approved Blue Cross Plans at a future date for their individual consideration for acceptance.

Mr. Helland stated that the need for more uniformity, as regards the rates and benefits of Blue Cross Plans, is becoming increasingly needed due to the fact that more and more national organizations are enrolling their employees in this non-profit hospital service. A large percentage of the more than 150,000 firms that have co-operated with their employees by permitting pay-roll allotment operate in more than one state, and it is necessary that Blue Cross Plans work together to provide a more unified protection for the employees of these firms. Unified procedure will simplify the mechanics of handling the service of employees of national accounts, and the ever increasing enrollment has resulted in a demand for unified thinking and concerted action on the part of Blue Cross directors. A committee for "National Enrollment and Reciprocity" has been appointed, with John R. Mannix of Detroit as Chairman.

The Approval Committee for Blue Cross Plans has established minimum quotas for each plan in an effort to increase the national enrollment from the present figure of 11,000,000 to 16,000,000 by the end of this year. It is felt that this minimum figure for 1943 will pacify, for the time at least, the Social Security Board, whose attitude has always been, "The voluntary system through the hospitals themselves is the ideal solution to this social economic problem." The only fault expressed by the Board is that Blue Cross Plans have thus far been unable to extend this protection to a great enough percentage of the population. Emphasis on new membership was given considerable discussion, due primarily to the ever present interest on the part of the Federal Government to enact legislation on a compulsory social security program based on the theme "Security from the Cradle to the Grave."

Physical ills are the taxes laid upon this wretched life; some are taxed higher, and some lower, but all pay something.—Lord Chesterfield, Letter to his son.

BOOK REVIEWS

"The chief glory of every people arises from its authors."—Dr. Samuel Johnson.

"ADVANCES IN PEDIATRICS." Adolph G. De-Sanctis, M.D., New York Post Graduate Medical School and Hospital, Columbia University, New York. Associate Editors: L. Emmitt Holt, M.D., Johns Hopkins Hospital; A. Graeme Mitchell, M.D., Children's Hospital, Cincinnati; Robert A. Strong ,M.D., Tulane University; Frederick F. Tisdall, M.D., Hospital for Sick Children, Toronto, Ontario. Illustrated. Pp. 306. Interscience Publishers, Inc., 215 Fourth Ave., New York. Price $4.50.

This book, Volume No. 1, represents a new effort to epitomize the advances in pediatrics which have occurred within the past year, and is perhaps best introduced by quoting from the preface. "It will be noted that 'Advances in Pediatrics' is in no sense a compilation of abstracts, but rather a collection of personalized monographs by outstanding authorities." This ,sentence very accurately describes the form of the book.

A glance at the list of contributors and the topics which they have discussed is convincing evidence of the value and the wide appeal which the book has. Men of scientific background and wide clinical experience have prepared monographs of varying lengths on new diseases, clinical procedure and advances in various conditions affecting pediatrics.

A complete bibliography appears at the end of each topic for those who wish to pursue that topic or any phase of it at more length. The contents include: Toxoplasmosis, A Recently Recognized Disease of Human Beings; Review of Virus Diseases; Chemotherapy in Diseases of Infancy and Childhood; Electroencephalography; The Role of Vitamin K in Hemorrhage in the New Born Period; Persistent Ductus Arteriosus and Its Surgical Treatment; The Premature Infant; Tuberculosis; Endocrinology; Other Short Abstracts on Influenzal Meningitis, Tetanus Toxoid, Casein, Hydrolysate in Nephrosis, etc.

This is a remarkable publication of current scientific information, analyzed, condensed and made available for practical application.—George H. Garrison, M.D.

"A VENTURE IN PUBLIC HEALTH INTEGRATION." (1941 Health Education Conference of the New York Academy of Medicine.) Columbia University Press.

This book is a compilation of addresses made at the 1941 Health Education Conference of the New York Academy of Medicine. The contents of the book are as follows:

Address of Welcome, by Malcolm Goodridge, M.D.

Introductory Comments by James R. Scott, M.D.

1. The Role of Health Education in the Promotion of Optimal Health and in the Retardation of Degenerative Diseases, by Edward J. Stieglitz, M.D.

2. Barriers to Health Education, by Edward L. Bernays.

3. Health Education by the Private Practitioner, the Voluntary Agency, and the Department of Health, by Allen Freeman, M.D.

Dr. Edward J. Stieglitz, in his discussion of "The Role of Health Education in the Promotion of Optimal Health and in the Retardation of Denegerative Diseases," attempts to define health. He is not satisfied with "health is the absence of disease," but calls attention to the fact that health has positive attributes, is not static, but is a kinetic state. He makes the interesting statement that health is relative, and that everyone has certain limitations within which it is wise to stay. These limitations may be either physical or mental. One interesting statement that is particularly for the layman is, "health and physical fitness are individual problems and cannot be standardized . . . . physical fitness includes not only the present status of the individual, but it also includes an impression of the future continuity of health and productiveness."

Dr. Stieglitz reminds us that it is not enough to increase the life span of humans, that with this longer life span there should be "group instruction in the hygiene of aging, of optimal diets in relation to age, and of the wise utilization of leisure and the limitations imposed by disease." This would eventually lead to a condition where lengevity would be paralleled by health in the later decades of life. He closes his talk by emphasizing the idea that the sense of personal responsibility toward health maintenance must be awakened to counteract the consequences of the many years of pampering.

Mr. Bernays gives some interesting figures regarding the economic phase of public health, the number of physicians, and the number of organized and volunteer groups promoting one or more phases of public health.

His premise is that in a democracy everyone must receive adequate health education, and suggests that we must educate public opinion. He lists as some of the "barriers": psychological attitudes, physical attitudes and habits, financial problems, fear, ignorance, superstition, and lethargy—a "let John do it" attitude.

He suggests that men in the medical profession are too often poor teachers and are more interested in the sick than in the well, which is what the public expects and demands. Health education is not given equal and proper emphasis in public schools, and teaching materials and methods are not on a parity with education in other fields.

Dr. Allen Freeman introduces his theme by saying that health education is not one but many things; it may be a mobile unit, an exhibit of food values at a country fair, a salesman selling paper cups, a nurse showing mothers how to sterilize nursing bottles, and various other activities.

Dr. Freeman commends most highly those people who make research and study possible by their endowments. At the same time, he .condemns the lack of knowledge of the most common diseases by the general public. This latter condition can be prevented only by better opportunities for health education for the public, and this requires appropriations for financing such an educational program; the securing of appropriations depends upon an educated public, which makes a vicious circle of our job—no beginning and no ending.—Medical Staff of Oklahoma State Health Department.

"THE AMERICAN ILLUSTRATED MEDICAL DICTIONARY, NINETEENTH EDITION." W. A. Newman Dorland, M.D., F.A.C.S., Lieutenant Colonel, M.R.C., U. S. Army, and E. C. L. Miller, M.D., Medical College of Virginia. Revised and Enlarged with 914 Illustrations, including 269 Portraits. Pp. 1647. W. B. Saunders Company, Philadelphia. Price $7.50.

Here is a faithful old friend in attractive flexible form, rejuvinated by the addition of all the youthful terms in a rapidly growing science.

The following paragraph from the preface of this Nineteenth Edition gives a brief but comprehensive account of its broad scope and its importance to students and doctors of medicine and to all those engaged in the allied sciences:

"In this nineteenth edition the Dictionary has received its usual thorough revision. Each page has been carefully scrutinized, and more than 2,000 new words have been added. These additions cover all departments of medicine and the related sciences. Among the most notable of these departments are Endocrinology, Physical Therapy, Biochemistry, Psychiatry, Drugs and Medicinal Preparations, Surgical Procedure and Clinical Syndromes, Signs and Symptoms of Disease. The student and practitioner will encounter these new terms in his daily reading and study. Hundreds of them are defined for the first time in the present edition of this book."

In addition to the carefully prepared definitions there is a great store of information in convenient tabular form. The text is supplemented by nearly a thousand illustrations including 269 portraits. The latter lend life and luster to the volume. It is refreshing and reassuring to find 1,647 responsive pages crowded into one volume so handy for reference.—Lewis J. Moorman, M.D.

"WAR GASES, THEIR IDENTIFICATION AND DECONTAMINATION." Morris B. Jacobs, Ph. D. Food, Drug and Insecticide Admin. U. S. Dept. of Agri. 1927. Chemist Department of Health, City of New York, 1928. Formerly, Lt. U. S. Chemical Warfare Service Reserve. Pp. 180. 7 Divisions . Interscience Publishers, Inc., New York, N. Y.—1942.

This book is the latest compilation of information to date disclosed in regard to the chemical agents which may be used against either military forces or civilian population. It is not practical to review such a book in the true sense because the book itself is a review, and a catalog of knowledge in detailed and technical form. It very adequately describes the physical, chemical, and physiological characteristics of all of the practical chemical warfare agents and evaluates their damaging proclivities, and gives the author's opinion as to the ones most likely to be used should the war reach that state of degredation. In addition to the characteristics of the gases, the amounts required for damage, the interval of exposure necessary, and the minimum lethal amounts of the gases, are given. Detailed methods of identification of the gases, both in the field and in the chemical laboratory are given, and recommended setup of materials necessary for testing are outlined. Methods of protection of materials, with a specific reference to foods and methods of cleansing and of decontamination of persons, areas, and materials are given, with specific instructions as to the preparation and evaluation of the decontaminating agents. The book is accompanied by a complete appendix and is extremely well indexed for aid in quick reference to the subject matter regarding tests, decontamination, and so on. Accompanying the various discussions of the gases is a most complete bibliography covering all of the published information regarding war gases up to the date of publication, 1942.—J. F. Messenbaugh, M.D.

"THE MIND AND ITS DISORDERS." By James N. Brawner, M.D., Smyrna, Georgia. 228 pages. Atlanta, Georgia: Walter W. Brown Publishing Company, 761 Peachtree St. Cloth. Price $3.50.

In the preface to this book, the author states that it has been produced in response to the requests of his numerous physician friends for an exposition of the problems involved in the field of neuropsychiatry in language that they can understand. Let it be said that he has most commendably lived up to his inspiration. As a matter of fact, the book is so simply written that it could even, with profit, be handed to anxious relatives or other lay individuals who had some occasion to inform themselves as to the exact nature of mental illness.

It is also with pleasure that one notes that the author has lived a sufficient number of years and worked in the field of neuropsychiatry during what one might say is its transition period. He reveals in an occasional passage and in the use of certain phrases and words that his experience goes back in this particular field to a period when we did not have psychoanalysis, shock treatments, etc. He is quite thoroughly an exponent of the doctrine that mental symptoms represent the clinical manifestation in most instances of some sort of physiological disturbance. An orthodox Freudian would hardly accept this statement without qualification which, after all, is for the most part an academic question except when the welfare of a patient is involved. His understanding of modern psychopathology, especially in the field of the neuroses, is that of the middle of the road attitude; therefore, conservative rather than being an ardent follower of what is commonly understood as the Freudian concept.

The book should find a wide acceptance among practitioners who wish to keep themselves in a working state of mind with respect to the problems of neuropsychiatry. The author can be excused for appending in the last few pages an article or two representing his personal opinions of Spencer and Freud.—Ned R. Smith, M.D.

"TUBERCULOSIS NURSING." Grace M. Longhurst, R.N. F. A. Davis Company, Publishers, Philadelphia. 1941. Price $3.00.

This is an interesting, well illustrated and informative text. It is a valuable guide for the nurse who works with the tuberculosis patient. The subject matter is well organized and emphasizes the following points: definitions, tests, modes of transmission, symptoms, diagnosis, classification, complications, medical management, aseptic techniques, collection of specimens, extra pulmonary tuberculosis, and all types of collapse therapy with surgical procedures. Other matters discussed are general nursing care, nursing care of complications, chest clinics, clinic routine, instruction to the patient and his family, behavior problems with case histories, rehabilitation, and the modern concepts in the field of tuberculosis and its implications in tuberculosis nursing.

The book is well adopted to its premise, that of nursing the whole patient which includes the fundamental factors of medical, surgical, communicable disease, and mental nursing. The selected references appearing at the end of each chapter should prove helpful in supplementing information on the various subjects discussed. Most noteworthy are the excellent illustrations in addition to the graphic sketches. They are clear, concise and pertinent.

The type is large which facilitates reading. Gloss finished paper is used. It is well bound in blue-grey cloth. This book is written primarily for the nurse who is interested in the institutional care of the tuberculous patient. However, many aspects of tuberculosis nursing in the field of Public Health are discussed. The book should prove helpful to physicians teaching in schools of nursing.—Golda B. Slief, A.B., R.N.

"CONSTITUTION AND DISEASE." Julius Bauer, M.D., Professor of Clinical Medicine, College of Medical Evangelists, Los Angeles, Calif. Grune & Stratton, 443 Fourth Avenue, New York City, 1942. Chapters VIII, Pp. 208.

A careful perusal of this interesting volume will help the clinician understand the varied personality patterns which are found cropping out when he examines a cross-section of his practice. It will enable him to more readily recognize and appreciate psychological conflicts and constitutional inadequacies. Furthermore, it will help to emphasize the limitations of medical science without the intricate are of medicine.

After an introduction dealing with the science and the art of medicine, one section is devoted to a detailed discussion of Constitutional Pathology, another to Constitutional Biological Inferiority. Considerable space is devoted to the integrative systems of individual constitution and to major diseases with chiefly constitutional etiology. Finally, there is a rich discussion of the principles of treatment with a consideration of pitfalls and errors.

Under a discussion of psychosomatic medicine, the author indicates that the good family doctor will not only choose a label for the existing disease but he will strive to analyze the disease and its effects in the light of both the physical and the psychic influence manifested in the clinical picture.

In the following paragraph, the author not only offers pertinent comment on diagnosticians as a specialty group, but he quotes two of our outstanding clinicians, to show that doctors must understand people as well as disease:

"I am in full accord with Houston concerning his statement: 'Diagnosis and treatment cannot be successfully divorced and must always go hand in hand.' The creation of diagnosticians as a specialty group is, in my opinion, one of the outgrowths of modern routine medicine attempting to accumulate as many tests as possible on a patient. 'Certainly, a sufficiently complete diagnostic survey should be made of each condition until its nature is clear, but the routine performance of needless tests indicates a lack of skillful observation and thinking, dulls clinical acumen, penalizes patients, wastes time and material, and gives the public an incorrect view of the cost of sound medical care' (Austrian)."

Attention is called to the fact that the human mind has been considered in modern medical schools only "as far as its obvious derangement calls for a psychiatrist" and that modern young physicians might learn much psychosomatic medicine from the old Greeks.

It is pointed out that the family physician should recognize the importance of "minor psychotherapy" and that more stress should be placed "upon re-education of a patient, on psychosymthesis rather than psychoanalysis, on re-adjusting him for the future rather than digging into his past."

The author approaches the philosophy of Robert Louis Stevenson when he says "It is the striving more than the achievement which makes a man happy and makes him fit."

Finally, the book makes clear the fact that the "concept of individual constitution is the basis of psychosomatic medicine in so far as it demonstrates the inseparable unity of body and mind," and that "the mechanistic trend in medical education, and the failure of academic medicine to indicate the need for a simple psychological approach as a supplement to physical and laboratory examination in all patients accounts for the fact that modern physicians have to learn about the true situation from recent publications."

The above brief review suggests the stimulating character of this small volume, and should recommend it to every young physician who is earnestly striving to supplement his exact science with the flexible art of medicine.—Lewis J. Moorman, M.D.

"WAR MEDICINE—A SYMPOSIUM." Editor Winfield Scott Pugh, M.D., Commander, (MC) U.S.N. Retired, Formerly Surgeon, City Hospital, New York. Associate Editor, Edward Podolsky, M.D., Technical Editor, Dagobert D. Runes, Ph.D., Printed in the U. S. by F. Hubner & Co., Inc., New York, N. Y. for The Philosophical Library, Inc., 15 East 40th St., New York, N. Y.

This book is exactly what its name indicates, a collection of some 57 papers, by a grand total of 67 authors and collaborators, that deals with medicine and war. The work is divided roughly into three groups under the headings of Surgery, Aviation and Naval Medicine, and General Medicine. Approximately three-fifths of the papers are devoted to surgery and one-fifth to each of the other principal sub-divisions. The acknowledgment page discloses that the papers have been sifted out from various books and magazines. Since so many of the active phases of war medicine are covered, the book is not capable of a critical review by any one mind. No claim is made for official status but it may be said that it could be read by anyone interested with profit. It is, in its surgical phases, quite up-to-date because many of the presentations are based upon actual experience of British war surgeons. The illustrations are mostly drawings with an occasional photographic reproduction. They are very informative when taken in conjunction with the text. To anyone interested in war medicine, especially in its surgical phases as practiced today, the book would prove interesting and valuable.—Ned R. Smith, M.D.

A Good Portrait Still Wanting in Literature and Movies

"Shakespeare has left us no finished portrait of a doctor. Moliere caricatured him. Thackeray failed to draw him, and generally in novels he is merely a man who is labelled 'Doctor.' The sole exception known to me is the marvellous delineation of Lydgate in 'Middlemarch.' He is all over the physician, his manner, his sentiments, his modes of thought, but he stands alone in fiction. How did that great mistress of her art learn all of physicians which enabled her to leave us this amazingly truthful picture? Her life gives us no clue, and when I asked her husband, George Lewes, to explain the matter, he said that he did not know, and that she knew no more of this than of how she had acquired her strangely complete knowledge of the low turf people she has drawn in the same book, and with an almost equal skill and truth to nature."—S. Weir Mitchell, Doctor and Patient, 1887.

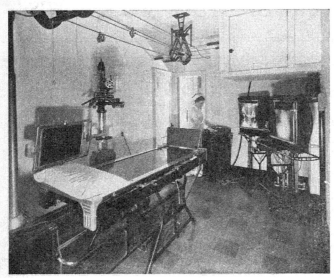

MEDICAL ABSTRACTS

"FRACTURES OF THE OS CALCIS." A. S. Blundell Bankard, The Lancet, 11, 175, August 15, 1942.

The author states, "The results of the treatment of crush fractures of the os calcis are rotten. They bear no relation to the accuracy with which the fractures are reduced." He points out that with few exceptions the results of the Bohler method of reduction and fixation is a permanently stiff and painful foot, due to immobilization in plaster for four months. Likewise, the results of subastragalar arthrodesis for fractures of the os calcis are often unsatisfactory, and he expresses belief that the best result to be obtained from fracture of the os calcis involving the subastragalar joint is a completely stiff, but painless, foot of good shape, and he recommends a complete triple arthrodesis as a primary measure. A slight modification in the operative procedure is offered, in that a short longitudinal incision is first made on the inner side of the foot over the navicular for excision of the navicular, as well as removal of the cartilage from the head of the astragalus and the base of the cuneform bone. The usual incision is then made on the outer side of the foot for the calcaneocuboid joint and the subastragalar joint.—E.D.M., M.D.

"FRACTURES OF THE OLECRANON PROCESS." D. Wainwright. The British Journal of Surgery, XXIX, 403, April, 1942.

The history of the treatment of fractures of the olecranon is reviewed. The general concensus of opinion is that closed reduction is rare lysuccessful and should be reserved for the younger patients. Open reduction with some form of internal fixation is used for the majority of patients. In the elderly, where there is a contra-indication for operation, a sling and early use of the arm is advocated, even though non-union usually takes place.

The writer has reviewed forty of his own cases. He concludes: (1) that a satisfactory reposition is seldom gained by closed reduction, and then only after prolonged fixation in extension; (2) that early motion with only a sling for protection is rarely worth while; and (3) that, while perfect results can be obtained by open operations, arthritic changes and permanent stiffness are so frequent that he has sought a better method of treatment.

He now advocates removal of the detached fragment and repair of the triceps tendon, claiming a more rapid recovery, freedom from arthritic changes, and freedom from non-union. The fragment is removed by a subperiosteal dissection, and the projecting sharp angle of the ulna is smoothed off. The triceps expansion is sutured firmly, and the arm is immobilized in extension. This operation is advocated for all middle-aged patients when the fracture is above the coronoid process, or for younger patients when early return to work is important, and whenever the fragments are badly comminuted.

Twenty cases have been studied after six months to four years. One patient has some lateral instability and two have limited extensions at the elbow. These results were better than from other methods which have been used.—E.D.M., M.D.

"THE ALLERGIC ASPECT OF VASOMOTOR RHINITIS." H. H. Telland, M.D., Archives of Otolaryngology, Volume 37, Page 1-14, January 1943.

In nonseasonal rhinitis the characteristic pathologic picture is that of a pinkish gray boggy mucosa with rhinorrhea and serous discharge, the bogginess resulting from epithelial hyperplasia. The patient complains of stuffiness of the nose with periods of complete obstruction, especially during the night, violent sneezing, often on getting up in the morning or going to bed. In its early stages, the condition may be mistaken for common cold, or even sinusitis by the patient.

If no signs of infection or other local pathologic changes such as deflected septums or spurs and polypi can be discovered, but the eosinophil cells in the blood and the nasal secretions are found to be increased and there is also a family history of allergy, the case may be regarded as one of vasomotor rhinitis of probable allergic origin.

The first step in further diagnosis of allergy will be an attempt to ascertain the causative agent by means of intradermal injections of all possible materials to which the patient may be allergic, using various concentrations of each material for the test. What these materials may be one may see from the observations of the author, who, among the patients studied in the outpatient department of Gouverneur Hospital, New York, distinguished the following groups:

1. Patients showing sensitivity to dust, animal epitheliums, orris root, insecticides, tobacco and miscellaneous inhalants. In this group, dust was found to be by far the most frequent cause. Treatment with the allergen and the removal of this factor from the patient's environment were effective in clearing up the symptoms.

2. Patients sensitive to occupational irritants. In this larger group the history showed onset of symptoms at varying periods after the patient's employment in a certain occupation. The sensitivity was present before the employment, or it gradually developed due to continued contact with the allergens. There are many occupations in which workers may become allergic to the materials of the trade. Furriers become sensitive to the undyed furs or to dyes and chemicals employed in the preparation of furs. Furs of raccoon, muskrat, and silver fox as well as dyes containing ursol D and ursol P are especially noted for causing allergy.

To upholsterers the chief excitants are feathers, cotton, kapok and animal hair. Clothing workers are affected by silk, wool, cotton, linen and shop dust. Hatmakers are exposed to silk, cotton, and rabbit fur, sometimes also a banana oil used in the process of bleaching. Cosmeticians may become allergic to orris root, also to acacia, tragacanth, karaya, linseed and quince seed, which substances are used in permanent wave lotions. Woodworkers have a long list of possible allergens, and even birch wood may be harmful. Jewelers are often sensitive to solder dust and cuttlefish bone. Chemists and druggists react to numerous drugs and chemicals, yet the cutaneous tests for sensitivity will remain negative unless the drug contains protein; the diagnosis depends more on the patient's occupational history and the presence of eosinophilia. Food handlers may be sensitive to any of the foodstuffs found in restaurants, grocery stores, and other places of business. Allergic rhinitis has been caused by the Mexican bean weevil as well as by the fumes of coffee, and the dust of cacao beans and chocolate. Paprika and other spices may also cause vasomotor rhinitis. Poultry handlers may be sensitive to feathers, to epithelium of chickens, or to the linseed meal in chicken feed. Bakers may be allergic to flours of all types, and paint workers are often irritated by fumes of turpentine.

3. Patients sensitized by ingested foods. The injurious food is ascertained by cutaneous tests and elimination diets. Various foodstuffs may act as allergens, such as milk, eggs, wheat, spices (onion, peppers, mustard, allspice, vinegar, tomato catsup), meats, fish, vegetables (asparagus, tomatoes, potatoes), fruits (grapefruit, pineapple, banana, melon, berries of various kinds).

4. Patients may be found who fail to show a cutaneous reaction to any inhalant or food. Such patients have to be referred to rhinologists for diagnosis and for specific or nonspecific methods of treatment.

Exhaustive and intensive therapy has helped in many of these cases to clear up vasomotor rhinitis which at first appeared to be intractable. Intensive therapy consists of rapidly working up to a dose of a particular allergen considered optimal for a particular patient by increasing the frequency of treatments to twice or three times a week, and then continuing with the maximum dose at short intervals. If a patient is found to be sensitive to cotton or horse hair from the bedding, wearing apparel and other articles of his environment, it is not enough to remove the allergen, but it is also necessary to immunize him to the substance by administering the optimal top doses.

The difficulty is in finding the causative allergens. Sometimes the allergen cannot be used for desensitization therapy, and the only possible treatment is avoidance, which in many cases means that the patient must give up his job.—M.D.H., M.D.

"ACUTE OTITIS MEDIA AND MASTOIDITIS." Ernest Seydell, M.D., Wichita, Kansas. Southern Medical Journal, Vol. 53, No. 7, July, 1942.

The author acknowledges nothing new in his paper but gives an excellent outline of his method of handling these cases. It is produced verbatim below.

Local Therapy.—The underlying philosophy of local therapy is to establish and promote drainage and to keep the auditory canal as free from secretion as possible. A culture should be taken at the time of paracentesis or as soon thereafter as possible.

General Therapy.—When constitutional, local, nasopharyngeal or tonsillar manifestations are marked, it is advisable to put the patient to bed, force fluids and institute such constitutional therapy as is indicated.

Sulfonamides.—An entire paper could be devoted to this phase of the subject. Time will not allow me to do more than touch a few of its high spots. There is as yet no unanimity of opinion in reference either to the value of the sulfonamides in the prevention of surgical mastoiditis or as to how and when they should be used. However, most investigators and clinicians agree that these drugs have little or no value when destruction of the mastoid cells has taken place. It is also a well established fact that sulfonamides frequently mask symptoms that are indicative of intracranial complications. Finally, it has been shown that the sulfonamides in some way change the normal roentgen ray picture in mastoiditis so that this otherwise important adjuvant in diagnosis is rendered more or less valueless.

There is a school of thought that believes that a sulfonamide should be given as soon as possible after the onset of an acute infection and should be continued for at least ten days after all symptoms have subsided. On the other hand, Champ Lyons and his associates have shown that the action of the sulfonamides is rendered ineffective unless the patient has been able to develop antibodies. They therefore advise that 24-48 hours be allowed to elapse between the onset of the patient's infection and the administration of the sulfonamides. They also have shown that much better results can be obtained where the sulfonamides are combined with immune serum therapy.

As a rule, I do not prescribe the sulfonamides to my ambulatory patients. I insist on a preliminary red, white and hemoglobin determination which should be repeated at least every 48 hours. The initial dosage that is necessary for a given case depends in a measure on the severity of the infection. The subsequent dosage depends not so much on the age and weight of the patient as on the sulfonamide blood level. I no longer have the courage to give these drugs for the prescribed ten days following the remission of symptoms, due to the fact that I have had three cases in which otitic sepsis developed which did not become manifest until the drug was withdrawn. In fact, I have no definite rule as to how long they should be continued. The drug is discontinued when surgical interference is decided upon.

Operative Therapy.—No hard and fast rules can be devised either as to the necessity of an operation or as to the opportune time to perform it. Each case presents an individual problem. Our final decision will depend upon our clinical experience, judgment, and quite often on intuition.—M. D. H., M.D.

"DIAGNOSIS AND TREATMENT OF MENIERE'S SYNDROME. M. Atkinson, M.D. Archives of Otolaryngology. Vol. 37, Page 40-53, January 1943.

Much of the failure in treatment of Meniere's syndrome is caused by incorrect diagnosis of this affection. Many cases of vertigo, without deafness and tinnitus, are called Meniere's disease, and even cases of vertigo caused by high blood pressure are treated as true Meniere's syndrome. The history of the patient may be very characteristic, and, if there is also deafness present, one may be tempted to make the diagnosis on history and deafness alone, which is a dangerous practice. Accurate diagnosis of Meniere's syndrome requires the most thorough examination and a process of exclusion.

Since paroxysmal vertigo with all the attributes of the syndrome can occasionally be the first, and for some time the only, symptom of a lesion in the cerebellopontile angle, a careful neurological examination has to be made in all cases, which occasionally may need repetition at regular intervals. An equally careful otologic examination is the next step, which has to include an appraisal of the relative patency of the eustachian tubes, but must not necessarily include the Barany tests. Stricture of the eustachian tube is the direct cause of Meniere's syndrome in an appreciable number of cases. From time to time complete obstruction from swelling of the mucosal lining may take place and so produce an acute alteration in pressure in the middle ear and labyrinth; the result is a labyrinth storm with deafness and tinnitus—a Meniere attack. Recurrence of such an attack can be prevented entirely by gradual dilatation of the stricture with a bougie. In many cases no other treatment is necessary.

The third step is a thorough general examination to determine the presence of any associated condition, in particular of any focus of infection, especially in the nose and throat. Blood pressure and disease of the gallbladder should be remembered among the possible associated conditions of Meniere's syndrome. A low blood pressure is as frequent a cause of vertigo as a high one, though neither is common. Gallbladder disease is a more frequent associate of Meniere's syndrome, and its treatment will at times have an appreciable effect on the attacks of vertigo. The author does not believe that focal infection is an important causative factor in producing the syndrome by setting up a so-called toxic labyrinthitis.

After elimination by these three steps there is left that large group of cases in which the disorder is the one commonly thought of as Meniere's disease and may be called idiopathic. Some of these cases own an allergic basis, and, therefore, it is necessary to eliminate allergy as a cause. Instead of trying a long series of allergens by cutaneous tests, one may investigate the patient's sensitivity to histamine. An intradermal test is performed by injection of 0.01 mg. of histamine hydrochloride.

In the normal person a wheal appears immediately, which begins to fade in 10 minutes and disappears in 20 minutes. Such a result is negative. In the sensitive person the wheal is large in size (½ to ¾ inch), with a surrounding flare of 2 to 2½ inches showing one or more trailing pseudopods. The pseudopod is definite at the end of five minutes and does not start to fade until the end of 15 to 20 minutes. Such a result is positive, and shows that the patient is sensitive to histamine.

By means of this histamine test patients with Meniere's syndrome can be divided into two groups: those who are sensitive, and those who are insensitive to histamine. The former can be treated with satisfactory results by desensitization to histamine, while the latter cannot. The desensitization is made by the so-called slow method. The test intradermal dose is repeated subcutaneously, and then at intervals of two to four days the dose is gradually increased as if one were giving a vaccine, and with the same consideration for general reactions. The maximum dose ever used in tolerant patients was 1 mg. of histamine dihydrochloride. When the maximum dose tolerated by the individual patient is reached, it is repeated at four weekly intervals. A second course is usually necessary after six months or so, and, as far as present knowledge goes, sometimes a third.

In patients insensitive to histamine, nicotinic acid has been the substance used for treatment, specifically on the grounds of its being a vasodilator. The author's practice has been to give as an initial dose an injection of 25 mg. intramuscularly. This usually produces no more than a transitory mild flush, lasting five to ten minutes, and even in the unduly sensitive patient does not give rise to an excessive reaction. The dose is then gradually increased to the limit of tolerance, maintained there for a month or more and eventually decreased by slow steps to a maintenance dose, which is continued for many months. Other vasodilatator drugs have been used, but none with such success as nicotinic acid.

Careful and accurate grouping of cases of Meniere's disease is very important. Each group should be treated by methods appropriate to it, Indiscriminate use of histamine in the histamine insensitive cases may result in actual harm to the patients. In the same way, nicotinic acid administered wrongly to the patients who are sensitive to histamine will increase symptoms. The results of treatment have been excellent in the histamine-sensitive group, though many patients improved also in the group treated by nicotinic acid. One should not forget, however, that only relief is to be regarded as the acme of success, and cure should not even be considered.—M.D.H., M.D.

"EMMETROPIA." E. S. Munson, M.D. Archives of Ophthalmology, Chicago, Vol. 29, Page 109-115, January, 1943.

About one hundred years ago the refractive errors of the eye were placed on a sound clinical basis by the work of Donders and Hemlholtz, whose writings have since been the guide of those who practice ophthalmology. It was Donders who called the normal refractive state of the eye by the term "emmetropia." He considered an eye normal, the principal focus of whose dioptric system is, in rest of accommodation, found in the retina. Of infinitely remote objects, which send out parallel rays, this retina receives accurate images, to be improved neither by convex nor by concave glasses, and by means of its accommodation it sees equally accurately at relatively short distances.

Besides accommodation, an important physiologic process also plays a part in placing the focus on the retina, and this is the normal tonus of the ciliary muscle. The existence of tonus of the ciliary muscle is proved by the changed refraction in paralytic conditions due to disease and to the effect of cycloplegics. The amount of tonus exerted by the ciliary muscle can be measured by its relaxation by a cycloplegic; it is about 1 dioptry,

being greater in hypermetropia and less in myopia. Tonus when normal is an ever present contraction of the ciliary muscle and involuntary in its action. It should be distinguished from accommodation, which is absent until called into play by a voluntary impulse. Accommodation fails with age, probably more from lenticular changes than from a weakening of the ciliary muscle. The activity of tonus may be also abolished by advanced sclerosis of the lens.

Under pathological conditions tonus changes may be caused by spasticity or atonia of the ciliary muscles, the first condition being sometimes incorrectly called spasm of accommodation, while the second is known as accommodative asthenopia.

Emmetropia is considered to be the perfect refractive state of the eye. It has no relation to vision. Whether the eye attains this perfection, or only rarely approaches it, it must be adopted as a standard for measurement of departures from the ideal normal. The refractive maturity of the eye is reached or approached only several years after birth. Some authorities place this age of eye maturity at about 10 years. Emmetropia depends on the correctness of such factors as the size and axial length of the eye, the curvature of the cornea and the lens, the refractive indices of the cornea, aqueous, lens and vitreous, and the tonus of the ciliary muscle. There is no exact method at present to establish the presence of emmetropia directly. Moreover, there are periods during the life of certain persons when emmetropia is only temporary. Even in an astigmatic eye one meridian may be emmetropic.

Most authorities believe that such a refractive state as emmetropia must be very rare, if it exists at all. But, if one considers as normal those persons who show a normal tonus under a cycloplegic and accept no spherical lens afterward, then the incidence of emmetropia may be considerably increased. Duke-Elder holds that emmetropia may be optically normal, but it is no more biologically normal than would be the universal attainment of a uniform height of five feet six inches.

A large group of young persons, such as college students, would provide a good statistical study of the incidence of emmetropia, and it would be probably detected that, after all, nature has not failed to approach the normal in the visual organ.—M.D.H., M.D.

"CYSTS OF THE FLOOR OF THE MOUTH." W. H. Johnston, M.D. The Annals of Otology, Rhinology and Laryngology, Volume 51, Page 917-927, December, 1942.

The multiform nature of the cysts of the floor of the mouth and their various ways of development are of interest. Some of them grow on or in the floor of the mouth, while others become, only secondarily, cysts of this region. Some are true cysts, while others should be considered ectasias of obliterated ducts, results of inflammatory processes or parasitic products. There seems to be no satisfactory classification available which includes all possible cysts of this region. It may be said, however, that they are either congenital or acquired. The congenital cysts are developmental errors.

These cysts are all characteristics, being of rather slow growth, and are mostly round or ovoid in shape. The subjective symptoms depend on the size. There may be difficulty in speech, mastication, swallowing, and even deformity of the neck or the mandible. The larger cysts may interfere with normal dentition; some of them may cause a marked swelling in the submental region. When infected, painful abscesses may result.

The rarity of these cysts accounts for many errors in diagnosis. A sublingual dermoid may be mistaken for a ranula. Only a histologic examination will show the true nature of these formations. Differential diagnosis from other types of tumors, or from cellulitis, should not be difficult. Even though the nature of a cyst of the floor of the mouth cannot always be recognized, an incorrect diagnosis is not a particular problem, since all cysts, regardless of their origin, have to be removed surgically.

The more important cystic tumors of the floor of the mouth are: (a) those originating from the Bochdalek ducts and the thyroglossal duct; (b) cystic degeneration of the sublingual or submandibular salivary glands; (c) dermoid cysts; (d) epidermoid cysts; (e) pseudocysts of the large mucous glands commonly called ranula; (f) cystic adenoma, which is a tumor of the mandible; (g) traumatic epithelial cysts.

Formerly, the term "ranula" meant any cystic swelling of the floor of the mouth. What cyst should be called ranula and what is the exact origin of such ranula is still a matter of discussion. Its classic site is sublingual; it is usually unilateral, and is mostly seen in women. By its content and general appearance it can be differentiated from dermoid cysts; ranula is generally of bluish color, and its content is clear and viscous. Recently, it has been stated that only a ranula lined with ciliated epithelium is a true cyst, and it develops from the plica fimbriata.

In the treatment it does not matter whether a cyst of the mouth floor is a true ranula or only a pseudocyst. The best method is to extirpate it in toto. The total removal may be performed either through the mouth, or from the neck. Hobert described a special operation consisting of partial excision and eventration of the inner wall of the cyst, and called this procedure by the fancy name of "batrakosioplastics." Blair recommended a permanent fistulization in place of total extirpation if the ranula has large parafaucial extensions.

Most observers feel that total extirpation, when possible, is the most satisfactory method of treatment. Ward recommends use of the endotherm knife for opening the cyst and destroying the epithelial lining by the desiccation current. There may follow various postoperative complications. Local anesthesia may predispose to local edema, which is very painful and may even endanger the patient's life. It has been suggested that the operation should be done under a block anesthesia of the lingual nerve, using as little anesthetic as possible.— M.D.H., M.D.

"MODERN TREATMENT OF PNEUMOCOCCIC PNEU- MONIA." Harrison F. Flippin, M.D.; Leon Schwartz, M.D., and Albert H. Domm, M.D., Philadelphia, Pa. The Journal of the American Medical Association, Vol. 121, Number 4, January 23, 1943.

This is a very timely report, summarized as follows: Within the period of this study, August 15, 1938 to April 1, 1942, 1,635 adults with pneumococcic pneumonia were treated with sulfapyridine, sulfathiazole or sulfadiazine with an averaged mortality of 10.6 per cent. This figure is to be compared to that of 40.1 per cent mortality obtained in 1,904 cases of this disease observed at the Philadelphia General Hospital during the five years prior to the introduction of these drugs. From the data presented in this report it appears that sulfadiazine is the drug of choice at the present time for the treatment of pneumococcic pneumonia. To obtain maximum therapeutic results with sulfadiazine in pneumonia, certain principles must be recognized and followed. Regardless of the effectiveness of sulfadiazine in pneumococcic pneumonia, it is not to be employed to the exclusion or neglect of other established therapeutic measures. The following plan of sulfadiazine treatment of pneumococcic pneumonia is suggested.

1. Early treatment.
2. Adequate chemotherapy:
    (a) Large initial dose.
    (b) Smaller doses at regular intervals.
    (c) Continuation of drug until convalescence is established.
3. Maintenance of adequate urinary output.

4. Routine use of alkalis.
5. Prompt recognition of drug toxicity.
6. Determination of specific pneumococcus type.
7. Employment of other therapeutic measures as necessary.
   (a) General supportive treatment.
   (b) Type specific serum.
   (c) Surgical procedures.

H.J., M.D.

"CLASSIFICATION OF BONE TUMORS." H. W. Myerding, M.D. Proceedings of the Staff Meetings of the Mayo Clinic. Vol. 18, Number 2, January 27, 1943.

A very comprehensive and yet simple classification of neoplasms of bone and lesions simulating them is recommended by this author as follows:

I. Lesions Simulating Neoplasms of Bone.
  A. Inflammatory lesions.
    1. Traumatic lesions (callus; ossifying hematoma).
    2. Infections (syphilis; tuberculosis; osteomyelitis; nonsuppurative osteomyelitis of Garre; Brodie's abscess; myositis ossificans; osteoperiostitis).
  B. Osteitis fibrosa cystica.
  C. Metabolic lesions.
    1. Hand-Shuller-Christian disease; Gaucher's disease; Niemann-Pick disease; hyperparathyroidism.
  D. Nutritional lesions.
    1. Rickets; scurvy.
II. Neoplasms of Bone.
  A. Benign osteogenic tumors.
    1. Osteoma (exostosis).
    2. Chondroma.
  B. Fibroblastic tumors.
    1. Benign fibroma.
    2. Malignant periosteal and cortical.
  C. Giant cell tumors.
    1. Benign giant cell tumor.
    2. Malignant giant cell sarcoma.
  D. Vascular neoplasms.
    1. Benign hemangioma (cavernous or plexiform); lymphangioma.
    2. Malignant hemangio-endothelioma (diffuse endothelioma or Ewing's tumor); lymphangio-endothelioma.
  E. Malignant osteogenic sarcoma (including chondrosarcoma).
  F. Multiple myeloma.
  G. Metastatic tumors.
  H. Miscellaneous group.
    1. Undifferentiated malignant neoplasms.
    2. Lymphosarcoma; liposarcoma; erythroblastoma; chloroma; adamantinoma.

—HJ.., M.D.

KEY TO ABSTRACTORS

E. D. M. .... Earl D. McBride, M.D.
H. J. .... Hugh Jeter, M.D.
M. D. H. .... Marvin D. Henley, M.D.

THE WHITE COAT

Here is a doctor who disdains the white coat. He hates it. He tells himself it is puerile. He thinks of it as the vestment of a dozen callings less honorable than his own. He regards the mind that sanctions it as the victim of a sort of exhibitionism that he cannot abide. He holds that the physician, his title won by years of hard work, approved and guaranteed by the legal statutes of his state, needs no such trapping to help him impress the public. You will never find this doctor wearing a white coat in his office. If you did the sky would fall.

What does the white coat connote? Is there a philosophy, a psychology, an economy, of white coats? There are doctors who wear them and doctors who refuse to wear them. Why such a violent difference of opinion on such a simple matter?

We might begin this serious investigation by asking ourselves how the custom of the doctor's wearing the white coat came about. Does it stem from his habit, all down through the centuries, of dressing in a manner distinctive of his profession? Does it have any relation to the long robe and the short robe that he wore in the Middle Ages? The present generation of physicians is probably the only generation that has eschewed a distinctive dress on public appearance. Who can tell a physician today from any other honest citizen on the street? Only a canny Sherlock Holmes with an uncanny eye for the most minute details. This was not true a generation ago. Then the physician's high hat and cutaway coat made him easily recognized.

We know very well when the vogue for white was started. When the Nightingale nurses rustled on to the stage with their emphasis on neatness, cleanliness, and decorum, when Lister and Pasteur made operating rooms the clean, germ-proof workshops of surgery, when hospitals began to look spick and span and to pride themselves on appearance, washable, sterilizable, white clothes became necessary. Orderlies, nurses, interns, and surgeons in the operating room donned white attire. When Lister's ideas finally filtered through to the public, and sanitation became a word the man on the street could understand, white was adopted as the emblem of the germless state. Barbers, butchers, hairdressers, dentists, druggists, even street cleaners, joined the army of white knights laboring to usher in a spotless world.

In hospitals white clothes became the symbol of aseptic medicine. White clothes became a uniform, a part of the hospital's *esprit de corps*. The fledgling physician found to his delight that his white clothes kept him from being confused with his patients' visitors. They achieved for him a certain respect that his youth, unaided, could not command. After two years of serving as a man in white, he usually sheds his white with a feeling of relief. He has outgrown the necessity of having to maintain his position by an external sign. He has come to realize that a physician should try to make his way by what he is and not by what he seems to be or what other people think he is.

But a strange thing happens. Before he knows it he is back again in white. If he becomes a surgeon he gets so busy that he forgets, or does not have the time, to exchange his operating gown for his plain clothes, and finds himself making his rounds dressed in the same white gown in which he appeared in the operating room.

If he becomes a full-time professor and is a researcher in the laboratory, he wears again a white coat to protect himself against blood, acids, and other noxious substances. When the time comes to make his ward rounds, he, like the surgeon, forgets to remove his work coat and discovers by chance the rarified atmosphere he creates, and the white coat becomes a matter of choice. If he becomes the less spectacular general practitioner and visits the hospital, he meets the surgeon and the professor in the corridor and thinks: "These birds with their flock of interns and nurses following in their train look pretty grand in their white coats," and so, not to be outdone by the gentlemen of the scalpel and the gentlemen of the stethoscope, the archangels of the profession, he returns to his little office with a new resolve. He is determined to bring glamor and drama into the quiet regime. He orders a change of white coats and is as punctilious in wearing them when about his business as any butcher, barber, or bartender of his acquaintance.

Perhaps the fashion has come to stay, for there are certain advantages accruing to it. It is a little like the carpenters' wearing overalls, the cook's wearing an apron—a matter of protection from wear and soil. It may be cool, and it makes a man feel professional, if it doesn't make him feel a fool.—*Editorial, Virginia M. Monthly.*

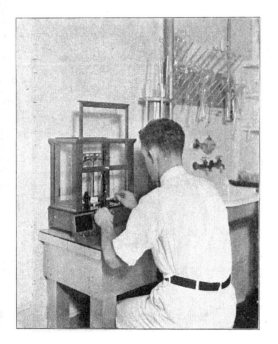

OFFICERS OF COUNTY SOCIETIES, 1943

COUNTY	PRESIDENT	SECRETARY	MEETING TIME
Alfalfa	H. E. Huston, Cherokee	L. T. Lancaster, Cherokee	Last Tues. each Second Month
Atoka-Coal	J. B. Clark, Coalgate	J. S. Fulton, Atoka	
Beckham	H. K. Speed, Sayre	E. S. Kilpatrick, Elk City	Second Tuesday
Blaine	Virginia Olson Curtin, Watonga	W. F. Griffin, Watonga	
Bryan	J. T. Colwick, Durant	W. K. Haynie, Durant	Second Tuesday
Caddo	F. L. Patterson, Carnegie	C. B. Sullivan, Carnegie	
Canadian	P. F. Herod, El Reno	A. L. Johnson, El Reno	Subject to call
Carter	Walter Hardy, Ardmore	H. A. Higgins, Ardmore	
Cherokee	P. H. Medearis, Tahlequah	James K. Gray, Tahlequah	First Tuesday
Choctaw	C. H. Hale, Boswell	E. A. Johnson, Hugo	
Cleveland	J. A. Rieger, Norman	Curtis Berry, Norman	Thursday nights
Comanche	George S. Barber, Lawton	W. F. Lewis, Lawton	
Cotton	A. B. Holstead, Temple	Mollie F. Seism, Walters	Third Friday
Craig	F. M. Adams, Vinita	J. M. McMillan, Vinita	
Creek	H. R. Haas, Sapulpa	C. G. Oakes, Sapulpa	
Custer	F. R. Vieregg, Clinton	C. J. Alexander, Clinton	Third Thursday
Garfield	Paul B. Champlin, Enid	John R. Walker, Enid	Fourth Thursday
Garvin	T. F. Gross, Lindsay	John R. Callaway, Pauls Valley	Wednesday before Third Thursday
Grady	Walter J. Baze, Chickasha	Roy E. Emanuel, Chickasha	Third Thursday
Grant	I. V. Hardy, Medford	E. E. Lawson, Medford	
Greer	G. P. Cherry, Mangum	J. B. Hollis, Mangum	
Harmon	W. G. Husband, Hollis	L. E. Hollis, Hollis	First Wednesday
Haskell	William Carson, Keota	N. K. Williams, McCurtain	
Hughes	Wm. L. Taylor, Holdenville	Imogene Mayfield, Holdenville	First Friday
Jackson	E. S. Crow, Olustee	E. W. Mabry, Altus	Last Monday
Jefferson	F. M. Edwards, Ringling	L. L. Wade, Ryan	Second Monday
Kay	Philip C. Risser, Blackwell	J. Holland Howe, Ponca City	Third Thursday
Kingfisher	C. M. Hodgson, Kingfisher	H. Violet Sturgeon, Hennessey	
Kiowa	B. H. Watkins, Hobart	J. William Finch, Hobart	
LeFlore	Neeson Rolle, Poteau	Rush L. Wright, Poteau	
Lincoln	H. B. Jenkins, Tryon	Carl H. Bailey, Stroud	First Wednesday
Logan	William C. Miller, Guthrie	J. L. LeHew, Jr., Guthrie	Last Tuesday
Marshall	O. A. Cook, Madill	Philip G. Joseph, Madill	
Mayes	Ralph V. Smith, Pryor	Paul B. Cameron, Pryor	
McClain	B. W. Stover, Blanchard	R. L. Royster, Purcell	
McCurtain	A. W. Clarkson, Valliant	N. L. Barker, Broken Bow	Fourth Tuesday
McIntosh	James L. Wood, Eufaula	William A. Tolleson, Eufaula	First Thursday
Murray	P. V. Annadown, Sulphur	F. E. Sadler, Sulphur	Second Tuesday
Muskogee-Sequoyah-Wagoner	H. A. Scott, Muskogee	D. Evelyn Miller, Muskogee	First and Third Monday
Noble	C. H. Cooke, Perry	J. W. Francis, Perry	
Okfuskee	L. J. Spickard, Okemah	M. L. Whitney, Okemah	Second Monday
Oklahoma	Walker Morledge, Oklahoma City	E. R. Musick, Oklahoma City	Fourth Tuesday
Okmulgee	A. R. Holmes, Henryetta	J. C. Matheney, Okmulgee	Second Monday
Osage	C. R. Weirich, Pawhuska	George K. Hemphill, Pawhuska	Second Monday
Ottawa	W. B. Sanger, Picher	Matt A. Connell, Picher	Third Thursday
Pawnee	E. T. Robinson, Cleveland	R. L. Browning, Pawnee	
Payne	L. A. Mitchell, Stillwater	C. W. Moore, Stillwater	Third Thursday
Pittsburg	John F. Park, McAlester	William H. Kaeiser, McAlester	Third Friday
Pontotoc	O. H. Miller, Ada	R. H. Mayes, Ada	First Wednesday
Pottawatomie	A. C. McFarling, Shawnee	Clinton Gallaher, Shawnee	First and Third Saturday
Pushmataha	John S. Lawson, Clayton	B. M. Huckabay, Antlers	
Rogers	C. W. Beson, Claremore	C. L. Caldwell, Chelsea	First Monday
Seminole	Max Van Sandt, Wewoka	Mack I. Shanholtz, Wewoka	
Stephens	W. K. Walker, Marlow	Wallis S. Ivy, Duncan	
Texas	R. G. Obermiller, Texhoma	Morris Smith, Guymon	
Tillman	R. D. Robinson, Frederick	O. G. Bacon, Frederick	
Tulsa	James C. Peden, Tulsa	E. O. Johnson, Tulsa	Second and Fourth Monday
Washington Nowata	J. G. Smith, Bartlesville	J. V. Athey, Bartlesville	Second Wednesday
Washita	A. S. Neal, Cordell	James F. McMurry, Sentinel	
Woods	C. A. Traverse, Alva	O. E. Templin, Alva	Last Wednesday
Woodward	C. E. Williams, Woodward	C. W. Tedrowe, Woodward	Second Thursday

THE JOURNAL
OF THE
OKLAHOMA STATE MEDICAL ASSOCIATION

| VOLUME XXXVI | OKLAHOMA CITY, OKLAHOMA, APRIL, 1943 | NUMBER 4 |

Treatment of War Gases

MAJOR R. E. GREER, M.C.

WILL ROGERS FIELD

OKLAHOMA CITY, OKLAHOMA

Regardless of treaties that exist between the belligerents of the world, no nation dares assume that preparation for chemical warfare can be neglected. The information we have concerning the amount of preparation by the Axis for chemical warfare urges us to promote our own efforts in that direction —just in case. Our enemies are well equipped with chemical agents and well prepared to use them; thus it is perfectly possible that gas warfare may burst into full intensity at any moment. In this connection, General Porter, Chief of the Chemical Warfare Service, states: "This war will never be really 'all out' until gases once more flood the battlefield."

Mindful of this fact, our Chemical Warfare Service plans to fight "fire with fire" if necessary. Representatives of this service are experimenting every day by adapting chemicals to aircraft. Their laboratories at Edgewood Arsenal have spent much time and money in equipment aboard aircraft for the discharge of smoke and for chemicals with greatest efficiency and safety to aircraft personnel.

Thus far in the European conflict, poison gas has not been used; but incendiaries and smoke have been extensively employed. The latter is an old trick, dating back centuries to Helen of Troy. "Several thousand years later, another fleet stood off Gallipoli within cannon shot of Troy. The Turks opposed the landing valiantly. At the first onset and at other bloody subsequent assaults, thousands of British troops were slain."

The passage of years has not lessened the problem which confronted the Greek and British in other wars. The landing of troops on a hostile shore is still one of the most dif-

ficult of operations, and if the defender adds chemical weapons to his inherent defensive advantage, the task of the attacking force becomes still more difficult.

In the Ethiopian campaign in Africa, Italians resorted to the use of mustard gas. In China, the Japs were reported to have used mustard gas. Up to the present time, the Germans have not considered it advantageous to them to use poisonous agents. Until the time of their great reverses in Russia, the Germans had been engaged in aggressive advances which were often made rapidly in a lightning-war manner that did not offer the prospects of gaining great advantages by using poisonous agents. The Germans were accomplishing their missions without poison gas. In Russia, they expect to advance again, perhaps under circumstances that will not be conducive to the use of poison gas. However, if Hitler sees an opportunity to make a gigantic, overwhelming stroke with gas, he can hardly be expected to hesitate.

Whether the present chemical agents and other new ones will be used in the present conflict will probably depend on whether the Axis groups take the initiative. If they do, the United States proposes to be ready. If Hitlerism is to be defeated, we must do more than follow its pace-making, we must plan to win by some greater application of technical means than is possible by the enemy and our research continues with this prospect in mind.

The First World War showed conclusively the effectiveness of chemicals. No nation has dared abandon them since. Gas will be used in the future, most likely in overwhelming amounts, to obtain a decisive result. We should prepare our minds for this idea — not by a mere squadron of two airplanes or a few chemical motor units, but by armies of airplanes dropping tons of mustard or Lewisite, or other gases, and by massed battalions of chemical troops organized and supplied to neutralize vast areas completely and effectively.

We, as medical men, should be vitally interested in the possibilities of gas attacks. Here are a few questions to think over: (1) Are we to see the populations of our cities choked and burned by the lethal fumes and sprays of war gases? (2) Is it necessary for every man, woman and child to be equipped with a gas mask? (3) Is there real danger in this terrible threat of such attack? These questions are being asked by a justifiably apprehensive public. Obviously this view is but one extreme.

War gases may be divided into five general classes. (1) Lacrimators, commonly called "tear gases." (2) The lung irritants, which have as their base such gases as chlorine, phosgene and combinations such as chlorpicrin. (3) Systemic toxic agents, usually based on the exceptionally dead hydrocyanic acid gas. (4) Vesicants, a type generally identified under the name of "Mustard Gas." (5) The sternutators, gases which cause sneezing.

Gas casualties offer a real problem both in their treatment and evacuation. Doctors are subject to becoming gas casualties while in the execution of their mission.

Here's what happens during and after a gas attack in the Army. The gas alarm sounds—the troops take cover in gas shelters. The type of chemical used is identified and sometimes brought back to the rear lines for further examination. After the gas attack is over, everybody is on the lookout for a second attack. As soon as possible, casualties are evacuated, and such degassing or decontamination measures as required are undertaken. At this point, it is imperative that gas casualties be given first aid.

THE LACRIMATORS: Men who are lacrimated do not require evacuation as casualties. It is important, however, that they leave the contaminated atmosphere and face the wind, allowing the wind to blow into their eyes. The clothes should be changed and thoroughly aired, if possible. If the individual has rubbed his eyes, which, in some instances is difficult to prevent, bathing the eyes with cold water or weak solution of boric acid or bicarbonate solution will relieve a good deal of the discomfort. The patient will also feel that something is being done for him, and the passage of time will improve his condition.

THE LUNG IRRITANTS: A lung irritant

casualty, in order to reduce his oxygen requirements to a minimum, should be made to lie down and not allowed to walk to an aid station, even though he insists he is able to do so. He should, as soon as possible, be removed from the contaminated atmosphere, his equipment removed, his clothing loosened, and he should be kept warm. In addition to wrapping him in blankets, non-alcoholic stimulants such as hot coffee or tea should be given and he should be evacuated as soon as possible.

Later, if available, oxygen therapy and venesection may be used to prevent pulmonary edema. If the grey pallor stage has developed, venesection is not indicated, but oxygen therapy will be found very beneficial. He is an absolute litter case and should be placed in a hospital bed. In the acute stages, supportive measures and medications are used. The period of convalescence will vary from a few weeks to several months.

THE SYSTEMIC TOXIC AGENTS: One of the most dangerous poisons known to man is hydrocyanic acid gas. Although used unsuccessfully in the World War, it may be tried again. In dilute concentration the patient has a sensation of constriction of the throat, an unpleasant taste in his mouth, senses an odor of almonds and has mental confusion, faintness, dizziness, palpitation and labored respiration. Because of the extreme rapidity with which it acts, only first aid treatment, immediately instituted, can be given. The patient must be quickly removed from the contaminated atmosphere. Artificial respiration should be given immediately, including the use of respiratory stimulants such as inhaling ammonia fumes. Amyl nitrite pearls should be crushed and inhaled, and caffein and intravenous respiratory stimulants used. If death does not occur within an hour, complete recovery can probably be anticipated. When the normal respiration is resumed, the ill effects will soon pass off. It should be remembered especially that removal of the patient to fresh air and the use of artificial respiration is the most valuable treatment.

THE VESICANTS: The two common vesicants are Mustard and Lewisite. Both are extremely toxic, and in addition to their action as vesicants will, if inhaled, act as powerful lung irritants. Therefore, the use of the masks is necessary against both. Lewisite, by releasing arsenic directly into the blood stream, acts as a powerful systemic poisoning. Mustard has not this action, and in this sense is not considered a poison. Mustard is a heavy, oily liquid, colorless in its pure state, and has the odor of garlic. During the World War, Mustard was the most effective chemical agent, and it produced more casualties than any other agent. It will penetrate ordinary clothing and affect any part of the body with which it comes in contact. The first effect noticed is the irritation and inflamation of the eyes and eyelids. Later, there occurs an irritation of the respiratory passages with cough, nasal drainage, nausea and pain in the epigastrium. In this manner it acts as a lung irritant.

In the case of a Mustard casualty, he should be taken immediately out of the contaminated area and his clothing removed. If only portions of the clothing have been splashed with liquid Mustard, these can be cut away. If the face has been exposed, wash the eyes and rinse the nose and throat with a saturated boric acid, a weak sodium bicarbonate or common salt solution. If the vapor has been breathed, he should be treated and handled as a lung irritant casualty. First aid must be prompt for little can be done later than 20 to 30 minutes after exposure. Vapor burns on the skin may be lessened or even prevented by thorough cleansing with soap and water (preferably hot) immediately after exposure. Cleansing the exposed parts with gasoline (not containing tetraethyl) or kerosene prior to the use of soap and water will facilitate the removal of all traces of gas.

Mustard burns or skin areas wet with liquid Mustard should be immediately and repeatedly swabbed with a solvent, such as kerosene, straight gasoline, any oil, alcohol or carbon tetrachloride. Fresh clothes should be used and the spreading of the contamination should be avoided. After cleansing with the solvent, the affected parts should be thoroughly washed with soap and hot water. Cloths used in removing the liquid Mustard will be contaminated and should be burned or buried after use. A weak, freshly prepared solution of chloride of lime in water may be used in place of the oil solvent. This solution is itself very irritating to the skin and must, therefore, be removed by subsequent washing with soap and water. All casualties should be evacuated as soon as possible.

Lewisite, the other common vesicant, was first isolated and described by Professor Lewis of Northwestern University. It was never manufactured in large quantities nor used during the World War. It is a heavy, oily liquid, colorless in its pure state. Irritation of the eyes, nose and throat commences immediately upon exposure, and its vesicant action is more rapid than that of Mustard. The vapor causes an inflammation of the entire respiratory tract, including the smaller bronchi, and a general congestion of the lungs with some edema. The patient will sneeze violently almost at once upon inhalation; the skin effects follow within an hour, and the victim has become a definite casualty within that period of time. To be of any value against Lewisite, first aid measures must be instituted almost immediately. The treament is similar to that for Mustard.

In Lewisite burns, whether from vapor or liquid, the danger of poisoning from absorbed arsenic far overshadows the effect of the actual burn. It is, therefore, imperative to neutralize, if possible, any arsenic present and not yet absorbed. This may be accomplished by the immediate application of some hydrolizing agent. A 5 per cent aqueous solution of sodium hydroxide has been found very efficient if applied soon enough. Following the hydroxide solution, and cleansing with soap and water, liquid burns should be repeatedly swabbed with some oily solvent and washed again with soap and water. Following this, or in the absence of the hydroxide solution, vapor burns should be thoroughly cleansed with soap and water and then dressed with a ferric hydrate paste. The paste should be spread on thickly, covered with gauze, and allowed to remain for 24 hours. Fresh clothing must be supplied where necessary and all casualties should be evacuated as soon as possible.

THE STERNUTATORS: Sternutators or irritant smokes usually cause an intense irritation of the eyes and nose, excessive lacrimation from the eyes and a profuse watery discharge from the nose, a feeling of suffocation and constriction of the chest, sneezing and coughing, nausea and vomiting, and a terrific headache. Occasionally, there is a feeling of pain in the stomach and numbness of the limbs. Patients develop such a state of mental despair that they would rather die than continue to suffer such extreme agony.

Treatment is this: Remove the patient from the stricken area, keep away from heat and remove outer clothing. Flush the nose and throat with a weak solution of sodium bicarbonate or ordinary salt. Breathing chlorine in low concentration tends to alleviate the irritation. In lieu of other facilities, this may be accomplished by breathing from a bottle containing bleaching powder or from a mixture of alcohol, chloroform and ether. The exposed surface of the body should be washed with soap and water.

For burns from incendiaries, other than white phosphorus, treatment and handling are the same as for ordinary heat or fire burns. For phosphorus burns, immerse the affected part into water to stop the burning of the phosphorus and pick out the solid particles from the flesh; wet clothes, mud or damp earth may serve the purpose if immersion in water is not possible. As phosphorus melts at 111 degrees F., if hot water is used, the melted particles may be removed with a cloth or sponge.

The prompt application of an approximate two or three per cent solution of copper sulphate in water will form a thin coating of copper phosphate on the phosphorus particles which will stop their burning at once. The coated particles can then be picked out from the flesh. The copper sulphate solution should be applied by soaking a pledget of cotton, a sponge, or a piece of cloth in the solution and then placing it on the phosphorus. A minute or two is sufficient time for the formation of the metallic covering coat. After removal of the phosphorus, the burns should be dressed. All severe cases should be evacuated.

The doctor who is not accustomed to the treatment of gas casualties in his daily practice might find the need to refer to these first aid principles until he has had time to acquaint himself with the specific and complete treatment of gas casualties.

It must be realized that the sooner first aid treatment is administered to those exposed, the better their chances for early recovery. There must be no delay. Quick action is necessary. Although each gas or chemical produces certain conditions requiring special treatment, there are certain first aid principles applicable to all, which, if applied early, will give relief. These principles are expressed in the following requisites and procedure.

Requisites are: Fresh air, rest, warmth, careful attention and neutralization of the chemical.

The procedure: Remove the patient immediately from the gas infected area to a pure atmosphere, preferably in open air. Remove the outer gas-infected clothing as soon as possible, and cover to keep the patient warm. Wash the exposed body surfaces with water to remove the chemical. If the patient is suffering from phosphorus burns, it is very important to keep the burned area covered with water. If the patient has inhaled large quantities of phosgene, chlorpicrin, chlorine, or any other of the lung irritants, keep him in a reclining position and do not permit him to talk.

Send the patient to a hospital or aid station where he can receive additional attention if necessary. Transportation will be by litter and by an ambulance which handles only gas casualties, the operating personnel being provided with the necessary protective clothing and masks.

Upon arrival at any hospital or decontamination center, gas cases go through a process of sorting, bathing, and assignment to the proper ward for gas patients. When pos-

sible the slightly gassed are separated from the more serious cases. Cases of Mustard patients are also separated from those suffering from pulomnary edema. In some instances the reception of cases might be of such numbers as to necessitate the designation of an entire clearing station for their care.

The clearing stations in the theater of operations are necessarily mobile and must follow the tactical forces; therefore, careful selection is made of the patients for disposition, each case being considered with judgment and discretion as to his prognosis. All slightly gassed cases who are expected to recover completely in a few days are kept in the mobile hospital and returned to the front on recovery. Cases which have been seriously gassed by Mustard are evacuated to the rear as soon as their temporary needs have been provided. They go through the evacuation hospital and then to a general hospital. When their recovery is assured, they are transferred to a convalescent camp. The early evacuation of the Mustard case is carried out because Mustard does not cause acute pulmonary edema and, therefore, does not present the difficulty of transportation as do phosgene cases.

Those cases which are the result of lung irritants must be kept at the sites of reception where possible for a period of 48 hours until their maximum illness is over and until they no longer require oxygen therapy. This site will normally be the clearing station.

Rail or water transportation is used whenever available for evacuating the pulmonary edema cases in order to provide them with the greatest comfort and avoid any unnecessary physical exertion on their part. Plane ambulances are to be generally avoided because of respiratory difficulty should it become necessary to seek a high altitude. It is difficult for the patient to realize his condition until he is out of breath and unable to carry on any physical activity; therefore, he must be informed about the danger of disobeying orders regarding his transportation. This type of case should remain on the litter from the time he becomes a patient until he arrives at the hospital where he is to receive permanent care.

The remainder of the cases can be transported and evacuated in the same manner as the traumatic cases resulting from the normal weapons of war. Evacuation of the strictly gas patient requires careful handling and classification of the patients, adding a very heavy burden to the evacuation system. Because of this fact, gas warfare will not be entirely welcome to the medical department personnel in the theater of operations, even though the actual deaths are less in proportion than those from other causes.

The United States is in a better position to produce combat chemicals and use them in war than any other nation in the world. It has been the feeling of our people, however, that we shall never be the ones to start a chemical war. It has been our plan to be prepared, but to leave the initiative, so far as this weapon is concerned, to the enemy.

Regardless of how we look upon the use of gas by our own forces, we certainly must know how our enemies might use gas against us; and we have long realized that we cannot be fully prepared against it unless we know these things.

"It is the common fate of the indolent to see their rights become the prey of the active. The conditions upon which God hath given liberty to man is eternal vigilance; which condition if he break, servitude is at once the consequence of his crime and the puishment of his guilt."

Hypertension in a Young Athlete Due To Coarctation of Aorta . . . Report of Case

JOHNNY A. BLUE, B.A., M.D.*

GUYMON, OKLAHOMA

This discussion with a case report is being presented because: 1. Such a case is relatively rare in an all-around athlete. A review of the literature for the past fifteen years failed to discover a case with similar physical activities. 2. The profession should be on the alert for such a condition and be able to diagnose it clinically rather than await the unpleasant post-mortem revelations. 3. Coarctation of the Aorta with high blood pressure must be differentiated from essential hypertension. 4. Having made the diagnosis, the attending physician must face the responsibility of determining to what extent physical activities should be restricted. 5. Hypertension in a youth should cause one to suspect coarctation of the Aorta. In the adult suffering from hypertension, this condition must be ruled out before the patient is informed as to diagnosis, prognosis and therapy.

CASE REPORT

A young high school athelete presented himself to me, not because he was ill, but because his coach and other school authorities demanded a statement indicating that he was physically fit for competitive sports. He stated that the school authorities refused to let him compete in athletics without a doctor's certificate because some eighteen months previously he had been denied an insurance policy by an examining physician because of a "bad heart and high blood pressure." His only other statement was "I feel good all the time but am scared of a doctor."

Being personally interested in sports, I had noted this boy's physique and had observed his activities on the play ground over a period of several years, and was impressed with his athletic possibilities.

His family history was essentially negative except that his mother, a young robust woman in her early forties, had a blood pressure of 190/100. His father, a well-developed man of the middle forties, had a normal blood pressure and passed a good physical examination. An older sister, examined two years previously, had a normal blood pressure and no demonstrable abnormalities. An older brother was an athlete, but he was not available for examination.

PHYSICAL EXAMINATION

A physical examination revealed a well-developed and well-nourished white male fourteen years of age, five feet ten and one-half inches tall, weighing 160 pounds and exhibiting massive shoulders and rather slender legs. Though manifesting average intelligence, he was extremely nervous and apprehensive.

The temperature was 98.6, pulse 90, rhythm normal, respiration 16. The systolic blood pressure could not be determined by a Baum Mercury manometer which registered to 265. On a Fouchet machine, a systolic pressure was 280, diastolic 120.

The head and neck were essentially negative. Examination with reference to the respiratory system was negative. Examination with reference to the circulatory system re-

*Since the preparation of this article Dr. Blue has entered the U. S. Navy as a Lieutenant and is stationed at Bainbridge Naval Training Station, Bainbridge, Md.

vealed the following: The P.M.I. was in the fifth interspace at the nipple line. There were no thrills or shocks, but a loud blowing systolic murmur was easily discernible over the entire precordial area and was transmitted to the axilla and to the back. There were no signs of any tortuous or pulsating superficial vessels of the thorax. The gastrointestinal and genitourinary systems were negative.

The lower extremities were not as well proportioned as the rest of the body, but the boy was very agile and manifested no defects in locomotion. The pulse in the vessels below the knee and in the feet were not demonstrable. Blood pressure in the lower extremities was 100/70. The reflexes normal.

This patient stated that another doctor had given medicine which reduced his systolic pressure to 150. He was told that, in all probability, athletic training under proper supervision would do him no more harm than the unsupervised play which he daily indulged in very strenuously. He was told, however, that the statement for his school authorities would have to be withheld pending further investigation.

On the insistence of the patient and his family, it was decided to give him a therapeutic test. His activities were restricted, and he was placed on bromides and sulphocyanates which reduced his systolic blood pressure to 190/100 in three weeks. The patient was then advised to have a complete diagnostic study with special reference to his neurocirculatory condition. This resulted in the following report from Dr. E. A. Webb, University Hospital, Michigan University, Ann Arbor, Michigan. (Permission to use this letter for publication was granted by Dr. Max M. Peet, Professor of Neurosurgery.)

"The patient was admitted with the history and systemic history were entension for three years, discovered incidentally on insurance examination. He had been entirely asymptomatic. There had been no demonstrable etiology for his hypertension. The past history and systemic history were entirely negative.

"Physical examination revealed temperature, pulse and respirations normal. Blood pressure 210/105. Funduscopic examination showed a slight increase in the arterial reflex stripe, O. U. Slight venous engorgement, O. U. Examination of the neck revealed bilateral cervical adenitis. The heart was not enlarged. The rate was rapid. The rhythm was normal. There was a sharp, systolic rub murmur in the mitral and pulmonary areas. The pulses were full and bounding. Examination of the gen-

italia revealed rather mild hypergenitalism, otherwise negative.

"Urine was entirely negative. Routine hematology was essentially normal. Electrocardiogram was entirely normal. Urea clearance was well within the normal range. Blood non-protein-nitrogen was slightly elevated, 38.7 milligrams per cent, with a total blood urea nitrogen of 17.2 milligrams per cent. Concentration test was entirely normal. The routine funduscopic examination by the Department of Ophthalmology revealed minimal early arteriosclerosis of the retinal vessels, O. U. The patient's admission blood Kahn was negative.

"Intravenous pyelograms were entirely normal. Orthodiagram revealed normal heart size. No signs of pulmonary disease.

"The patient was referred to the Department of Internal Medicine and examination by the Medical Consultant prompted him to believe that the patient might very well have a coarctation of the aorta because of decreased blood pressure in the lower extremities, compared with the hypertension in the upper extremities. The examiner felt that there was no gross cardiac enlargement and no signs of myocardial insufficiency. X-ray examination, re-evaluation of orthodiagram films, showed only a suggestion of rib notching. However, since pulsation could not be felt in the feet, it was the examiner's oipnion that the diagnosis of coarctation of the aorta was fairly certain. Therefore, the balance of the routine hypertensive studies was not carried out and the patient was informed as to the type of illness which he has, also informed of the prognosis, was told not to limit his activity whatsoever and discharged home without further recommendations.

"Diagnosis: Coarctation of aorta."

Since the date of my first examination, the patient has had a full year of competitive athletics in high school, excelling in football, basketball, baseball and, to some extent, tennis and swimming. During his vacations, he engages in normal labor. His blood pressure has ranged from 210/100 to 265/120.

DISCUSSION

The word "coarctation" is derived from the Latin words "crum" (together) and "arcta're" (to make tight).

Coarctation of the Aorta is a congenital anomaly or mal-development which causes a narrowing of this vessel. The most common site of this narrowing is just distal to the communication of the ductus arteriosus with the Aorta.

There are two types depending on the degree of constriction of the Aorta; namely, the infantile type which always proves fatal before the ninth month, and the adult type which is often asymptomatic and undetected, according to the degree of localized constriction of the Aorta.

More than three hundred cases have been reported. It has been noted that the adult type occurs three times as often in males as in females. Levine states that 0.1 per cent of the entire population have this anomaly.

In a series of two hundred cases of the adult type reported by Abbott, the average age at death was 32 years. Sixty died of congestive heart failure, two of sudden heart conditions, thirty-eight of ruptured Aorta, twenty-six of Cerebral complications and fourteen of bacterial endarteritis.

The diagnosis is arrived at by keeping the condition in mind, by the presence of an elevated blood pressure in the upper extremities and a lowered blood pressure in the lower extremities, and in most cases a loud blowing systolic murmur over the precordium. Other findinigs may be signs of collateral circulation between the upper and lower extremities by the way of the intercostal, mammary, deep epigastric and scapular arteries, decrease in or absence of the shadow of the Aortic knob by X-ray, notching of the ribs by the dilated collateral vessels, enlargement of the heart, weakness of the lower extremities, flushing of the face, profuse sweating in the upper portion of the body, headaches, tinnitus and dizziness.

As a rule, the adult type of Coarctation of the Aorta terminates in heart failure, rupture of the Aorta, cerebral accident, bacterial endarteritis or valvular disease.

The life expectancy of the patient is dependent upon the severity of the case and the degree of collateral circulation between the upper and lower extremities.

The difficulties are those accompanying vascular hypertension. The treatment generally consists of advice along lines customarily given to patients with hypertension; namely, protection against physical and mental strain and infections.

CONCLUSION

Although this patient, whose blood pressure is very high, has suffered no apparent ill effects from prolonged and very strenuous athletic competition, the prognosis is guarded.

BIBLIOGRAPHY

White, Paul D: Heart Disease, Second Edition, Macmillan Company, 1937.

Leaman, William G.: Management of Cardiac Patient, J. B. Lippincott Company, 1940.

Levine, Samuel A.: Clinical Heart Disease, W. B. Saunders Company, 1942.

Yater, Wallace M.: Fundamentals of Internal Medicine, D. Appleton-Century Company, 1940.

King, J. T.: Annals of Internal Medicine, 10: 1802-1827, June, 1937.

Parks, W. K.: Causes of Hypertension in Young, South, M. J., 30: 1009-1012, October, 1937.

Wichster, N. F., and Gustofson: Coarctation—Adult Type, American Heart Journal, 14: 107-112, July, 1937.

Goodson, Jr., W. N: Coarctation—Two Unusual Cases, New England Journal of Medicine, 216: 339-345, February, 1937.

Flexner, J.: Coarctation—Adult Type, Clinical and Experimental Study, American Heart Journal, 11: 572-580, May, 1936.

Uhrick, N. L.: Coarctation—Adult Type, American Heart Journal, 7: 641-657, June, 1932.

Strary, G. F.: Coarctation—With Report of Three Cases, Canada M. A. J., 27: 15-19, July, 1932.

Page, I. H.: Blood Pressure in Dogs—Attempt to Produce Coarctation, American Heart Journal, 19: 218-232, February, 1940.

Steckney, J. M., and Dry, T. I.: Coarctation—Case With Slight Aortic Constriction, Staff Meeting Mayo Clinic, 14: 265-268, April, 1939.

Hallock, P., and Hibbel, R: Coarctation—Non-Clinical Type, American Heart Journal, 17: 444, April, 1939.

Wilson, M. G.: Coarctation—Adult Type with Hypertension, American Journal Diseases of Children, 44: 390-393, April, 1932.

Love, Jr., W. S., and Halem, J. H.: Coarctation with Associated Stenosis of Right Subclavian Artery, American Heart Journal, 17: 628, May, 1939.

Shapiro, M. J.: Coarctation—Ten Years Observation of Patient, J. A. M. A., 100: 640, 1942.

Walker, Livingston: Coarctation—Two Cases, Lancet, 2: 660-663, September, 1938.

Eisenberg, G.: Coarctation Recognized During Childhood, Journal of Pediatrics, 13: 303-308, September, 1938.

Rytand, D. A.: Renal Factor in Coarctation, Journal of Clinical Investigation, 17: 391, July, 1938.

Troutman, W. B.: Coarctation—Case, Kentucky Medical Journal, 35: 398, August, 1937.

Gitlow, S.: Coarctation—Report of Living Case, New York State Journal of Medicine, 37: 155, January, 1937.

Stewart, J. H., and Bailey, Jr., R. L.: Cardiac Output and Other Measures of Circulation in Coarctation, Journal of Clinical Investigation, 20: 145, March, 1941.

Grishman, A., Stunberg, M. F., and Sussman, M. L.: Contrast Roentgen Visualization, American Heart Journal, 21: 365, March, 1941.

Gitlow, S., and Senmer, R. I: Complete Coarctation: Case, American Heart Journal, 20: 106, July, 1940.

Woodbury, R. A., Murphy, E. E., and Hamilton, W. F.: Blood Pressure in Coarctation, Arc. Int. Med., 65: 752, April, 1940.

Nicholson, G. H. B.: Coarctation in Child with Arrested Subacute Bacterial Endocarditis and Calcified Mycotic Anurism, Medical Woman's Journal, 48: 159, June, 1941.

Boyd, C. E.: Coarctation, Tri-State Medical Journal, 14: 2570, November, 1941.

Sangster, C. B.: Coarctation: Case, Medical Journal Australia, 1: 733, May, 1937.

Coarctation, American Journal Diseases of Children, 62: 1224, December, 1941.

Coarctation, British Heart Journal, 3: 121, April, 1941.

Haverhill Fever
(A Case Report)

WILLIAM K. ISHMAEL, M.D.*

OKLAHOMA CITY, OKLAHOMA

Haverhill Fever is an acute infectuous disease, usually appearing in epidemics, characterized by an abrupt onset of the usual symptoms of sepsis. In addition to chills, malaise and fever, most patients present a skin rash and an acute polyarthritis. In most instances these symptoms are severe; however, the disease is usually self-limited and rarely terminates fatally.

This disease syndrome was first reported in 1925 by Levaditi, Nicolau and Poincloux.[1] These authors described the symptom complex accurately and in detail. They obtained blood cultures and described the organism, a gram negative streptobacillus. In addition to this, they demonstrated the peculiar affinity of the organism for mice, and described the typical joint involvement. They named this bacillus, "Streptobacillus moniliformis," and classed the disease in the infectuous polymorphous erythemas. The question of this organism playing an etiological role in arthritis was discussed.

Kirkwood and Stall[2], in discussing both types of rat-bite fever, state that probably the first case of Haverhill fever described was that reported by Schottmuller in 1914 which occurred in Germany. They also cite the case reported by Blake in 1916 in this country.

This syndrome was next reported in February, 1926, by Place, Sutton and Willner.[3] Their report described an epidemic of around 60 cases which occurred in Haverhill, Massachusetts, in January of the same year. The disease name was gained from this city. In addition to "Haverhill fever," the disease has since been known as, "acute septicemic polymorphous erythema," "erythema arthriticum epidemicum," and "rat-bite fever." The etiological agent also is known by several names, "Streptobacillus moniliformis," "Haverhillia moniliformia," "Streptobacillus muris ratti," "Actinomyces muris," and "Haverhillia multiformis."

These authors described the disease accurately, obtained positive blood cultures, but apparently erred in their observations in

regard to etiology. They concluded that the epidemic was transmitted by contaminated milk.

Subsequent reports on Haverhill fever have appeared from time to time. Parker and Hudson, in 1926[4], reported on the etiology of the disease. Levaditi and Selbie in 1929[5]. Levaditi, et al, also have reported on the disease in 1930[6], 1931[7], and 1932[8]. Winifred Strangeways, in 1933[9], discussed the reaction in mice and rats. He found that rats can carry the organisms in their nasopharynx, acting as carriers, not manifesting evidence of the disease themselves. Many cultural characteristics were described also.

In 1940, Allbritten, et al[10], reported on the characteristics of the two types of rat-bite fever, and clarified many points in regard to their differentiation.

In 1941, three papers were found on Haverhill fever. Kirkwood and Stall[2] summarize our present knowledge of the disease. Andrew Hart, Jr.[11] reported a case from Virginia, and Carl T. Larson[12] reported two cases of Haverhill fever in Washington, D. C.

From these reports, it is known that Haverhill fever is an infectuous disease caused by the Streptobacillus moniliformis, usually gained by the bite of an infected rat which carries the organisms in the nasopharynx. The disease is characterized by the following:

1. Incubation period of three to seven days.

2. Abrupt onset of severe symptoms of chills, malaise, nausea and vomiting, generalized muscular pain and headache. The initial fever usualy reaches from 104 to 106 degrees and frequently ends abruptly after three or four days. It may then persist for several weeks at a lower level.

3. A skin rash, appearing on the third or fourth day, characteristically a maculopapular erythema, having a red center, sometimes petechial, surrounded by a pale ring. This usually appears on the extensor surfaces, frequently over the joints. The rash usually lasts four or five days and may be followed by desquamation.

*Doctor Ishmael is now a Captain in the Medical Corps, stationed at Harding Field, La.

4. Polyarthritis, usually appearing between the fourth to the fourteenth day of the disease. The arthritis is usually acute and severe and persists for a period of seven to fourteen days. In many instances, however, the joints become chronic and persist for months. The fever in this latter group runs a course comparable to a mild typhoid fever but is apt to be more variable in the daily curve.

5. Epidemiology: It is difficult to estimate the distribution of Haverhill as the two types of rat-bite fever were not differentiated until recently. Kirkwood and Stoll[2], in 1941, stated that the disease had been reported in sporadic form in only two states at that time. Since then, Hart[11] has reported a case in Virginia, and Larson[12] has reported two cases in Washington, D. C. No previous reports could be found from the State of Oklahoma.

CASE HISTORY

This patient, a white male, thirty-nine years of age, was seen in the Arthritis Clinic of the Bone and Joint Hospital, Oklahoma City, on June 20, 1942. He complained of multiple joint pain, stiffness and swelling, associated with moderate generalized malaise.

History revealed that he was in normal health until the onset of his present illness. On April 13, 1942, he received a rat bite on his nose. There was free bleeding and the wound healed satisfactorily. About ten days following the rat bite, he developed a sudden chill which was followed with high fever. He stated that chills occurred daily for five consecutive days. The temperature remained quite high throughout this period. During this time he developed a skin rash "something like measles" but had small "blood blisters" in many of the eruptions. The rash persisted only five or six days. He stated that where the rash was severe over his knuckles, infected areas developed and continued draining.

Sometime during the latter part of the period in which the fever was present, he developed rather severe aching in his legs. This soon progressed to localized tenderness and swelling in the knees which migrated to the elbows and the joints of the hands. After a period of two or three weeks the joints subsided in severity but became chronic, and had persisted to the time of examination. He stated that he continued to run a mild fever for three or four weeks after the acute symptoms subsided.

The past history revealed no evidence of rheumatic disease, and was otherwise essentially negative. The family history was negative.

Examination revealed the patient to be a well developed and nourished man but apparently chronically ill. Oral temperature 99.2 degrees. The skin had a healthy appearance in general but there were lesions over the dorsum of the first interphalangeal and metacarpal joints of both hands and also the elbows. These lesions resembled ordinary "boils" in the various stages of induration, suppuration, drainage and healed areas.

The head and neck were negative. X-rays of the teeth revealed no evidence of infection. The chest was normal and the vascular and lymph systems revealed no evidence of disease. No changes were demonstrated in the nervous system.

The deformities in the hands resembled those seen in rheumatoid arthritis except for the presence of the skin lesions over the joints. A rather marked effusion was present in the first interphalangeal joints and the elbows. Tenderness to compression was present in these joints. Motion was limited about 50 to 60 per cent, no total ankylosis being present in any. The feet and ankles had no swelling, but motion was slightly limited and caused pain when forced. Both knees had a mild effusion, were tender to local pressure, and were limited about 15 degrees in motion.

Laboratory results: C.B.C. — negative. Wassermann — negative. Blood uric acid — 2.1 mg. per cent. Blood culture — immobile streptobacillus, three microns long, gram negative. There were filaments with filaform enlargements present on some. This culture was made by the Oklahoma State Health Laboratories and the organism was identified as the Streptobacillus moniliformis (Haverhillus). A blood culture was repeated one week later and was again positive, similar organisms being obtained. Cultures

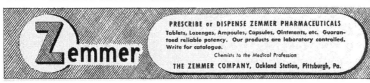

from the discharge from the skin lesions revealed a mixed growth, but no evidence of the Streptobacillus moniliformis. Synovial fluid culture negative.

The diagnosis of Haverhill fever was made on the patient on the basis of the history, joint findings, and the identification of the Streptobacillus moniliformis in the blood stream.

Treatment consisted of, in addition to ordinary supportive measures, nine weekly injections of .4 grams of neoarsphenamine. The patient made an uneventful recovery during the first four weeks of therapy. The joints returned to normal and regained full function.

In the two weeks observation period before therapy was started, the patient ran a daily temperature of around 99 to 100.5 degrees. In the second week of therapy, the temperature returned to normal and the symptoms of malaise and weakness disappeared. It should be noted here that the patient had received an eight day course of sulfathiazole prior to his admission. He stated that he was unable to note any change in his course as result of the sulfathiazole.

The patient returned to work after the second week of therapy and remained symptom-free until October, 1942. At that time he developed two ulcerated areas, one on the anterior surface of the right leg and one similarly located on the left leg. These areas drained a sero-sanguinous material similar to the previous lesions on the hands and elbows. The areas were painless and the joints were not involved. Hot saline fomentations and local sulfathiazole failed to improve these areas. Neoarsphenamine was again given and the lesions healed in about fourteen days. To date, no new exacerbations have occurred.

DISCUSSION

This case of Haverhill fever is reported in view of the fact that there is no evidence of previous cases being reported in the State of Oklahoma. This patient was living near Earlsboro when the bite occurred. No other similar cases have been reported from that area.

It should be noted that, whereas this patient apparently responded satisfactorily to arsenicals, there is no known specific therapy for this infection. The vast majority of cases are self-limited and according to the literature, heal spontaneously after several months.

BIBLIOGRAPHY

1. Levaditi, C., Nicolau, S. and Poincloux, P.: On the Etiologic Role of Streptobacillus Moniliformis in Acute Septicemic Polymorphus Erythema, Compt. rend. Acad. d. Sc., 180: 1188, 1925.

2. Kirkwood, Tom and Stoll, C. G.: "Rat-bite and Haverhill Fevers," Ill. Med. Jour., 80: 141 (August) 1941.

3. Place, Edwin H., Sutton, Jr., Lee E. and Willner, Otto: "Erythema Arthriticum Epidemicum," The Boston Medical and Surgical Jour., 194: 285, (February 18) 1926.

4. Parker, Frederick, Jr. and Hudson, N. Paul: "The Etiology of Haverhill Fever (Erythema Arthriticum Epidemicum)," American Jour. of Path. 2: 357 (September) 1926.

5. Levaditi, C. and Selbie, F. R.: "Mode of Transmission of Acute Epidemic Polymorphaus Erythema," Compt. rend. Acad. d. Sc., Par., 189: 1332, 1929.

6. Levaditi, C., Selbie, F. R. and Schoen, R.: "Myocarditis in the Polyarticular Rheumatism of Mice caused by the Streptobacillus Moniliformis," Compt. rend. Soc. de biol., 103: 463 (February 21) 1930.

7. Levaditi, C., Selbie, F. R. and Delorme, M.: "Mode of Spontaneous Transmission of Infectuous Polyarticular Rheumatism of Mice caused by the Streptobacillus Moniliformis," Compt. rend. Soc. de biol., 107: 501 (June 5) 1931.

8. Levaditi, C., Selbie, F. R. and Schoen, R.: "Spontaneous Infections Rheumatism of the Mouse caused by the Streptobacillus Moniliformis," Ann. Inst. Pasteur, 48: 308 (March) 1932.

9. Strangeways, Winifred I.: "Rats as Carriers of Streptobacillus Moniliformis," Jour. of Path. and Bact., 37: 45, 1933.

10. Allbritten, F. F., Sheely, R. F., and Jeffers, W. A.: "Haverhilla Multiformis Septicemia, its Etiologic and Clinical Relationship to Haverhill and Rat-bite Fevers," J.A.M.A., 114: 2360 (1940).

11. Hart, Andrew D., Jr.: "Haverhill Fever following Rat Bite," Virginia Med. Monthly, 68: 582 (October) 1941.

12. Larson, Carl L., "Rat-bite Fever in Washington, D. C. due to Spirilum munus and Streptobacillus Moniliformis," Public Health Reports, 56: 40 (October 3) 1941.

Ether As the Anesthetic of Choice in Prolonged Operations

On a certain occasion after I had removed the greater portion of the lower jaw as a sequestrum, walking back into the operation room after washing my hands I noticed a swelling under the chin which indicated that there was a pocket which required external drainage. The ether anesthetic had been stopped for some time so I had the attendants hold him firmly while I made a quick incision, expecting the patient to try to jump off the table, but he did not budge. I was greatly impressed with this fact but attached no particular importance to it until some years afterward when I had occasion to explore the right cerebral cortex, turning down an osteoplastic flap and opening the dura. I remember feeling that I wanted to be sure that this patient did not get too much anesthetic, so I instructed the anesthetist, who was giving drop ether on an open mask, to get the patient completely under surgically and then stop the anesthetic until she heard further from me. I got busy with my operation and forgot all about the anesthetic and when I got through I found out that I had been working for over two hours and that the patient had received no more anesthesia after once being deeply anesthetized. I began to feel then that there must be something different about ether, and now and then instructed the anesthetist to stop the anesthetic sometime before the end of the operation. More recently, I have been making it a rule in operations that I expect to last for much more than an hour to have the anesthetic discontinued after giving it for 45 minutes or one hour. I found that we could work for at least another hour without difficulty. Still more recently, I cut the period of anesthesia after the operation was started to 20 minutes and later again to 15 minutes, and I found that we could still continue to operate for an hour or more after the anesthetic had been stopped. I further found that we could continue to operate while the patient recovered consciousness to the extent of being able to converse with the operator or the assistants during the operation.

The ether is administered on the open cone in the usual way, deep surgical anesthesia induced and maintained during the period of administration. In patients who object to ether, with or without their knowledge ethylene has been given till the patient becomes unconscious, then the ether started. The mask has in some instances been left on the patient's face, in others removed.—Joseph A. Danna, M.D., New Orleans Medical and Surgical Journal, September, 1942.

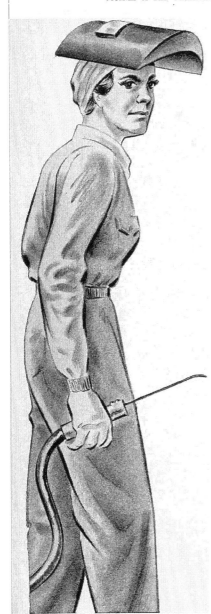

"MANPOWER"...
and the Menopause

"MANPOWER" in industry is rapidly changing to "womanpower." And, with so many women on production and assembly lines, the problem of absenteeism and lowered efficiency, particularly among women in their forties, deserves consideration.

It has been estimated that 80 per cent of women in this age group experience menopausal symptoms of varying intensity. Efficiency demands that these workers be physically and emotionally fit. Clinical investigations show that, in a large percentage of cases, they can be kept "on the job" through the use of adequate estrogenic therapy.

The high clinical effectiveness of Amniotin in relieving the distressing vasomotor symptoms of the menopause has been amply demonstrated by numerous clinical reports published during the past 12 years. The product has likewise proved valuable in treating other conditions related to a deficiency of estrogenic substances.

Two New Advantages ... The new economy-size vials of Amniotin offer two distinct advantages. They provide a substantial saving over the cost of Amniotin in ampuls and they facilitate the use of fractional doses without waste of material.

Differing from estrogenic substances containing or derived from a single crystalline factor, Amniotin is a highly purified, non-crystalline preparation of naturally occurring estrogenic substances derived from pregnant mares' urine. Its estrogenic activity is expressed in terms of the equivalent of international units of estrone. In addition to the economy-vial packages and the ampuls (both of which are for intramuscular injection) you can secure Amniotin in capsules for oral administration and in pessaries for intravaginal use.

ECONOMY-SIZE VIALS
10 cc..........20,000 I. U. per cc.
10 cc..........10,000 I. U. per cc.
20 cc.......... 2,000 I. U. per cc.

For literature address Professional Service Department, 745 Fifth Avenue, New York

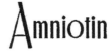

A SQUIBB PREPARATION OF ESTROGENIC SUBSTANCES OBTAINED FROM THE URINE OF PREGNANT MARES

· THE PRESIDENT'S PAGE ·

There can be little doubt among either the lay public or the medical profession that during the present world emergency medicine, as a profession, is on scientific trial.

Congregation of large masses of people in newly constructed industrial centers, attendant with inadequate living facilities in both rural and urban communities, is simply inviting the creation of medical problems. To combat effectually the effort of disease to conquer the normal, healthy person, calls for a constant vigil by the doctor of medicine. He must at all times preach and practice preventive medicine, and use the most modern of treatment methods commensurate with the needs of his patients.

It is for the above reasons that the medical profession has believed in and sponsored scientific meetings for the purpose of medical education. The Annual Meeting of the Association, to be held in Oklahoma City May 11 and 12, is designed to give an opportunity to physicians to refresh and add to their professional knowledge. Every member should immediately start making arrangements to attend at least one day of the meeting. You owe this time not only to yourself, but to your patients.

A healthy nation is a safe nation. This charge is your responsibility. What will be the verdict of the public? What part will you have played in bringing about the verdict? Will you have appeared for the defense or the prosecution in the eyes of your patients and the public?

Sincerely yours,

James D Osborn

President.

The JOURNAL Of The
OKLAHOMA STATE MEDICAL ASSOCIATION

EDITORIAL BOARD
L. J. MOORMAN, Oklahoma City, Editor-in-Chief

E. EUGENE RICE, Shawnee

NED R. SMITH, Tulsa

MR. R. H. GRAHAM, Oklahoma City, Business Manager

CONTRIBUTIONS: Articles accepted by this Journal for publication including those read at the annual meetings of the State Association are the sole property of this Journal.

The Editorial Department is not responsible for the opinions expressed in the original articles of contributors.

Manuscripts may be withdrawn by authors for publication elsewhere only upon the approval of the Editorial Board.

MANUSCRIPTS: Manuscripts should be typewritten, double-spaced, on white paper 8½ x 11 inches. The original copy, not the carbon copy, should be submitted.

Footnotes, bibliographies and legends for cuts should be typed on separate sheets in double space. Bibliography listing should follow this order. Name of author, title of article, name of periodical with volume, page and date of publication.

Manuscripts are accepted subject to the usual editorial revisions and with the understanding that they have not been published elsewhere.

NEWS: Local news of interest to the medical profession, changes of address, births, deaths and weddings will be gratefully received.

ADVERTISING: Advertising of articles, drugs or compounds unapproved by the Council on Pharmacy of the A.M.A. will not be accepted. Advertising rates will be supplied on application.

It is suggested that members of the State Association patronize our advertisers in preference to others.

SUBSCRIPTIONS: Failure to receive The Journal should call for immediate notification.

REPRINTS: Reprints of original articles will be supplied at actual cost provided request for them is attached to manuscripts or made in sufficient time before publication. Checks for reprints should be made payable to Industrial Printing Company, Oklahoma City.

Address all communications to THE JOURNAL OF THE OKLAHOMA STATE MEDICAL ASSOCIATION, 210 Plaza Court, Oklahoma City.

OFFICIAL PUBLICATION OF THE OKLAHOMA STATE MEDICAL ASSOCIATION
Copyrighted April, 1943

EDITORIALS

THE STATE MEETING

One of the major evils of long continued war is the retardation of civil medical science and its application to individual and community needs. In the State of Oklahoma the members of the medical profession must do every thing possible to minimize the evil effects of the present world-wide conflict. The cancellation of plans for nearly all the national scientific meetings makes it incumbent upon us to have the best possible program for our coming state meeting, and to employ every legitimate means to secure a full attendance.

In view of the existing circumstances, only a matter of life and death should interfere with attendance at this meeting. Though the time required may represent an immediate sacrifice, it offers rich rewards—at least it will bear a handsome rate of interest. In fact, a doctor's right to practice medicine implies a liberal knowledge of current diagnostic and therapeutic methods. Let's stock up, speed up and keep up. Let's surprise our fellows at the front by securely holding their heritage at home through the adequate application of both the science and the art of medicine in the care of their patients.

Please do not fail to show your shining face at the meeting.

AN ILLUSTRIOUS ALUMNUS

The homing instinct brought back our former student, "Bill," who as Major Oscar W. Stewart with the Royal Canadian Army Medical Corps, gave a talk at the Medical School auditorium on his experiences during the past two and one-half years in England. He was among the first to volunteer when Great Britain entered the war, and went overseas with Dr. Penfield's Neurological Unit from the Montreal Neurological Institute.

In addition to his introductory remarks, which had a significant bearing upon the importance of cooperation with proper integration of all services from first aid to final hospitalization, he presented striking pictures of varied casualties, some of which were new to military surgery and therefore handled with alarm and reticence by first aiders, but ultimately demanding only good surgical management along accepted lines.

The victims of air raid bombing were among those arriving with little or no first aid. Many of them were brought in limp and livid, covered with the cement-like dust and plaster of bomb debris, and exhibiting fresh or dried blood over their heads and faces in gruesome patterns. But through the magic of medicine and surgery, they were soon rehabilitated and clamoring for action so characteristic of the indomitable English.

Out of the discussion on scalp, skull and intracranial injuries comes one significant lesson for all doctors: namely, the importance of scalp wounds. It was pointed out that the intimate inter-communication of the extra and intra-cranial circulation favors serious infection, making it necessary to be very thorough in the application of first aid, or to apply the simplest dressings while speeding up transportation to the point of ultimate surgical care. In one picture after another it was shown that scanty scalp shaving, hasty cleansing and premature suturing without searching for concealed missiles, resulted in serious infections. Attention was called to the fact that in World War I eight hours after injury was considered the maximum time for safe primary closure of such wounds, but recent experience based upon Dieppe cases when the casualties came in with only dry gauze dressings and otherwise little or no first aid, indicates that primary closure may be safe after 20 to 40 hours. This statement must be supplemented by the fact that the local use of the sulfonomides is materially influencing results. The high note of the discussion was the insistence upon the best possible surgical principles from the first aid to the final effort, and that "the exigencies of war" or "the best under the circumstances" should never be accepted as an excuse for poor surgery.

Major Stewart graduated from the University of Oklahoma School of Medicine in 1934. His studies were continued at the Massachusetts General Hospital, the Johns Hopkins Hospital, and at the Montreal Neurological Institute where he was pursuing a four year scholarship in neuro-anatomy and neuro-physiology when he went overseas. When Lord Tweedsmuir was in the Institute suffering from a fatal neuro-surgical condition, Major Stewart was assigned to special duty on his case, and after his death Lady Tweedsmuir presented him with a set of Lord Tweedsmuir's monogramed cuff links as a token of esteem and appreciation.

"THE GLEN WUDNA DAE WEEL WITHOOT WELLIUM MacLURE"

The above title is quoted from "A Doctor of the Old School," one of the most moving chronicles in the English language. This statement should give some comfort to those who decry the loss of so many young doctors for military service and fear that civilian medicine is going to the dogs .

The word "choice" implies an alternative, and it may be said that the selection of doctors for military service has been made with care and discrimination. The young have been chosen because they have reserve energy and endurance. They are ardent and courageous, endowed with imaginative passions well adapted to war. The old have been left at home because through the expenditure of reserves and experience they are limited in endurance, and have learned to calmly mix their wine with reality.

Without casting any reflections upon the young, we may say that it is fortunate for the people who are left at home and the young doctors who have gone to war, that the older doctors remain to take care of civilian practice. Fortunately, man may grow old chronologically without losing intellectual acuity. In this alert age, with its unusual facilities for rapid dissemination of knowledge, many doctors who have grown old are relatively well informed as to scientific advances and technical procedures.

Increasing age gives rise to experience; out of experience comes knowledge and, perchance, wisdom. What, after all, is so stimulating and informative as the practice of medicine? The young doctor, well grounded in the scientific principles of modern medicine and fired with energy and enthusiasm, is peculiarly fitted for military service. The older doctor, seasoned by experience, is equally well suited for civilian practice. This is particularly true in time of war when people's souls are distraught because of mental and physical strain. The experience and equanimity which have been evolved through the doctor's contact with human trials compliments individual and community needs, inspires faith, and resolves psychological conflicts. No doctor can live long with his patients without discovering that "practice is science touched with emotion."

The nation will be surprised to learn how much the older doctors can do. If their wings had been made of wax, they would have fallen in the sea long ago. The inevitable increase in morbidity and mortality in this country will depend largely upon the exigencies of war, rather than upon the want of medical care. The education of the special senses and the accumulation of knowledge through experience have taught them how to work with both deliberation and dispatch. With their accustomed unlimited hours, they will get the job done. With their ethical traditions and training, they will welcome the return of the young doctors, no matter how long the war may last.

There should be no wasted energy through worry about the additional burdens placed upon the shoulders of elderly doctors. As the record will show, they have a yen for dying in their boots. Apparently the gods have granted them a special dispensation through coronary disease. If the excitement of battle should hasten the end, may the God of Peace give them an easy crossing.

HEMOPTYSIS

Thirty years ago blood spitting was considered pathognomonic of tuberculosis, provided mitral disease could be ruled out. Today our knowledge of the various causes of hemoptysis and modern methods of investigation make presumption inexcusable.

When a patient presents himself for examination because of blood spitting, or when it occurs in a patient under management, it is the doctor's duty to recognize such an episode as only a symptom and to initiate diagnostic studies with a view of determining the source and the cause of the bleeding. Having eliminated the upper respiratory tract, the gums, and the varicose veins at the base of the tongue as probable sources, hematemesis must be considered. It may be said that the mode of expulsion is suggestive, and that blood from the bronchopulmonary system during active hemorrhage is bright red and often accompanied by air bubbles, while blood from the stomach is dark and may contain fragments of food. If hemorrhage of the stomach is massive, pallor and even fainting may precede hematemesis. While hemorrhage from the respiratory tract may be very profuse and occasionally may cause sudden death, the above described picture seldom, if ever, occurs.

Tuberculosis must be recognized as the most common cause of blood from the bronchopulmonary system. It usually comes from ulceration in the lungs, but may arise from tuberculous lesions in the bronchi or trachea, including irritation from a tuberculous broncholith. If tuberculosis can be eliminated as the cause, still the doctor is faced with serious differential diagnostic difficulties. The non-tuberculous causes of blood from the bronchopulmonary system are numerous, and a definite diagnosis may depend upon methods which are supplementary to the usual diagnostic procedures. These include exhaustive x-ray studies with bronchography if indicated, and bronchoscopic examinations. The latter should not be made for several days after a frank and profuse hemorrhage.

Jackson and Diamond[1], after careful diagnostic studies, reported 436 nontuberculous cases with hemoplysis as follows: Bronchiectasis, 138; primary carcinoma of bronchus, 82; tracheobronchitis, 74; pulmonary abscess, 51; no evidence of disease, 34; nonsuppurative pneumonitis, 15; suppurative pneumonitis, 11; adenoma of bronchus, 11; secondary cancer of lung, 6; lobar atelec-

tasis, 4; primary carcinoma of trachea, 2; suppurating pneumoconiotic lymph node discharging into bronchus, 1; nonspecific granuloma of bronchus, 1; streptothricosis, 1; chondroma of bronchus, 1; osteoma of trachea, 1; dermoid cyst communicating with bronchus, 1; broncholithiasis, 1; neurofibroma involving wall of bronchus, 1.

1 Jackson, C. L. and Diamond, S.: Haemorrhage From the Trachea, Bronchi and Lungs of Nontuberculous Origin. American Review of Tuberculosis. Vol. XLVI, 1942, p. 126.

REGIONAL MEETING OF THE COLLEGE OF PHYSICIANS

A regional meeting of the College of Physicians will be held in Kansas City, Missouri, on Saturday, May 8, 1943. This will comprise the states of Missouri, Kansas and Oklahoma.

This is in keeping with the policy of the College, since the general annual meeting will not be held this year, but groups of states and individual states are planning these smaller meetings in deference to the congested railroad traffic, and to give doctors in these areas a chance for refresher courses. The Surgeon General of the Army and Navy, the A.M.A., College of Surgeons and like societies are whole hearted in backing and abetting these meetings.

Meetings of this type have a very definite value since those left on home duty are unable to get away for any length of time due to increased work and diminished transportation facilities. Especially is this true of the men who have been drafted back to work in their respective communities, and who feel the need of a little "brushing up." It also gives valuable service to those in uniform as there will be a seminar held in Leavenworth, Kansas, and Kansas City the evening before, which will be of a military-medical nature.

It is quite unfortunate that this meeting is to be held just on the eve of our State Medical Meeting (May 11 and 12), but it is to be hoped that Oklahoma will be well represented at this Kansas City meeting, as an excellent program will be presented.—Lea A. Riely, M.D.

Opium

There is a popular idea that opium gives pleasant dreams, and that it takes us away into the land of poetry, to which it is supposed to have conducted Coleridge and DeQuincey. As a matter of fact, there are but few persons who get more out of opium than relief of pain, sense of comfort, and next day's remorses. The opium dream is not for all. I have known only four or five cases of habitual and distinct opium dreamers. There was more of Coleridge than of opium in "Kubla Khan," and more of DeQuincey than of the juice of poppies in the "Vision of Sudden Death." When it came to the telling of these immortal dreams, we may well suspect that the narrative gained in the literary appeal from the poet opium-drunk to the poet sober.—S. Weir Mitchell, Doctor and Patient, 1887.

GUEST SPEAKER

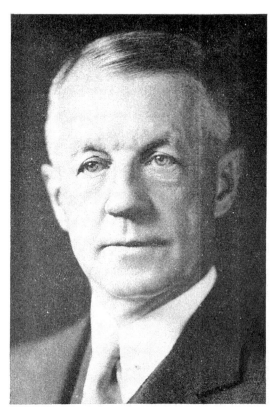

FRANK H. LAHEY, M.D.,
Boston, Mass.
Chairman, Directing Board
Procurement and Assignment Service

PROGRAM

Fifty-first Annual Session of the Oklahoma State Medical Association
Oklahoma City, May 11, 12, 1943

GREETINGS FROM THE OKLAHOMA COUNTY MEDICAL SOCIETY

The Oklahoma County Medical Society is again privileged to be the host society for the Annual Meeting of the State Association. Its membership is fully aware of the responsibilities of a host society, and pledges itself to make the stay of the visiting physicians as pleasant and entertaining as possible in view of wartime restrictions.

The program of the meeting, while being streamlined for obvious reasons, still gives an opportunity for an exchange of medical knowledge that cannot help but be of benefit to all physicians who attend.

The Oklahoma County Medical Society is pleased to invite you to a complimentary buffet supper on Tuesday evening, May 11, in the Venetion Room, Skirvin Hotel.

The Oklahoma County Society is looking forward to having you as their guests, and will strive to maintain the hospitality of past years.

The Auxiliary of our society has planned entertainment for your wife, so, of course, plan to bring her along.

We are keenly anticipating a visit from you on May 11 and 12.

> Walker Morledge, M.D., President
> Oklahoma County Medical Society.

General Information

HEADQUARTERS
Skirvin Hotel

REGISTRATION
Fourteenth Floor, Skirvin Hotel

All physicians, except visiting guests and members of the military forces, must have membership cards for 1943 before registering. Dues will not be accepted at the registration desk except from County Secretaries.

GENERAL SESSIONS AND SECTION MEETINGS

All meetings will be held in either the Venetian Room or the Rose Room on the fourteenth floor of the Skirvin Hotel. Section meetings will start at 9.00 A.M., and the formal papers at 11.00 in the morning and 4.00 in the afternoon. Roundtable section discussion will be on the Mezzanine floor, Skirvin Hotel at 12:15 P.M.

HOUSE OF DELEGATES

The House of Delegates will meet Monday, May 10, at 8:00 P.M. and at 8:30 A.M. Tuesday in the Crystal Room, Mezzanine Floor, Skirvin Hotel.

COUNCIL

The Council will meet at 4.00 P.M., Monday, May 10, in Room 741, Skirvin Hotel, and thereafter on the call of the President.

ROUNDTABLE LUNCHEON DISCUSSIONS

An innovation for this year's meeting will be the holding of scientific section roundtable luncheons during the noon hour for the purpose of discussing the papers presented in the sections during the morning. The luncheons will be held on the Mezzanine floor of the Skirvin Hotel. You must purchase your ticket at time of registering due to food rationing.

RESOLUTIONS—AMENDMENTS TO CONSTITUTION AND BY-LAWS

Resolutions and amendments to the Constitution and By-Laws for the consideration of the House of Delegates must be submitted at the first meeting of the House of Delegates.

WOMEN'S AUXILIARY

Registration will be on the Mezzanine floor of the Skirvin Hotel. The complete program will be found on this page.

OKLAHOMA UNIVERSITY MEDICAL ALUMNI LUNCHEON

The annual meeting of the alumni has been postponed due to war conditions. Dr. J. William Finch of Hobart, President, desires that all alumni continue as members of the Alumni Association. Dues should be sent direct to Dr. Finch. If feasible, a meeting will be held during the Oklahoma City Clinical Society meeting in the fall of the year.

BUFFET SUPPER

Tuesday evening, May 11, there will be a complimentary buffet supper at 6:30 in the Venetian Room, fourteenth floor, Skirvin Hotel, given by the Oklahoma County Medical Society. Highlighting the meeting will be Frank Lahey, M.D., Boston, Massachusetts, Chairman of the Directing Board of Procurement and Assignment Service, and Colonel W. Lee Hart, Surgeon General of the Eighth Service Command, Dallas, Texas.

PRESIDENT'S INAUGURAL DINNER DANCE

The dinner dance will be held on Wednesday evening, May 12, at 7.00 o'clock in the Venetian Room, fourteenth floor, Skirvin Hotel. The Honorable Robert S. Kerr, Governor of Oklahoma, will be the guest speaker. Ticket reservations must be made at the time of registering due to food rationing.

GOLF TOURNAMENT

The golf tournament will be held at the Oklahoma City Golf and Country Club, and will be medal play over 18 holes. Those wishing to compete may play any time during the meeting. Hugh Jeter, M.D. is chairman of the tournament.

Women's Auxiliary Program

State Auxiliary Officers

President Mrs Frank L. Flack	Secretary Mrs. James Stevenson
President-Elect Mrs. F. Maxey Cooper	Treasurer Mrs. H. Lee Farris
Vice-President Mrs. Jim L. Haddock	Historian Mrs. Clinton Gallaher

Parliamentarian
Mrs. Edward D. Greenberger

Mrs. Henry H. Turner, Convention Chairman

Tuesday, May 11, 1943

9.00 A M. Registration ....Skirvin Hotel

4:00 P M. Pre-convention Executive Board meeting and tea in the home of Mrs. F. Maxey Cooper, 248 NW 34th Street, Oklahoma City.

6.30 P.M. Buffet Supper ....Skirvin Hotel

Wednesday, May 12, 1943

9.00 A.M. Registration.

10:00 A.M. General Meeting ....Venetian Room, Y.W.C.A.

12.00 Noon Coffee ....Venetian Room, Y.W.C.A.

1:00 P.M. Post-convention Executive Board Meeting ....Venetian Room, Y.W.C.A.

7:00 P.M. Dinner Dance ....Skirvin Hotel

OFFICERS

of

Oklahoma State Medical Association
1942-43

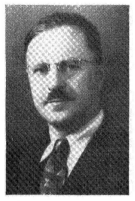

James Stevenson, M.D., Tulsa
President-Elect

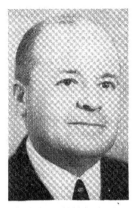

J. D. Osborn, M.D., Frederick
President

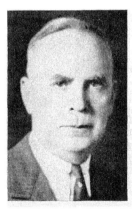

Lewis J. Moorman, Oklahoma City
Secretary-Treasurer

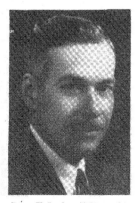

George H. Garrison, Oklahoma City
Speaker, House of Delegates

Scientific Program

Oklahoma State Medical Association

May 11, 12, 1943
Fourteenth Floor, Skirvin Hotel
Oklahoma City

All Sections will meet in either the Rose or Venetian Rooms, Fourteenth Floor, Skirvin Hotel. All Session meetings will be in the Venetian Room.

Tuesday, May 11

Venetian Room
Fourteenth Floor, Skirvin Hotel

General Chairman, Ben H. Nicholson, M.D., Oklahoma City

9:00—11:00 A.M.

SECTION ON PUBLIC HEALTH

Grady F. Mathews, M.D., Commissioner of Health, Oklahoma City, Chairman
Mack I. Shanholtz, M.D., Wewoka, Secretary

9:00 Chairman's Address, "Public Health in War Time"—Grady F. Mathews, M.D.

9:20 "Syphilis in Industry"—David V. Hudson, M.D., Tulsa.

9:40 "The Rapid Treatment Method for Syphilis"—Udo J. Wile, M.D., Professor of Dermatology and Syphilology, University of Michigan School of Medicine, Ann Arbor, Michigan.

10:00 "The Child in the Local Health Program"—Captain Glidden Brooks, Mayes County Health Superintendent, Pryor. (*By invitation.*)

10:20 "Sanitation in War Time"—Mr. H. J. Dorcey, Director of the Bureau of Public Health Engineering, State Health Department, Oklahoma City. (*By invitation.*)

10:40 "The County Health Department in Oklahoma"—John W. Shackelford, M.D., Public Health Department, Oklahoma City.

11:00 Adjournment to Venetian Room for presentation of formal paper.

(*Discussion of papers will be conducted at roundtable luncheon.*)

Rose Room

Fourteenth Floor, Skirvin Hotel

General Chairman, Elmer Musick, M.D., Oklahoma City

9:00—10:00 A.M.

SECTION ON PEDIATRICS

David J. Underwood, M.D., Tulsa, Chairman
Clark H. Hall, M.D., Oklahoma City, Secretary

9:00 Chairman's Address, "The Rh Factor"—David J. Underwood, M.D.

9:20 "Common Orthopedic Conditions in Childhood"—D. H. O'Donoghue, M.D., Oklahoma City.

9:40 "Intramedullary Transfusions of Blood in Infancy"—Charles M. Bielstein, M.D. University Hospital, Oklahoma City. (*By invitation.*)

10:00 Adjournment for Section on Neurology, Psychiatry and Endocrinology.

(*Discussions of papers will be conducted at roundtable luncheon.*)

10:00—11:00 A.M.

SECTION ON NEUROLOGY, PSYCHIATRY AND ENDOCRINOLOGY

Rose Room, Fourteenth Floor, Skirvin Hotel
John L. Day, M.D., Fort Supply, Chairman
James A. Willie, M.D., Oklahoma City, Secretary

10:00   "Demonstration of Minimum Neuropsychiatric Examination for Inductees"—Coyne H. Campbell, M.D., Oklahoma City.

10:20   "Some Neuropsychiatric Problems Arising in New Army Recruits"—Major Lester D. Borough, M.D., Neuropsychiatric Division, Cantonment Hospital, Fort Sill.

10:40   "Neuropsychiatric Problems Arising in the Civilian Population"—James A. Willie, M.D., Oklahoma City.

11:00   Adjournment to Venetian Room for presentation of formal paper.

(Discussion of papers will be conducted at roundtable luncheon.)

Venetian Room
Fourteenth Floor, Skirvin Hotel

11:00 A.M.

FORMAL PAPER

Ben H. Nicholson, M.D., Chairman

"Tuberculosis in the State Sanatorium" (Illustrated)—Forrest P. Baker, M.D., Director, Eastern Oklahoma State Tuberculosis Sanatorium, Talihina.

12:00 Noon

ROUNDTABLE LUNCHEONS

(Luncheon programs will be discussions of the papers presented during the morning sessions of the Sections.)

SECTION ON NEUROLOGY, PSYCHIATRY AND ENDOCRINOLOGY

John L. Day, M.D., Chairman

Green Room, Mezzanine Floor, Skirvin Hotel

Discussions

"Demonstration of Minimum Neuropsychiatric Examination for Inductees'—Charles E. Leonard, M.D., Oklahoma City.

"Some Neuropsychiatric Problems Arising in New Army Recruits"—Major Moorman Prosser, M.C., Camp Gruber.

"Neuropsychiatric Problems Arising in Civilian Population"—Felix Adams, M.D., Vinita.

SECTION ON PEDIATRICS

David J. Underwood, M.D., Chairman

Parlor G, Mezzanine Floor, Skirvin Hotel

Discussions

"Common Orthopedic Conditions in Childhood"—Maurice J. Searle, M.D., Tulsa.

"Intramedullary Transfusions of Blood in Infancy"—W. B. Mullins, M.D., Shawnee.

SECTION ON PUBLIC HEALTH

Grady F. Mathews, M.D., Chairman

Wilson Room, Mezzanine Floor, Skirvin Hotel

Discussions

"Syphilis in Industry"—Captain John A. Cowan, M.D., Public Health Department, Oklahoma
.   City. (By invitation.)

"The Child in the Local Health Program"—C. W. Arrendell, M.D., Ponca City.

"Sanitation in War Time"—Captain A. W. Green, M.C., Fort Sill.

"The County Health Department in Oklahoma"—Mack I. Shanholtz, M.D., Wewoka.

Venetian Room
Fourteenth Floor, Skirvin Hotel

General Chairman, James Stevenson, M.D., Tulsa, President-Elect
Oklahoma State Medical Association.

2:00—4:00 P.M.

SECTION ON GENERAL MEDICINE

Paul B. Cameron, M.D., Pryor, Chairman

Bert F. Keltz, M.D., Oklahoma City, Secretary

2:00   Chairman's Address, "The Negro Diabetic"—Paul B. Cameron, M.D.

2:30   "Neutropenias"—Colonel William H. Gordon, M.C., Borden General Hospital, Chickasha. (By invitation.)

2:50   Discussion—Hugh Jeter, M.D., Oklahoma City.

3:00   "Unusual Findings in Coronary Disease"—H. A. Ruprecht, M.D., Tulsa.

3:20   Discussion—Harry A. Daniels, M.D., Oklahoma City.

3:30   "Androgenic Therapy in the Female"—J. William Finch, M.D., Hobart.

3:50   Discussion—D. M. McDonald, M.D., Tulsa.

4:00   Adjournment to Venetian Room for presentation of formal paper.

Rose Room
Fourteenth Floor, Skirvin Hotel

General Chairman, J. D. Osborn, M.D., Frederick, President
Oklahoma State Medical Association

2:00—4:00 P.M.

SECTION ON GENERAL SURGERY

A. Ray Wiley, M.D., Tulsa, Chairman
Oscar White, M.D., Oklahoma City, Secretary

2:00   Chairman's Address, "Use of Blood Plasma in the Rural Community"—A. Ray Wiley,
M.D.

2:30   "Carcinoma of the Breast"—Gregory E. Stanbro, M.D., Oklahoma City.

2:50   Discussion—John H. Robinson, M.D., Oklahoma City.

3:00   "Acute Surgical Abdomen"—V. C. Tisdal, M.D., Elk City.

3:20   Discussion—Louis H. Ritzhaupt, M.D., Guthrie.

3:30   "Modern Aids in the Treatment of Appendicitis"—F. M. Lingenfelter, M.D., Oklahoma City.

3:50   Discussion—C. E. Northcutt, M.D., Ponca City.

4:00   Adjournment to Venetian Room for presentation of formal paper.

Venetian Room
Fourteenth Floor, Skirvin Hotel

4:00 P.M.
FORMAL PAPER

James Stevenson, M.D., Chairman

"Naval Medicine"—Captain Leslie B. Marshall, M.C., U.S.N.R., Commanding Officer United State Naval Hospital, Norman.

Wednesday, May 12
Venetian Room
Fourteenth Floor, Skirvin Hotel

General Chairman, Maurice J. Searle, M.D., Tulsa

9:00—10:00 A.M.

SECTION ON EYE, EAR, NOSE AND THROAT

F. R. Vieregg, M.D., Clinton, Chairman
Leo F. Cailey, M.D., Oklahoma City, Secretary

9:00   "Surgical Indications in Glaucoma"—Donald V. Crane, M.D., Tulsa. (*By invitation.*)
9:20   "The Role of Short Wave Therapy in Otolaryngology"—E. H. Coachman, M.D., Muskogee.
9:40   "Clinical Importance of Refractive Errors"—A. C. McFarling, M.D., Shawnee.
10:00   Adjournment for Section on Dermatology and Radiology.
        (*Discussion of papers will be conducted at roundtable luncheons.*)

10:00—11:00 A.M.

SECTION ON DERMATOLOGY AND RADIOLOGY

Venetian Room, Fourteenth Floor, Skirvin Hotel
John H. Lamb, M.D., Oklahoma City, Chairman
M. M. Wickham, M.D., Norman, Secretary

10:00   Chairman's Address, "A Case of Dermatomysitis With Autopsy"—John H. Lamb, M.D.
10:20   "Fractional X-Ray Treatment of Skin Cancer"—Marque O. Nelson, M.D., Tulsa.
10:40   "Spontaneous Gastro-Colic Fistula—Report on Two Cases" (Illustrated)—P. E. Russo, M.D., Resident Radiologist, University Hospital, Oklahoma City. (*By Invitation.*)
11:00   Adjournment to Venetian Room for presentation of formal paper.
        (*Discussion of papers will be conducted at roundtable luncheons.*)

Rose Room
Fourteenth Floor, Skirvin Hotel

General Chairman, C. R. Rountree, M.D., Oklahoma City

9:00—10:00 A.M.

SECTION ON UROLOGY AND SYPHILOLOGY

E. Halsell Fite, M.D., Muskogee, Chairman
J. W. Rogers, M.D., Tulsa, Secretary

9:00   Chairman's Address—E. Halsell Fite, M.D.
9:20   "Verumontanitis and the Uses of the Sex Hormones"—Robert H. Akin, M.D., Oklahoma City.
9:40   "Management of Late Syphilis"—C. P. Bondurant, M.D., Oklahoma City.
10:00   Adjournment for Section on Obstetrics and Gynecology.
       (*Discussion of papers will be conducted at roundtable luncheons.*)

10:00—11:00 A.M.

SECTION ON OBSTETRICS AND GYNECOLOGY

Rose Room, Fourteenth Floor, Skirvin Hotel

Charles Ed. White, M.D., Muskogee, Chairman
Edward N. Smith, M.D., Oklahoma City, Secretary

10:00   Chairman's Address, "Obstetrical Deaths in Oklahoma"—Charles Ed. White, M.D.
10:20   "Surgical Complications During Pregnancy"—Gerald Rogers, M.D., Oklahoma City.
10:40   "Lower Abdominal Pain in the Female"—Lt. Commander Clyde M. Longstreth.
       M.C., U.S.N.R. Naval Base, Norman. (*By invitation.*)
11:00   Adjournment to Venetian Room for presentation of formal paper.
       (*Discussion of papers will be conducted at roundtable luncheons.*)

Venetian Room
Fourteenth Floor, Skirvin Hotel

11:00 A.M.

FORMAL PAPER

Maurice J. Searle, M.D., Chairman

"Brain Tumors With X-Ray as a Diagnostic Aid"—Harry Wilkins, M.D., Oklahoma City.

12:00 Noon

ROUNDTABLE LUNCHEONS

(*Luncheon programs will be discussions of the papers presented during the morning sessions of the Sections.*)

SECTION ON EYE, EAR, NOSE AND THROAT

F. R. Vieregg, M.D., Chairman
Wilson Room, Mezzanine Floor, Skirvin Hotel

Discussions

"Surgical Indications in Glaucoma"—Clinton Gallaher, M.D., Shawnee.
"The Role of Short Wave Therapy in Otolaryngology"—L. C. Kuyrkendall, M.D., McAlester.
"Clinical Importance of Refractive Errors"—F. Maxey Cooper, M.D., Oklahoma City.

SECTION ON DERMATOLOGY AND RADIOLOGY

John H. Lamb, M.D., Chairman
Parlor G, Mezzanine Floor, Skirvin Hotel

Discussions

"Fractional X-Ray Treatment of Skin Cancer"—W. A. Showman, M.D., Tulsa.
"Spontaneous Gastro-Colic Fistula—Report on Two Cases"—Ralph E. Myers, M.D., Oklahoma City.

SECTION ON UROLOGY AND SYPHILOLOGY

E. Halsell Fite, M.D., Chairman
Blue Room, Mezzanine Floor, Skirvin Hotel

Discussions

"Verumontanitis and the Uses of the Sex· Hormones"—Henry S. Browne, M.D., Tulsa.
"Management of Late Syphilis"—Joe Fulcher, M.D., Tulsa.

SECTION ON OBSTETRICS AND GYNECOLOGY

Charles Ed White, M.D., Chairman
Green Room, Mezzanine Floor, Skirvin Hotel

Discussions

"Obstetrical Deaths in Oklahoma"—J. T. Bell, M.D., Public Health Department, Oklahoma
City.
"Surgical Complications During Pregnancy"—James F. Murray, M.D., Sentinel.
"Lower Abdominal· Pain in the Female"—Milton J. Serwer, M.D., Oklahoma City.

Venetian Room
Fourteenth Floor, Skirvin Hotel

General Chairman, James D. Osborn, M.D., Frederick

2:00—4:00 P.M.

SECTION ON GENERAL MEDICINE

Turner Bynum, M.D., Chickasha, Vice-Chairman
Bert Keltz, M.D., Oklahoma City, Secretary

2:00 "Some Observations on Coronary Disease"—Wann Langston, M.D., Oklahoma City.
2:20 Discussion—Joe Phelps, M.D., El Reno.
2:30 "The Private Physician and War Industry"—Donald Macrae, M.D., Claremore.
2:50 Discussion—Paul B. Rice, M.D., Oklahoma City.
3:00 "Rocky Mountain Spotted Fever"—Paul Sizemore, M.D., Durant,.
3:20 Discussion—Lea A. Riely, M.D., Oklahoma City.
3:30 "Chronic Digestive Disturbances in the Elderly Patient"—D. D. Paulus, M.D., Okla-
      homa City.
3:50 Discussion—Minard F. Jacobs, M.D., Oklahoma City.
4:00 Adjournment to Venetian Room for presentation of formal paper.

Rose Room
Fourteenth Floor, Skirvin Hotel

General Chairman, James Stevenson, M.D., Tulsa

2:00—4:00 P.M.

SECTION ON GENERAL SURGERY

Ralph A. McGill, M.D., Tulsa, Vice-Chairman
Oscar White, M.D., Oklahoma City, Secretary

2:00 "Some Observations Relative to Surgery of the Thyroid"—H. M. McClure, M.D.,
      Chickasha.
2:20 Discussion—R. M. Howard, M.D., Oklahoma City.
2:30 "Management of Concussions, Lacerations and Compound Fractures"—M. A. Connell,
      M.D., Picher.
2:50 Discussion—Lt. Commander C. F. Ferciot, M.C., U.S.N.R., Naval Hospital, Norman.
3:00 "Comparative Symptoms in Peptic Ulcers and Cholecystitis in Two Hundred Cases"
      —Andre B. Carney, M.D., Tulsa.
3:20 Discussion—A. S. Risser, M.D., Blackwell.

3:30   "Congenital Defects of the Sternum with Case Report"—John F. Burton, M.D., Oklahoma City.
3:50   Discussion—George H. Garrison, M.D., Oklahoma City.
4:00   Adjournment to Venetian Room for presentation of formal paper.

Venetian Room
Fourteenth Floor, Skirvin Hotel

4:00 P.M.

FORMAL PAPER
James D. Osborn, M.D., Chairman
"Problems of Induction"—Colonel Monti L. Belot, M.C., Medical Liaison Officer, Eighth Service Command, Dallas, Texas.

Entertainment Program
Tuesday, May 11
Venetian Room
Fourteenth Floor, Skirvin Hotel

6:30 P.M.

BUFFET SUPPER
Presiding—Walker Morledge, M.D., President, Oklahoma County Medical Society.

Program

Introduction of Guests ....Walker Morledge, M.D.
"Activities of the Medical Department in the Eighth Service Command"—Colonel W. Lee Hart, Surgeon General, Eighth Service Command, Dallas, Texas.
"The Continuing Obligation of Medicine in the War"—Frank H. Lahey, M.D., Boston, Massachusetts, Chairman Directing Board Procurement and Assignment Service.
(*Tickets must be purchased at time of registering due to food rationing.*)

Wednesday, May 12
Venetian Room
Fourteenth Floor, Skirvin Hotel

7:00 P.M.

PRESIDENT'S INAUGURAL DINNER DANCE
Presiding—Walker Morledge, M.D., President Oklahoma County Medical Society.

Program

Installation of President-Elect—James D. Osborn, M.D., Frederick, President, Oklahoma Sttae Medical Association.
President's Response and Introduction of Guest Speaker—James Stevenson, M.D., Tulsa.
Address—Honorable Robert S. Kerr, Governor, State of Oklahoma.
Dancing 10:00-12:00   Venetian Room

Welcome To . . . . .

Skirvin Hotel

Oklahoma City

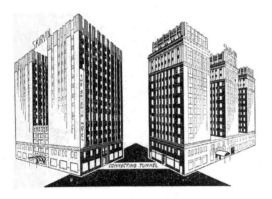

Official Headquarters

Oklahoma State Medical Association
1943 Annual Meeting

HENRY C. DICKSON, Manager   Rates $2.50 up

COMMITTEE REPORTS

ANNUAL REPORT OF DISTRICT NO. 1

To the President and House of Delegates
Oklahoma State Medical Association
Gentlemen:

As you are aware the First District is one of magnificent distances, and under present conditions it is impossible for me to cover the entire district.

Besides meetings of the Woods County Society, I have attended meetings at Cherokee, Woodward, and Supply. A meeting was held in Alva on January 26, in which members from Alfalfa, Harper, and Woodward counties were present. Dr. Mathews, State Health Commissioner, Dr. E. A. Gillis, and Dick Graham were present. The film "Syphilis" was put on by the State Health Department. A district wide meeting was held at Supply, December 3, at which members from eight counties were present. Dr. James Stevenson, President-Elect, of Tulsa, was present and gave an inspiring address. Dr. J. D. Osborn was to be present, but pressure of other duties prevented his coming.

A Crippled Children's Clinic was held in Alva, November 23, with children from four counties of the district present.

I have attended three Council meetings in Oklahoma City, and by writing many letters have tried to assist in collection of dues, settling of minor differences and keeping up the general morale of the membership. I have cooperated with the Medical Department of the U. S. Army and the Procurement and Assignment Service in securing physicians to go into active military service.

Respectfully submitted,
O. E. TEMPLIN, M.D.
Councilor District No. 1.

ANNUAL REPORT OF DISTRICT NO. 8

To the President and House of Delegates
Oklahoma State Medical Association
Gentlemen:

When Doctor S. D. Neely joined the armed forces of the United States Government, he resigned his place on the council. The council saw fit to appoint me to carry on in his absence. It has been a pleasure to serve again.

I have visited each active county society and found them in very good condition, especially considering the large number of doctors who have been taken into the armed forces. This district has been hit rather hard because of the war industries which have been located in and around this section, which has greatly increased the population. This, with the reduction of the number of doctors in the district, has worked rather a great hardship on those remaining. However, I find them all taking it in their stride and happy to do what they can to keep American medicine on an even keel during this war.

Respectfully submitted,
FINIS W. EWING, M.D.
Councilor District No. 8.

ANNUAL REPORT OF DISTRICT NO. 9

To the President and House of Delegates
Of the Oklahoma State Medical Association
Gentlemen:

The Ninth Councilor District Societies have been rather inactive this year, meeting only occasionally and making every effort to carry on under most trying and difficult conditions. Interest has not lagged, but with so many doctors in the service and the increase in population, there has been difficulty in obtaining programs as well as attendance.

The postgraduate course conducted in the fall of 1942 at McAlester was enthusiastically received, and more than 20 doctors attended. All expressed their appreciation of the postgraduate committee's work and wish these courses continued.

An effort is being made to amalgamate Latimer with Pittsburg County into the Pittsburg-Latimer County Medical Society because of their being so few doctors in Latimer County.

A District meeting of County Chairmen of Procurement and Assignment was held in McAlester on March 21, 1943, at which time the rules governing Procurement and Assignment were outlined. This meeting was attended by the State Chairman as well as the District Chairman and the Executive Secretary of the Oklahoma State Medical Association.

Respectfully submitted,
L. C. KUYRKENDALL, M.D.
Councilor District No. 9.

REPORT OF COMMITTEE ON MEDICAL EDUCATION AND HOSPITALS

The Committee on Medical Education and Hospitals submits the following report to the House of Delegates:

While your committee has not been confronted with any immediate problems as it pertains to medical education in Oklahoma, it cannot refrain from offering an observation concerning the future. During the present world emergency there will probably be many changes made in medical education, designed primarily to produce additional physicians for the armed forces. While this is a necessary exigency, it is the opinion of the committee that the needs of the military forces should not completely obliterate the very real and necessary situation that will develop with regard to replacement of civilian physicians who will be protecting the home front.

Medical schools and teaching hospitals, in cooperation with the federal government, should immediately take steps to see that sufficient physically disabled for military service and women students are accepted in medical schools to take care of civilian replacements.

The federal government should be admonished that in medical education, as well as in other situations, the maxim, "haste makes waste," is still true, and that inadequately trained physicians cannot be created by legislation or governmental decree. There has never been a time in the history of our nation when there has been a greater need for well trained physicians, yet it is difficult for your committee to believe that the federal government is more capable of determining the minimum requirements in medical education to produce a finished physician than those who have spent their lives in this field. Your committee recommends that the House of Delegates go on record as approving the accelerated teaching program in medical schools, but opposing the decreasing of the number of hours of study and the prerequisites necessary for entrance into a medical school.

Hand in hand with medical education goes the problem of medical licensure by state boards. The right of the state to set its own standards has as yet not been broken, though it is badly bent. Periodically the newspapers of the nation carry releases from Washington in regard to communities in need of additional physicians and the necessity for relocation of physicians from

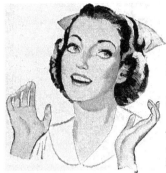

Some men
are so clever!

Take my boss for instance . . .

Yesterday, I overheard him talking to another doctor about infant feeding.

"Jim," he said, "I'll tell you why you never have any time to spare. You get yourself tied up with a lot of unnecessary work.

"You believe in prescribing plain cow's milk modified. Haven't you found out that S-M-A* will save you a lot of unnecessary questions? Cut out a lot of bothersome arithmetic?

"Heaven knows, we're busy enough as it is. I'll bet you a couple of tickets for the big game that with S-M-A on the job—your patients won't have to telephone you so often to ask about their baby's formula."

Well, you can see why I think my boss is so clever. Why don't you try S-M-A in your own practice, doctor? See if you don't like it better.

BUSY DOCTORS TODAY— PRESCRIBE S-M-A !

With the exception of Vitamin C . . . S-M-A is nutritionally complete. Vitamins B₁, D and A are included in adequate proportion . . . ready to feed. Their presence in S-M-A prevents the development of subclinical vitamin deficiencies . . . because the infant gets all the necessary vitamins right from the start.

S-M-A has still another highly important advantage not found in other modified milk formulas. It contains a special fat that resembles breast milk fat . . . resembles it chemically and physically—according to impartial laboratory tests. S-M-A fat is more readily digested and tolerated by most infants than cow's milk fat.

S-M-A IS EASIER TO PREPARE. ONE MEASURE OF POWDER TO EACH OUNCE OF WARM, BOILED WATER, COMPLETES THE FORMULA . . . TWENTY CALORIES TO THE OUNCE

The infant food that is nutritionally complete

*REG. U. S. PAT. OFF.

SMA

S. M. A. Corporation
8100 McCormick Boulevard
Chicago, Illinois

S-M-A, a trade-mark of S.M.A. Corporation, for its brand of food especially prepared for infant feeding—derived from tuberculin-tested cow's milk, the fat of which is replaced by animal and vegetable fats, including biologically tested cod liver oil; with the addi-tion of milk sugar and potassium chloride; altogether forming an antirachitic food. When diluted according to directions, it is essen-tially similar to human milk in percentages of protein, fat, carbohydrate and ash, in chemical constants of the fat and physical properties.

one state to another. Your committee does not deny that such communities may exist, but it cannot believe that relocation cannot be accomplished within the borders of the respective states, and without a complete destruction of the medical practice acts of the states. It commends the Oklahoma State Board of Medical Examiners for its stand in this respect.

As to hospitals, your committee is of the opinion that the Procurement and Assignment Service is well aware of the need of continuing to make adequate hospital facilities available to the public. At the same time, your committee does not believe that ownership of a hospital should preclude a physician's serving in the armed forces if he is of military age so long as there are sufficient other hospitals in the community to care for the population, or if there are other physicians in the community who could administer the hospital in the absence of the owner.

The maintenance of adequate intern and resident staffs is, of course, a necessity. At the same time, your committee is of the opinion that the number of interns and residents needed in the hospitals should be determined by the patient load rather than for the convenience of the staff. Your committee does not mean to infer that this condition exists in Oklahoma, but it does make the observation as a recommendation for the Procurement and Assignment Committee and hospital administrators for future guidance.

In closing its report, your committee feels that it cannot too strongly emphasize that the success or failure of medical education and hospital administration will be in ratio to the leadership developed by the medical profession. This leadership will in the end determine the future of medicine.

Respectfully submitted,
Galvin L. Johnson, M.D., Chairman
Roscoe Walker, M.D.
Sam A. McKeel, M.D.

REPORT OF THE COMMITTEE ON PUBLIC POLICY

The Committee on Public Policy submits the following report to the House of Delegates:

The nineteenth session of the Oklahoma legislature, which concluded its deliberations on April 1, was one of the shortest on record. Under the able leadership of Governor Robert S. Kerr, its health program was sound and constructive, though one important health measure introduced was not enacted into law. This measure was the immunization bill which would have made it mandatory for all persons attending public schools to be vaccinated against smallpox and diphtheria except those religiously opposed.

Your committee particularly wishes to commend the work of the Public Health and Sanitation Committee of the Senate headed by Senators Clinton Braden of Wilburton and Louis H. Ritzhaupt, M.D., and the Public Health and Sanitation and Practice of Medicine Committees of the House of Representatives under the leadership of Raymond Lucas, Spiro, Orange W. Starr, M.D., and Elbert "Pete" Weaver of Stillwater, respectively. Had it not been for the cooperation of these legislators, the work of your committee would have been much more difficult.

A complete analysis of all health measures passed by the legislature will be carried in the May issue of the Journal. For the purpose of this report, your committee believes it sufficient to give only a brief resume of these measures.

House Bill 222 amends the Medical Practice Act with reference to the appointment of the board, suspension and revocation of licenses, and the manner of conducting examinations.

House Bill 236 makes it mandatory that the names appearing upon birth or death certificates be either typewritten or hand printed.

House Bills 37-38-39 strengthens and broadens the power and scope of the statutes relating to venereal diseases.

House Bills 252 and 373 amend the Crippled Children's Law and the State Social Security Act to modernize its provisions in relation to payments to hospitals.

Senate Bill 98 clarifies the statutes with reference to the liability of physicians and hospitals in the performance of caesarian sections.

Senate Bill 90 makes certain provisions for the deduction of medical and hospital expenditures in compilation of state income taxes.

Your committee desires to express its appreciation to all county societies and individual physicians who assisted in the work of the committee during the year. This help was sincerely appreciated.

While it will be two years before the legislature again convenes, your committee believes that now is the time for the House of Delegates to instruct the Public Policy committee to be working. In the consideration of this suggestion, the House of Delegates' attention is directed to two public health proposals that would, in the opinion of the committee, be beneficial to public health. One deals with compulsory immunization, and the other with the establishment of a public health commission. The latter suggestion would tend to bring under one head the state administration of all hospitals, sanatoria, and the State Health Department. Should the House of Delegates believe these suggestions merit its consideration, it is suggested that the Resolutions Committee be directed after consultation with the Public Health Committee, to prepare proper resolutions for the deliberation of the delegates.

There is little doubt that in the immediate year to come the activity of both the Association and the committee will be amplified in reference to health legislation emanating from the National Congress. If the practice of medicine and the health of the public is to be maintained on its present high plane, the profession must take the lead in the education of both the public and the members of Congress. There is no doubt that to accomplish this there must be a united effort of the American Medical Association, its component state associations and their individual members. It is doubtful if there has been a time in the history of our country when there was a greater responsibility on the medical profession, both scientifically and economically.

The public policy of the physician must continue to be solely in the interest of his patient and in the preservation of the American way of life.

Respectfully submitted,
J. T. Martin, M.D., Chairman
Frank W. Boadway, M.D.
Harper Wright, M.D.

REPORT OF COMMITTEE ON JUDICIAL AND PROFESSIONAL RELATIONS

Your Committee on Judicial and Professional Relations desires to report that during the year 1942-43 there was one request made for assistance from the medical defense fund. Of two cases previously filed, one has been settled and the other has not come to trial.

Your committee has not been called upon to intercede in compensation cases said to have arisen from malpractice except as requested by application for assistance from the medical defense fund.

As of April 1, there was on deposit in the medical defense fund $586.34 augmented by the bonds as shown in the audit report of the Association.

Respectfully submitted,
A. S. Risser, M.D., Chairman
J. M. Bonham, M.D.
Claude S. Chambers, M.D.

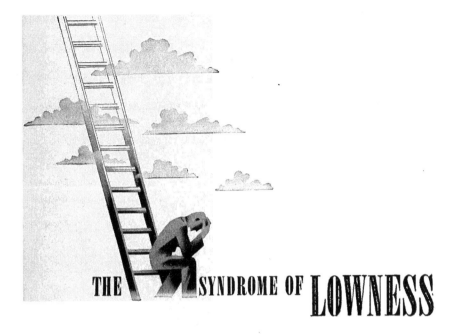

THE SYNDROME OF LOWNESS

LOW MUSCLE TONE, LOW BLOOD PRESSURE LOW RESISTANCE are part of a syndrome characteristic of adrenal cortical insufficiency.

Adrenal Cortex Extract (Upjohn) is a most potent specific therapy now available for alleviation of these typical symptoms, when due to adrenal cortex insufficiency. Adrenal Cortex Extract (Upjohn) is a potent natural complex representing steroids which influence carbohydrate metabolism, capillary tone, vascular permeability, plasma volume, body fluids and electrolytes. "No one of these substances and no synthetic substance has yet been shown to possess all of the effects of a potent cortical extract." N. N. R. 1942

ADRENAL CORTEX EXTRACT (UPJOHN)

Sterile Solution in 10 cc. rubber-capped vials for subcutaneous, intramuscular and intravenous therapy.

REPORT OF BENEVOLENT FUND COMMITTEE

Your committee, after studying the subject of the creation of a benevolent fund from the accumulated medical defense fund, has arrived at the conclusion that there is no real demand for a relief fund to be established to assist indigent doctors, but that a real constructive and beneficial use could be made of this fund in the establishment of a revolving fund to make loans to deserving junior and senior medical students who are pursuing their studies in the University of Oklahoma School of Medicine.

It is the recommendation of the committee that a committee be appointed to work out details for setting up and administering a revolving loan fund for the purpose of aiding deserving junior or senior medical students of the University of Oklahoma, and that their report should be made to the House of Delegates for their consideration at the meeting in 1944.

Repectfully submitted,
Finis W. Ewing, M.D., Chairman
A. W. Pigford, M.D.
S. B. Leslie, M.D.

REPORT OF THE COMMITTEE ON MEDICAL ECONOMICS

The Committee on Medical Economics submits the following report to the House of Delegates:

During the past year your committee has again been faced with the problem concerning cooperation between the Farm Security Administration and the county medical societies. At the last meeting with the F.S.A. officials, your committee invited Mr. N. D. Helland, Director of the Oklahoma Blue Cross Plan, to participate in the discussion, it being felt by the committee that the Blue Cross Plan was the logical organization to carry a hospitalization program. The results of this conference were highly satisfactory, and there is every reason to believe that a hospitalization plan will be developed.

Your committee is well aware that the solution of the hospital program does not cover the entire field, and that it is in reality the minor problem There is still the issue of medical and surgical care. On this point, your committee did not feel that it could circumvent the action of the House of Delegates taken in 1942 when it adopted the report of this committee with reference to this question, by stating that co-operation with the F.S.A. should be left to the discretion of the local county societies after careful and complete study.

While your committee has no desire to usurp the rights and privileges of the county societies and individual physicians with reference to the practice of medicine, it does not feel that it would be fulfilling its duties if it did not draw to the attention of the House of Delegates the necessity for calm and deliberate consideration of the changes taking place in the economic field of medicine as it pertains to prepayment plans for low income groups. There is no intention on the part of your committee to advocate the immediate establishment of a prepaid plan of surgical or medical care for two reasons. First, your committee has not given study to the problem; and secondly, this Association has a special committee on prepaid medical care that will submit its own report. Nevertheless, each delegate is admonished in his deliberations to consider the activities of world leaders and recent reports that have been made in relation to the so-called health problem.

It is also the opinion of your committee that the State Association and the county societies should concern themselves with the economic rehabilitation of the physician who will return from the present world war. Just how far this program should reach or be developed is not for this committee to decide, but it does recommend that either through this committee or the appointment of a special committee, a study of the problem be started.

In closing this report, your committee sincerely hopes that as physicians there will not be a single one of you who will so seclude yourself in your practice that you will not recognize the need for medicine to lead the way in the future planning of the health of the nation irrespective of its approach, whether it be economic or scientific.

Respectfully submitted,
McLain Rogers, M.D., Chairman
James Stevenson, M.D.
H. M. McClure, M.D.

REPORT OF COMMITTEE ON MEDICAL TESTIMONY

The Chairman of the Committee on Medical Testimony has been assisted in reviewing procedures and opinions by the legal department of the American Medical Association, by the reprints which have been furnished from the Harvard Law School, but especially by Dr. E. M. Hammes who is Chairman of the Committee on Medical Testimony for the Minnesota State Medical Association.

Your chairman now wishes to submit for your consideration the following items:

1. It appears desirable to find some method of avoiding, as much as possible, the inexcusable divergence in expert medical testimony which often appears in the records of cases which are appealed to the Oklahoma Supreme Court.

2. The suggestion has been made that if there were some committee of the State Medical Association to which they could refer cases in which testimony is so contradictory that one of the witnesses seems to be deviating from the truth, it would do much to remedy this condition.

3. The chairman of your committee respectfully suggests that a resolution similar to the immediately following sentence be incorporated in the report which we are requested to make to the House of Delegates. "The Committee on Medical Testimony of the Oklahoma State Medical Association most respectfully recommends to the House of Delegates that the Council, or the President, of the Oklahoma State Medical Association be instructed to appoint a committee of a suitable number, perhaps five or seven, as is proper under the circumstances, the said committee to be empowered to review those court cases in which medical testimony appears to the court to have been so contradictory as to indicate that one or more of the medical witnesses appears to be deviating from the truth.''

4. It would seem that a review of the medical testimony in such cases including a discussion of the matter with those physicians who have testified, would undoubtedly have a beneficial effect in the quality of future medical testimony. It seems that where the facts indicate a willful disregard for the truth, the matter should be referred to the Oklahoma State Board of Medical Examiners for suitable action in regard to the license of the physicians concerned, and that appropriate disciplinary action be taken by the local component medical society in respect to those physicians who are members of the Oklahoma State Medical Association. It should be emphasized that medical testimony investigation should not be confined to any particular type of legislation, nor to any particular court.

5. It has been suggested that the medical advisory committee as appointed should be without any legal authority and should act in a purely advisory capacity. It should be the intention of the State Medical Association to inform its members of the existence and nature of this committee, and to assist and cooperate in every way possible to promote favorable publicity throughout the State, and especially among the members of the Okla-

The
Menninger Sanitarium

For the Diagnosis and Treatment
of Nervous and Mental Illness.

The
Southard School

For the Education and Psychiatric
Treatment of Children of Average
and Superior Intelligence.

Boarding Home Facilities.

Topeka, Kansas

homa Bar Association and all those who may be interested in the purposes of this committee.

It is our opinion that the objects of this committee are worthy of careful consideration of every member of the Oklahoma State Medical Association. We are quite aware of the many obvious difficulties which may be encountered but we are convinced that if sincere approval and honest cooperation is given by every member of the Medical Association we shall find no lack of assistance from other desirable sources.

Respectfully submitted,
Clinton Gallaher, M.D., Chairman
James Stevenson, M.D.
Finis W. Ewing, M.D.

REPORT OF COMMITTEE ON POSTGRADUATE MEDICAL TEACHING

The Committee on Postgraduate Medical Teaching submits the following report to the House of Delegates:

The postgraduate internal medicine program, conducted by L. W. Hunt, M.D., Chicago, Illinois, has been a success from every viewpoint. Five circuits, comprising 25 teaching centers in central and eastern Oklahoma, have been completed with a total enrollment of 621 physicians with an average attendance of 85 per cent. Doctor Hunt has held 655 consultations with physicians and conducted clinics with a total of 331 patients.

The sixth circuit opened March 22, with the teaching centers Chickasha, Ardmore, Duncan, Frederick, Lawton and Fort Sill. A total of 139 have enrolled thus far in this circuit, making a grand total to date of 760 physicians taking the course. It is expected that more than 1,000 doctors will have taken advantage of Doctor Hunt's lectures by the close of the program, January 31, 1944. This, we believe, is excellent considering the fact that many actual and potential registrants have been called to military duty.

Total receipts for the first year's instruction amounted to $16,343.50. Total disbursements were $12,525.51, leaving a reserve of $3,817.99. At the present rate of expenditures and receipts there will be a reserve at the completion of the program which will be prorated back to the participating agencies according to the percentage of their contributions.

The Committee desires to thank The Commonwealth Fund of New York, the Oklahoma State Health Department, the United States Public Health, and the Oklahoma State Medical Association for their financial assistance, and further recommends that the House of Delegates, by resolution, express its appreciation to these contributing agencies.

The response to questionnaires indicates a definite desire of the members of the State Medical Association for a course in Surgical Diagnosis beginning in February, 1944. The Committee recommends that the House of Delegates approve the participation of the State Medical Association in such a course and the appropriation of $2,000.00 per annum for such participation.

In cooperation with the Committee on Industrial and Traumatic Surgery and the Oklahoma State Health Department a two-day Institute on Wartime Industrial Health, financed by the State Health Department, was held in Tulsa and Oklahoma City on March 18 and 19, respectively, with a total attendance of 240. Nationally known speakers representing industrial medicine, surgery, public health and plant management took part in the program. The increasing number of wartime industrial plants in the state evidenced the need of such programs, and it is our opinion that similar institutes should be arranged by the County Medical Societies at their regional medical meetings.

Respectfully submitted,
Henry H. Turner, M.D., Chairman
M. J. Searle, M.D.
H. C. Weber, M.D.

REPORT OF THE COMMITTEE ON PUBLIC HEALTH

The Committee on Public Health submits the following report to the House of Delegates:

Your Committee on Public Health desires to submit a three point program. One part of the program should be immediately activated, and the other two parts should have preliminary preparation made. This program is as follows:

1. An immediate educational program directed to both the public and the profession for the complete immunization of all persons within the age limits of susceptability for at least smallpox and diphtheria.

2. The creation of a State Public Health Commission which would have full and complete control of all state owned hospitals and sanatoria and the Public Health Department.

3. The passage of a state law to cover section one of this suggested program.

These recommendations are general in character, and should be worked out in cooperation with all other interested organizations. It is suggested that the Public Policy Committee be requested to ask for a conference with Governor Robert S. Kerr and the Commissioner of Health concerning this program, which, in the opinion of the committee, is particularly vital during the present war. The present members of your committee pledge their full cooperation.

During the past year the advancements that have been made in public health in Oklahoma, in the opinion of your committee, are directly a result of the cooperation that has been developed by the activities of the Public Health Department, and a better understanding of its objectives and methods on the part of the medical profession. Your committee desires to especially commend Dr. Grady F. Mathews for the manner in which he has conducted the affairs of the Public Health Department, as well as all other members of his administrative staff.

There can be no doubt that during the present emergency the medical profession will be called upon to function in the field of preventative medicine as never before, and it is a charge and obligation that must be met.

Respectfully submitted,
Carroll M. Pounders, M.D., Chairman
G. S. Baxter, M.D.
H. K. Riddle, M.D.

REPORT OF THE COMMITTEE ON THE STUDY AND CONTROL OF CANCER

The Committee on the Study and Control of Cancer submits the following report to the House of Delegates:

Your committee during the past year has continued its cooperation with the Women's Field Army of the American Society for the Control of Cancer. Active work in the field of cancer control has been limited due to necessary reorganization of the Women's Field Army, but it is expected that a complete program will be placed in operation during the last quarter of 1943 and the first quarter of 1944.

County medical societies and individual physicians should continue to give full and complete cooperation in conducting lay and professional meetings in the interest of cancer control. Statistics continue to show that cancer remains one of the major causes of death in the United States, and unless through education the public can be educated that early diagnosis is necessary, there can be little hope of reducing its mortality rate.

Your committee urges every county society to devote at elast one meeting each year to cancer control and treatment, and the entire facilities of the committee are available to the county societies. Available for distribution to lay groups is an unlimited supply of educational literature, as well as color and sound movies.

County societies are also urged to take the initiative

in conducting cancer education in the high schools and colleges of Oklahoma.

Respectfully submitted,
Carl L. Brundage, M.D., Chairman
Ralph A. McGill, M.D.
Wendell Long, M.D.

REPORT OF COMMITTEE ON STUDY AND CONTROL OF TUBERCULOSIS

The Committee on the Study and Control of Tuberculosis submits the following report to the House of Delegates:

The committee has assisted in the preparation of a booklet describing the Oklahoma tuberculosis control agencies and their activities. Oklahoma has made definite progress in controlling tuberculosis during the past year. This is reflected in the death rate for 1942, which showed a definite decrease. To combat the expected increase in tuberculosis due to the war, we urge that present sanatoria facilities and case finding facilities be maintained, and where at all possible, that they be expanded.

We recommend. (1) Unification of tuberculosis control under the State Health Department. (2) Adequate appropriations for properly maintaining the state sanatoria. Their present bed capacity should not be reduced any further. (More sanatorium beds are needed especially for Negroes, but this must wait until after the war). (3) Expansion of the case finding program of the State Health Department so that all counties are provided with regular tuberculosis clinics. At present this is not possible except in some 40 counties supporting full-time county health units. (4) Assistance should be extended to state mental institutions for the control of tuberculosis. (5) More active measures should be taken to control tuberculosis in Northeastern Oklahoma. (6) Expansion of the rehabilitation program for the tuberculous.

Respectfully submitted,
Richard M. Burke, M.D., Chairman
R. M. Shepard, M.D.
Carl Puckett, M.D.

REPORT OF COMMITTEE ON VENEREAL DISEASE CONTROL

The Committee on Venereal Disease Control wishes to submit the following report:

Since the War Emergency has become a reality, a wide interest has been taken in the apparent flare-up in all venereal diseases, such as is seen in all wars. Venereal diseases in this war have assumed a role of vast importance, both in civil and military life. The public and medical personnel are more aware of this problem than heretofore.

Methods of control are systematized and treatments are standardized. Special attention is called to the House Bills passed by the present legislature. House Bill 37: an act amending Section 548, Title 63, Oklahoma States, 1941, relating to the examination and treatment of persons confined to public and private institutions or any person arrested by lawful warrant, the patient still retaining his right to choose his physician but making treatment and examination mandatory under the penalty of quarantine for such purpose. House Bill 39: an act providing penalties for aiding, participating in or providing premises for prostitution, defining prostitution and aiding law enforcement officers greatly in handling this problem. (The other bill I cannot get a copy of.)

Another step forward and one highly approved by the committee is the manner in which industry has met the problem of syphilis. We are gratified to find it a widely accepted practice to not penalize those with lues but to allow them to retain their jobs and stay under observation and treatment of competent medical supervisors. This urges routine Wassermann tests on all workers, and when positives are found, follow-ups in their families, urging above all routine Wassermanns on all pregnant women. The committee feels there should be no persecution of the syphilitic and that he should be treated with the same respect and care as one with other disease.

Respectfully submitted,
C. P. Bondurant, M.D., Chairman
Joe Fulcher, M.D.
C. B. Taylor, M.D.

Delegates and Alternates Selected For Annual Meeting

The following listed delegates and alternates have been certified to the Executive Office as representatives of their respective counties at the annual meeting.

Credential cards have been mailed to the delegates and alternates, who in turn must present their credentials to the Credentials Committee prior to the first meeting of the House of Delegates on Monday evening, May 10. This date, which is the evening before the first day of the meeting, has been set due to the streamlining of the convention.

COUNTY	DELEGATE	ALTERNATE
Alfalfa	G. G. Harris, Helena	Forrest Hale, Cherokee
Atoka-Coal	H. C. Huntley, Atoka	T. H. Briggs, Atoka
	R. C. Henry, Coalgate	J. B. Clark, Coalgate
Beckham	H. K. Speed, Sayre	
Blaine	Virginia Olson Curtin, Watonga	
Bryan	J. A. Haynie, Durant	A. J. Wells, Durant
Caddo	G. E. Haslan, Anadarko	C. B. Sullivan, Carnegie
Canadian	J. T. Phelps, El Reno	M. E. Phelps, El Reno
Carter	F. W. Boadway, Ardmore	G. E. Johnson, Ardmore
Cherokee		
Choctaw	R. L. Gee, Hugo	E. A. Johnson, Hugo
Cleveland	J. A. Rieger, Norman	Curtis Berry, Norman
Comanche	W. F. Lewis, Lawton	Donald Angus, Lawton
Cotton	George A. Tallant, Walters	George W. Baker, Walters
Craig	F. M. Adams, Vinita	Lloyd McPike, Vinita
Creek	J. B. Lampton, Sapulpa	O. C. Coppedge, Bristow
	C. R. McDonald, Mannford	Frank H. Sisler, Sr., Bristow
Custer	McLain Rogers, Clinton	C. H. McBurney, Clinton
	Ellis Lamb, Clinton	C. Doler, Clinton
Garfield	V. R. Hamble, Enid	
	D. S. Harris, Drummond	
Garvin	G. L. Johnson, Pauls Valley	M. E. Robberson, Jr., Wynnewood
Grady	H. M. McClure, Chickasha	L. E. Woods, Chickasha
Grant	E. E. Lawson, Medford	
Greer	J. B. Hollis, Mangum	R. W. Lewis, Granite

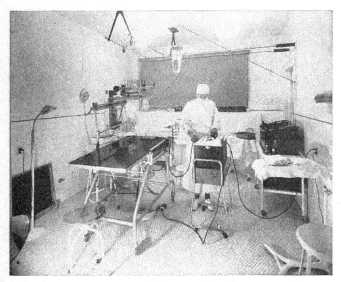

Harmon	W. G. Husband, Hollis	L. E. Hollis, Hollis
Haskell	J. C. Rumley, Stigler	Wm. S. Carson, Keota
Hughes	W. L. Taylor, Holdenville	
Jackson	E. S. Crow, Olustee	
Jefferson	L. L. Wade, Ryan	John R. Reid, Altus
Kay	A. S. Risser, Blackwell	J. C. Wagner, Ponca City
	Dewey Mathews, Tonkawa	L. H. Becker, Blackwell
Kingfisher	C. M. Hodgson, Kingfisher	A. Meredith, Kingfisher
Kiowa	J. M. Bonham, Hobart	
LeFlore	F. P. Baker, Talihina	
Lincoln	U. E. Nickell, Davenport	Ned Burleson, Prague
Logan	L. A. Hahn, Guthrie	
Marshall	J. L. Holland, Madill	J. F. York, Madill
Mayes	Carl Puckett, Oklahoma City	
McClain		
McCurtain	R. D. Williams, Idabel	J. T. Moreland, Idabel
McIntosh	W. A. Tolleson, Eufaula	D. E. Little, Eufaula
Murray	W. D. DeLay, Sulphur	F. E. Sadler, Sulphur
Muskogee-Sequoyah-	C. E. White, Muskogee	L. S. McAlister, Muskogee
Wagoner	E. Halsell Fite, Muskogee	J. R. Rafter, Muskogee
	John A. Morrow, Sallisaw	
	H. K. Riddle, Coweta	J. H. Plunkett, Wagoner
Noble	Jesse W. Driver, Perry	T. F. Renfrow, Billings
Okfuskee	W. P. Jenkins, Okemah	A. S. Melton, Okemah
Oklahoma	W. F. Keller, Oklahoma City	W. K. West, Oklahoma City
	Walker Morledge, Oklahoma City	R. Q. Goodwin, Oklahoma City
	L. C. McHenry, Oklahoma City	K. J. Wilson, Oklahoma City
	C. R. Rountree, Oklahoma City	W. J. Thompson, Oklahoma City
	O. A. Watson, Oklahoma City	Clark H. Hall, Oklahoma City
	D. H. O'Donoghue, Oklahoma City	Floyd Moorman, Oklahoma City
	C. M. Pounders, Oklahoma City	Vern Musick, Oklahoma City
	Neil W. Woodward, Oklahoma City	Charles M. O'Leary, Oklahoma City
	W. E. Easlaud, Oklahoma City	Harvey O. Randel, Oklahoma City
	Minard F. Jacobs, Oklahoma City	Ralph A. Smith, Oklahoma City
	Harper Wright, Oklahoma City	Alvin R. Jackson, Oklahoma City
Okmulgee	J. G. Edwards, Okmulgee	G. Y. McKinney, Henryetta
	J. C. Matheney, Okmulgee	G. A. Kilpatrick, Henryetta
Osage	G. I. Walker, Hominy	Roscoe Walker, Pawhuska
Ottawa	W. B. Sanger, Picher	L. P. Hetherington, Miami
	M. A. Connell, Picher	J. P. Cunningham, Miami
Pawnee	R. E. Jones, Pawnee	J. L. LeHew, Sr., Pawnee
Payne	John W. Martin, Cushing	
Pittsburg	L. S. Willour, McAlester	F. J. Baum, McAlester
	T. H. McCarley, McAlester	W. C. Wait, McAlester
Pontotoc	R. E. Cowling, Ada	E. M. Gullat, Ada
	Sam A. McKeel, Ada	C. F. Needham, Ada
Pottawatomie	G. S. Baxter, Shawnee	C. C. Young, Shawnee
	W. M. Gallaher, Shawnee	E. E. Rice, Shawnee
Pushmataha	D. W. Connally, Antlers	E. S. Patterson, Antlers
Rogers	B. F. Collins, Claremore	R. C. Meloy, Claremore
Seminole	Claude Chambers, Seminole	L. R. Pace, Seminole
Stephens	A. J. Weedn, Duncan	W. Z. McClain, Marlow
Texas		
Tillman	T. F. Spurgeon, Frederick	C. C. Allen, Frederick
Tulsa	W. S. Larrabee, Tulsa	James D. Markland, Tulsa
	M. J. Searle, Tulsa	M. O. Hart, Tulsa
	W. A. Cook, Tulsa	Monte V. Stanley, Tulsa
	W. A. Showman, Tulsa	A. W. Pigford, Tulsa
	Marvin D. Henley, Tulsa	E. O. Johnson, Tulsa
	Ralph A. McGill, Tulsa	Roy W. Dunlap, Tulsa
	John C. Perry, Tulsa	David V. Hudson, Tulsa
Washington-Nowata	K. D. Davis, Nowata	S. A. Lang, Nowata
	H. C. Weber, Bartlesville	E. E. Beechwood, Bartlesville
	L. D. Hudson, Dewey	Thomas Wells, Bartlesville
Washita	A. H. Bungardt, Cordell	James F. McMurry, Sentinel
Woods	D. B. Ensor, Hopeton	W. F. LaFon, Waynoka
Woodward	John L. Day, Fort Supply	D. W. Darwin, Woodward
	Hardin Walker, Buffalo	F. Z. Winchell, Buffalo

AMENDMENTS TO CONSTITUTION AND BY-LAWS TO BE ACTED UPON AT ANNUAL MEETING

At the 1942 annual meeting two amendments to the constitution and one amendment to the by-laws have been submitted, and must be acted upon at the coming annual meeting.

One amendment to the constitution and the amendment to the by-laws pertain to the same subject, and provide that the delegate elected at the annual meeting shall take office the January following his election rather than immediately following the session at which he is elected.

The amendment and by-law submitted on this subject are as follows:

Amendment To Constitution

Article VIII, Section 3. All of the above officers shall assume the duties of their respective offices immediately upon the close of the annual session at which they were elected to serve and shall serve until their successors have been elected and installed with the exception of Delegate to the American Medical Association who shall take office the first of January succeeding his election.

Amendment To By-Laws

Chapter V, Section 4. Installation: All officers elected at the final session of the House of Delegates shall assume office at the close of the annual session, except the President-Elect who shall assume the duties of President at the close of the next annual session and Delegate to the American Medical Association who shall assume office the first of January succeeding his election. The terms of office shall be as herein provided or until their successors have been elected and qualified.

The effect of these amendments would mean that a delegate would not serve for one year following his election unless there was a special meeting of the House of Delegates of the American Medical Association called after January 1 of the year following his election. At the present time the Delegate elected at any annual meeting attends the House of Delegates of the A.M.A. the following month.

The second amendment to the constitution brings into conformity Article VIII, Section 4 of the constitution with Chapter VI, Section 4 of the by-laws. This change concerns the filling of the unexpired term of the Speaker of the House of Delegates, and is merely a corrective amendment. The wording of the amendment is as follows:

Amendment To Constitution

Article VIII, Section 4. Vacancies created by the death, resignation, or removal of the above-named officials shall be filled by temporary appointment of the Council, such appointment being effective until the next annual meeting of the House of Delegates, which shall elect a successor to complete the unexpired term, if any, except the President, whose place shall be filled by the Vice-President, and the Speaker of the House of Delegates, whose unexpired term shall be filled by the Vice-Speaker.

HONORARY MEMBERSHIP APPLICATIONS

The following names have been submitted to the Executive Office, in compliance with the By-Laws, for election to Honorary Membership:

L. W. Cotton, M.D., Enid

R. W. Holbrook, M.D., Perkins

J. T. Frizzell, M.D., Clinton

Should any member know of any reason why this honor should not be afforded these physicians, his objections should be presented to the House of Delegates.

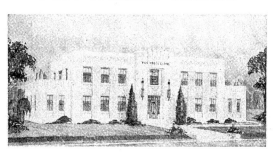

DR. L. J. MOORMAN TO BE INSTALLED AS PRESIDENT NATIONAL TUBERCULOSIS ASSOCIATION

Dr. L. J. Moorman, Oklahoma City, Secretary of the Oklahoma State Medical Association, who for the past year has served as President-Elect of the National Tuberculosis Association, will be installed as President at the annual meeting of the Association to be held in St. Louis, Missouri, May 5 and 6.

Dr. Moorman previously had held the office of Vice-President, and has received additional recognition in the field of tuberculosis, having served in 1941 as President of the American Trudeau Society. For the last 25 years Dr. Moorman has been the director of the Oklahoma County Tuberculosis Dispensary, and in recognition of this service he was awarded the National Tuberculosis Association 25-year service pin. His recent publication, ''Tuberculosis and Genius,'' has been accepted as one of the finest works of its kind ever published. The Oklahoma State Medical Association is justly proud of Dr. Moorman not only for the contribution he has made in the field of tuberculosis, but for his sterling qualities as a gentleman and a scholar. It is regretted that every member of the Association cannot be present at his installation as President.

BASIC SCIENCE BOARD GIVES EXAMINATIONS

Sixty-three applicants were present to take the Basic Science examinations given in Oklahoma City on April 5 at the University of Oklahoma School of Medicine. This is the largest class ever to take the examinations.

At a meeting of the Board prior to the examinations the following officers were re-elected. H. W. Orr, Ph.D., Stillwater, President; R. J. Kaufmann, Ph.D., Tulsa, Vice-President; J. D. Osborn, M.D., Frederick, Secretary.

Dr. Osborn has recently been reappointed by Governor Kerr for an additional five years.

ANNUAL AUDIT REPORT

Mr. R. H. Graham, Executive Secretary
Oklahoma State Medical Association
210 Plaza Court
Oklahoma City, Oklahoma

Dear Sir:

We have completed the audit of the financial records of

THE OKLAHOMA STATE MEDICAL ASSOCIATION
Oklahoma City, Oklahoma

for the period from January 1, 1942, to December 31, 1942, and submit herewith the following Exhibits:

EXHIBIT ''1''—BALANCE SHEET
EXHIBIT ''2''—STATEMENT OF CASH RECEIPTS AND DISBURSEMENTS
EXHIBIT ''3''—OPERATING STATEMENT
EXHIBIT ''4''—BANK RECONCILIATION

We wish to thank you for this audit, and if we can be of further service, please feel free to call upon us.

Respectfully submitted,

H. E. COLE COMPANY

OKLAHOMA STATE MEDICAL ASSOCIATION
Oklahoma City, Oklahoma

EXPLANATION

Since the Association operates on a Cash Receipts and Disbursement basis, the disbursements for December, which are paid in January, are included in the report for the following year.

OKLAHOMA STATE MEDICAL ASSOCIATION
Oklahoma City, Oklahoma

EXHIBIT I

BALANCE SHEET
Dec. 31, 1942

ASSETS

	Total	Membership Fund	Journal Fund	Medical Defense Fund	Annual Meeting
Petty Cash	$ 11.37	$ 11.37	$............	$............	$............
Bank	6,076.43	4,069.46	1,321.63	685.34	....
U. S. Treasury Bonds	6,178.88	1,235.78	....	4,943.10	....
U. S. Defense Bonds	3,220.00	....	....	3,220.00	....
TOTAL ASSETS	$15,486.68	$ 5,316.61	$ 1,321.63	$ 8,848.44	$............

LIABILITIES & RESERVES

Operating Reserve	$15,486.68	$ 5,316.61	$ 1,321.63	$ 8,848.44	$............
	$15,486.68	$ 5,316.61	$ 1,321.63	$ 8,848.44	$............

OKLAHOMA STATE MEDICAL ASSOCIATION

Oklahoma City, Oklahoma

EXHIBIT 2

STATEMENT OF CASH RECEIPTS & DISBURSEMENTS

January 1, 1942 to December 31, 1942

	Total	Fund Membership	Fund Journal	Medical Fund Defense	Meeting Annual
Cash Balance—January 1, 1942	$ 3,930.30	$ 2,126.54	$ 834.42	$ 309.34	$ 660.00
Petty Cash Balance—January 1, 1942	14.94	14.94			
Transfer from Membership Fund*	1,862.66		1,500.00		362.66
RECEIPTS:					
1942 Membership Dues	13,861.50	12,500.50		1,361.00	
1941 Membership Dues	54.00	49.00		5.00	
1940 Membership Dues	20.00	18.00		2.00	
Miscellaneous Income	107.97	101.47	6.50		
Journal Advertising & Subscriptions	7,509.34		7,509.34		
U. S. Government Bond Interest	135.00	27.00		108.00	
Annual Meeting Income	1,901.65				1,901.65
Total Cash to be Accounted for	$29,397.36	$14,837.45	$ 9,850.26	$ 1,785.34	$ 2,924.31
DISBURSEMENTS:					
National Defense Bonds Purchased	$ 1,000.00	$............	$............	$ 1,000.00	$............
Transfer	1,862.66	1,862.66	$............	$............	$............
Expenses for 1942	20,446.90	8,893.96	8,528.63	100.00	2,824.31
TOTAL DISBURSEMENTS	$23,309.56	$10,756.62	$ 8,528.63	$ 1,100.00	$ 2,924.31
Bank Balance—December 31, 1942	$ 6,076.43	$ 4,069.46	$ 1,321.63	$ 685.34	$............
Petty Cash Balance—December 31, 1942	11.37	11.37			
	$ 6,087.80	$ 4,080.83	$ 1,321.63	$ 685.34	$............

*NOTE—Transfer of $1,500.00 was made from Membership Fund to Journal Fund, to take care of publication deficit.

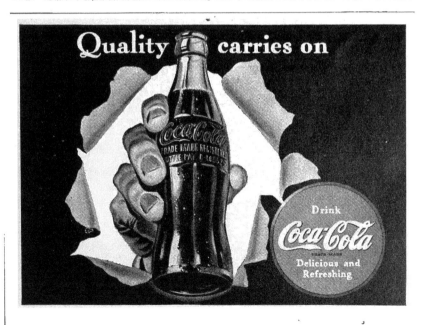

OKLAHOMA STATE MEDICAL ASSOCIATION
Oklahoma City, Oklahoma

EXHIBIT 3

OPERATING STATEMENT
1942

REVENUE:	Total	Fund Membership	Fund Journal	Medical Fund Defense	Meeting Annual
1942 Membership Dues	$13,871.50	$12,509.50	$............	$ 1,362.00	$............
1941 Membership Dues	54.00	49.00	....	5.00	....
1940 Membership Dues	20.00	18.00	....	2.00	....
Journal Advertising & Subscriptions	7,509.34	....	7,509.34	....	....
U. S. Government Bond Interest	135.00	27.00	....	108.00	....
Annual Meeting	1,901.65	....	....	....	1,901.65
Miscellaneous Income	107.97	101.47	6.50	....	....
TOTAL REVENUE	$23,599.46	$12,704.97	$ 7,515.84	$ 1,477.00	$ 1,901.65
EXPENSES:					
Salaries	$ 7,729.10	$ 3,889.00	$ 3,840.10	$............	$............
Journal Printing & Mailing	4,225.03	....	4,225.03	....	....
Press Clipping Service	7.40	....	7.40	....	....
Journal Engraving	135.83	....	135.83	....	....
Telephone & Telegraph	567.59	565.19	2.40	....	....
Postage	486.42	401.21	85.21	....	....
Office Rent	300.00	150.00	150.00	....	....
Printing & Stationery	471.25	471.25	....	....	....
Office Supplies	325.22	325.22	....	....	....
Traveling Expense	460.70	460.70	....	....	....
A.M.A. Delegate Expense	531.00	531.90	....	....	....
Annual Meeting Expense	3,214.37	285.46	4.60	....	2,924.31
Post Graduate Committee	1,319.39	1,319.39	....	....	....
Certificate Frames	30.60	30.60	....	....	....
Sundry	47.87	44.81	3.06	....	....
Secretaries' Conference	137.07	137.07	....	....	....
Auditing & Legal	287.50	112.50	75.00	100.00	....
Express	11.58	11.58	....	....	....
American Red Cross	12.00	12.00	....	....	....
Chamber of Commerce	25.00	25.00	....	....	....
Surety Bond Premium	58.48	58.48	....	....	....
Safety Deposit Box Rental	6.00	6.00	....	....	....
A.M.A. Directory	15.00	15.00	....	....	....
Flowers	41.60	41.60	....	....	....
TOTAL EXPENSES	$20,446.90	$ 8,893.96	$ 8,528.63	$ 100.00	$ 2,924.31
Revenue Over Expenses	$ 3,152.56	$ 3,811.01	—$1,012.79	$ 1,377.00	—$1,022.66

OKLAHOMA STATE MEDICAL ASSOCIATION
Oklahoma City, Oklahoma

EXHIBIT 4

BANK RECONCILLIATION
December 31, 1941

MEMBERSHIP FUND—Liberty National Bank
Balance per Bank Statement .... $ 4,429.78
Outstanding Checks:
    Voucher No. 945 ....$ 37.50
    Voucher No. 946 .... 3.57
    Voucher No. 947 .... 319.25   360.32

Balance per Books .... $ 4,069.46
JOURNAL FUND—Liberty National Bank
Balance per Bank Statement .... $ 1,621.63
Outstanding Checks:
    Voucher No. 949 ....$ 100.00
    Voucher No. 950 .... 200.00   300.00

Balance per Books .... $ 1,321.63
MEDICAL DEFENSE FUND—Liberty National Bank
Balance per Bank Statement .... $ 1,685.34
Outstanding Checks:
    Voucher No. 951 ....$ 1,000.00 $ 1,000.00

Balance per Books .... $ 685.34

TOTAL MONEY ON DEPOSIT .... $ 6,076.43

GOVERNOR KERR APPOINTS MEDICAL BOARD OF EXAMINERS

Governor Robert S. Kerr has appointed the following physicians as members of the Medical Board of Examiners: C. E. Bradley, M.D., Tulsa; Galvin L. Johnson, M.D., Pauls Valley; S. B. Leslie, M.D., Okmulgee; Sam A. McKeel, M.D., Ada; O. C. Newman, M.D., Shattuck; J. D. Osborn, M.D., Frederick; Henry C. Weber, M.D., Bartlesville.

As provided in House Bill 222, which was enacted into law by the last legislature, the Oklahoma State Medical Association, through the Council, nominated 14 physicians to Governor Kerr for his consideration in the appointment of the Board. In addition to the seven physicians appointed, the Council submitted the following names: Finis W. Ewing, M.D., Muskogee; David S. Harris, M.D., Drummond; H. M. McClure, M.D., Chickasha; L. J. Moorman, M.D., Oklahoma City; George H. Niemann, M.D., Ponca City; George Stagner, M.D., Erick; O. E. Templin, M.D., Alva.

The Board will meet and elect officers May 10, at which time it will also conduct examinations.

University of Oklahoma School of Medicine

Dr. George N. Barry, Medical Director State University and Crippled Children's Hospitals, attended the meeting of the New Orleans Graduate Medical Assembly, Seventh Annual Meeting, in New Orleans, on March 15 to 18.

Miss Clare M. J. Wangen, Superintendent of Nurses and Director of the School of Nursing, has resigned effective April 1, 1943.

Dr. Tom Lowry, Dean of the School of Medicine, is now making occasional visits to the school and we are extremely happy to see him recovering his health, and look forward to having him take an active part in the affairs of this school at an early date.

Dr. Donald B. McMullen, Associate Professor of Hygiene and Public Health, is giving a short course to medical technologists on parasitological technique.

A large group of women is working at the School of Medicine folding dressings for the Red Cross, under the direction of Miss Jeanne Green, Instructor in Pathology.

OFFICERS OF COUNTY SOCIETIES, 1943

★

COUNTY	PRESIDENT	SECRETARY	MEETING TIME
Alfalfa	H. E. Huston, Cherokee	L. T. Lancaster, Cherokee	Last Tues. each Second Month
Atoka-Coal	J. B. Clark, Coalgate	J. S. Fulton, Atoka	
Beckham	H. K. Speed, Sayre	E. S. Kilpatrick, Elk City	Second Tuesday
Blaine	Virginia Olson Curtin, Watonga	W. F. Griffin, Watonga	
Bryan	J. T. Colwick, Durant	W. K. Haynie, Durant	Second Tuesday
Caddo	F. L. Patterson, Carnegie	C. B. Sullivan, Carnegie	
Canadian	P. F. Herod, El Reno	A. L. Johnson, El Reno	Subject to call
Carter	Walter Hardy, Ardmore	H. A. Higgins, Ardmore	
Cherokee	P. H. Medearis, Tahlequah	James K. Gray, Tahlequah	First Tuesday
Choctaw	C. H. Hale, Boswell	E. A. Johnson, Hugo	
Cleveland	I. A. Rieger, Norman	Curtis Berry, Norman	Thursday nights
Comanche	George S. Barber, Lawton	W. F. Lewis, Lawton	
Cotton	A. B. Holstead, Temple	Mollie F. Seism, Walters	Third Friday
Craig	F. M. Adams, Vinita	J. M. McMillan, Vinita	
Creek	H. R. Haas, Sapulpa	C. G. Oakes, Sapulpa	
Custer	F. R. Vieregg, Clinton	C. J. Alexander, Clinton	Third Thursday
Garfield	Paul B. Champlin, Enid	John R. Walker, Enid	Fourth Thursday
Garvin	T. F. Gross, Lindsay	John R. Callaway, Pauls Valley	Wednesday before Third Thursday
Grady	Walter J. Baze, Chickasha	Roy E. Emanuel, Chickasha	Third Thursday
Grant	I. V. Hardy, Medford	E. E. Lawson, Medford	
Greer	G. P. Cherry, Mangum	J. B. Hollis, Mangum	
Harmon	W. G. Husband, Hollis	L. E. Hollis, Hollis	First Wednesday
Haskell	William Carson, Keota	N. K. Williams, McCurtain	
Hughes	Wm. L. Taylor, Holdenville	Imogene Mayfield, Holdenville	First Friday
Jackson	E. S. Crow, Olustee	E. W. Mabry, Altus	Last Monday
Jefferson	F. M. Edwards, Ringling	L. L. Wade, Ryan	Second Monday
Kay	Philip C. Risser, Blackwell	J. Holland Howe, Ponca City	Third Thursday
Kingfisher	C. M. Hodgson, Kingfisher	H. Violet Sturgeon, Hennessey	
Kiowa	B. H. Watkins, Hobart	J. William Finch, Hobart	
LeFlore	Neeson Rolle, Poteau	Rush L. Wright, Poteau	
Lincoln	H. B. Jenkins, Tryon	Carl H. Bailey, Stroud	First Wednesday
Logan	William C. Miller, Guthrie	J. L. LeHew, Jr., Guthrie	Last Tuesday
Marshall	O. A. Cook, Madill	Philip G. Joseph, Madill	
Mayes	Ralph V. Smith, Pryor	Paul B. Cameron, Pryor	
McClain	B. W. Slover, Blanchard	R. L. Royster, Purcell	
McCurtain	A. W. Clarkson, Valliant	N. L. Barker, Broken Bow	Fourth Tuesday
McIntosh	James L. Wood, Eufaula	William A. Tolleson, Eufaula	First Thursday
Murray	P. V. Annadown, Sulphur	F. E. Sadler, Sulphur	Second Tuesday
Muskogee-Sequoyah-Wagoner	H. A. Scott, Muskogee	D. Evelyn Miller, Muskogee	First and Third Monday
Noble	C. H. Cooke, Perry	J. W. Francis, Perry	
Okfuskee	L. J. Spickard, Okemah	M. L. Whitney, Okemah	Second Monday
Oklahoma	Walker Morledge, Oklahoma City	E. R. Musick, Oklahoma City	Fourth Tuesday
Okmulgee	A. R. Holmes, Henryetta	J. C. Matheney, Okmulgee	Second Monday
Osage	C. R. Weirich, Pawhuska	George K. Hemphill, Pawhuska	Second Monday
Ottawa	W. B. Sanger, Picher	Matt A. Connell, Picher	Third Thursday
Pawnee	E. T. Robinson, Cleveland	R. L. Browning, Pawnee	
Payne	L. A. Mitchell, Stillwater	C. W. Moore, Stillwater	Third Thursday
Pittsburg	John F. Park, McAlester	William H. Kneiser, McAlester	Third Friday
Pontotoc	O. H. Miller, Ada	R. H. Mayes, Ada	First Wednesday
Pottawatomie	A. C. McFarling, Shawnee	Clinton Gallaher, Shawnee	First and Third Saturday
Pushmataha	John S. Lawson, Clayton	B. M. Huckabay, Antlers	
Rogers	C. W. Beson, Claremore	C. L. Caldwell, Chelsea	First Monday
Seminole	Max Van Sandt, Wewoka	Mack I. Shunholtz, Wewoka	Third Wednesday
Stephens	W. K. Walker, Marlow	Wallis S. Ivy, Duncan	
Texas	R. G. Obermiller, Texhoma	Morris Smith, Guymon	
Tillman	R. D. Robinson, Frederick	O. G. Bacon, Frederick	
Tulsa	James C. Peden, Tulsa	E. O. Johnson, Tulsa	Second and Fourth Monday
Washington-Nowata	J. G. Smith, Bartlesville	J. V. Athey, Bartlesville	Second Wednesday
Washita	A. S. Neal, Cordell	James F. McMurry, Sentinel	
Woods	C. A. Traverse, Alva	O. E. Templin, Alva	Last Tuesday Odd Months
Woodward	C. E. Williams, Woodward	C. W. Tedrowe, Woodward	Second Thursday

THE JOURNAL
OF THE
OKLAHOMA STATE MEDICAL ASSOCIATION

VOLUME XXXVI   OKLAHOMA CITY, OKLAHOMA, MAY, 1943   NUMBER 5

A Study of Trachoma With A Report Of 318 Cases, 233 Treated With Sulfanilamide

CLINTON GALLAHER, M.D., F.A.C.S.

SHAWNEE, OKLAHOMA

DEFINITION

The name Trachoma is derived from a Greek word which means "rough." Trachoma is defined as a rough granular conjunctivitis, characterized by a sub-epithelial cellular infiltration with a follicular distribution, the natural resolution of which is cicatrization. The latter is associated with great potential visual disturbance and gross deformity. The importance of the disease as the cause of human grief, because of loss of vision and from economic loss, is probably secondary to no other illness of man. Coston reports that 501 cases in Oklahoma receive blind pension aid from the State Welfare Board because of loss of vision in which the examining physicians state that the etiology is trachoma or the complications of trachoma. This represents 23.3 per cent of the total number of cases who receive aid because of blindness.

INTRODUCTION

No physician living in this area who is in any way interested in eyes can fail to be aware of the problems of trachoma. We had a considerable increase of interest in the fall of 1938. This was occasioned by the fact that we attended the session of the Southern Medical Association in Oklahoma City and visited the section in Ophthalmology. There was heard a discussion of the treatment of trachoma. The speakers were men who merit respect for the knowledge of the subject; but the wide variety of opinions expressed, as to the best means of securing relief for the trachoma patient, was such that one could hardly believe them discussing the same topic, had not the subject been announced. One doctor was persuaded that

treatment with copper sulphate sticks was always the method of choice. His opinion is upheld by Duke-Elder. Another believed that a weak solution of copper sulphate was more effective. A third physician expressed the opinion that all trachoma could be ultimately healed or at least greatly improved if adequate cleansing could be accomplished. In fact he stated he believed he could effect as much benefit by placing the patient's head under a tap and flushing the eyes repeatedly with plain water, as with any other method. The opinion was also expressed that all cases of trachoma ultimately become surgical, and that much time, money and suffering may be avoided by early surgical treatment. We cannot help believing that there is something to be said for every method discussed, but that no one has yet found the ultimate answer for the simple reason that the essential cause and nature of the disease is not sufficiently understood. We cannot be satisfied with the results from treatment with sulfanilamide or the combination of sulfanilamide with any number of other methods. We cannot be satisfied with the bland statement that trachoma is caused by a filtrable virus. We do not dispute this latter statement, but we do believe there is some evidence in support of the contention that there are other factors which cannot be dismissed.

From the year 1938 our interest in trachoma was renewed and we began reviewing the cases we had seen. From that time we began to look more carefully for trachoma, and especially among our Indian patients.. About three years ago Doctor Charles Haygood became the Director of the Pottawatomie County Health Unit, and I at once learned that he was also greatly interested in the disease. To him I am grateful for the fact that he has found a large number of cases among children in the public schools of this county, many of whom have ultimately found their way to this office for observation and care.

It appears that we live in an area where there are an unusual number of cases of trachoma. With few exceptions they occur among the poor. We feel that the failure to recognize a large number of cases in many adjacent communities is simply due to the fact that the examination of school children, and others, does not include eversion of the upper lids. This procedure is necessary in order to make a diagnosis. We suspect another reason is found in the fact that the early stages of trachoma are not severe enough to bring these patients to any physician, especially to an eye physician. In this paper we propose to submit a statistical analysis of a series of cases, most of which have been treated within the last 48 months in this office. The interval of treatment and the response which we have seen, can in no wise justify any definite conclusions as yet, but it is our feeling that the results are somewhat unique and should be recorded. We are impressed with the apparent fact that our results do not compare favorably with reports from various series in the Indian Department. We are, of course, of the opinion that sulfanilamide possesses certain advantages heretofore unknown in the treatment of trachoma, and we should like to be of some assistance in determining the relative merits of this method.

CLASSIFICATION

In order to simplify the classification of cases and to prepare an average of results, which may be compared with others, we have adopted a system as recommended by Doctor J. G. Townsend in the office of Indian Affairs. Our cases are classified as follows:

TABLE No. 1

Grades	1	2	3	4	
No. of cases	211	64	39	4	Total: 318

Grade One represents the primary stage of trachoma. In this stage the conjunctiva is usually hyperemic and slightly congested, or swollen. A small amount of muco-purulent material may be noted in the mornings. When the upper lids are everted there may be seen small subepithelial follicles under the conjunctiva. They dot the surface over the tarsus and are particularly apt to be prominent at the transitional folds. The everted lower lid will often present a similar, though less marked appearance. One

may rarely see the reverse of this situation, with signs more prominent in the everted lower lids. Superficial observation gives the impression of a velvety surface, but closer examination usually discloses the presence of distinct follicular congestion. It is necessary to this classification that there be an early involvement of the cornea. This involvement begins at the upper limbus as a slight dilation and extension of the vessels beyond the limbus, together with an early gray infiltration of the corneal substance. Until this corneal change has appeared (panus), cases presenting such pictures as those presented above must be classified as grade five, which is suspected trachoma.

Grade Two presents at least a few bleb-like excrescences which protrude above the surface of the rest of the conjunctiva. They form what might be called vegetative pedunculated masses and contain a gelatinous substance. Their distribution is more prominent in the retrotarsal folds, but they are usually scattered over the mucosa of both lids. This stage may also be described as being a papillary hypertrophy, raspberry like in its appearance. The corneal changes of grade one are somewhat more advanced in grade two. The panus is also essential to the diagnosis.

Grade Three is characterized by cicatrization. The conjunctiva may be rather thick, but there is apt to be little or no hyperemia. The conjunctival surface begins to show an irregularity because of the development of connective tissue bands. Contraction of the scar now begins, resulting in eversion or inversion of the lids, usually the latter (entropion).

Grade Four is the classification assigned to healed trachoma. If any active process is present it is secondary. This stage is characterized by layers of panus and the various sequelae incident to cicatrization.

RACE AND SEX DISTRIBUTION

In the present series the distribution as to sex was male 188, female 130. We are unable to explain why it happened that in this series there is a preponderance of males in contrast with the usual number of females affected. It is probable that the small number of cases is as adequate as any explanation.

Distribution as to race is as follows: White: 209; Indian: 108; Colored: 1.

It is generally agreed that the Indian race in this country seems more susceptible than others. In spite of the large number of white patients seen, the per capita population still gives a large preponderance of involvement among the Indians. The Shawnee Indian Agency population is about 5,000, where as the total population of the county is about 75,000. It may be of some significance to remark that practically every Indian in this county has been examined for trachoma, has been advised to have treatment, and has had his treatment in this office, if at all. Although many of them refuse to have adequate treatment, these cases are observed and recorded when the Indian reports for other complaints. A survey of the white population has never been made, except as hereafter described. About December 1, 1940, Doctor Charles Haygood began his survey of all school children in the county. In each school visited from that time to the present, examination of the children included eversion of the upper lids and inspection in good light. Although Doctor Haygood is not an eye physician, his interest in the disease and his experience in diagnosis is such that I believe we are justified in assuming that no cases of trachoma which have been inspected have been overlooked. We are even more inclined to believe this is true since there have been several cases of simple follicular conjunctivitis sent to the office on the suspicion that they might have trachoma. We have tried to be very careful to exclude all such cases from this series. We have required the presence of a panus as a distinguishing characteristic necessary to the diagnosis of trachoma.

It is generally thought that trachoma rarely appears among colored people. The reason for this relative immunity is obscure. Certainly there are many colored people in this community who are as poor as the Indians. In general they are much poorer than our white population. I am not aware if they are more particular about personal cleanliness. We do not see many negro children but in our small experience it appears that this is the only eye disease to which they have any appreciable immunity. The one negro child which we report had a definite panus, a gross velvety appearance with subepithelial infiltration, having a follicular distribution. Both of our eye physicians saw this child and agreed that it was a typical case of trachoma, grade one, early, acute.

HOSPITALIZATION

Three-hundred-fifteen of these cases were ambulatory, three were hospital cases, Indians who were being treated for tuberculosis in the Shawnee Indian Sanitorium. In two of these hospital cases we have the only severe febrile reactions observed in the entire series. One of these patients sustained a severe anemia. The red cell count and hemoglobin were restored in a reasonable length of time during the administration of ade-

quate diet and supplementary Lextron. This patient did not show agranulocytosis at any time. The routine therapy was stopped when the fever first appeared. With few exceptions all ambulatory patients we treated with sulfanilamide. When sulfanilamide was advised the parents or the patients were warned of the possible toxic effects of the drug and instructed to stop the treatment and report to the office as soon as possible if any signs of poisoning should occur. There were specific instructions to watch for possible nausea, vomiting, fever, rash, headache, or any gastrointestinal disturbances. In spite of the somewhat hazardous nature of this method which we freely admit, we have had no serious secondary effects except the one previously noted. We have been obliged to decide whether we should treat our ambulatory patients with sulfanilamide, and attempt to make them comfortable by this means, or to advise hospitalization which for most of them would have been entirely impossible.

AGE

Of these 318 cases, 134 were adults of 18 years or more, and 184 were children. Ages of the children are charted below:

TABLE NO. 2

Up to 2 years of age	8 cases
Age 3 years	7 cases
Age 4 years	7 cases
Age 5 years	11 cases
Age 6 years	15 cases
Age 7 years	15 cases
Age 8 years	21 cases
Age 9 years	18 cases
Age 10 years	27 cases
Age 11 years	13 cases
Age 12 years	12 cases
Age 13 years	6 cases
Age 14 years	8 cases
Age 15 years	6 cases
Age 16 years	9 cases
Age 17 years	1 case

It will be seen that the greater number of cases are reported among children of ages five to twelve. We feel there is no peculiar significance attached to this fact. These are the cases which are discovered in the public schools and children above and below these ages are not examined. It is possible, however, that the contagious nature of the disease will show that young school children are more apt to acquire it than pre-school children. We are not aware if it is true that any age is immune. It appears that children are more susceptible than adults. We are inclined to think that trachoma is acquired first of all from mothers and it is usually found that the incidence of trachoma among infants is relatively high when the mothers are diseased. The next large group usually occurs in early school age.

GEOGRAPHICAL

The distribution as to climate is of course beyond our scope of investigation, but the large number of cases in this community is entirely compatible with the impression that Oklahoma is in the so-called "trachoma zone" of the United States. I would like to comment briefly on the observation which has been made by Doctor J. N. Alley of Lewiston, Idaho, which is to the effect that Coastal Indians seem to be immune to trachoma. Indians who live east of the Divide are often affected. At least one difference in these tribes is the fact that the former are notably fish eaters, principally salmon fish. It is therefore possible that the iodine content of sea foods may bear some direct relation to the incidence of trachoma. I am unable to learn if this theory has been investigated but suggest that the administration of small amounts of iodine or the introduction of sea foods in the diet might be found to exert a protective influence. The idea should at least be considered.

TREATMENT METHODS

There has been good authority for the recommendations of treatment by use of copper sulphate sticks. This method we have had the temerity to abandon entirely because of the amount of pain associated with its use. In our practice it is necessary to find some method which is relatively painless, or we find that our patients refuse to return. We assume no critical attitude against the use of copper sulphate sticks, but find its use inadvisable for the type of patients with whom we are concerned. Patients who submit to copper sulphate stick treatment must be made of sterner stuff. Maybe this is an admission of a small "friction hold" on our patients. In any event we have been greatly pleased with the number of patients who continue to return, a condition we would not expect if our method were painful, especially in children. The same may be said of silver nitrate treatment, although it has been used on some occasions. It is now prescribed for use in cases which are primarily, or are complicated by, Neisserian infections. Even in these infections we feel that silver nitrate is largely a prophylactic or early treatment measure. We use it one time as a rule, when the diagnosis of a Neisserian infection is first made. It is not usually repeated. It is our experience that sulfapyridine or sulfathiazole is more effective than any other drugs we have used.

In our series of cases one or more of the following methods of treatment have been used in every case. Usually two or more drugs are used. The report of patients who have received the various types of treatment is charted below:

TABLE No. 3

Sulfanilamide by mouth	199
Grettage	26
Brossage	2
Zinc Sulphate	58
Copper Sulphate (solution)	46
Sulfanilamide (1% in Ringers)	40
Sulfathiazole, 3% ointment	9
Vitamin A (U. 25,000 or more daily)	4
Neo Silvol	2

Sulfanilamide by mouth is recommended for every patient in our clinic, wherein the diagnosis of active trachoma is made. The number of patients thus treated now totals 199. The remainder of the cases in the total of 318 are not considered in relation to treatment or results for the simple reason that the period of observation was too brief for any value to be attached. Most of the cases not considered were advised to have sulfanilamide therapy. We feel justified in assuming that a certain number actually had the treatment, but did not return again because of satisfactory improvement. Of this we are, of course, uncertain. In not more than one-half dozen cases was treatment actually refused or denied.

Our routine treatment of sulfanilamide consists in the administration of one-half grain per pound of body weight per day for a period of ten days. Our patients are instructed to divide the total daily dosage in four parts, equal if possible, larger toward the latter part of the day if this cannot be done. The tablets are washed down with a small amount of soda water which is made by adding one teaspoonful of baking soda to a glass of drinking water. Parents or adult patients are always cautioned to note the appearance of any toxic effect such as fever, rash or gastrointestinal disturbance and to stop the treatment and report as soon as possible to the office, if these or other disturbing symptoms occur. They are told that some patients are unable to continue this method of treatment, that this is the method of preference, but it may be impossible to continue with safety. It is explained that they are asked to report immediately in order that some other form of treatment, less effective but more safe, may be started. Thus far we have found parents highly cooperative and we have observed no serious complications. When our patients come from an appreciable distance out of town, we recommend that the family physician be advised of the fact that the patient is using sulfanilamide, and consulted if necessary. The toxic effects which we have encountered, we will list in another paragraph. We realize that hospitalization is extremely desirable if the patient is to have sulfanilamide therapy. It is impossible for us to arrange hospitalization for most of our patients. We are therefore obliged to choose between using a drug which appears to be highly beneficial without hospitalization or insisting upon an unreasonable and apparently unnecessary expense.

In Grade Two trachoma we have found that grettage appears to be an essential part of treatment in a certain number of cases. The patients are told of this fact on the occasion of the first office visit. The routine sulfanilamide treatment is first given and most of the patients are observed for a period of four to six weeks before grettage is done. We are still somewhat surprised to see the large granular trachoma bodies fade and melt away with sulfanilamide treatment. We still feel that we cannot expect this to occur in many of the Grade Two cases, although with few exceptions relief of the itching and other distress is the rule. When grettage is done it is usually followed by the administration of sulfanilamide locally, one per cent in Ringer's Solution. Grettage is usually performed under local anesthesia in children as young as eight or nine years of age. If the child is younger we cannot expect to have adequate cooperation. Brossage is rarely necessary. We believe this is due to the fact that grettage is quite thorough.

More and more we are inclined to use zinc after sulfanilamide therapy or during the time of its administration. Zinc is used in the form of one-half per cent sulphate ointment. The parent or patient is instructed to place a small amount of the ointment in the lower cul de sac at bed time. The procedure is actually shown to some one who will be responsible for seeing that it is done each night. The ointment is washed away with normal saline in the morning, and local sulfanilamide is then used in most cases. The zinc appears to exert a beneficial influence on the follicles per se. In this particular circumstance we have used weak solution of copper sulphate but generally find the results are disappointing.

Following the administration of sulfanilamide by mouth our routine more and more includes the use of sulfanilamide drops locally for intervals varying from one to three months. This is the rule in spite of the fact that improvement seems as likely to occur within the first ten days as any time thereafter. It appears that if sulfanilamide therapy is to be effective in a given case, the results will be definitely apparent within a very few days. Our druggist is instructed as to the manner in which sulfanilamide may be dissolved in Ringer's solution. This is accomplished by the use of heat, agitation, and with care to avoid boiling. The supersaturated solution is thus prepared, cooled and filtered. This will usually produce a clear fluid with a few fine granules settling out after a day or two. When the prescription is filled the druggist is careful to pour off supernatant fluid so that the patient receives a perfectly clear solution.

For the past several months we have also used Vitamin A locally in the form of Afaxin in Oil (Winthrop) in cases with the complications of phlyctenules or acute keratitis, with or without ulcerations. When Vitamin A is given by mouth we use from 25 to 50,000 units daily for a brief interval of five to seven days. Unless there is some apparent benefit we feel that continuation is futile. We are impressed with the greater importance of instructing these patients about adequate diet with special attention to foods high in Vitamin A content.

Epilation is a routine treatment in Grades Three and Four trachoma with entropion. Surgical treatment is not considered in this paper.

The various collodial silver salts, such as argyrol and neosilvol, we have discontinued altogether. It is our feeling that they may be of some benefit, but that the other drugs mentioned elsewhere in this paper have superior advantages. One reason we do not like the use of silver salts, except in the office, is that we have seen several patients with argyrosis. It is our experience that when some simple remedy is suggested the patient may assume on his own responsibility, an unusual continuation of its use. Even though patients may be warned of the possibility of argyrosis they are apt to forget or disbelieve.

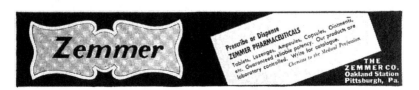

It is also true that the suggestion that argyrol is a good treatment for the eyes, may be passed on to a friend or neighbor and adequate treatment delayed because of misinformation or ignorance.

As a routine wash in all cases of trachoma, as well as other debris producing conditions of the eyes, we feel that normal saline is without an equal. Although saturated solutions of boric acid satisfies our condition for a wash in most cases, we have observed a few wherein it seemed irritating. We have yet to see any patient whose eyes appeared to manifest a harmful effect which could be assigned to normal saline.

We are aware that there are other drugs and other procedures which should be considered in the treatment of trachoma. We are not persuaded that sulfanilamide per se, is the most beneficial azosulfonamide. We are inclined to believe that even sulfanilamide might be more effective or equally so, if used as a routine locally. At present we are concerned with the serious attempt to evaluate this particular routine. We do not intend to change it until such time as some adequate authority leads us to believe that another method is superior. We were very interested to note the experience of Doctor Fred Lowe with the local use of powdered sulfanilamide. We feel that the findings of Luo and P'an in aqueous humor concentrations of sulfanilamide may bear some direct relation to the trends of treatment of trachoma. If concentrations in the aqueous are so greatly increased by the local instillation of the powdered drug, it seems reasonable to suspect that concentrations in the tissues of the lids will be correspondingly great. When this can be accomplished without danger from the strong irritant local effects we may have advanced somewhat in the treatment of trachoma.

TOXIC EFFECTS

In 199 patients receiving routine sulfanilamide therapy by mouth, there were 40 who sustained toxic effects of one kind or another. These are: Nausea, 9; Dizziness, 8; Fever, 5; Headache, 6; Rash, 7; Nervousness, 2; Diarrhea, 1; Anemia, 1; Urinary Frequency, 1.

None of our patients have been affected by such toxic effects as vomiting, psychosis, neuritis, acidosis, hepatitis, leukopenia, jaundice, agranulocytosis, or any more than a mild cyanosis. It appears that nausea is less apt to occur when the sulfanilamide tablets are washed down with soda water. Our patients are instructed that if neausea only occurs the treatment should be discontinued for a period of 24 hours and resumed thereafter as if no toxic effect had occurred. The

symptom of dizziness is usually associated with weakness and a moderate tachycardia, sometimes in cases of anemia and other conditions of more serious consequence.

Patients who sustain febrile reactions during the course of treatment are advised to stop immediately and sulfanilamide is not again used by mouth in these cases. When a rash occurs the drug may be temporarily discontinued or stopped according to the severity of the reaction. We do not advise that sulfanilamide be stopped because of headache or nervousness. Diarrhea or any other serious gastrointestinal disturbance is interpreted as a warning that sulfanilamide should be stopped.

The one patient who had a secondary anemia during and following sulfanilamide by mouth, was a patient in the Shawnee Indian Tuberculosis Sanitorium. This young women was restored again to a normal red cell count and hemoglobin while taking a liberal diet and Lextron. Both the tuberculosis and trachoma were arrested and have remained so for more than three years. Of the 199 patients, 159 denied any toxic effects at all.

OBSERVATION INTERVAL

Our present report is considered preliminary because of the limited period of observation. Thirteen have been observed for less than six months; 13 have been observed for six to twelve months; and 292 have been observed for more than twelve months.

RESULTS

It is impossible to make an accurate chart of results, but our impression with these patients whom we have been able to follow, are charted below:

Worse during treatment 4
Unchanged 6
Symptoms relieved 190
Signs gone 37
Considered arrested 120
Unable to follow 101

In 67 of these cases all treatment has been discontinued, but we continue to exert pressure to maintain periodic observations of progress and changes if any. We have not felt that we could as yet be justified in assuming a cure, regardless of the degree of improvement. These cases have shown the most favorable response and all signs and symptoms have disappeared. We would like to continue to handle these cases until such time as we are able to list them as "five year cures."

We would be much more inclined to credit the value of the routine if it were not for the fact that three cases we were permitted to observe rather closely, had an increase in both signs and symptoms during the periods of active treatment. On the other hand it was most gratifying to have so many patients tell us that the symptoms of itching, burning and other irritations were completely relieved within five to ten days after the treatment was started. Most of the patients in whom all signs disappeared were in Grade One. The patients now classified as arrested have had a complete remission of all symptoms and exhibit only what we considered minimal signs. These minimal signs are characterized as minimal congestion of the follicles with no hyperemia and no other signs of the disease. In 152 such cases we have felt justified in advising that all treatment be stopped. Every patient is requested to return at intervals of no more than three months. They are also advised to return at any time should any signs or any symptoms recur. In spite of this request we have been unable to follow 101 patients.

SUMMARY

One hundred ninety-nine patients with active trachoma, in various stages, have had sulfanilamide therapy and have been observed for an appreciable period. The methods of classification and modes of treatment are described. Preliminary results of treatment and toxic effects are related.

CONCLUSION

1. The results of sulfanilamide therapy are such that the drug must be included among those considered in the treatment of trachoma. All methods of treatment with or without sulfanilamide, do not yet give reasonable assurance of the ability to produce beneficial changes in every case. Well over 90 per cent of cases can be assured of some improvement.

2. The sulfanilamide therapy, in combination with other drugs, affords a method which may be used with reasonable safety without hospitalization and without the necessity of prolonged daily treatment and observation. One or more courses of sulfanilamide alone is apt to produce disappointing results.

3. The specific remedy for trachoma is not yet found. The essential nature of the disease, its cause, and its treatment, remain a problem to be solved by the aler tophthalmologist who continues to study trachoma. Nothing can delay the answer so much as the complacent satisfaction with our present knowledge of the disease and its treatment.

BIBLIOGRAPHY

Coston, Tullos O., "Causes of Blindness in Oklahoma," J. Okla. State Med. Assoc., Vol. XXXV, No. 11, Nov. 1942.

Allen, E. A., Sulfanilamide and its derivatives, J.M.A Geroria, XXIX, 429, Sept, 1940

Brown, A. E, The sulfamido compounds; their practical application in clinical medicine, Minnesota Med., XXIII, 572, Aug. 1940.

Brown, A E., Sulfanilamide, Neoprontosil and Sulfapyridine; their clinical application, Wisconsin M. J., Jan. 1940.

Cosgrove, K. W., The local use of Sulfanilamide in trachoma. A. J. Ophth., 911, Aug. 1940.

Cooper, William Legrande, Management of Recurrent Trachoma following sulfanilamide treatment, Archives of Ophth., Sept. 1940.

Doane, J. C. Blumberg, N. & Teplick, J. G. Sulfanilamide therapy. . M. Rec., cl. 439, Dec 20, 1939.

Foster, Wesley G., Treatment of trachoma with sulfanilamide, Fort Apache, Ariz., Am. J. Ophth., May 1940.

Harley, R. D, Brown, A. E. & Herrell, W. E., Sulfanilamide in the treatment of trachoma, Am. J. Opth., XXII, 299, March 1939.

Hirschfelder, M., Treatment of trachoma with sulfanilamide and its derivatives sulfapyridine and azosulfamide, J.A.M A., CXV, 107, July 13, 1940.

Harley, Brown & Herrell, Proceedings of Staff of Mayo Clinic, "Sulfanilamide and Neoprontosil in the treatment of trachoma, Oct. 11, 1939.

Harley, Brown & Herrell, Sulfanilamide and Neoprontosil in the treatment of trachoma, Am J. Ophth., Nov. 1939.

Julianelle, Lane and Whitted, Effect of Sulfanilamide in the course of trachoma, Am. J. Ophth., Nov. 1939.

Julianelle, Gamet, Sulfanilamide Therapy in trachoma, Missouri Trachoma Hospital, Rollo, Mo., Am. J. Ophth., Nov. 1939.

Keller & Rutherford, Sulfanilamide in old trachoma, J. Indiana State Med. Assn., May 1940.

Lee, O S., Jr. & Rottenstein, H. Trachoma treated with sulfanilamide and its derivatives sulfapyridine and azosulfamide, J.A.M.A., CXV, 107, July 13, 1940.

Lone, P. H., The clinical use of sulfanilamide and its derivatives in the treatment and prophylaxis of certain infections. Bull. New York Acad. Med., XVI, 782, Dec. 1940.

Luo, T. H & P'an, S. Y. Concentration of sulfanilamide in the aqueous humor of human eyes. Chinese M. J., IVIII, 167, Aug 1940.

Long, Haviland, Edwards & Bliss, Clinical evaluation of the use of sulfanilamides, John Hopkins, Mississippi Doctor, March 1940.

Lee and Rotenstein, Trachoma treated with Sulfanilamide and its derivatives, J.A.M A., July 13, 1940.

MacCallan, A F., Sulfanilamide treatment of bacterial and trachomatous conjunctivitis, F.E.C.S British Medical Journal, March 23, 1940

Smith, J. E. Director of Trachoma Hospital at Rollo, Missouri, Report of Committee on Conservation of Vision to the State and Provincial Health Authorities of North American, Washington, D. C, May 1941.

Spining, W. D, Observation of Sulfanilamide in Trachoma and associated ocular conditions, Am., J. Ophth., March 1940

Thygeson, Phillip, Treatment of trachoma with Sulfanilamide, Archives of Ophth., Nov. 1939.

Townsend, J G., Trachoma control in the Indian service, Sight Saving Review, Dec. 1939.

The Terrible Patient

S. Weir Mitchell once said, "The terrible patients are nervous women with long memories, who question much where answers are difficult, and who put together one's answers from time to time and torment themselves and the physician with the apparent inconsistencies they detect."

Case Report: Lithokelyphopedion
(Lithopedion With Calcified Membranes)

With Some Remarks on Ectopic Pregnacy in General

GRIDER PENICK, M.D., F.A.C.S.

Department of Gynecology
University of Oklahoma School of Medicine

OKLAHOMA CITY, OKLAHOMA

It is estimated that extra uterine implantation of the fertilized ovum takes place in approximately 1.25 per cent of all pregnancies. It is indeed surprising that it does not occur more frequently. Theoretically, it is possible for it to occur at any point of its course from the ovary to the uterine cavity, and cases illustrating all these locations have been reported.

By far the most frequent site of all extra uterine pregnancies is in the tube. Any portion of the tube may be involved from the fimbriated end to the interstitial portion. All of us are more or less familiar with the classical description of that exceedingly dramatic chain of events which occurs when a tube ruptures suddenly and the patient loses an alarming amount of blood into her own peritoneum. Many of us are not aware, however, of the fact that these classical cases are not so numerous as those which rupture more gradually, producing symptoms of only moderate severity and urgency, from which the patient may apparently completely recover, and which may be repeated in a few days, due to leakage of a little more blood into the pelvis or peritoneal cavity.

If the implantation has been at the fimbriated end, usually the tube does not rupture as the ovum enlarges, but stretches and allows the clot and ovum to escape at the end of the tube—the so-called "tubal abortion;" if the pregnancy is early and the pelvis clean, absorption occurs with no serious after effects. If infection is present, the hematoma may abscess and thus produce symptoms of peritoneal irritation. However, if the fetus and the placenta are viable, the villi may invade some other structure with which they are in contact and continue to live. Cases have been reported

in which the placenta was attached to the posterior surface of the uterus, the broad ligament, the amentum, liver, stomach, anterior parietal peritoneum, etc. This chain of events is called secondary abdominal pregnancy to differentiate it from primary abdominal pregnancy, in which condition the fertilized ovum is implanted before entering the tube.

When abdominal implantation occurs, either primary or secondary, if the fetus continues to live till term, or near term, spurious labor occurs. This is characterized by uterine cramps, with passage of some blood and decidual tissue per vagina. If by this time a correct diagnosis has not been made and the abdomen opened, the fetus dies. This is caused by loosening of the placenta in places, from its attachment, due, in turn, to hemorrhagic changes in the placenta. This interferes with the circulation to the fetus, so death ensues.

When the fetus dies it usually becomes macerated and the soft parts absorbed, leaving only the bony skeleton. If infection occurs, suppuration may follow with an attempt on the part of nature to expel the bones through sinuses. Fistulae may develop into the bowel or bladder, which may in turn be followed by generalized sepsis, hemorrhage and death.

If infection does not occur, mummification of the fetus may occur. The tissues lose their fluids by absorption, and remain well preserved. After a number of years calcium salts are deposited, producing a "lithopedion" (stone child). If the membranes are intact and are included in the mass a "lithokelyphopedion" results. These masses may remain for a long time in the abdomen, frequently 20 or 30 years. One extremely interesting case was reported by a Dr. Lye, of Singapore, in the Lancet (1936). The patient, a Chinese woman, was delivered of a normal child at the age of 30. At the age of 40, she again became pregnant and went nine months when severe abdominal pain developed. The abdomen was massaged and at the end of the day, fetal movements ceased. Pain continued for one month; she did not menstruate for one year. At the age of 41 the periods were resumed and continued regularly till the age of 70. At the age of 100, a lithopedion was found by X-ray during an examination to determine the cause of a vague distress in the abdomen.

CASE REPORT

Only the relevant facts pertaining to the history, physical, surgical and pathological reports will be included.

Mrs. Nettie Graham, a colored para III, grav. IV, was admitted to the hospital September 13, 1942, complaining of "lumps in her stomach." In January, 1939, her menstrual period was only two days in duration and scant. Ordinarily the duration of her periods was four days and she flowed rather profusely. Soon she thought she was pregnant and was sure of this later when she felt movement. She progressed satisfactorily until September, 1939, when she developed abdominal cramps and a bloody vaginal discharge. She consulted a doctor who told her the fetus was dead and that she would soon pass it. An X-ray was taken at this time (Fig. 1). She went home and continued to have a bloody vaginal discharge for one month. Meanwhile the pain in the abdomen diminished and soon she was able to attempt to do her work. In November, 1939,

she menstruated normally and has had a normal menstrual history until her admission to the hospital (three years later).

General physical examination (including laboratory work) showed her to be in good physical condition. Examination of the abdomen revealed a mass which almost filled the cavity. This mass seemed to lie transversely and could be felt about four inches above and the same distance below the umbilicus. The head could be definitely palpated and identified on the right side of the abdomen. The entire mass was movable, but not freely so. Bimanual vaginal examination revealed the presence of a Fibroid uterus (about four inches in diameter). Behind the uterus, and occupying the right posterior part of the pelvis was a smooth, fixed, stony hard mass about six inches in diameter. This was thought to be the calcified placenta (Fig. 2).

With the tentative diagnosis of lithopedion, calcification of the placenta and Fibroid uterus, surgery was advised and accepted. The abdomen was opened and the lithopedion immediately came into view. It was free everywhere except on the right side of the abdomen where the fetal head was densely adherent to the anterior parietes. When these adhesions were loosened the lithopedion was lifted out of the abdomen. Next the pelvis was explored. The Fibroid uterus was found to be pushed upward by the rounded hard mass previously described. This mass was intimately attached to the posterior surface of the right board ligament and posterior surface of the uterus, so in order to remove it with the greatest ease a right sal-

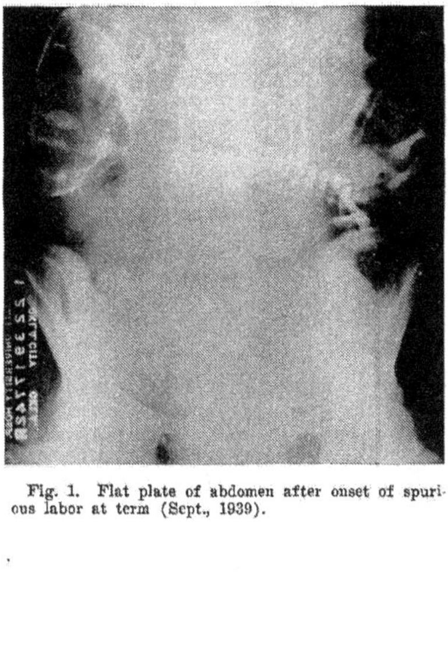

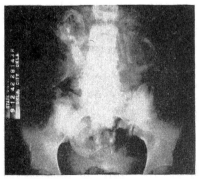

Fig. 1. Flat plate of abdomen after onset of spurious labor at term (Sept., 1939).

Fig. 2. Flat plate of abdomen on admission to hospital (Sept., 1942). Notice rounded shadow in right pelvis which is not present in Fig. 1. This is calcified placenta.

pingo-oophorectomy and supravaginal hysterectomy were done. No technical difficulty was encountered and the patient left the operating room in good condition. Her post-operative course was uneventful and she was dismissed from the hospital two weeks later.

GROSS PATHOLOGICAL DESCRIPTION
(DR. BELA HALPERT)

The specimen (Fig. 3) consists of a fetus, uterus with right fallopian tube and a globular mass. The fetus measures 25 cm, in length and is enclosed in a delicate membrane which follows the body contour and can be peeled off. The face is distorted, is fairly smooth with the contours only outlined. The extremities are tightly adhered to the body. They are distorted and folded in abnormal positions. The right hand is missing. Outlines of the left hand with some fingers missing are discernible. The left hand is placed over the dorsum of the left foot as if it were being held by it. The right leg is folded anteriorly at right angles parallel with the thigh. The toes, foot and ankle are missing. After the membrane is peeled off, the face is black brown and firm.

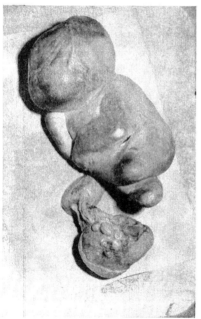

Fig. 3. Photograph of specimens removed—litho-pedion, fibroid uterus and calcified placenta.

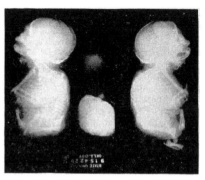

Fig. 4. X-ray of the specimens after removal, to show comparative densities. Two views of fetus, calcified placenta and uterus in center.

The extremities and the body also feel stony hard and are gray and yellow .

Dr. Halpert then dscribes the uterus and tube in some detail.

DIAGNOSIS

Lithopedion.

Uterus with right fallopian tube, and attached calcified placenta.

DISCUSSION

Lithopedion is a rare formation. No statistics are available as to its relative frequency. The first mention in the literature was in 1626. Since that time a total of 235 cases have been reported. P. Brooke Bland, in 1930, collected all the known cases and added 14 new ones, making at that time, a total of 221. Since that time 14 cases have been reported. Bland made the categorical statement that in these cases "when mummification of the fetus occurs, no trace can be found of placenta or placental tissue." In the case I report, the placenta was not only calcified and found at operation, but was strongly suspected before operation. Apparently, this is the first case to be reported in which it has been possible to arrive at the above conclusions through physical examination and X-ray findings.

Another interesting point in regard to this case is the fact that if we can place reliance in the history this patient gave (and I believe we can), we are almost forced to consider the case as one of primary abdominal pregnancy. There was nothing at all suggestive of symptoms (pain, vaginal bleeding, etc.) which she should have had early in her pregnancy if she had had a tubal abortion.

A third interesting point is that this patient was a negress. In this locality, ectopic pregnancy in a negress is rare. Out of 55 consecutive cases at the University Hospital, only three have been negresses. Out of 41 cases at St. Anthony Hospital, only one was a negress.

SUMMARY

1. Brief remarks are made in regard to ectopic pregnancy.

2. A case of lithokelypedion is reported in which it was possible to dagnose a calcified placenta before operation.

BIBLIOGRAPHY

1. Case, P.: Note with Report of Case. Brit. M. J., 1: 383-384, Feb., 1937.
2. Laconture, J.: Abdominal Pregnancy with Retention of Fetus 22 years; Ablation during Laparotomy for Ovarion Tumor. Case: Bull. of Society of Obstetrics & Gynecology, 26: 56-57, Jan., 1937.
3. Masson, J. C. & Simon, H. E: Lithopedion Surg. Gynecology & Obstetrics, XLVI: 500-508, 1928.
4. Recklin: Case in a Native: Annals of Society of Tropical Medicine; 17: 130-131, March 20, 1937.
5. Schmitt, F. J.: Lithokelyphopedion: Case. Bull. of Belgian Society of Gynecology & Obstetrics, 28: 383-386, May, 1939.
6. Smith, Wm. P. & Bolton, J. P.: Lithopedion. International Clin., Vol. 3, Series 46, Sept., 1936.
7. Reeves, T. K., and Lipman, G. S.: Lithopedion. Report of Case and Review of Literature. Penn. Medical Journal, 1548-1549, Sept., 1941.

Early Diagnosis of Tuberculosis[*]

THOMAS C. BLACK, M.D.[**]

CLINTON, OKLAHOMA

The National Tuberculosis Association, the parent organization of all tuberculosis workers, has had as it's slogan for many years the early diagnosis of tuberculosis. While there has been a marked reduction in the mortality rate in tuberculosis in the United States, the fact remains—tuberculosis is still the leading cause of death in the age group, 21-45.

In Oklahoma there are over 1,100 deaths annually from tuberculosis. Despite the splendid work that has been done and the progress that has been made, it is essential that we have a clear understanding of the problem in order to find early tuberculosis. This is especially pertinent at this time while we are all concentrating on the war effort and paying less attention to public health matters. It is a well established fact that during war time mortality rates increase, and very likely present conditions will prove to be no exception.

In 1938, 11 per cent of the patients admitted to the Western Oklahoma Tuberculosis Sanatorium had minimal disease, and 57 per cent had far advanced disease. These figures

have since gradually changed until in 1941-42 only 5 per cent of the patients admitted had minimal disease, and 76 per cent had far advanced disease. Therefore, during this four year period there has been a decrease in the cases admitted with early tuberculosis, and an increase in patients admitted with far advanced disease. This situation usually results from the amount of money available and effort spent in case finding. It is to be hoped that the next few years will see a reversal of this trend with the discovery and subsequent admission to the Sanatorium of a larger percentage of patients with early tuberculosis. Therefore, the purpose of this paper is to call attention to the necessity of finding early tuberculosis in order to better cope with this problem.

Because of the insidious onset of tuberculosis, the average individual does not present himself to his physician until symptoms are fairly well established. In the very earliest stage of the disease, tuberculosis produces no symptoms and can only be diagnosed by a chest x-ray. Later as the disease spreads and becomes more extensive, symptoms make their appearance.

Fatigue is one of the earliest symptoms. The individual finds that work he has been doing regularly tires him when it formerly

*Read before the Custer County Medical Society, Jan. 19, 1943.
**Superintendent and Medical Director Western Oklahoma Tuberculosis Sanatorium.

did not. The tired feeling is out of proportion to the amount of work done. Indigestion or a gastro-intestinal disturbance is often an early symptom. The so called nervous indigestion may be secondary to pulmonary tuberculosis. The tuberculous patient frequently becomes very nervous and irritable. Because of the extreme nervousness present in tuberculosis, a diagnosis of nervous breakdown often has been made previously. Any individual who has had a nervous breakdown should be thoroughly examined with the possibility of tuberculosis kept in mind. Loss of appetite in an individual with a previously normal healthy appetite and the resultant gradual loss of weight should certainly be investigated. Indifference to food is quite often a symptom of early tuberculosis. Loss of appetite and loss of weight should be explained before tuberculosis is eliminated.

Cough is one of the most frequent symptoms of tuberculosis. At first it may be a clearing of the throat or occasionally described as a cigarette cough; later it may become more pronounced and productive causing the patient to raise sputum. Usually cough is not an early symptom unless it follows an acute respiratory condition. Quite often tuberculosis will be in advanced condition by the time a cough is well developed. Any patient with a cough that continues for three or four weeks after an acute cold is supposed to be over should be examined for tuberculosis.

Pleurisy should be considered as a warning of tuberculosis. In approximately 85 per cent of patients with pleurisy, tuberculosis can be demonstrated as the underlying cause. Therefore, any individual with pleurisy should be investigated from the tuberculosis standpoint. In a very few patients pleurisy with effusion is one of the earliest symptoms causing pain, fever and shortness of breath. Fortunately for them, these symptoms suggest a chest examination, and as a result their disease may be diagnosed in an early stage.

Hemorrhage, or blood spitting or hemoptysis as it is more technically called, is occasionally the first symptom that makes its appearance in an apparently healthy person and should suggest tuberculosis. Of course, all patients with tuberculosis do not cough up blood, but any bleeding of a teaspoonful or more from the lung should be considered as due to tuberculosis until proven otherwise.

Rectal fistula is very often of a tuberculous nature. Any individual with this condition, or one who has had this condition, should have a very careful chest examination.

Fever or an afternoon elevation of temperature is frequently present in the tuberculous individual. Therefore, it would be perfectly logical to consider the possibility of tuberculosis in anyone having a chronic elevation of temperature.

An individual who gives a history of frequent chest colds or so called "Flu," or one presenting any one or more of the above symptoms, should be examined for tuberculosis. This is especially true if the individual has had exposure to tuberculosis in the family or among friends. Patients complaining of cough, sputum, fever, hemorrhage, loss of weight, strength and appetite will in the great majority of instances have advanced tuberculosis with it's unfavorable prognosis. If these individuals could have had a diagnosis made in the early stages of their disease the period of treatment would have been materially shortened and the prospects of complete recovery materially improved. If we are to find early tuberculosis, therefore, we must confine ourselves to case finding among apparently healthy individuals. Several methods of doing this are at our disposal.

Tuberculin testing of selected groups is perhaps best known. For some years testing of large groups of school children has been carried out, resulting in the decision that this procedure has considerable educational value, but yields few cases in comparison with selected adult groups. For this reason tuberculin testing of groups of school children has largely been discontinued.

Case findings among contacts and suspects is also well known. Annual chest films of all individuals known to have had contact with an open case of tuberculosis is recommended for several years after the contact has been broken. This group probably yields the greatest number of new cases. This contact group includes relatives and close friends of the patient, as well as others associated with him at work or school. Experience has shown that many cases of early tuberculosis are found upon routine tuberculin testing and subsequent annual roentgen ray examination of all positive reactors among college students. Soper of Yale has shown that the yield is much greater among the older college students.

The chest x-ray is the most important diagnostic method for finding early tuberculosis. If the cost could be materially reduced to permit routine x-raying of the entire population, we could soon materially increase the number of cases of early tuberculosis discovered. This would permit x-raying of the general public especially between the ages of 15-35 with or without a preceeding tuberculin test and irrespective of the presence or absence of symptoms or physical signs. This would especially apply to athletes and those people who continue to work regularly to a mild degree of exhaustion either mental or physical.

It is necessary, in order that early tuberculosis may be discovered, that the services of a roentgenologist be available for those who can and those who cannot pay. This service should be provided by the public health department in cooperation with the local medical societies.

Another common method of case finding, but less widely known in some sections and one that in some sections of our country is the main procedure in use at present, is the fluorograph. This 35 mm. film, made of the fluoroscopic image, is made by · equipment easily transported. It is quite possible to take 400-500 films per day by this method by having the selected group at a specified time and location. By routine checking not only all contacts and suspects, but certain occupational groups in their entirety, we are able to detect many cases of early tuberculosis. These groups may be divided into (1) food handlers, including cooks, waiters, and grocers, (2) barbers and beauty operators (3) school personnel, including lunch room workers, teachers, and janitors (4) women following delivery (5) industrial workers of various occupations, to name only a few.

Unless we are more aggressive in our efforts to find the early cases of tuberculosis, we will never reduce the number of patients with advanced tuberculosis entering our sanatoria. The methods at our disposal should warrant an increased tuberculosis budget compared with that available in the past for case finding purposes. We must place great stress on finding early tuberculosis because early discovery plus early treatment means early recovery.

Intestinal "Decompression" . . . A Review of Methods

A. S. RISSER, M.D., F.A.C.S.

BLACKWELL, OKLAHOMA

In spite of the great advance which has been made in our knowledge of surgical diagnosis, surgical pathology and operative technique, obstruction of the intestine remains one of our most serious and harassing problems. The high mortality and morbidity of intestinal obstruction has not been lowered in comparison with surgical progress in other serious conditions. Enterostomy, once advocated as a universal panacea, has frequently failed to give the relief desired. Hence, the forward looking surgeon is ever searching for newer and better means of combatting the dangerous complications resulting from mechanical obstruction of the bowel and from other forms of intestinal incompetence. Intestinal intubation combined with suction has recently shown a wide field of usefulness in many abdominal conditions. Hence, it seems worth while to review briefly the advantages of non-surgical decompression; to note its possible application in diagnosis in pre and post-operative treatment, and as a valuable adjunct to surgical treatment.

This paper will not be concerned greatly with controversial subjects — such, for instance, as the nature or exact method of production of the toxins and resultant toxemia, which in severe intestinal obstruction are found in the gut lumen, nor the cause of the characteristic local tissue changes and systemic blood alterations which occur in protracted obstruction. For our purpose it is sufficient to know that such changes do occur and that they must be recognized early and combatted promptly in order to conserve health and life. Briefly, these changes are a decrease in the chloride content of the blood, a rise in the carbon dioxide combining power of the plasma (causing alkalosis), and in protracted obstruction, an increase of the non-protein nitrogen in the blood. These changes are frequently spoken of as a loss of the electrolytes of the body. How serious these blood and tissue changes are which result from intestinal incompetence may be seen by a reference to the mortality from intestinal obstruction. Treves, in his book on Intestinal Obstruction published in 1884, page 461, gave the mortality as from 60-70 per cent. Miller, T. G. and W. A. Abbott, Am. J. Med. Sc. 187: 895-899, May 1934, gave the mortality in 1929 as 61 per cent. McIver (Monroe A. Arch. Surg. 25-1098-1134, 1932) estimated the mortality as 44 per cent.

In face of conditions so frequently fatal, it is only natural that surgeons have been diligently seeking means and methods of overcoming the dangers incident to intestinal obstruction. The various means employed form an interesting and enlightening, not to say encouraging, chapter in the history of surgical research and progress. The multiplicity of drugs and instruments which have been fashioned, tried and discarded, would furnish a small museum. It is the surgeon's instinct that having tried and found efficient a certain method, he should advocate that proceeding which is capable of enlarging our diagnostic skill and our surgical and therapeutic efficacy, especially as it is more generally appreciated, and its indications and contraindications are understood. So this paper aims to review briefly the methods of gastric and intestinal "decompression."

It is in order to make a brief summary of the local pathological processes instituted in the bowel by obstruction. Thus we may understand the possible seriousness of the conditions and the factors necessary to combat them. There is time in a brief paper for only an outline, but the main facts are these: Acute obstruction of the small intestine leads quickly to the establishment of a vicious circle which is dependent upon or related to the distention of the bowel and to the influence of the distention (per se) in causing altered intestinal motility and absorptive power. The first result of mechanical obstruction is perhaps accelerated secretion and accumulation of the normal gas and fluids within the lumen, and consequent distention of the intestine. There is evidence that in severe cases the normal gas content is increased by fermentation within the bowel, and perhaps by swallowed air (aerophagia). Thus, since nitrogen is only very slowly absorbed by the gut wall, the consequent dilation is increased and prolonged. The distention of the gut results in abnormal stretching and pressure upon the blood and lymph vessels of the bowel wall, and the disturbances of the blood and lymph circulation causes an increased secretion of plasma-like but very toxic fluid into the bowel and a greatly lessened absorption from the gut lumen. On farther dilation of the intestine with gas and fluids, the vessels within the bowel wall become still further stretched and compressed, the veins with their thinner walls first yielding to the pressure, the arteries somewhat later. Thus, the blood supply of the gut wall (both arterial and venous) is still further compromised; absorption is prevented; the stretching and fatigue of the intestinal muscle results in intestinal (muscular) paralysis; complete vascular occlusion may result, with anoxemia of the bowel; hemorrhagic infarcts may form; the intestinal wall becomes oedematous and friable, necrosis may ensue, first in the submucosa and inner muscular coat, later in the outer. Ulceration and perforation may finally result, even gangrene of a segment of the gut.

Added to the systemic intoxication, this is a serious condition in any abdomen. Small wonder that surgeons from the earliest beginnings of the science have been seeking for a means of prevention and cure of these daugerous conditions. Of the various means and methods employed it can be said their name is legion. Time is not sufficient to discuss them. Spinal anesthesia has been advocated and used, but to the writer it seems a dangerous remedy, particularly in the presence of great abdominal distention and the frequent accompanying respiratory and cardiac embarrassment. Pituitrin, Pitressin and Prostigmine have their advocates, but the wrtier is tempted to say their general use is mentioned only to be condemned. Morphine in large doses is generally credited with being an intestinal stimulant, but this drug also should be employed intelligently, and its sedative effect should not be permitted to mask the symptoms and true status of the patient.

Enterostomy has for years been employed as an emergency measure when the patient's condition did not warrant a complete or prolonged operation. It can be done under local anesthesia with no added risk. Ideally the opening should be made in the distended loop of the gut just proximal to the obstruction, but technically there are frequently many difficulties. Often the exact site of the obstruction can not be known—and there may be multiple sites of obstruction— as in paralytic ileus which may have become in effect real obstruction because of adhesions of angulated and distended loops of gut. Because of the fact that a single enterostomy so frequently fails to afford adequate drainage, multiple enterostomies have been advocated and employed, but here again the added trauma of handling already damaged intestine, the added operative time, and the increased danger of peritoneal soiling and peritonitis are factors which make many surgeons unwilling to accept this as a routine procedure.

The presence of air or gas with the fluid in the distended bowel, particularly if the intestinal muscle has become paretic, is prone to cause "air lock," and so make enterostomy of no avail. This fact has led some surgeons to combine "stripping" or milking of the intestinal contents out of the distended gut during the performance of the enterostomy. Unfortunately, common surgical experience indicates, and scientific observers have proved, that such manipulation is accompanied by very definite undesirable and damaging effects. It would seem inevitable that the manipulation of an already overdistended gut, with intramural strangulation of the circulation and tissues friable in consequence, would cause still further tissue damage and absorption of toxins. Furthermore, it has been definitely proven by competent experimenters that the process of "stripping" in itself may cause a fall in blood pressure and produce true surgical shock. Moreover, the intestine so treated showed a lowered absorption rate, and a lowered peristaltic activity for as long as twenty-four hours after such manipulation. The experimenters concluded, in view of these undesirable effects and the increased danger of peritonitis, that stripping is dangerous, and should not be performed except when evacuation is necessary to permit replacement of the small intestine and closure of the abdomen, or to prevent kinks of "water hose" type.

Cecostomy and appendicostomy have often been utilized to secure decompression. Neither operation is of avail in high obstruction. Both can readily be done under local anesthesia. Appendicostomy has the advantage that in chronic obstruction the opening can be progressively enlarged by inserting drain tubes of increasing calibre, so that ultimately it may serve as practically an artificial anus.

The stomach tube as invented probably by John Hunter was for years our best non-surgical method of abdominal decompression. Frequent gastric lavage was of value in emptying the stomach of accumulated gas and liquids and so tending to reduce the general abdominal tension.

When in 1921, almost a hundred years after the invention of the stomach tube, Levine described the duodenal tube, which could be introduced through the nose, it was recognized that we had a new and more efficient instrument for securing abdominal decom-

pression, so that now the duodenal tube is as much a part of the progressive physician's armamentarium as the sphygmomanometer and the stethoscope. Since some twenty-five years ago Westerman and Karpis advocated its use for the relief of the distention resulting from peritonitis, the general employment of the duodenal tube dates back only about seven years, and increased employment has greatly widened its field of usefulness.

Its application requires not too much skill. The well lubricated tube is passed through the more roomy side of the nose — (Only rarely is local anesthesia required) and to the depth sufficient to extend well into the duodenum. The tube is then connected to the suction apparatus and a competent nurse continued in charge.

Recently the principle of this method has been greatly extended by the invention of the ingenious Miller-Abbott double lumen intestinal tube. By means of this tube, intelligently and skillfully employed, any part of the intestinal tract, including even the large bowel, may be subjected to continuous drainage and decompression. The aim is to introduce the tube into the intestine to such a depth that the opening lies just above the point of obstruction in the gut, after which continuous suction can be maintained to secure decompression.

Also, if operation is not urgent, by means of the Miller-Abbott tube, barium suspension may be introduced for the purpose of diagnostic X-ray study, after which the barium can be siphoned off. Without this means of removal, the giving of barium to patients suspected of having obstruction of the small bowel is not without danger, nor often diagnostically efficient.

The technique of employment of the Miller-Abbott tube is not always without difficulty, and its proper application may be time-consuming (but to a good purpose). Vomiting, reverse peristalsis, extreme dilatation of the stomach, or pylorospasm may interfere with its passage, especially in advanced cases of intestinal obstruction, but time and patience usually overcome these difficulties. The well-lubricated tube with the bulb deflated is swallowed by the patient, for whom the right lateral position is recommended. It usually requires some six hours for the bulb to reach the third portion of the duodenum. The bulb is then inflated with air, or some 30 cubic centimeters of an 8 per cent sodium iodide solution may be used, for aid in X-ray studies. In favorable cases peristaltic action carries the tube further into the bowel, some 5 ccs every ten minutes, though not always "according to schedule," so that in many cases intelligent cooperation on the part of surgeon, house officer and nurses can subject any part of the intestinal tract to drainage and decompression. It gives to date the most efficient means of removing excess intestinal fluid and gas from the distended bowel, thus improving the circulation of the bowel wall and relieving the heart and lungs embarrassed by the abdominal distension. Vomiting may be relieved and thereby much needed rest for the patient obtained.

By means of the tube we can provide food and fluids as indicated. Both intake and output of fluids can be measured, so that we have an added check on the condition and progress of the patient. In many recorded cases the relief of the distention by this means alone has been sufficient to cause return of peristaltic action and ultimate relief without operation.

However, and this is to be emphasized, the contraindications for non-surgical treatment must be understood and recognized, else a method which promises to satisfy a greatly enlarged field of usefulness may be brought into disrepute. Before relying on tube decompression alone we must exclude total mechanical obstruction. First, and perhaps most easily recognized of the contraindications, are strangulated external hernias. To treat such conditions conservatively is to confess ignorance of the most primary surgical principles. Exception might be made of mesenteric embolism and thrombosis, but these are comparatively rare and are usually fatal regardless of the treatment instituted.

More difficult to diagnose, and hence the more important to determine, are cases of internal hernia, volvulus and intussusception. Small Richter's hernias are rather common, and should not be overlooked. The importance of early recognition and proper treatment of these dangerous conditions has been stressed by McIver (Arch. Surg. 25: 198, 1932) quoted by Johnston (C. G. Johnston: J. Michigan State Med. Soc. 37: 623 July 1938) in a group of cases reported by him: Intussusception, volvulus, internal hernia, inflamed Meckel's diverticulum, and rare congenital anomalies formed only 11.1 per cent of the total number of cases, or 19.1 per cent of all the cases except external hernia, and the mortality in this group (except external hernia) was 44 per cent. Such figures make an eloquent appeal to utilize early surgery in cases where strangulation of the gut is suspected, where there is evidence of complete mechanical closure of the gut lumen, and in obstruction of the colon, for in this portion of the intestinal tract malignancy is usually the cause of the obstruction.

If indications for immediate operation are not present, if the contraindications as outlined are understood and none of them are in evidence, tube suction may be used for purposes of diagnosis, preoperative treatment, post operative treatment, or therapeutically, not only in frank surgical conditions but in such cases of marked distention occasionally encountered in severe pneumonia, uremia, severe accidental wounds and crushing injuries of chest or abdomen, and certain fractures. In paralytic ileus or peritonitis, intubation and suction provide relief of the gastric and intestinal distention which in itself may threaten life. As glucose intravenously seems to stimulate peristalsis, it should be given (perhaps best with normal saline solution) as the individual patient requires. Since one of the dangerous results of intestinal incompetence is the marked dehydration and loss of electrolytes of the body, these substances must be replaced. This may be done hypodermically, by means of the Levine or Miller-Abbott tube, or intravenously, and it is suggested that a total of at least 3,000 cc. of fluid be given in the 24 hours. The glucose should total at least 100 grams. Care should be exercised as to the amounts of glucose and salt given. Hyperglycemia and hyperchloremia are both harmful, but they can be avoided by careful observation of the patient and the use of the proper laboratory tests. We must not be deceived by temporary signs of improvement which often follow decompression and the administration of intravenous fluids. Apparent improvement may occur even with impending gangrene of the gut.

We need to remember that the mortality of obstructive and perforative lesions increases tremendously with delay (just as in perforated peptic ulcer), and not allow signs of temporary improvement to camouflage an underlying frank obstruction or acute inflammatory process or a perforative lesion.

In the treatment of intestinal incompetence we have the choice of the various methods of decompression mentioned. Their advantages and disadvantages, the indications and contraindications for their employment must be kept in mind. Of all the non-surgical methods available, continuous intestinal suction with the Miller-Abbott tube has most successfully reduced the mortality in this dangerous condition. Hence, the extended employment of this method is recommended.

Special Article

The Doctor of Medicine and His Responsibility*

ALFRED W. ADSON, M.D.
ROCHESTER, MINNESOTA

Members of the North Central Medical Conference, representing the states of North Dakota, South Dakota, Minnesota, Wisconsin, Nebraska, and Iowa, have entrusted me with the responsibility of addressing this National Conference on Medical Service concerning medical problems that are of both local and national interest.

It is the duty of every doctor of medicine to prevent illness, to supply adequate medical care to those who are ill, to perpetuate the science of medicine and to encourage medical investigation. It is true that the average physician would prefer to go unregimented among his sick and administer to their needs, irrespective of race, color, creed, or financial status, rather than busy himself with administrative and political problems. However, since the courts have ruled that group health is a business and have found that medical societies are guilty of restraining trade when attempting to maintain the standards of the practice of medicine, a challenge has been issued to the medical profession: Is there a necessity for lay groups and the Federal Government to take over the control of the practice of medicine.

Has the Science of medicine reached its zenith? Have the men and women of medicine become so decadent that they are unable to assume their responsibilities? Are the doctors of medicine no longer able to conduct their practice without government control? Do they lack ability to appreciate their problems? Or are they incapable of constructive leadership in the solution of the numerous responsibilities that are confronting the medical profession today? The reply is, "No."

The science of medicine has been nurtured by men and women who have advanced the knowledge of relieving pain, correcting deformities, lowering infant mortality, prolonging life and preventing illness by sanitary and public health measures. This progress must continue if civilization is to survive.

The medical profession is conscious of social and economic changes and stands ready to cooperate with, and offer leadership to, state and federal agencies in the solution of medical problems. It further believes that better medical service can be rendered by offering advice and leadership to welfare agencies than by serving as a tool under political bureaus.

The medical profession recognizes the necessity of state and federal control of communicable diseases and medical services to inmates of state and federal institutions. It appreciates its responsibility to the Armed Forces and expects to supply the needed personnel. It is willing to cooperate with welfare agencies in providing adequate medical care for the low income and indigent groups of the population; but in providing this care, it believes that the medical service is augmented when the patient-physician relationship can be maintained by permitting the patient, whenever possible, to choose his own physician. In order to protect the public from

worthless, so-called medical procedures and unnecessary operations by unscrupulous individuals, it likewise believes that high standards of medical education and practice must be maintained. This applies not only to the practice of medicine in the office; it applies to the practice of medicine in the humble home or in the most modern hospital.

Although medical education begins in the medical school, it is never completed as long as the physician continues his practice. Medical schools have adopted standards of education and have required certain courses of study in order that the public might avail itself of the best practices of medicine. Medical licensing boards have further protected the public by requiring of their candidates for licensure prescribed courses of study. State laws governing the practice of medicine and conduct of physicians further protect the public from irregular practices and charlatans.

Medical societies, county, state, and national, have been organized to further the education of the physician by acquainting him with the advances and new discoveries in the science of medicine. They likewise serve as administrative units in the consideration and solution of medical problems. It is obvious that the responsibilities of the respective state organizations are greater than those of the county organizations, and that the national organization is charged with greater responsibilities than those of the state organizations. However, it is also obvious that the activities of all groups must be integrated if medical problems are to be solved effectively. In some states, such as Minnesota, the administrative and the legislative bodies have the confidence of the medical profession. Likewise the medical profession has the confidence of the state administrative and legislative bodies. This confidence has made it possible for representatives of both groups to attack and solve the medical problems which are of mutual interest.

The national organization, through its respective bodies and committees, has conducted an excellent program in furthering medical education. It has crystallized the standards of medical education for the medical student as well as for the practitioner of medicine; it has investigated the claims of new and nonofficial remedies, foods and therapeutic measures and has further protected the public by approval or disapproval of the articles investigated. It has taken active steps through its Procurement and Assignment Committee in providing medical men for the Armed Forces without robbing communities of adequate medical personnel and has made provisions for relocation of physicians where more medical service is needed. It has acquainted the public with the important role that the science of medicine plays in their daily lives, but apparently it has not gained the confidence of the national administrative and legislative bodies that some of the state medical societies have attained. The National Physicians' Committee has made some progress in acquainting the public with the necessity of medical science, but it too had

*Read at the meeting of the National Conference on Medical Service, February 14, 1943.

not obtained the confidence of the national administrative and legislative branches of our Government. Therefore, the recent court decision has emphasized the weakness of conducting a program of education to acquaint the public, the administrative and legislative bodies of certain states, and the national institutions with the important function of the science of medicine in our civilization. It is our duty, as physicians and citizens, to assure those in administrative positions and legislative bodies that we are familiar with the social and economic changes that have thrown greater responsibilities on the medical profession and that we stand ready to cooperate with these agencies in offering leadership in the solution of the numerous problems which nonmedical personnel are trying to solve.

The chief medical problem that concerns doctors of medicine and welfare agencies is that of providing adequate medical care to those who are financially unable to procure this care. This group includes those who are indigent and those with low incomes. Medical care, in its true sense, embraces more than emergency treatment for a particular illness, since it should include a rehabilitation program, such as the correction of deformities and ailments that impair the efficiency of individuals. The rehabilitation program also should include adequate and proper diets, physical training, recreation, protective clothing and housing. In most of the cities the indigent are provided with proper medical care through the charity hospitals, where competent physicians give of their services. This same group in the rural districts is not always so fortunate, since local welfare boards are reluctant to provide this care. It is in these situations that the physicians have been overburdened in assuming all of the responsibilities in providing the necessary medical care. Prior to the more recent economic changes, physicians were willing to assume this obligation because those who could afford to pay for professional services attempted to meet their obligations. However, as a result of the recent social and economic changes, the Government has taken over more and more control of the civilian's activities, and those with moderate and low incomes have been less willing to assume their obligations of medical care and are insisting that it is the Government's duty to provide medical care and that it is the individual's privilege to squander his extra change.

The problems of this group cannot be solved by physicians alone or by federal, state, and local welfare agencies alone. Ours is a joint responsibility. Conscientious leadership by physicians working in cooperation with county, state and federal agencies can and will bring forth a solution of the problem. Medical service must be rendered, and the physician is willing to give a good portion of his services. But the Government must provide reasonable funds for the care of its indigent, as it must provide for catastrophic illness in the low income group. Nevertheless, those who come within the low income group should likewise be made to realize that they too owe a responsibility to their local, state and federal governments and should be encouraged and advised in budgeting their income and expense.

Industrial compensation has accomplished much in providing proper medical care and the necessities of life, during illness, for those employed in industrial institutions. However, there still remain a large group of individuals who receive moderate or low incomes and are desirous of securing the assurance of adequate medical service in the event of illness. Insurance companies have offered this protection through policies covering accident and illness disabilities, but again this protection only partially solves the problem, since many an insuree expects more for his premium than the insurer is able to give. In several states medical societies have attempted to develop medical service plans whereby the insuree may purchase from the doctors within the group full medical protection or medical protection for unexpected, serious illnesses. In some states under the

farm security program, experimental medical service plans are being tested out by use in an attempt to find the solution of the problem of supplying medical care to the farmers and their families who are being rehabilitated. In some instances physicians are hired to render medical service to indigent and cooperative groups. Even though physicians, welfare agencies and low income groups are struggling with the problems of medical service plans, as yet a satisfactory plan for all classes has not been developed. The recipients expect more than the vendors can supply for the premiums paid.

These controversies give rise to discussions on the necessity of compulsory medical insurance. Should such a program evolve, results would be disappointing from the patient's as well as the physician's points of view if placed under the control of political bureaus, and the patient would be deprived of his free choice of physician.

Therefore, we as physicians believe that a more equitable solution of the perplexing medical problems referred to will be reached if we are permitted to consult and advise administrative officials, legislative bodies, and welfare agencies, since we are more familiar with the medical needs of our respective communities than are those who have a casual knowledge of the medical necessities.

It is befitting to quote the statement found in the opinion written by Justice Miller, of the United States Court of Appeals, of the District of Columbia, in the case of the United States of America versus the American Medical Association, and the case of the United States of America versus the Medical society of the District of Columbia. The italics are mine.

"It may be regrettable that Congress chose to take over in the Sherman Act the common law concept of trade, at least to the extent of including therein the practice of medicine. Developments which have taken place during recent decades in the building up of standards of professional education and licensure, together with self-imposed standards of discipline and professional ethics, have, in the belief of many persons, resulted in substantial differences between professional practices and the generally accepted methods of trade and business. As we pointed out in our earlier decision, the American Medical Association and other local medical associations have undoubtedly made a profound contribution to this development. *However, our task is not to legislate or declare policy in such matters, but rather, to interpret and apply standards and policies which have been declared by the legislature. That Congress was not otherwise advised was perhaps because of the failure of the professional groups to insist upon the distinction and to secure its legislative recognition.*"

Does the medical profession of this country need a stronger invitation, or a more direct challenge to take an intelligent, helpful and fair stand in the enactment of legislation that not only concerns the public welfare but the welfare of medicine itself? Does not the medical profession of this country, as citizens and tax payers, have a right to express its opinion in these matters before legislation is enacted and rules and regulations adopted by some bureau? I do not share the opinion that the time for the medical profession to speak up is after such things have taken place. Neither do I have the opinion that Congress would be resentful of intelligent, courageous and fair advice on such matters. What better proof can be asked than the quotation from Justice Miller's opinion that the Court is not responsible for the absence of advice from the medical profession when Congress is drafting a law.

It is not the purpose of this paper to criticize the efforts of our national medical organization nor to criticize the efforts of the National Physicians' Committee, but it is the desire of the members of the North Central Medical Conference to express a wish that a more active program be conducted to acquaint the public, government officials, and legislative bodies with the necessity of medical science and the important role it plays in our civilization. It is essential that we as physicians dispel the fear that government administrative agencies and legislative bodies have of our medical organizations and that they be assured of our cooperation in solving the social and economic problems that confront us as a nation.

The functions of acquainting the public on matters of medical interest, assisting bureau in formulating plans on medical care and offering constructive advice on proposed medical legislation rightfully belong to the national organization known as the American Medical Association. They could be assigned to the National Physicians' Committee, or they might even be undertaken by unifying the activities of the various state committees on public policy and legislation. Representative committees could be appointed for each of the component societies, county, state, and national. These could all be so integrated that national opinion and advice could be obtained and made available for committee hearings on legislation within a few hours' time. Through the national, state, and county committees the entire profession could be informed of proposed medical legislation. Thus, the local constituents of the respective state and federal legislators could express their views before legislation is enacted. Some states already have medical advisory committees from each county. They also have state medical committees on public policy with a physician as part-time executive chairman assisted by legal counsel. A national committee constructed on the same plan as these state committees would have to be created. A physician who has practised medicine should be chosen as the executive chairman. Both he and his legal counsel would need to be stationed in our national capital. The expense of the national committee on public policy could be financed by one of three agencies, the American Medical Association, the National Physicians' Committee, or the respective state organizations bearing the expense jointly. It would appear more equitable if each physician would be assessed each year for the specific purpose of maintaining a national committee on public policy and legislation.

Our problems are not unlike those of dentists and hospital associations. Therefore, unified effort of medical, dental and hospital associations should further the welfare of the patient.

Dividens in Man Power

A very considerable part of our fighting and productive force is the direct result of reduced mortality since the beginning of the century; and this in turn is to be credited to our organized public health effort and the remarkable advances of medical science in past decades. This effort has saved millions of babies, children, and young adults, so that now the numbers available for the fighting forces to defend the country, and for production in factory and field, are much larger than would have been possible under health conditions prevailing among us 40 years ago.

To obtain a numerical measure of what the improvement in our health conditions means in terms of man power, an estimate was made of the number of men of draft age present among us today, who owe their existence to the improvement in mortality since the beginning of the century. Taking into account on the one hand the survival rates which actually operated in the intervening years, and on the other the survival rates that prevailed at the beginning of the century (when men now 40 years old were born) it is found that 11 percent of men between the ages of 20 and 44 are among us simply because of improvement in mortality experienced since 1900.—Statistical Bulletin, Metropolitan Life Insurance Company.

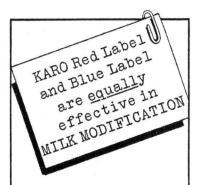
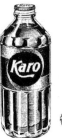

· THE PRESIDENT'S PAGE ·

Physicians thrive on excitement and hard work. An epidemic is something to groan about, but to work at very cheerfully. In leisure time, in happier days, the doctor sought relaxation in more excitement—hunting, fishing and golfing. There is less time for these diversions now, and much hope for America when a good citizen discourses on his vegetable garden instead of his golf score.

Reading in bed can be exciting, and better for the next day's work than barbiturates. Try Trueta's "Treatment of War Wounds and Fractures," a small book which will keep you awake all night, and haunt your days. The "smelly little Spanish Doctor's" work is as stimulating as Sherlock Holmes.

Also put on your bedside table "Miracles of Military Medicine" by Albert O. Maisel. Written in popular style, it tells of the triumphs of modern military medicine in a most interesting way—a very helpful book to those of you who give radio talks, or otherwise address lay audiences, as most of you should.

A third must is "Tuberculosis and Genius" by L. J. Moorman. Too few of us recognize that we have a great classical scholar in our midst. The editorials of your State Journal—for their variety of thought, the beauty and simplicity of the language used, are unequalled by those of any journal in the United States.

Sincerely yours,

James Stevenson

President.

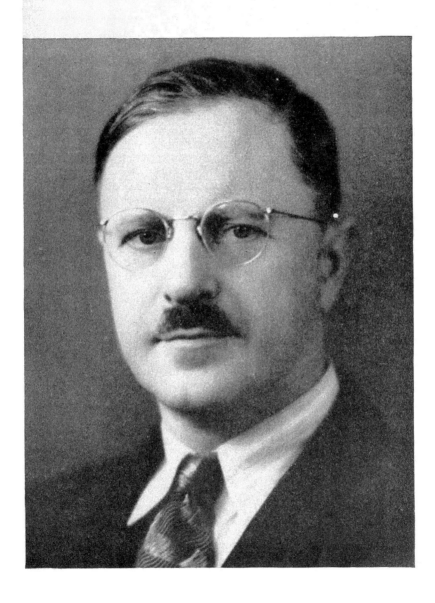

The JOURNAL Of The
OKLAHOMA STATE MEDICAL ASSOCIATION

EDITORIAL BOARD
L. J. MOORMAN, Oklahoma City, Editor-in-Chief

E. EUGENE RICE, Shawnee

NED R. SMITH, Tulsa

MR. R. H. GRAHAM, Oklahoma City, Business Manager

CONTRIBUTIONS: Articles accepted by this Journal for publication including those read at the annual meetings of the State Association are the sole property of this Journal.

The Editorial Department is not responsible for the opinions expressed in the original articles of contributors.

Manuscripts may be withdrawn by authors for publication elsewhere only upon the approval of the Editorial Board.

MANUSCRIPTS: Manuscripts should be typewritten, double-spaced, on white paper 8½ x 11 inches. The original copy, not the carbon copy, should be submitted.

Footnotes, bibliographies and legends for cuts should be typed on separate sheets in double space. Bibliography listing should follow this order: Name of author, title of article, name of periodical with volume, page and date of publication.

Manuscripts are accepted subject to the usual editorial revisions and with the understanding that they have not been published elsewhere.

NEWS: Local news of interest to the medical profession, changes of address, births, deaths and weddings will be gratefully received.

ADVERTISING: Advertising of articles, drugs or compounds unapproved by the Council on Pharmacy of the A.M.A. will not be accepted. Advertising rates will be supplied on application.

It is suggested that members of the State Association patronize our advertisers in preference to others.

SUBSCRIPTIONS: Failure to receive The Journal should call for immediate notification.

REPRINTS: Reprints of original articles will be supplied at actual cost provided request for them is attached to manuscripts or made in sufficient time before publication. Checks for reprints should be made payable to Industrial Printing Company, Oklahoma City.

Address all communications to THE JOURNAL OF THE OKLAHOMA STATE MEDICAL ASSOCIATION, 210 Plaza Court, Oklahoma City.

OFFICIAL PUBLICATION OF THE OKLAHOMA STATE MEDICAL ASSOCIATION
Copyrighted May, 1943

EDITORIALS

EQUALITY, LIFE, LIBERTY AND THE PURSUIT OF HAPPINESS

1. All Men Created Equal: Of all the professions, groups and agencies in this country, it is doubtful if any can match medicine in the interpretation of the term "created equal" when applied to the art of living. It is eminently our business to speculate upon the creative forces and to come as close to the secrets of life as science will permit. Granting a comparable environment, we agree that in the light available to the majority of the signers of the Declaration of Independence, all men are created equal. But we now know better than ever before that life (personality constitution)is composed of two sets of factors, the hereditary and the environmental, and that the influence of environment depends upon the character and quality of the transmitted genes.

In spite of this knowledge, medicine insists that all people, regardless of rank, moral, religious, social, or economic position, are entitled to all that medicine can give whether in the slums or in palaces. Without regard to rank and with tolerance for all, medicine takes broken bodies and strives to mend them, with a little medicine for the soul thrown in. Many would lose their equal chance in time of need if it were not for medicine.

2. Life: Medicine has been evolved to meet the insistent needs of society since the first painful cry of primative man. It has grown to its present magnitude and efficiency with the sole purpose of helping to initiate the normal life and to foster and sustain the normal processes of the body while fending the individual and the community against disease and accident. The guidance of the expectant mother, the saving of life in infancy, and the fostering of health in childhood and adolescence, have achieved results which find expression throughout the life cycle, culminating in the mounting old age group. It now becomes medicine's function to fathom the causes of degenerative processes, and to stay their progress as far as possible in order that longevity may be increased with added comfort and efficiency.

Medicine has made invaluable contributions toward the security of life through the voluntary initiation of nearly all the fundamental principles upon which our public health organizations are based. What would life be worth without the service which has been provided by voluntary medicine?

3. Liberty: Without life and reasonable health, the word "liberty" would have little meaning. Yet how significant it is in the development of our American way of life. If it were not for liberty, the above mentioned achievements of American medicine would be of no purpose. Through this priceless attribute of our democratic government, voluntary medicine integrated with the voluntary response of a free people, has made the principles of liberty ever more desirable, and its blessings, when understood in the light of medicine, increasingly obvious. Rob medicine and the people of their liberty through any plan of regimented practice and the spirit which has made American medicine rise above that in any comparable nation will sicken under the lash of bureaucracy, pine for liberty and initiative, and die of inertia. If the guardians of liberty value the commendation of future generations, they had better deliver the people from the threat of socialized medicine.

4. The Pursuit of Happiness: Thank God! Our forefathers had the wisdom to vouchsafe to us the privilege of the pursuit of happiness, and not the annulling thought of the gift of happiness. Already, with unwonted paternalism, we have robbed a good section of our citizenry of the main sources of happiness by stultifying their spirit of self-expression and their desire for p h y s i c a l self-sufficiency. Paternalism, which requires no initiative and little or no physicial effort, gnaws at the vitals of conscience and preys upon character and self-respect. It will require generations of individual initiative and industry to live down the influence of these wounds.

Medicine understands human nature too well to approve such a dangerous remedy as wholesale paternalism, which at best can be only paliative. Happiness depends upon the normal initiation of life with equality of opportunity as conditioned by environment, and the liberty of personal freedom in the development of hereditary endowments under available conditions. If the chief aim of life is happiness, the chief aim of voluntary medicine is to make happiness possible through the preservation and stabilization of life.

Considering the common weal, we plead that American medicine may be permitted to continue its evolutionary development to meet the shifting needs of a changing world as provided by the Declaration of Independence.

THE CONTAGIOUSNESS OF PUERPERAL FEVER (CENTENNIAL)

The year 1943 is the centennial commemoration of one of the milestones in medical progress. To be more specific, it was 100 years ago that Dr. Oliver Wendall Holmes, through his essay on the contagiousness of puerperal fever, promulgated the idea that childbed fever was not the act of God, but due to the fact that his servants on earth had carried an infection from one patient to another.

In March, 1843, he discussed the subject in the Boston Society for Medical Improvement, and in April he published his essay in the New England Quarterly Journal of Medicine and Surgery. This journal had a very small circulation and quit publication the next year. The article was reprinted in 1850 with very little change, but with the following addenda: "This paper was written in a great heat and with passionate indignation. If I touched it at all, I might trim its rhetorical exuberance, but I prefer to leave it all its original strength of expression. I could not, if I had tried, have disguised the feelings with which I regarded the attempt to put out of sight the frightful facts which I brought forward and the necessary conclusions to which they led. Of course, the whole matter has been looked at in a new point of view since the microbe, as a vehicle of contagion, has been brought into light and explained the mechanism of that which was plain enough as a fact to all who were not blind or who did not shut their eyes." This paper had such a wealth of bibliography of a personal nature from doctors in this country, as well as in England and Europe, as to put to shame some of the articles appearing in our magazines at this present time. These facts were established in Holmes own mind without the question of a doubt as to the saneness of his thesis. The more positive knowledge we gain, the more we incline to question all that has been received without positive proof, and this philosophy of doubting has been the basis of all original thinking. In this manner alone has medicine attained its present high position.

Semmelweiss in 1853, a recent medical graduate, sustained his contention that the cause of puereral fever was conveyed by the examining finger of the doctor, the midwife's sponges, or, more rarely, by air.

Holmes deplored the teachings of the medical schools which did not hold his views: "Any violent impression on the instructor's mind is apt to be followed by some lasting effect on the pupil. No mother's mark is more permanent than the mental naevi and moles and excrescenses and mutilations that students carry with them out of the lecture rooms if once the teeming intellect, which nourishes theirs, has been scared from its propriety by any misshapen fantasy."

"The students naturally have faith in their instructors, turning to them for truth and taking what they may choose to give them; babes in knowledge, not yet able to tell the breast from the bottle, pumping away the milk of truth at all that offers, were it nothing better than a professor's shrivelled finger." Thus, Holmes keeps on with his trenchant pen against those professors who had opposed his teachings.

Not until 1867 did Lister give the world his essay, "On The Antiseptic Principles in the Practice of Surgery," and in 1879, Pasteur published his observations that the streptococcus was the organism causing puerperal fever. Thus, the basis for the prevention of puerperal infection was established.

It is said that Holmes never could become indifferent to the painful scenes of the sick room and, of course, when his friends and neighbors were the sufferers, he did not find his heart hardened. He later said he did not make any strenuous effort to obtain business, but that the best thing about practicing medicine was that he had to keep a horse and a chaise.

For two years he was Professor of Anatomy at Dartmouth, and then Professor of Anatomy at Harvard for 35 years, where he did not only have the Chair of Anatomy, but a settee covering other subjects. Holmes' interest in microscopy accompanied his anatomical research. He was a poet, an essayist, a lecturer and a humorist. The two former accomplishments would give him a place among the immortals.

We, as members of the medical profession, can be justly proud of Oliver Wendell Holmes. He practiced medicine for awhile, but that was not his forte. Hoimes studied under Louis in Paris after graduating from Harvard. His inspiration was quickened by the contact with this exceptional man who had influenced so many of our American students.—L.A.R.

FOR THE DURATION

Because of the war certain plans formulated by the Editorial Board for the improvement of the Journal have been impeded, and it has become necessary to defer changes and to accept limitations imposed by the exigencies of war. Our readers are reminded of the fact that the induction of so many of our wide awake young men into military service has materially reduced our scientific resources; that our limitations in quantity and quality of paper will continue to exert an unfavorable influence upon the size and appearance of the Journal; and that our dwindling income brings the inevitable inhibitions of economy.

In view of these handicaps, the members of the Editorial Board wish to urge those who write scientific papers to say clearly and succintly what they have to say in as few words as possible. Robert Louis Stevenson, who made a science of artistic writing, once said, "If there is any where a thing said in two sentences that could have been as clearly and as engagingly and forcefully said in one, then it is amateur work."

Finally, the members of the Board desire that you should know they are striving to maintain creditable scientific and editorial standards, and that they invite your cooperation, whether it be through constructive criticism or commendation.

What S. Weir Mitchell Thought of His Profession

"As a profession, it is my sincere conviction that in our adherence to a high code of moral law, and in the general honesty with which we do our work, no other small and large, negative and positive, are many and constant, and yet I am quite sure that no like group of men affords as few illustrations of grave moral weakness. It is commonplace to say that our lives are one long training in charity, self-abandonment, all forms of self-restraint. The doctor will smile at my thinking it needful to even state the fact. He begins among the poor; all his life, in or out of hospitals, he keeps touch of them always. He sells that which men can neither weigh nor measure, and this sets him over all professions, save one, and far above all forms of mere business. He is bound in honor to profit by no patent, to disclose all he has learned, and to give freely and without reward of his best care to all others of his profession whom may be sick. What such a life makes of a man is largely a question of original character, but in no other form of occupation is there such constant food useful to develop all that is best and noblest."—Doctor and Patient, Lippincott, 1887.

Minimum discomfort and
inconvenience to patients from . . .

SOLUTION LIVER EXTRACT
[PARENTERAL]
Lederle

BECAUSE OF ITS SMALL VOLUME, low concentration of solids and high concentration of anti-anemic substances, a minimum of discomfort and inconvenience to the patient may be expected from the administration of concentrated "Solution Liver Extract (Parenteral) *Lederle*," (15 U.S.P. Injectable Units per cc.).

For physicians who prefer to give fewer units of active material at more frequent intervals, there is "Refined Solution Liver Extract (Parenteral) *Lederle*," 5 U.S.P. Injectable Units per cc. and 10 U.S.P. Injectable Units per cc. In addition, there is "Solution Liver Extract (Parenteral) *Lederle*," 3.3 U.S.P. Injectable Units per cc. A palatable oral solution containing not less than 1 U.S.P. Oral Unit per 60 cc. is also available.

All Lederle's Liver extracts conform to the United States Pharmacopoeia Twelfth Revision. In the treatment of Pernicious Anemia with Liver Extract—

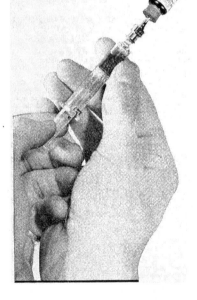

Specify *Lederle*

LIVER PRODUCTS *Lederle*

"CONCENTRATED SOLUTION LIVER EXTRACT (PARENTERAL) *Lederle*"
PACKAGES:
    3—1 cc. vials (15 U.S.P. Injectable Units each)
    1—10 cc. vial (150 U.S.P. Injectable Units each)

"REFINED SOLUTION LIVER EXTRACT (PARENTERAL) *Lederle*"
    1—10 cc. vial 5 U.S.P. Injectable Units per cc. (50 units)
    1—5 cc. vial 10 U.S.P. Injectable Units per cc. (50 units)
    1—10 cc. vial 10 U.S.P. Injectable Units per cc. (100 units)

"SOLUTION LIVER EXTRACT (PARENTERAL) *Lederle*"
    3—3 cc. vials (10 U.S.P. Injectable Units per vial)

"SOLUTION LIVER EXTRACT ORAL *Lederle*"
    8 fluid ounce bottle (4 U.S.P. oral units)
    1 pint (16 fluid ounce) bottle (8 U.S.P. oral units)

ASSOCIATION ACTIVITIES

FIFTY-FIRST ANNUAL MEETING WELL ATTENDED

FOUR HUNDRED NINETY-FIVE REGISTER

The Fifty-first Annual Meeting of the Association was unprecedented from the standpoint of attendance. With one-third of the state under water, and with 332 members in the armed forces, registration still bordered the 500 mark. Four hundred and ninety-five physicians registered.

Outstanding physicians appearing on the program included Frank H. Lahey, M.D., Boston, Massachusetts, Chairman of the Directing Board of the Procurement and Assignment Service; Colonel W. Lee Hart, Surgeon General of the Eighth Service Command; Captain Leslie B. Marshall, U. S. N., Commanding Officer Station Hospital, Norman; Colonel William H. Gordon, Executive Officer, Borden General Hospital, Chickasha; Commander Clyde M. Longstreth, Station Hospital, Norman; Harry Wilkins, M.D., Oklahoma City; and Forrest P. Baker, M.D., Talihina.

The Oklahoma County Medical Society was host at a buffet supper Tuesday night with Dr. Lahey as speaker, and the President's Inaugural Dinner Dance was held the following evening with Governor Robert S. Kerr, as speaker.

House of Delegates

The actions of the House of Delegates dealt mainly with the Association's participation in the war effort.

Dues for the coming year are unchanged with the exception of members serving in the armed forces on record this year, who will be carried for the duration without the payment of dues.

The Medical Defense Fund was stabilized at the present amount of bonds and cash on hand.

Delegates to the American Medical Association were instructed to support or introduce necessary action in the House of Delegates of the A. M. A. for the establishment of a bureau of information in Washington, D. C., in order that Congress and the Federal bureau dealing with health and welfare might have the advice of organized medicine.

House of Delegates Approves Experimental Prepaid Medical and Surgical Plan

The House of Delegates in a far reaching decision, approved the inauguration of an experimental prepaid medical and surgical plan to be operated in connection with the Blue Cross Plan, and authorized President James Stevenson of Tulsa to appoint a committee to work out the details for the activating of the plan. The report of the Committee on Prepaid Medical and Surgical Plans, as adopted, appears in this issue of the Journal.

Election of Officers

Officers of the Association elected by the House of Delegates are as follows: C. R. Rountree, M.D., Oklahoma City, President-Elect; J. G. Edwards, M.D., Okmulgee, Vice-President; L. J. Moorman, M.D., Oklahoma City, Secretary-Treasurer; and J. V. Athey, M.D., and C. W. Arrendell, M.D. were re-elected Councilors for their respective districts. A Councilor for District No. 9, which includes Haskell, Latimer, LeFlore, McIntosh and Pittsburgh Counties, was not elected as there were no delegates present from that district due to the flood conditions. Dr. L. C. Kuyrkendall will therefore hold over until the next annual meeting. Dr. A. S.

Risser of Blackwell was elected to succeed himself as Delegate to the A.M.A., and Dr. J. D. Osborn of Frederick, the out-going President, was selected as Dr. Risser's alternate.

Tulsa was selected as the meeting place for 1944.

PLANS FOR 1944-45 POSTGRADUATE COURSE BEING FORMULATED

Dr. Gregory E. Stanbro, Oklahoma City, Chairman of the Postgraduate Teaching Committee, will leave May 20 for Washington and New York in the interest of the postgraduate course that will start in February, 1944. The Postgraduate Committee, following a survey of the questionnaires received from physicians completing the present Internal Medicine course, have selected Surgical Diagnosis as the subject for 1944-45.

Enrollments in the present course are running over 200 ahead of the previous programs, and well exemplify the growing interest of Oklahoma physicians in postgraduate education.

Dr. Stanbro and Mr. L. W. Kibler urge that all members of the Association feel free to communicate with the committee on any suggestions they may have concerning the program on Surgical Diagnosis.

EXPERIMENTAL PREPAID MEDICAL AND SURGICAL PLAN APPROVED BY HOUSE OF DELEGATES

In adopting the report of the Prepaid Medical and Surgical Service Committee of the Association, the House of Delegates authorized President James Stevenson of Tulsa to appoint a special committee to work out the details of the program, and place it in operation through the Blue Cross Hospital Plan. Dr. Stevenson's appointments to this committee will be announced as soon as they are made in order that the members of the Association may participate in the working out of the details.

The following is the report as adopted by the House of Delegates. The attention of all members of the Association is directed to Sections 3, 4 and 5 of the report, which outline the restrictions placed on the plan.

REPORT OF THE COMMITTEE ON PREPAID MEDICAL AND SURGICAL SERVICE

On April 22, 1942, during the State Medical Association meeting, the following resolution, pertaining to prepaid medical and surgical care plans, was passed by the House of Delegates of the Oklahoma State Medical Association:

"First, that the State Association establish a permanent committee to handle these problems. That this committee should be composed of members whose term of membership should be staggered so as to preserve its continuity.

"Secondly, that the State Medical Association instruct its various county societies to establish committees for the study of prepaid medical and surgical care, and to urge them to start immediately upon the consideration of their individual local problems, and if possible, to work out a plan suitable to their locality.

"Thirdly, that these county committees would be in close liaison with the State Committee and the Council, seeking advice and counsel, and that before they put any local plan into operation, they would have the approval of the State Committee.

In accordance with this resolution, your committee has made considerable study of various plans. Several counties have considered the possibility of establishing such plans, but to date nothing has been definitely done. Your committee feels that the county societies are somewhat hesitant in setting up any plan of this nature without more definite approval of specific basic principles by the State Association.

For these reasons, the committee is submitting definite recommendations for your careful attention and discussion in directing the State Association in formulating a policy upon prepaid medical and surgical care. The committee recommends the following:

1. That some type of prepaid medical and/or surgical care under the guidance of the medical profession should be made available to the citizens of Oklahoma.

2. Investigation convinces us that the start should be made with a limited plan which must be of a progressive nature, gradually expanding its services until all phases of medicine and surgery are covered.

3. That the plan be made available to groups enrolled in the Blue Cross Plan in certain income brackets, namely, single persons making up to $1,800.00 per year; a person with one dependent (spouse or child) making up to $2,400.00 per year; and a person with two or more dependents (spouse and/or one or more children) making up to $3,000.00 per annum.

4. That the plan adopt the unit system of compensation for its participating physicians.

5. That a committee be appointed composed of a representative from each branch of medicine, who, after having conferred with all other members of his group, would meet and work out the schedule for the unit system.

6. That it be operated initially only on selected groups which are now enrolled with the Blue Cross Plan for actuarial purposes.

7. That the operation of this plan be delegated to Group Hospital Service with a stipulation that they receive not to exceed 10 per cent of gross income to compensate them for expenses; that an additional 10 per cent be set aside for reserve to provide a cushion for expanding future services.

The committee further recommends that the President with the approval of the Council immediately appoint a committee to take the necessary steps to activate this program. The Council should be authorized to provide necessary funds to put this program in action. It is suggested that this appropriation not exceed $500.00, and it is to be set up as a loan if the expenses cannot be borne by Group Hospital Service, and that this money would be repaid from the operating fund.

Respectfully submitted,
John F. Burton, M.D., Chairman
V. C. Tisdal, M.D.
C. W. Arrendell, M.D.
Benjamin Davis, M.D.

COMMITTEE REPORTS ADOPTED BY HOUSE OF DELEGATES

The following committee reports not previously published were adopted by the House of Delegates at the 51st Annual Session. The report of the Prepaid Medical and Surgical Service Committee is printed elsewhere in the Journal.

REPORT OF COMMITTEE ON MALPRACTICE INSURANCE

Your Committee on Malpractice Insurance makes the following report:

The master policy under which malpractice insurance is made available to the members of this Association was transferred from the Tulsa County Medical Society to the State Association on February 3, 1942.

On the anniversary date of the policy there was on record with the insurance carrier, London and Lancashire Insurance Company, 296 certificates spread over only 39 of the 77 counties. These are listed as follows:

Alfalfa, 1; Beckham, 2; Blaine, 1; Bryan, 3; Caddo, 4; Canadian, 4; Carter, 6; Cleveland, 9; Comanche, 9; Craig, 1; Creek, 6; Custer, 7; Garfield, 13; Garvin, 3; Grant, 1; Hughes, 2; Kay, 9; Kingfisher, 2; LeFlore, 1; Logan, 2; Major, 1; Marshall, 1; Mayes, 2; Muskogee, 6; Okfuskee, 3; Oklahoma, 77; Okmulgee, 9; Osage, 5; Ottawa, 3; Payne, 6; Pittsburg, 9; Pontotoc, 5; Pottawatomie, 6; Rogers, 2; Stephens, 2; Tulsa, 54; Wagoner, 1; Washington-Nowata, 10; Woodward, 8. Total, 296. Total premium, $10,209.49.

This, the committee feels, is not a sufficient number of policies to be in force, and it recommends to the House of Delegates that the committee be authorized to put into immediate effect a campaign of education among the members of the Association.

Six cases have been filed under the policy during the past year, of which only one has been disposed of by either judgment or settlement.

Your committee further recommends to the House of Delegates that it be authorized to review, and, if necessary, decline to approve the application of any physician who has at least two suits filed against him in any one year, which upon impartial investigation prove to be undefendable.

It is also the request of the committee that it be authorized to contact the county societies for the purpose of establishing a procedure whereby the members of the county society may be approved either by the secretary, as is now being done, or by a specially appointed committee.

The committee further recommends that it be authorized to rewrite the present master policy to extend the period of time limit of the master policy to cover a three year period in order that a three year policy may be issued. This three year policy is to be obtainable at ten per cent reduction. The applicant may continue to elect the one year policy if he so desires.

Respectfully submitted,
V. K. Allen, M.D., Chairman,
Claude S. Chambers, M.D.
A. S. Risser, M.D.
L. J. Starry, M.D.
O. C. Newman, M.D.

REPORT OF THE MEDICAL ADVISORY COMMITTEE TO THE DEPARTMENT OF PUBLIC WELFARE

The Medical Advisory Committee to the Department of Public Welfare has now functioned for two years. The original committee was composed of five members. As the work progressed, the committee requested that a Psychiatrist be added in order to have the benefit of his services in regard to those persons who are reported to have mental condition. Dr. Moorman P. Prosser, Central State Hospital, Norman, was appointed and served as consultant until August of 1942, when he went into the Army. Dr. Hugh M. Galbraith, Oklahoma City, was then appointed to fill the vacancy. Dr. Walker Morledge was appointed in May, 1942, to replace Dr. F. Redding Hood, now in the armed forces.

The present membership of the Committee includes: Dr. C. R. Rountree, Oklahoma City, Chairman; Dr. Walker Morledge, Oklahoma City, Vice Chairman; Dr. Alfred R. Sugg, Ada; Dr. Clinton Gallaher, Shawnee; Dr. R. M. Shepard, Tulsa; Dr. Hugh M. Galbraith, Oklahoma City; and Miss Olivia Hemphill, Assistant Supervisor, Division of Public Assistance representing the State Department of Public Welfare.

The necessity for curtailing travel has forced the committee to discontinue monthly meetings and we are now meeting every three months. In order to expedite the work of the committee and to insure current reports on cases being studied, a sub-committee, composed of the Chairman, Vice Chairman and the department representative, was agreed upon to meet as often as necessary for the purpose of reviewing those cases in which eligibility is questioned by the individual member. This arrangement has seemed to function satisfactorily and we propose to continue the plan.

In July of 1942 we recommended to the Oklahoma Public Welfare Commission that fees be paid to physicians who examine applicants for aid to dependent children in which physical or mental incapacity must be established in order to qualify for this type of assistance. It was suggested that a fee of $3.00 be allowed for the first examination; $3.00 for an examination by a consultant or a physician named by a member of the committee, and $2.00 each for re-examination. Laboratory fees were provided for an a basis comparable to those charged by the U. S. Veteran Administration. All laboratory work, including X-ray films and fluroscopic examinations, must be authorized by the committee before the work is done in order to come in line for payment. The Commission accepted the recommendation of the committee and the payment of fees by the Department of Public Welfare became effective August 1, 1942.

The department reports that for the period of 8-1-42 to 4-27-43, 323 physicians submitted claims for 823 examinations amounting to $2,398.50. The department has paid $1,744.00 of this amount and fees in the amount of $654.00 are still outstanding.

Considerable confusion and some dissatisfaction has arisen in regard to the preparation of the physicians examination order (Form BC-16) and the filing of claim for fees. Please remember that it is necessary to attach to the claim the original BC-16 covering each examination listed on the claim. The original and one copy of the claim must be signed and attested to by a Notary Public or other qualified public official. We regret that these claims must be notorized before payment can be made, but the committee has gone into the matter thoroughly and finds that this is the law and there is no way to get around it.

The committee has again revised the form used by the physicians to report the findings of their examinations, a copy of which is attached to this report. This revised form, when filled out in entirety, gives the committee a comprehensive picture of the condition of the applicant. We beseech you, therefore, to complete the form in detail so as to give us a better opportunity to render sounder opinion as to incapacity.

The Department is preparing to make a study of cases involving incapacity. This study may give the committee more accurate information relative to the facilities throughout the state for medical care and treatment. The committee has recognized the need for planning with families, where the breadwinner is incapacitated, to make it possible for them to receive the care necessary for rehabilitation. In many instances it is found that although the disability which makes it impossible for the parent to follow his usual occupation is of a minor nature and repairable, facilities to care for him are lacking.

In considering this problem of incapacity and the family's need for assistance because of it, the committee is of the opinion that, if assistance were available to needy families, when the parent may be incapacitated for less than six months, it might prevent the parent from developing a chronic condition. With this in mind the committee is planning to recommend to the Oklahoma Public Welfare Commission that they reduce their present requirement (that applicant be incapacitated for at least six months before being eligible) to three months.

From 3-8-42 to 4-9-43 the committee members have had referred to them by the department 1,689 cases. Of this number 1,119 were new cases; 278 were reviews to establish continued eligibility; 190 were re-examinations made at the request of the committee; 50 were cases in which the applicant had appealed for a Fair Hearing; and 52 were cases in which the county department submitted further information. There were 108

cases carried over from the last period, making a total of 1,797 cases reviewed. The committee was of the opinion in 1,083 cases that the parent was incapacitated. In 600 cases the committee did not consider the applicant disabled. The county departments disposed of 50 cases prior to final review by the committee "for other reasons" such as death, moved out of the State, etc. There are 62 cases pending recommendation as to disability at this time.

This report will not be complete without adding a word of praise for the splendid cooperation and help which we have had from the Department of Public Welfare and also the Oklahoma Public Welfare Commission. Our recommendations have been favorably received and promptly considered.

We are also deeply grateful for the valuable service which Miss Hemphill has rendered. Last, but not least, we desire to express our appreciation to the physicians of the State, who have given of their time and otherwise cooperated most thoroughly in this program.

There is no doubt that the rolls of the ADC program are being reduced. Factors such as availability of work, higher wages, etc. undoubtedly play a considerable part in this reduction, but the fact remains that the work of the Medical Advisory Committee has no doubt been responsible for a more careful selection of cases placed on the rolls and a certain decrease that would not otherwise be possible.

Respectfully submitted,

C. R. Rountree, M.D., Chairman
Walker Morledge, M.D., Vice Chairman
Alfred R. Sugg, M.D.
Clinton Gallaher, M.D.
R. M. Shepard, M.D.
Hugh M. Galbraith, M.D.

REPORT OF COMMITTEE ON MATERNITY AND INFANCY

Last year this committee announced that preparations had been made to instigate a survey of all maternal deaths occurring in this state.

The committee now reports on the progress of this survey, and suggests certain plans for future attacks on the problems of maternal health which this survey has uncovered.

The response to the questionnaires, which are mailed to each physician signing a death certificate, have been very gratifying indeed. Instead of finding these questionnaires too lengthy and cumbersome, many physicians added personal reports in the form of letters, and some even refused the fee which was offered, saying that they were only too glad to have the chance to clarify the facts surrounding a maternal death.

The results of this survey will be published in the State Journal in complete form and in due time. The salient points are the same as have been brought out in so many other reports from so many other states; namely, the abortion problem, the toxemia problem, and the hemorrhage problem.

For the first time in the history of this state, there is accurate information as to why, how and when our women are dying in childbirth. This information is interesting and vital, but its collection would serve no real purpose unless the facts were utilized to prevent in the future the 79 per cent of deaths which this survey found were preventable.

On the evils here uncovered, this committee proposes a systematic and sustained attack, working through two channels. The first concerns the enlightenment of the public, through the regular educational, social, and religious channels; and the second concerns a program of publicity through individual county medical society meetings. Subsequent progress of this committe will be duly reported.

Respectfully submitted,

Charles Ed White, M.D., Chairman
J. B. Eskridge, Jr., M.D.
J. T. Bell, M.D.

NEWS FROM THE COUNTY SOCIETIES

The Beckham County Medical Society held their regular meeting in Elk City on April 27, with about ten members in attendance. There was no planned program, and the time was spent in general discussion of current topics.

Dr. R. C. Newkirk of Joplin, Missouri, was the guest speaker of the Ottawa County Medical Society at their meeting held in the Miami Baptist Hospital at Miami on April 15. His subject pertained to the various types of trichitis seen in children and their treatment.

A general business meeting was held in addition to the program.

A dinner meeting was held in Clinton by the Custer County Medical Society on April 20, with 11 members in attendance.

Dr. K. D. Gossom, Medical Director of the Field Hospital for Dunning, James, Patterson, contractors for the construction of the Naval Air Base near Clinton, presented a very interesting paper on "Types and Treatment of Industrial Accidents." The topic of Dr. J. O. Asher, Superintendent of the Western Oklahoma Charity Hospital, was "Shock and its Treatment."

Several nurses from the Field Hospital of the Naval Base construction project were guests of the society.

The Muskogee-Sequoyah-Wagoner County Medical Society met on April 5 at the Baptist Hospital in Muskogee.

"Gold Treatment in Arthritis" was the topic selected for presentation by Dr. Brown Oldham, and Dr. E. H. Coachman gave a paper on "The Role of Short Wave Diathermy in Otolaryngology."

Dr. Udo J. Wile will be the guest speaker at the next meeting of the society.

The Woods-Alfalfa Medical Society met at the Bell Hotel in Alva on March 30 for a dinner meeting, with the wives and several nurses as guests.

Dr. D. B. Ensor of Hopeton presented a paper on "The Medical Treatment of Peptic Ulcer," and "The Surgical Treatment of Peptic Ulcer" was discussed by Dr. W. F. LaFon of Waynoka. An interesting motion picture, "Peptic Ulcer," in color and sound was shown by Mr. A. W. Williams, representing John Wyeth and Brother.

Sugar, unknown to the Greeks and Romans, was introduced into Europe as a medicine.

"Simplicity and clearness are the eloquence of science."—Macaulay.

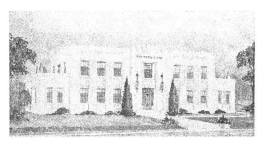

WOMEN'S AUXILIARY NEWS

A MESSAGE FROM OUR PAST PRESIDENT

I wish to thank our very efficient Executive Board for their cooperation throughout the year. Their enthusiasm for Auxiliary work has been an inspiration and stimulant to encourage me to find an ever wider field for our efforts.

I wish to thank each County President for her valiant service in this, a trying year. I know she has worked early and late to hold her organization together. I wish to commend her for her loyalty to our Auxiliary and to the purposes for which it was organized.

No executive could be a success if it were not for the support of the membership. The faithful member, who is willing to serve on committees and in various ways relieve the burdens of the executives, is indeed an asset to our Auxiliary. We salute her.

Mrs. Maxey Cooper, Oklahoma City, will be your leader for the coming year. I urge you to assist her, as your President, and make the year of 1943-44 a successful one.

Mrs. Frank L. Flack, President.

The sixteenth Annual Convention of the Auxiliary to the Oklahoma State Medical Association will be history by the time this issue of the Journal is printed. The meeting was held in Oklahoma City with Mrs. Henry H. Turner as Convention Chairman and Oklahoma County Auxiliary as the hostess county, on May 11th and 12th with headquarters in the Skirvin Hotel. The following officers have served the State Organization during the past year and now have turned over their responsibilities to the newly elected executives: President, Mrs. Frank L. Flack, Tulsa; President-Elect, Mrs. Maxey Cooper, Oklahoma City; Vice-President, Mrs. Jim L. Haddock, Norman; Secretary, Mrs. James Stevenson, Tulsa; Treasurer, Mrs. H. Lee Farris, Tulsa; Historian, Mrs. Clinton Gallaher, Shawnee; Parliamentarian, Mrs. Edward D. Greenberger, McAlester.

Standing Committees: Public Relations and War Work, Mrs. S. J. Bradfield, Tulsa; Program-Health Education, Mrs. Rush Wright, Poteau; Hygeia, Mrs. Maxey Cooper, Oklahoma City; Student Loan, Mrs. C. F. Needham, Ada; Press and Publicity, Mrs. Carl Hotz, Tulsa; Exhibits, Mrs. Joseph Kelso, Oklahoma City; Convention, Mrs. Henry H. Turner, Oklahoma City; Tray, Mrs. Carroll M. Pounders, Oklahoma City; Organization, Mrs. Jim L. Haddock, Norman; Legislative, Mrs. George Garrison, Oklahoma City; Printing, Mrs. Thomas B. Coulter, Tulsa.

We feel that the officers of 1943-44 will have the same splendid cooperation from the County Auxiliaries which we have experienced in the past year. Our congratulations are extended to those who will follow us during the ensuing year, and if there is any way that we can be of service, we will be only too happy to do so.

We are publishing a summary of the annual reports from three of our counties and expect to use the remainder of the reports in the successive Journals, as we have the space available.

Pontotoc County

The Pontotoc County Medical Auxiliary, with 13 active members, meet on the third Wednesday of each month. Luncheon is served, a business meeting held, followed by a social hour, after which surgical dressings are made at the Valley View Hospital. During the past year many of the organization have spent one afternoon a week assisting at the hospital wherever needed. Many members have actively engaged in Red Cross work, Mrs. C. F. Needham, being Chairman of the Surgical Dressings, and Mrs. W. F. Dean, Vice-Chairman. Mrs. Alfred R. Sugg, Hygeia Chairman, reports 16 subscriptions.

Oklahoma County

Oklahoma County Medical Auxiliary, under the leadership of Mrs. W. Floyd Keller, as president, reports 109 paid members, with the names of the wives of service men, who have temporarily moved from Oklahoma City, carried on the roster without dues. Their average attendance at the luncheon meetings has been 35, at which time a business meeting is held. Forty-one scrap books have been completed and given to the Crippled Children's Hospital, and 12 layettes, consisting of 26 pieces, made from material purchased by the auxiliary, and given to the hospitals for the use of needy patients. Forty subscriptions to Hygeia were obtained during the year. At one meeting a talk was made by one of the local doctors on the subject, "Attitude of Children Concerning the War." The Auxiliary has been very busy with war activities. A grand total of 32,448 hours of volunteer service has been reported. Aside from assisting in all phases of Red Cross work, the Troop Transit Committee has met trains and buses, taking candy, cigarettes, matches, postcards, etc., to inductees. It has been a very busy and interesting year for the members of Oklahoma County Auxiliary.

Tulsa County

Mrs. J. W. Childs, president of Tulsa County Auxiliary, in reviewing the activities and accomplishments of the organization which she, with the help of her officers, has directed, speaks of the wholehearted response she has received from the membership. One hundred and twenty-six active and 10 honorary members were listed in the Year Books which were distributed at the first meeting of the year in October. Two purely social meetings were held. An Executive Board meeting preceded all regular meetings.

Talks were made during the year on a variety of subjects such as "Our Responsibilities at the Polls," "Tightening up the Home Front," "Your Diet and Your Health, Madame," "Victory Garden Roundtable," and "Our Flower Garden in Wartime." A Public Health Forum was presented by the Public Relations Committee in the Y.W.C.A. Clubroom to which the general public was invited. Many representatives of various city-wide organizations attended. Subjects discussed were, "Our Concern Every Child," "Community Cooperation in the Local Health Program," "A Wartime Program for Physical Fitness," "Nutrition Today," and "Immunization Facts." This Forum was initiated last year, this being the second time it has been held, and the leadership of the doctor's wives in promoting good health has been given the approval of the general public throughout the city.

The Auxiliary, through the Hygeia Committee, placed 60 school-year subscriptions in the Tulsa county and city schools, and 19 one-year subscriptions were obtained.

The Philanthropic Committee distributed toys to the various hospitals at Christmas, 24 articles were contributed to Needle Work Guild, a new edition of Pharmacopeia and several books on the sulpha drugs were given to the Tulsa County Medical Society, and a wheelchair was purchased and presented to the Tulsa County Clinic.

The Public Relations Committee placed in the County Courthouse a rack containing health education pamphlets. This has required frequent refilling.

Three dayrooms were furnished at Camp Gruber with chairs, tables, pianos, ping pong tables, etc. Thirty-eight Christmas boxes were sent to the Camp Gruber soldiers.

Practically all members have given many hours of volunteer service in the Red Cross. Two members are Nurse's Aids. One member has taught over 500 pupils Home Nursing. Several First Aid instructors are kept busy. The Auxiliary membership is represented in all phases of the war activities in the community.

DO YOU HAVE ANY EARLY DAY OKLAHOMA MEDICAL JOURNALS?

The librarian at the University of Oklahoma School of Medicine would like to have a complete file of the medical journals published in the state and in Oklahoma and Indian territories before statehood. The following are needed to complete files already started:

Journal of Oklahoma State Medical Association, vol. 5, No. 1-7, June-Dec. 1912.

Oklahoma Medical Journal, vol. 1-8, 1893-1900; vol. 9, No. 1-3, 7, 12, Jan.-Mar., Jul., Dec. 1901.

Oklahoma Medical News, vol. 1, No. 1-3, 5, Jul.-Sep., Nov. 1901.

Oklahoma Medical News-Journal, vol. 10, No. 3, Mar. 1902; vol. 12, No. 11-12, Nov., Dec. 1904; vol. 15, No. 4, 11, 12, Apr., Nov., Dec. 1907; vol. 16, No. 1, 3-12, Jan., Mar.-Dec. 1908; vol. 17, No. 2-12, Feb.-Dec. 1909; vol. 18-20, 1910-12.

Southwest Journal of Medicine and Surgery, vol. 21-22, 1913-14; vol. 28, 1920 to last volume published.

If you know of any other journals published in Oklahoma, she would be very glad to hear of them or to receive gifts of any volumes which you would care to donate.

The School, of course, will pay the postage or express charges on any journals sent. Address all communications to Librarian, University of Oklahoma School of Medicine, 801 East 13th Street, Oklahoma City, Oklahoma.

Advertising News

Vitamin Films in Color-Eli Lilly and Company, Indianapolis, announces the release of three sixteen-mm. silent motion pictures in color descriptive of vitamin deficiency diseases. The films are available to physicians for showing before medical societies and hospital staffs. One deals with thiamine chloride deficiency, one with nicotinic acid deficiency and the third with ariboflavinosis. The major part of all films concerns the clinical picture presented by the patient with reference to treatment by diet and specific medication. They do not contain advertising of any description, nor is the name of Eli Lilly and Company mentioned.

The films were made at the Nutrition Clinic of the University of Cincinnati at the Hillman Hospital, Birmingham, Alabama, where studies were initiated in 1935, under the joint auspices of the Department of Internal Medicine of the University of Cincinnati and the University Hospitals of Cleveland. Subsequently these investigations became a cooperative project between the Departments of Medicine of the University of Cincinnati and the University of Alabama and the Department of Preventive Medicine and Public Health of the University of Texas.

Blue Cross Reports

America will be the "Arsenal of Democracy" only if her workers, the men and women who stand behind the machines that stand behind the guns, maintain their productive efficiency at a peak. A sick employee slows up production of defense necessities.

The Blue Cross Plan can help in two ways: (1) If you are a member and never become ill, never need the service, perhaps some of your good health is due to the security you enjoy, to the knowledge that if you became ill or are injured, you won't delay going to the hospital if you are a Plan Member. The doctor usually finds that early treatment at the hospital releases you that much sooner to active life.

The hospitals of America symbolize our national desire to assure freedom and personal participation for every individual in America. The community's resources are coordinated in an effort to maintain each person's health at the highest possible level of efficiency.

The mere existence of fine hospitals in a community does not guarantee that a sick person will receive sufficient and proper hospital care, any more than the existence of well stocked grocery stores and restaurants mean that a hungry person will receive sufficient and proper food. Good hospital care costs money, which must ultimately be paid by the people for whom the service is rendered or held in readiness. No one can tell when he will need hospital care or what the cost of that hospital care will be. This uncertainty has created a problem for hospital patients, not all of whom can meet the costs from their private resources at the time of sickness. As a result many hospitals have faced difficulty in obtaining the money with which to pay for the professional services and supplies which combine to make hospital care.

But the hospitals, through their administrators and trustees, have done more than provide facilities to which an individual might come for personal service. They have also exemplified American tradition by joining forces to make it easier for families to gain access to their professional facilities and service which the communities have provided. This method is the Blue Cross plan, by which millions of Americans have removed the uncertainty of hospital bills by making regular payments equal to a few cents a day per family into a common fund, which is used to provide hospital care for those who need it.

The distinctive feature of Blue Cross plans in the provision of hospital care is the voluntary participation by American citizens of several classes. These include: (a) the 10,000,000 workers and dependents who budget their hospital bills through payments equal to a few cents per day; (b) the 2,200 member-hospitals, the administrators and trustees of which support the Blue Cross plan through guaranteeing the all-important service benefits of plans; (c) the 1,800 civic, industrial, labor, professional, and religious leaders who, as trustees, guide the broad policies and procedures which make the Blue Cross movement a success; (d) the 150,000 employed groups whose management and representatives have encouraged and facilitated enrollment of members and collection of subscriptions.

The Blue Cross movement is an American "success story," the counterpart of the spirit of initiative and cooperation which has characterized the settlement and growth of the United States during the past generations. It now gives promise of being the example for greater expansion and service in the distribution of health service to the American people. The specific developments of Blue Cross plans are merely manifestations of the underlying objectives and methods which have just been described.

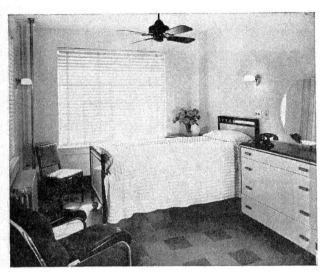

FIGHTIN' TALK

(Editor's Note: Each month the Journal office receives many notices of change of address of our members in Service, letters from the men themselves, and bits of news about them. We feel that all of these would be of great interest to our readers, and thus we are initiating a new monthly column, ''Fightin' Talk.'' We strongly urge all members in Service to send us any news, for we on the home front are vitally interested in where you are, and what you are doing).

The following letter was recently received from Dr. John Y. Battenfield, formerly located in Oklahoma City with the State Health Department:

551st Parachute Infantry,
APO 832 New Orleans, La.
April 18, 1943.

Secretary,
Oklahoma State Medical Association
Oklahoma City, Okla.

Dear Sir:

In Mr. Graham's absence I am writing this letter to no specific individual. The last I heard he was in Washington and I presume he is still there.

None of my Journals have arrived at my present address and I miss them very much. News of our friends is certainly welcome in a place like this.

You may be interested to know that since I left Sheppard Field, Texas, I have attended the Medical Field Service School at Carlisle Barracks and the Parachute School at Ft. Benning, Georgia. For some time I have been on overseas duty as Surgeon for this organization. We are allowed to say only that we are in the tropics.

Our time has been occupied from early to late with jungle training. As parachutists in these dense jungles we have certainly had some good laughs at our predicament when we land in swamps or high up in some of these very tall trees. Our most interesting problem by far has been the study of those men who become emotionally unstable and are unable to jump. We have coined the term ''jump-fear'' which fairly well describes the condition but fails to express its intensity. Lately my activities have been considerably hampered by a fractured ankle, received during a very windy night jump. At present the ankle is practically well.

Give my regards to my friends in your office and please send my Journals to the above address.

Sincerely,
John Y. Battenfield, Capt. M.C.

Captain John M. Allgood, M.C., formerly of Altus, has recently been transferred from the U. S. Army Recruiting and Induction Station, New Orleans, Louisiana, to Camp Bowie, 315 Station Hospital, Brownwood, Texas.

Lieutenant Colonel Fenton Sanger, of Oklahoma City, has been transferred to Camp Barkley as Commanding Officer of the 32nd Evacuation Unit.

Captain Glenn S. Kreger of Tonkawa, who has been stationed at Fort Bliss, Texas as Battalion Surgeon, now reports his address as: 447 C. A. B. N. (A. A.), A.P.O. No. 439 c/o Postmaster, Los Angeles, California.

A most interesting letter and newspaper clipping has been received concerning the work of Major Hervey A. Foerster, formerly of Oklahoma City, as Venereal Disease Control Officer of Camp Maxey, Texas. In addition to his venereal disease work, he is Chief of the Dermatology and Syphilology Service of the Station Hospital.

Lieutenant John Philip Haddock, M.C. of Norman is now over seas. His address is 58th Medical Bn. Co. C., A.P.O. 3792, c/o Postmaster, New York, N. Y.

The Pontotoc County Medical Society has recently furnished the present addresses of five of their members now in service, all of them being former residents of Ada. They are: Major John B. Morey, M.C., 0239873, Field Hospital No. 2, A.P.O. 923, c/o Postmaster, San Francisco, California; Major Glen W. McDonald, 54 White Place, Brookline, Massachusetts; Dr. Harrell Webster, 745 North Main Street, Shelbyville, Tennessee; Dr. Ivan Bigler, M.C., Lou Foote Flying Service, Stamford, Texas; Dr. E. D. Padberg, 442 Royston, San Antonio, Texas.

Word has been received that Lt. Logan A. Spann, M.C., formerly of Tulsa, has safely reached his destination overseas. His present address is H&S Btry., 3d Spl. Wea. Bn., 3d Mar. Div. FMF, c/o Fleet Post Office, San Francisco, California.

E. M. Harms, M.D., of Blackwell is now located at the Army Air Base Hospital, Casper, Wyoming.

Lieutenant O. H. Box, Jr., reports that he has been transferred from Greenwood, Caddo Parrish, La., to Headquarters, 4th Army Air Force, San Francisco, Calif. Prior to entering the service, Dr. Box practiced at Grandfield.

Colonel Wallace N. Davidson, formerly of Cushing, has recently been transferred from the Headquarters, 3rd Army, San Antonio, Texas, to 73rd Evacuation Hospital, A.P.O. No. 3492, care Postmaster, New York City.

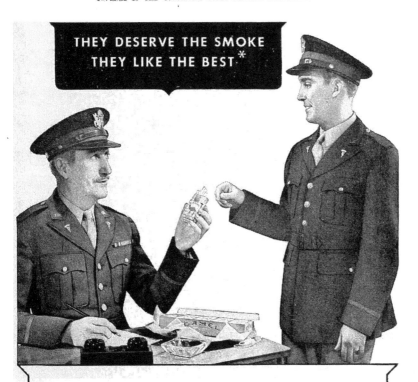

THEY DESERVE THE SMOKE
THEY LIKE THE BEST*

YOUR gift of cigarettes to men in service is the most welcome of all remembrances. And the preferred brand, according to actual survey, is Camel.*

Send Camel—the cigarette noted for mellow mildness and appealing flavor. It's one way, and a good way, to express your appreciation of the sacrifices being made by our fighting forces.

Camels in cartons are featured at your local tobacco dealer's. See or telephone him—today—while you have the idea in mind.

*With men in the Army, Navy, Marine Corps, and Coast Guard, the favorite cigarette is Camel. (Based on actual sales records in Post Exchanges and Canteens.)

. . .

Remember, you can still send Camels to Army personnel in the United States, and to men in the Navy, Marines, or Coast Guard wherever they are. The Post Office rule against mailing packages applies only to those sent to men in the overseas Army.

CAMEL COSTLIER TOBACCOS

BUY WAR BONDS AND STAMPS

News From The State Health Department

Rheumatic Fever

Rheumatic fever, one of the major enemies of child health in America today, and a leading cause of heart disease, may become an even greater menace as conditions favoring its spread now exist in many boom towns throughout the nation. This warning was recently expressed by the Metropolitan Life Insurance Company, whose studies show that over-crowding. makeshift housing, and general unhygienic conditions may be responsible for explosive outbreaks of the disease.

In Oklahoma, mortality rates of rheumatic fever are somewhat below the average for the country as a whole. Nevertheless, the death rate in this state from heart disease of all types has steadily increased from 140.5 per 100,000 population in 1937 to 182.9 in 1941.

The importance of the disease and its crippling heart complications is shown by the fact that among children between the ages of five and fourteen in Oklahoma, rheumatic fever and rheumatic heart diseases cause more deaths than tuberculosis, and almost as many as diphtheria, whooping cough, measles, and scarlet fever combined. Infantile paralysis has, in recent years, caused less than one-fourth as many fatalities among Oklahoma's children in this age group.

A nation-wide educational campaign is now under way to reduce the mortality from this disease.

While the family physician occupies the key position in the attack on rheumatic fever he needs the cooperation of the family, teachers and others who have daily supervision of the child in order to prevent, as far as possible, subsequent recurrences. Parents and others need to know the essential facts about the disease in order to be of greatest assistance.

A rheumatic child whose case is diagnosed and treated early may be able to escape heart damage. Most children who have recovered from the active phase of the disease need not be restricted from ordinary activities, even though heart damage has occurred. Many children have been made invalids because this fact has not been fully appreciated. Suitable educational and vocational guidance will assist children with severe heart damage to lead useful and relatively normal lives.

Classified Advertisements

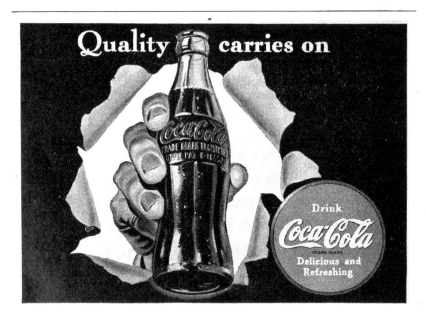

• OBITUARIES •

A. D. Bunn, M.D.
1879-1943

Dr. A. D. Bunn died February 10 at his home in Savanna, Oklahoma, after an illness of only a few days.

He was born at Rowell, Arkansas, on July 22, 1879. He attended the University of the South at Sewanee, Tennessee, graduating in 1901. Following his graduation from medical school, he practiced medicine with the late Dr. Harry E. Williams, Sr., for a short time, later moving to Humphrey where he practiced medicine for about 18 years. For the past 22 years Dr. Bunn and his family have resided at Savanna, Oklahoma, where he had continued his practice of medicine.

He was a member of the State and County Medical Associations, a member of the Masonic Lodge and the Methodist Church of Savanna.

In addition to his widow, he is survived by a son, Dudley Bunn of Savanna; three sisters, Mrs. Ora Kesterson of Pine Bluff, Arkansas; Mrs. C. J. Davidson of Little Rock, Arkansas; and Mrs. Ida Kavanaugh of Bakersfield, California.

O. O. Dawson, M.D.
1885-1943

Dr. O. O. Dawson was born March 26, 1885 at Sherman, Texas, and died April 20, 1943.

He moved with his parents to Guthrie, Oklahoma, in 1893, and received his grade and highschool education there, making an outstanding record scholastically and as an athlete. He graduated from the Medical School at the University of Oklahoma, and was a member of Beta Theta Pi social fraternity. Upon his graduation he went directly to Wayne, and began the practice of medicine. He was widely known throughout that area, and took a great interest in Wayne's civic affairs. He was a member of the Oklahoma State Medical Association, Masonic Lodge and American Legion. He was a Lieutenant in the first World War, and was stationed at Cody, New Mexico.

He is survived by his wife, Gladys L. Dawson; one son, Wilfred; one daughter, Mary Lou; one sister, Mrs. Will Van Meter; and two brothers, William and LeRoy.

John Elwood Cullum, M.D.
1859-1942

Dr. J. E. Cullum died at the home of his daughter in Tulsa, Oklahoma, on December 6, 1942.

He was born September 7, 1859 on a farm in Tippecanoe County, Indiana. He began studying medicine under his father-in-law, Dr. J. D. Freeman, at Mountain View, Missouri, and later studied and graduated from Gate City Medical College, Texarkana, Texas. In 1904 he moved to Earlsboro, Oklahoma, where he practiced medicine until his retirement in 1939.

Dr. Cullum was a public spirited man, and was devoted not only to his practice, but to the town and community in which he lived, serving in many public offices. A special pleasure was attending the weekly meetings of the Pottawatomie County Medical Society, and particularly did he enjoy being host to the Society at his home in Earlsboro.

He is survived by his widow; a daughter, Vera Cullum Moore, a son, Clifford E. Cullum of Kermit, Texas; eight grandchildren and four great grandchildren.

BOOK REVIEWS

"The chief glory of every people arises from its authors."—Dr. Samuel Johnson.

THE PATHOLOGY OF TRAUMA. Alan Richards Moritz, M.D., Professor of Legal Medicine, Harvard Medical School; Lecturer in Legal Medicine, Tufts College Medical School; Lecturer in Legal Medicine, Boston University School of Medicine. Lea & Febiger, 1942. Pp. 386. Price $6.00.

Due to the great increase in the incidence of injuries by violence as a result of the increase in industrial and automobile accidents and from the spread of armed conflict over the world, this work on the Pathology of Trauma is very timely.

The entire subject of the pathological changes due to trauma, including the pathogenesis of their complications and sequellae, has been adequately covered with a good discussion of the principal causes of mechanical injuries, the resulting manner by which they cause the general functional or organic changes, and the medico-legal aspects of such changes.

Chapter I, "General Considerations of Mechanical Injuries," covers in detail the reaction of the tissues to injury, the types of wounds most commonly encountered, with an excellent discussion of the dynamics, types of wounds inflicted, and the medico-legal aspects of bullet wounds.

Chapter II presents the effects of mechanical injury augmenting a previously existing disease and its exacerbation as a result of the injury. Infections of traumatic wounds, both immediate and delayed, from the usual bacterial and the less frequent invaders, is well presented in a way easily understood.

Chapter III presents the effects of trauma upon normal and abnormal cell growth, with a complete discussion on the relationship of tumors to trauma.

The pathological effects of trauma upon the various systems of the body is taken up in detail, with particular attention to the medico-legal angle of the injuries.

The injuries of the circulatory system is divided into neurogenic, such as shock and reflex from peripheral stimuli; hemogenic, including thrombosis, hemorrhage contusions and lacerations of the heart and blood vessels.

Asphyxia is the most important respiratory pathological condition considered. It may be caused by obstructive means such as strangling, with its important legal angle, by foreign bodies, by drowning, by the gases and from mechanical injuries of the chest and pleura.

Mechanical injuries of the alimentary canal may involve any portion including the esophagus, the stomach, the duodenum, and intestine, liver, gall-bladder, pancreas and spleen. Foreign bodies, rupture, penetrating wounds, non-penetrating wounds, and acute or chronic inflammatory disease resulting from the pathological changes, may be the etiological factor, and are adequately covered with a very excellent discussion of the changes due to the application of blunt force when applied to the abdominal viscera.

The injuries of the kidneys are well covered with a discussion of the mechanics of injury and the typical resulting pathology.

The pathological changes due to injury to the female genitalia is of importance from a medico-legal standpoint, particularly in relation to the diagnosis of rape and attempted rape and to criminal abortion. The various tests and means of diagnosis are well explained and adequate for any type.

Cerebral injury by mechanical violence is one of the commonest forms of pathological changes due to both accident and assault, and it is here that very severe injuries may be sustained without external evidence of violence. The discussion of epidural, subdural hemorrhage, and the mechanics of contralateral injury is excellent and comprehensive, and the discussion of all types of injuries to the brain and its covering is very adequate, with a discussion of the injuries of the spinal cord and meninges.

Fractures are probably the most common lesions resulting from trauma and the pathological anatomy and histology are probably the most complex, and is adequately and typically explained in relation to fractures of the skull. The most common mechanical cause of death is head injury. The mechanics in relation to the injury produced is very excellently presented. The pathology of fractures in general and of the specific bones are well covered.

This book can be recommended for the large number of very fine illustrations, many of which are unusual, and all are very interesting.

The Table of Contents has been divided adequately so that easy reference may be made to the particular subject wanted.

The author has shown by the way he has handled his material that his experience in medico-legal work has been very extensive and that he has had the opportunity to examine the pathological changes produced by trauma in a very large number of cases. Every physician should have the information contained in this volume at hand. Although the opportunity to use this knowledge in the case of the general practitioner or surgeon is not very frequent, its importance from a medico-legal standpoint cannot be overemphasized. By having this volume available the physician will be able to make an intelligent diagnosis of the pathology present, the probable means of injury, and give an adequate opinion of the legal angle of the injury.—E. Eugene Rice, M.D., F.A.C.S.

DISABILITY EVALUATION. By Earl D. McBride, B.S., M.S., F.A.C.S. Third Edition Revised. 1942. J. B. Lippincott Co., Philadelphia, London and Montreal. Price $9.00.

This represents the Third Edition of a work which was first offered in 1936, and presents many valuable additions and enlargements to the First and Second Editions which have already been reviewed in this department. Anyone who is at all familiar with the problem of disability evaluation knows that it has been one of the most mooted subjects in the field of medicine. Medicine itself being an inexact science, and the adjudication of the court, being of necessity non-standardized, brings together a combination of two variables which often result in decisions which appear to be wide of of the mark. The author of the book has attempted to clarify many of the abstruse points which are always subject for discussion, and indeed to the court, along the direction toward standardization of ratings. One of the notable additions to this Third Edition has been the "blue section" included in the work, in which the author has given his composite schedule for evaluation of partial permanent disability. At first glance this appears to be extremely complicated, and of necessity it must be intricate in detail. However, it will be of extreme value for study by those who are familiar with the routine of the courts and disability evaluation, and is also an extremely good guide for those who have to evaluate the occasional case. The author has broken down the subject of disability evaluation into its many different components and then advises reaching a sum total of the whole to cut down somewhat the margin of error due to individual observation. Obviously, the summation of inconstants cannot make a constant; however, by individual consideration of each separate factor in causation of the disability, it should be apparent that more accurate figures should be reached than by casual examination of the disability as a whole.

The various editions of this work represent augmented missionary effort to obtain more standardized procedures and to minimize the wide variation of disability estimates which can be noted in any Industrial Commission or any Court of Law where evaluation of physical disability is an integral part of the adjudication. The author has gone into great detail in the discussion of each individual type of disability and in many instances has covered not only the estimation of disability but the ideal type of treatment which would serve to prevent disability. His ideas are sound, and if there is any criticism to be made, it is that the author is perhaps somewhat ahead of the profession in his desire to add to the intricacy and hence to the accuracy of disability evaluation. True it is that it will require careful study of the part and careful evaluation of each of the factors to use the tables well. This, however, is more to be commended than condemned, for obviously it is impossible to make accurate disability estimation without careful and detailed study of each of the various factors which, combined, mean disability. This book is extremely interesting reading and merits close study by anyone interested in this branch of medicine. Surely anyone who will work to minimize the discrepancies between various "expert witnesses" deserves to be commended. This book should be a welcome addition to the shelves of the industrial surgeon and will be of especial value to one whose experience is of necessity somewhat limited in this field.—D. H. O'Donoghue, M.D.

A PRIMER ON THE PREVENTION OF DEFORMITY IN CHILDHOOD. By Richard Beverly Raney, B.A., M.D., in collaboration with Alfred Rives Shands, Jr., A.B., M.D. National Society for Crippled Children in the United States of America, Inc., Elyria, Ohio. Price $1.00.

The prevention of deformity should be a major aim for anyone who is treating a disease that may be crippling, and it is fundamental because it dams the source of supply at its origin and thus prevents the later flood. The authors have in a small volume covered a very large field and by the use of simple language and lucid illustrations have given us a primer which should be of considerable help to anyone who treats either the crippled child, or crippling diseases.

The first chapter deals concisely with the common affections of childhood which may result in deformity, and thus calls to mind those conditions which should be specifically watched for their secondary effect on the skeleton, or its related structures.

In the following three chapters, the authors then take up each of the extremities, their related skeletal structures, and the neighboring joints, describing all the affections of each point at the same time, thus, making easy reading and quick differential diagnosis. Each sub-title is divided into "Characteristics," "Causes," and "Methods of Prevention."

Anyone who has had any experience in the handling of such cases as those described, will appreciate the authoritative and concise manner in which the recommendations for treatment are given. The line drawings are typical, readily recognized, and concisely titled. This volume should be of particular value to doctors and nurses doing public health work and to social workers whose interests lie in the treatment and prevention of the crippling diseases of childhood.—L. Stanley Sell, M.D.

SAFE DELIVERANCE. By Frederick C. Irving, M.D., Boston, Houghton Mifflin Company, Price $3.00.

This interesting book is one of the Houghton Mifflin Company's Life-in-America Series. Its inclusion in this group of only four publications is a compliment to the author and to the medical profession.

In part one, "Apprenticeship of a Doctor," we find a brief but striking biographical sketch of the author's grandfather, who was a remarkable country doctor, and who unwittingly inspired the young grandson with an ambition to study medicine. The remaining chapters in part one are devoted to a moving story of the author's life with interesting reminiscences of student life and teaching at Harvard Medical School. The language is chaste, the style engaging, and the story intriguing. The text contains many interesting experiences and humorous anecdotes. In addition, there are numerous constructive reflections on medical education. The author's experiences as house pupil at the Massachusetts General Hospital are well told and his reflections upon the history and traditions of the Hospital, including his charming personality sketches of faculty members, are well worth the reading. After a short turn at the war in Europe, he came back to Boston in 1919 to take up his career at the Boston Lying-in Hospital and as professor of obstetrics at Harvard Medical School.

Part two, "The Biography of a Hospital," is devoted to the history of the Boston Lying-in Hospital. The story of this institution is of interest not only to obstetricians, but to all doctors and laymen as well. It is crowded with the undercurrents from the sea of life, bearing strange clues as to "how the other half lives. '

Part three, "Aspects of a Professor," deals with a number of medical questions couched in language which makes them intelligible to the average lay reader. Childbearing, in and out of wedlock, receives much attention, with an instructive excursion into the history of the subject from the earliest mythological fantasies to the well established modern facts.

The book is worthy of a careful reading by every doctor interested in the history of medicine, and particularly by every obstetrician.—Lewis J. Moorman, M.D.

ARTHRITIS IN MODERN PRACTICE. Otto Steinbrocker, M.D., Assistant Attending Physician and Chief, Arthritis Clinic, Belleview Hospital, Fourth Medical Division, New York City. With chapters on Painful Feet, Posture and Exercises, Splints and Supports, Manipulative Treatment and Operations and Surgical Procedures by John G. Kuhns, M.D., Chief of the Orthopedic and Surgical Service ,Robert Breck Brigham Hospital; Assistant Visiting Orthopedic Surgeon, Boston Children's Hospital. 606 Pages. Philadelphia and London: W. B. Saunders Company, 1942, Price $8.00.

"Rheumatism represents a heterogenous group of conditions arising from many causes." With this broad concept of rheumatic diseases, the author has prepared a text embracing the entire field and has accomplished it in such a manner so as to be highly acceptable by both the student and the practitioner.

The subject matter is quite comprehensive and is handled in a conservative manner, yet all the newer developments are presented in their true light. In addition to the "regular" types of arthritis, such syndromes as backache, the painful shoulder, sciatica, neuralgias, painful feet and pain are very adequately discussed. The chapter on local and regional anesthesia injections is well worth the price of the book and serves as a ready office reference in such cases.

Dr. Kuhns contributed the chapters dealing with the orthopedic management of arthritis, and no text on rheumatic disease is complete without this phase. His views are well accepted and he has summarized well many controversial subjects.

It is possible that the author has neglected somewhat the subject of gouty arthritis. The concept of gout has changed considerably the past several years, and is due to change even more in the future.

The chapter on physical therapy is adequate and serves as an excellent guide in the use of physical therapy in the treatment of rheumatic disorders. Its use is not over emphasized as is frequently the case, but its beneficial effects are well presented.

It is apparent that this text was not hastily written, but was prepared by a man well grounded in the subject who gave each fact and idea presented ample thought. This book is, at the present time, our most comprehensive, up to-date text on the subject of rheumatic disease.—William K. Ishmael, Capt., Medical Corps.

DISEASES OF THE BREAST. By Charles F. Geschickter, M.A., M.D., Lieut. Commander Medical Corps, United States Naval Reserve; Director of the Francis P. Garvin Cancer Research Laboratory; Pathologist, St. Agnes Hospital, Baltimore. J. P. Lippincott Company, Philadelphia, 1943. Price $10.00.

The author presents a comprehensive treatise that is readable and yet almost encyclopedic in scope. An excellent bibliography and summary concludes almost every chapter. A large amount of clinical material from the surgical wards of Dean Lewis at the Johns Hopkins Hospital and Laboratories as well as data from Doctor Bloodgood and his predecessors, Doctors Halsted and Welch, have been carefully analyzed and presented in tabular form in such a manner that the reader can form his personal judgments concerning the conclusions and recommendations made.

The material is organized in seven parts. The first section deals with mammary development, physiology of the breast is included with sections on postnatal hypertrophy, growth during adolescence, the mammary gland of maturity with special reference to the effects of pituitary, ovarian and placental hormones.

Part two covers a very complete description of the breast in pregnancy and lactation, and pathology associated with these conditions. Chronic cystic mastitis or mammary dysplasia is covered in an excellent manner. The altered physio-pathology is clearly described, and therapeutic measures definite. The relationship of these conditions to mammary cancer has been afforded special consideration.

Section four includes a comprehensive study of benign mammary tumors. The two common types of benign tumors, namely, the benign fibro adenomas and the benign intracystic papillomas are discussed. Space is also given to the benign tumors of the areola, nipple and non-indigenous tumors of the breast. Beautiful micro-photographs illustrate all lesions discussed, as well as in section five, which incorporates mammary malignancy. Particular stress is placed on diagnosis and values of biopsy.

The section on treatment is prepared in collaboration with Dr. Murray M. Copeland, Instructor in Surgery at the Johns Hopkins Medical School. The indications given for surgery are definite, and the technique concise and easy to follow with excellent illustration of each operative procedure described.

One of the present paramount questions—to what extent does roentgen or radium therapy supplement or replace radical surgery, is clearly answered. A careful evaluation of results obtained by each form of therapy is given. A special section covers measures to combat complications resulting from therapy, such as edema of the arm, pleural effusions, painful contractures, the relief of pain, etc.

The style of this book makes for pleasant reading, and there is admirable balance between the presentation of the underlying anatomy and physiology and their correlation with clinical pathology and associated symptoms, diagnosis and treatment. It is the opinion of

this reviewer that this book will be a valuable addition to the library of the general practitioner as well as the surgical specialist.—Gerald Rogers, M.D., F.A.C.S.

ADVANCES IN INTERNAL MEDICINE. Edited by J. Murray Steele, M.D., Welfare Hospital, New York University Division, Welfare Island, N. Y. Seven associate editors and ten contributors. Volume 1. Interscience Publishers, Inc., 215 Fourth Avenue, New York. 1942. Price $4.50.

This volume is the first of a contemplated series to record some of the recent advances in internal medicine. It is the purpose of the editor to present the material simple enough to be intelligible to those individuals whose main interest lies outside the scope of the particular subject, and at the same time, sufficiently detailed to be of use to those persons working in the field. The background of each essay is intended to furnish an understanding of the problem whose partial solution represents advancement. Each article is written by one who has contributed to the advances of which he writes.

Ten subjects are presented in the first volume. These include: 1. The Use of the Miller-Abbott Tube in the Diagnosis and Treatment of Disorders of the Gastro-Intestinal Tract; 2. The Use of Insulin and Protamine Insulin in the Treatment of Diabetes; 3. Sympathetic Nervous Control of the Peripheral Vascular System; 4. The Antibacterial Action of the Sulfonamide Drugs; 5. The Choice of the Sulfonamides in the Treatment of Infection; 6. Infections of the Urinary Tract; 7. Present Trends in the Study of Epidemic Influenza; 8. Hypertension: A Review of Humoral Pathogenesis and Clinical Treatment; 9. Nephrosis; 10. Riboflavin Deficiency.

Most of the articles are well written, clear, concise, not too detailed, and show the rapid advances that are being made in solving some of the problems in internal medicine. The articles on "The Use of Insulin and Protamine Insulin in the Treatment of Diabetes," "The Choice of the Sulfonamides in the Treatment of Infection" and "Infections of the Urinary Tract" will be found of great value to the internist and general practitioner.

Each article contains a summary of the material presented, and an extensive bibliography. The latter will be of special value to research workers and others who desire more information. Students and practitioners will find this volume valuable in keeping abreast of the advances that are being made in the subjects discussed.—L. W. Hunt, M.D.

SHOCK: DYNAMICS, OCCURRENCE, AND MANAGEMENT. Virgil H. Moon, A.B., M.Sc., M.D., Professor of Pathology, Jefferson Medical College, Philadelphia. Lea & Febiger, 1942. Pp. 324. Price $4.50.

Dr. Moon as a pathologist, is probably more competent to discuss the difficult phenomena of shock than either an internist or surgeon as his outlook is broader and he has accumulated a very large amount of physiologic, experimental and clinical data.

To conserve the time of the busy physician who lacks time for extensive reading, most of the chapters in the book close with a short summary covering the significant matter and the author's interpretation.

Dr. Moon has divided his book into two parts. The first, or Part I, titled "Vascular Dynamics of Shock," deals very extensively with the physiology and pathology of the capillary system. The explanation of the great importance of the capillary endothelium is very excellent, and with an adequate knowledge of the functions of the capillary endothelium the cause of shock is more easily understood. An adequate discussion of the physiological disturbances is given, and the importance of hemoconcentration as a means of the very early diagnosis of shock is emphasized, and this condition is present even before there are any changes in the blood pressure readings.

The definition, "Shock is a disturbance of fluid balance resulting in a peripheral circulatory deficiency which is manifested by a decreased volume of blood, reduced blood flow, hemoconcentration, and by renal functional deficiency," is very comprehensive and is probably the most adequate to explain the phenomena in a few words.

Chapter IV gives adequate explanation of the association of endothelial damage and anoxia, and how the reciprocating effects of these two conditions act as a vicious circle which leads to irreversible changes and precipitate a condition of fatal shock.

Traumatic shock, or toxemia, is discussed, and it is concluded that this type of shock results from a combination of causes including exhaustion, exposure, pain, anxiety, hemorrhage, infection, and the absorption of products of tissue autolysis from the area of injury. The latter was regarded as the most important of these factors. Adequate experiments with many substances confirm the fact that this statement is true, and that the mode of their action is by damage to and in increasing the permeability of the capillary endothelium.

The importance and the difficulty in differentiating between shock and the effects of hemorrhages is emphasized, and the many points of contrast have been adequately discussed and are so numerous and apparent that they should not be confused even though each evokes the same mechanism of compensation.

It is emphasized that many believed that shock is purely a physiologic disturbance, unaccompanied by significant morphologic changes, but here the definite pathologic changes are discussed under two important headings: (a) those which have a direct causative relationship to the mechanism of the circulatory disturbance, and (b) those which are regarded as secondary or as resulting from inefficient circulation. The direct changes seen in the lungs, liver, kidneys and spleen are of congestive, edematous, and hemorrhagic nature, while the occurence of parenchymatous degeneration may be considered as secondary.

Chapters XII, XIII and XIV give a very excellent discussion of the occurrence of shock in burns with an explanation of the mechanism and the importance of the toxic factor. The occurrence of shock in other conditions such as anaphylaxis, transfusions, abdominal emergencies, obstetrics, and infections are very well discussed and explained on a rational basis that have a good experimental background.

The importance of impaired renal function that always occurs whenever a severe degree of shock develops is well explained under the headings of "Extrarenal Uremia," and the occurrence and mechanism are discussed and their importance ephasized, although the exact mechanism is not fully understood and there is a requirement that further investigation is necessary.

The relationship of the adrenals to shock is well known, and the relation to circulatory deficiency is discussed and compared with the condition of traumatic shock and their similarity emphasized, with a good discussion of the condition of status lymphaticus, and Addison's disease.

Chapter XVII gives a very brief but adequate resume of Part I, which is very helpful in integrating the entire material in this part, and gives the reader a clearer picture of the detailed and experimental work done for the author to reach his conclusions and interpretations of this part. There is also a discussion of the mechanics of death in this chapter.

Part II, "The Prevention, Recognition and Management of Shock," takes up in detail the clinical application of the experimental studies of Part I.

The prevention of shock is very excellently presented, with due emphasis placed on the selection of anaesthesia with a discussion of the newer methods including spinal, regional, intravenous and the gases, and the prevention of the loss of blood and fluids is stressed .

The importance of the prevention of absorption by debridement in open wounds, the immediate local treatment of burns by coagulation, and the newer methods of prevention of absorption of toxins from the intestinal tract in obstruction by decompression are adequately presented in a few words.

Hemoconcentration is again emphasized, and the methods of determination are given. Its importance in the early diagnosis of shock and in the differential diagnosis from hemorrhage is very excellent.

The discussion of the therapeutic agents used in the treatment of shock are considered under the title of "Symptomatic," such as the use of stimulants, mechanical aids, oxygen therapy, the use of morphine, and the importance of the newer drug which has demonstrated its value, adrenal cortical hormone.

Chapter XXIII presents the all important subject of the replacement of fluids in the treatment of shock with a good discussion not only of the transfusion of whole blood, but the use of plasma and serum, both fluid and dessicated, and of the use of blood substitutes including saline and glucose, acacia, pectin, gelatin, hemoglobin-Ringer solution, Bovine plasma and serum.

Dr. Moon's book shows years of experimental study of the difficult subject of shock, and is a worthy successor of his former treatise on "Shock and Related Capillary Phenomena." Every surgeon or physician who attempts to treat the acutely injured should have the principles of the dynamics and the treatment of shock as presented in this excellent book available.—E. Eugene Rice, M.D., F.A.C.S.

MEDICAL PARASITOLOGY. By James T. Culbertson, Assistant Professor of Bacteriology, College of Physicians and Surgeons, Columbia University, New York. 285 Pages. 1942. Price $4.25.

The authors have compiled information such as is remarkably convenient to read, and arranged in a very practical manner. It contains the type of information that is useful for any practitioner of medicine. It is particularly adaptable to the use of those confronted with diagnostic problems where parasites are suspected. Several tables contain certain condensed information from which summaries and conclusions may be readily drawn.

Gems such as the following are scattered throughout: "As yet, with no parasitic infection has the vaccination of man been tried significantly."

"Malaria is the only protozoan disease of man in which immune serum therapy has been tried as a means of treatment. In the hands of a few investigators, favorable results have been obtained, but even in these the results of such treatment have not been strikingly successful."

The book contains sixteen figures and seven tables and an ample number of illustrations. It is cloth bound, the printing is satisfactory and the paper used, in keeping with that of the times. Several pages contain details of techenical methods in connection with the identification of the various types of parasites, and two pages list book references—Hugh Jeter, M.D.

A New Approach to the Treatment of Snoring

On the basis of the theory that the true functional snoring is caused by the vibrations of the soft palate, uvula and posterior pillars, and that the sound produced is related to the natural periodic vibrations of the tissue involved, it is suggested that the "fluttering" factors be modified by producing a controlled fibrosis in the vibrating soft tissues through the injection of a sclerosing solution, such as sylnasol (a 5 percent solution of the sodium salts of certain of the fatty acids of the oil extracted from a seed of the psyllium group).—Jerome F. Straus, M.D., Arch. of Otolaryng., Sept., 1942.

MEDICAL ABSTRACTS

"CLINICAL IMPORTANCE OF THE LIPOID RING OF THE CORNEA." Rintelen, F. (Basel) Schweizerische Medizinishe Wochenschrift, Vol. 72, No. 32, page 881-882, 1942.

Many investigators pointed out the importance of ocular symptoms in general medical diagnosis. Their studies included also the problem of whether the presence of a lipoid ring of the cornea may be considered the manifestation of a general pathological process (P. Marie-Laroche, Virchow, Listo Vollaro, Rohrschneider).

In case of the lipoid ring, or so-called senile ring, one has assumed that it is an old age phenomenon inherited as a dominant character; that it is a senile character present already in the germ plasma. Rohrschneider, who made a special study of the senile ring, stated that the presence of a senile lipoid ring of the cornea makes it probable that the person is arteriosclerotic.

In view of the great practical importance of the problem, the present author examined the eyes of 600 cadavers at the Basel Pathological Institute for the presence of corneal lipoid ring. The examination showed the following:

In 214 cases there was a distinct lipoid ring, or at least an arc in the upper circumference of the cornea, which could be observed without the aid of any optical instrument even by doctors who were not ophthalmologists.

Examining the entire cardiovascular system of the 214 cadavers, there was no arteriosclerosis detectable in 66, or in 31 per cent of the cases; 97 cadavers or 45 per cent of the cases showed moderate sclerosis of the whole or of a part of the arterial vascular system, in 51 cadavers or in 24 per cent of the cases the arteriosclerosis was very much advanced, especially in the large blood vessels.

In 39 cadavers of persons past 60 there was no lipoid ring or arc to be found yet in 13 of these, or in 33 per cent of the cases, there was a very severe arteriosclerosis present, which in seven cases was the immediate cause of death (apoplexy, heart infarctation, etc.).

Lipoid ring was also found in four cadavers of persons below 30 years of age; but there was neither macroscopic nor microscopic evidence of arteriosclerosis in these cases.

The investigation of Rintelen lead to the conclusion that there is no close relationship between lipoid infiltration of the cornea and arteriosclerosis. Such a conclusion is not at all surprising. The lipoid arc or ring is a senile character determined already by the genotype, while arteriosclerosis is an exceedingly complex pathological process. The word arteriosclerosis is a generic name for many variations of vascular disease which greatly differ from each other as to their pathogenesis, localization in the vascular wall, and in their clinical course. Contrary to the origin of lipoid arc, the pathogenesis of arteriosclerosis includes, besides endogenous constitutional factors, also important exogenous moments such as syphilis, rheumatism, lead, nicotin, etc. It should not be denied, however, that certain exogenous factors, as a previous keratitis or catarrhal ulcer, may quicken the development of lipoid rings in the cornea.

The practitioner should, therefore, remember that the lipoid arc of the cornea is not a "signum mali ominis," and a patient with a corneal senile ring is not necessarily arteriosclerotic. One may reach a ripe old age with a senile ring in his eye, while another with normal cornea may die early form an arteriosclerosis not manifested by any lipoid ring.—M.D.H., M.D.

"THE PERIOSTEAL FLAP IN MASTOID SURGERY." Ogilvy, Reid W. (Hereford). The Journal of Laryngology, and Otology. Vol. 57, No. 9, Page 405-410, 1942.

The ideal in aural surgery is the eradication of disease with as little disturbance of the anatomy and physiology of the region as possible. On this criterion the radical mastoid operation stands immediately condemned if anything short of it can be adequate. The establishment of a good conservative procedure, is therefore, much to be desired. The author describes a good operation, the essential points of which are: (1) complete clearance of the mastoid air cells, (2) enlargement of the aditus and removal of disease in the ear involving, if necessary, the incus, (3) the closure of the enlarged aditus by a well cut periosteal flap, (4) no permanent enlargement of the external meatus by perichondreal flaps.

An incision is made from the tip of the mastoid to about half an inch above the attachment of the pinna down to the subcutaneous plane. The wound is undercut forwards to the level of the posterior meatal wall and dorsum pinnae. Undercutting is then carried backwards to beyond the posterior margin of the mastoid process and upwards over the surface of the temporal muscle fascia well above the supra mastoid ridge. This dissection exposes the attachment of the sternomastoid muscle to the periosteum covering the process. The flap is now cut as follows:

An incision is made through the muscles and periosteum from the tip of the process upwards and backwards just in front of the posterior margin of the process as far as the posterior superior angle of the mastoid. A horizontal incision is then made through the fascia and periosteum at the lower margin of the temporal muscle just below the supra mastoid ridge from a point level with the posterior meatal margin to meet the first incision in the region of the posterior superior angle of the mastoid.

The flap thus outlined should be carefully raised with a sharp periosteum elevator, any bruising of the tissue being avoided. Next take hold of the tip of the flap with tissue forceps and gently pull it forward. The mastoid retractor is now introduced with its anterior blade in front of the flap to avoid damage to the latter. The flap is then gently laid aside with the tissue forceps still attached until it is required later.

The usual cortical mastoidectomy is now carried out, all diseased bone being thoroughly eradicated. The roof and outer wall of the aditus are now removed as far forward as possible without weakening the bony tympanic ring. To achieve this satisfactorily, the posterior meatal wall is removed to a varying extent. The incus can now be readily inspected and its removal depends upon whether or not it appears to be diseased. It is sometimes a difficult and tedious procedure and care must be taken not to remove the malleus. An incus hook is used, and the instrument is introduced between the incus and the inner wall of the middle ear and hooked on to the body and descending process of the ossicle. When the latter has been removed there is freer access for the removal of diseased mucous membrane in the posterior part of the middle ear cavity.

It is important to remove all the mucous membrane especially on the inner wall of the antrum. The cavity is now syringed out with hydrogen peroxide followed by alcohol, these being forced through the aditus and out through the meatus by way of the perforation in the tympanic membrane. This results in a very adequate attic cleanout. The whole exposed surface of the wound (bone and soft parts) should be smeared with Bisform, and when this procedure is completed the cavity should be quite dry. The flap must now be firmly placed in position and before doing so, its tip, which was held in forceps, should be cut away as it is traumatized. It should be placed gently, but firmly, with its tip in the enlarged aditus and care must be taken in all subsequent manipulation to avoid moving it.

One or two mattress sutures are employed, the object being to bring together large surfaces of tissue in order to obtain sound healing and, also, to act as a splint. Removal of these sutures is facilitated by introducing a small piece of rolled gauze under the loop and tying the knot over a similar small pad. The remainder of the wound is now closed by fine silk-worm gut or horse-hair sutures. A dressing of gauze, impregnated with the iodoform preparation, is then placed over the suture line and a dressing of the same material is placed in the meatus down to the tympanic membrane. In this way the whole operation field is completely sealed off. Primary healing is practically certain, therefore, it is not necessary, nor even advisable, to disturb the dressing under ten days.

In cases of acute inflammation and cholesteatoma the operation is contraindicated. Otherwise it may be performed in all cases in which a conservative operation would appear to be adequate, i.e., where the disease is more or less localized in the antrum and aditus, posterior parts of the tympanic cavity, attic and possibly incus.

In the majority of the author's cases a subtotal or large perforation was present in the drum so that it was possible to determine beforehand whether or not the descending process of the incus was diseased. This would appear to be the most commonly diseased part of the incus and, of course, it cannot be examined when the incus is viewed from the attic aspect at operation. Such evidence is vital, therefore, in deciding when to remove the ossicle.

It should be emphasized that in all cases eradication of nasopharyngeal infection likely to be a factor in the production of the disease was undertaken prior to a decision to operate. This applies especially to removal of septic tonsils and adenoids. In 12 of 18 cases operated on by this method, a completely dry ear was obtained. The length of time required for this cure to be manifest varied from 15 days to over four months, but on the whole the time required compares satisfactorily with that generally required when other recognized operative procedures are employed. There were but two failures.—M. D. H., M.D.

"THE GENERAL CONCEPT OF ALLERGY IN OTORHINOLARYNGOLOGY." Marinho, J. (Rio de Janeiro) Revista Brasileira de Oto-rino-laringologia, Vol. 10. No. 4. Page 395-423. 1942.

Darier was the one who said that allergy is life itself. Though life cannot be properly defined, its material basis is well known. There are indispensable physical constituents of life found in all living beings. The structure of life is based on the combination of C. N. O. H. S. P. into protids, lipids and glucids. The minerals of the organism exercise a catalytic function. The basis of any living being is the cell, and cells unite into tissues, tissues into organs, and organs into the organism. The basic element of the organized cell substance is protein, the essential conditions of life. Protein is a combination of amino acids; ingested proteins are built up and modified in the organism by the metabolic process. The residues of metabolism are eliminated from the body. One of the residues is amine, and the amine of the tissues is histamine.

If histamine is not eliminated, it will act, like any other catabolic substance, as a poison. According to experimental and clinical studies, the allergic shock is usually attributed to the toxic action of histamine. The author states that allergy is a form of indigestion, or abnormal protein metabolism. Antigen is any substance which is poorly digested. Antibody is any substance which promotes protein digestion.

In certain organisms certain proteins are not well digested. The organism is, therefore, intolerant or sensitive to those indigestible proteins. Proteins are also produced by bacteria which enter the body in infection. In breaking down bacterial protein there will be also histamine produced, which is either eliminated or retained, producing allergy. In normal organisms, bacterial protein produces antitoxins before its final breaking down. Allergy may be, therefore, considered as an immunity which has gone astray. Though allergy is not identical with immunity. even the abnormal reaction of an allergic shock serves the purpose of freeing the tissues from histamine and of establishing a normal proteic digestion. Thus, a spontaneous desensitization may take place. In persons who always fall back into the original allergic state there is a marked predisposition for allergy.

In rhinology it has been observed that some acute sinusitic infections become chronic even after operation, while others rapidly cure under identical conditions. LaCarrere and Del Carril explain this phenomenon by the hypothesis that chronic sinusitis, resisting even surgical treatment, is caused on the one hand by local infection which leads to allergy, and on the other hand allergy itself maintains the infection. This cycle of infection allergy and allergy infection is broken by bacterial therapeutics, or by desensitization by means of histamine. These are the two fundamental methods of treatment of any allergic condition.

Recently, Meniere's disease and the functional labyrinthitis of seasickness are also explained on the basis of an allergic upset of the sympathetic-parasympathetic nervous system. The success of desensitization therapy by means of histamine in both conditions is a sufficient proof of this hypothesis. Desensitization by histamine starts with a minimal dose (one-tenth of a milligram), which is gradually increased to the limit of tolerance. The top dose, usually one milligram, is injected once a week for four weeks in succession—M. D. H., M.D.

"UNILATERAL INVOLVEMENT OF THE OPTIC NERVE IN HEAD INJURIES." Rodger, F. C. (Glasgow) The British Journal of Ophthalmology. Vol. 27, No. 1, Page 23-33. January, 1943.

Cases of traumatic optic atrophy are to be found in every surgical ward. Types of accident most frequently producing it are motor accidents; falls or blows on the head received in industry; and, in these days, war injuries such as blunt injuries sustained in air attacks from falling timber and masonry. The lesion is uniocular and, therefore, prechiasmal. The degree of violence may be so great that the patient suffers a fractured skull and lies unconscious for some weeks, or may be so slight that the patient is only momentarily dazed, with perhaps no external signs of violence at all. One case has been mentioned in which optic atrophy resulted from a knock on the eyebrow with a potato.

The clinical picture is a simple one. Soon after the accident each patient complained of a reduction of vision in one of his eyes. The pupils of the affected eyes reacted to light directly, more or less according to the degree of damage to the nerve fibers, while in all of them the consensual reaction remained. In the cases showing partial optic atrophy, central vision was depressed, and in a few patients there was a contraction of the field with an insular scotoma. Externally, apart from the pupillary anomaly, nothing could be seen. Internally, on the other hand, the nerve head sooner or later revealed a pathological state, in from four to seventeen days.

The earliest phenomenon observed ophthalmoscopically is paller of the disc, in whole or in part. The papilla retains its sharp border, the pigment and scleral rings being unchanged, and the lamina cribrosa in many cases easily discernible. The change of the disc does not depend entirely upon a degeneration of the optical fibers. There develops also a change in the vessels, or rather in the arteries. The tiny central vessels begin to disappear; the larger arteries become narrower and straighter than in the sound eye. The vascular changes may be caused by organic changes in the neuroglia of the injured optic nerve, or they may be due to vasomotor action. The changes described are those typically found in simple or primary optic atrophy.

In studying the optic bony canal by x-ray, it was found that the canal is not necessarily injured in these cases. Even in those cases in which fracture of the optic canal was evident, there is the role of associated hemorrhage to be considered. In some cases the hemorrhage alone can explain the changes in the optic nerve. The optic nerve is similar in structure to the white matter of the brain. The axis cylinders have no sheaths and there are no cells of Schwann, so that there can be no regeneration. And yet the truth is that many of these cases show improved vision and fields. This can only mean one thing: the nerve fibers have not been destroyed after all, but their conductivity in some degree only temporarily suspended. Like the rest of the brain the optic nerve is surrounded by the three meningeal sheaths. With this knowledge the following explanations are possible in cases of unilateral involvement of the optic nerve in head injuries: (1) subvaginal hemorrhage with pressure on or tearing of the nutrient vessels of the optic nerve; (2) intraneural hemorrhage; (3) fracture with perhaps tearing, or pressure on, the nervous tissue.—M. D. H., M.D.

"HEREDITARY DEFORMING CHONDRODYSPLASIA."
B. T. Vansant and Frances R. Vansant. The Jr. A.M.A. CXIX. 786. 1942.

Hereditary deforming chondrodysplasia, a relatively rare condition, is a term used in preference to many others which are mentioned, although it is noted that the Standard Nomenclature of Disease, in a recent revision, prefers the term dyschondroplasia to chondrodysplasia, and multiple cartilaginous exostoses is not considered an identical disease. The authors, however, believe that they are merely different manifestations of the same clinical entity.

In a description of the disease, the different manifestations and the deformities they produce are pointed out. The disease is distinctly one of growth and age. Sarcomatous changes may be found in a relatively small percentage of the cases, probably less than five per cent. The theories of both Keith and Geschickter as to the origin of the disease are mentioned, but it felt that neither theroy completely explains the phenomena. The authors believe that there is an inherited defect in the primitive anlage for both cartilaginous and membranous bone, which produces disturbances of bone formation; these disturbances are expressed as growth, and hence are most pronounced at the points at which growth is more active—namely, at the growing ends of long bones. A rather complete differential diagnosis deals with Ollier's disease, Albers-Schonberg disease, Voorhoeve's disease, et cetera.

Heredity plays an important part in the etiology of this disease, which is believed to be transmitted as a mendelian dominant. In five generations of one family of 78 members, 36 persons are known to have had this disease. It has repeatedly stated that the disease is more common in males than females by a ratio of three to one, but the authors point out that this ratio is probably too high; they believe it is more nearly one and one-half to one. An interesting sociological discussion as to the origin of the disease and the final outcome by dissemination is added.—E.D.M., M.D.

"TOXOPLASMIC ENCEPHALOMYELITIS." CLINICAL DIAGNOSIS OF INFANTILE OR CONGENITAL TOXOPLASMOSIS; SURVIVAL BEYOND INFANCY. By David Cowen, M.D., Abner Wolf, M.D. and Beryl H. Paige, M.D., New York. Archives of Neurology and Psychiatry. Vol. 48. No. 5. November. 1942.

Cases of protozoon disease have been found to affect the human race in many instances and new diseases have recently been reported, particularly anaplasmosis and toxoplasmosis. The authors, in this, have reviewed cases of toxoplasmic encephalomyelitis and their own summary, which follows, seems appropriate.

A review of the symptoms in nine cases of infantile, or congenital toxoplasmic encephalomyelitis recognized at necropsy permitted the formulation of a clinical picture of the disease. The children all died during infancy, usually in the early weeks or months of life, in the acute or subacute stage. The outstanding feature of the syndrome was the concomitant occurrence in infants at or soon after birth of striking ocular lesions and neurologic symptoms and signs. The ocular signs consisted of multiple focal, bilateral areas of chorioretinitis, almost invariably involving the macula, with less constant microphthalmos, nystagmus and ocular palsies. The neurologic findings included convulsions, hydrocephalus and, as the most striking sign, multiple foci of intracerebral calcification.

On this basis, the first six clinically identified cases have been diagnosed and are reported here. In the majority of these the patients are children who have survived beyond infancy, indicating that, contrary to our previous experience, the infection is not uniformly fatal and may become chronic, healed or latent. An analysis of the findings in these six cases reveals that at this stage the clinical picture consists chiefly of the residual effects of the lesions occurring in the acute or the subacute stage. In these older children the outstanding symptom is usually diminution in vision due to the effects of multiple foci of healed chorioretinitis, which are readily identifiable ophthalmoscopically. Strabismus, microphthalmos and minor congenital ocular defects may also be present. Generalized convulsions or petit mal attacks may persist or later make their appearance. Internal hydrocephalus may become chronic and progressive. Foci of intracerebral calcification persist, and may at first increase in number and size. Retardation in the development of speech and minor degrees of mental deficiency occur.

The intrauterine inception of the disease in many, if not all, of these patients is stressed. The fact that these children often survive into the juvenile period would make it desirable to refer to this form of toxoplasmosis as infantile, or congenital, toxoplasmic encephalomyelitis to distinguish it from toxoplasmosis which may be acquired during the juvenile and in adult life. These forms might be termed juvenile and adult acquired toxoplasmosis respectively. It may be that a type of acquired infantile toxoplasmosis exists.

Infantile, or congenital, toxoplasmic encephalomyelitis is evidently not a rare disease. It is believed that many cases may have been erroneously classified as instances of congenital malformation of the brain, cerebral birth injury, epilepsy, congenital hydrocephalus, etc. The identification of additional cases may yield some knowledge as to the epidemiology of the disease. In any event, the present indications are that the infection is widespread in the United States, and cases have been encountered in South America and Europe as well. Various mammals, and perhaps birds, are probably the animal reservoirs of the infection, but the mode of transmission to man is not yet known.

The use and limitations of a serologic method as a diagnostic aid are discussed.—H. J., M.D.

KEY TO ABSTRACTORS

OFFICERS OF COUNTY SOCIETIES, 1943

★

COUNTY	PRESIDENT	SECRETARY	MEETING TIME
Alfalfa	H. E. Huston, Cherokee	L. T. Lancaster, Cherokee	Last Tues. each Second Month
Atoka-Coal	J. B. Clark, Coalgate	J. S. Fulton, Atoka	
Beckham	H. K. Speed, Sayre	E. S. Kilpatrick, Elk City	Second Tuesday
Blaine	Virginia Olson Curtin, Watonga	W. F. Griffin, Watonga	
Bryan	J. T. Colwick, Durant	W. K. Haynie, Durant	Second Tuesday
Caddo	F. L. Patterson, Carnegie	C. B. Sullivan, Carnegie	
Canadian	P. F. Herod, El Reno	A. L. Johnson, El Reno	Subject to call
Carter	Walter Hardy, Ardmore	H. A. Higgins, Ardmore	
Cherokee	P. H. Medearis, Tahlequah	James K. Gray, Tahlequah	First Tuesday
Choctaw	C. H. Hale, Boswell	E. A. Johnson, Hugo	
Cleveland	J. A. Rieger, Norman	Curtis Berry, Norman	Thursday nights
Comanche	George S. Barber, Lawton	W. F. Lewis, Lawton	
Cotton	A. B. Holstead, Temple	Mollie F. Seism, Walters	Third Friday
Craig	F. M. Adams, Vinita	J. M. McMillan, Vinita	
Creek	H. R. Haas, Sapulpa	C. G. Oakes, Sapulpa	
Custer	E. R. Vieregg, Clinton	C. J. Alexander, Clinton	Third Thursday
Garfield	Paul B. Champlin, Enid	John R. Walker, Enid	Fourth Thursday
Garvin	T. F. Gross, Lindsay	John R. Callaway, Pauls Valley	Wednesday before Third Thursday
Grady	Walter J. Baze, Chickasha	Roy E. Emanuel, Chickasha	Third Thursday
Grant	I. V. Hardy, Medford	E. E. Lawson, Medford	
Greer	G. P. Cherry, Mangum	J. B. Hollis, Mangum	
Harmon	W. G. Husband, Hollis	L. E. Hollis, Hollis	First Wednesday
Haskell	William Carson, Keota	N. K. Williams, McCurtain	
Hughes	Wm. L. Taylor, Holdenville	Imogene Mayfield, Holdenville	First Friday
Jackson	E. S. Crow, Olustee	E. W. Mabry, Altus	Last Monday
Jefferson	F. M. Edwards, Ringling	L. L. Wade, Ryan	Second Monday
Kay	Philip C. Risser, Blackwell	J. Holland Howe, Ponca City	Third Thursday
Kingfisher	C. M. Hodgson, Kingfisher	H. Violet Sturgeon, Hennessey	
Kiowa	B. H. Watkins, Hobart	J. William Finch, Hobart	
LeFlore	Neeson Rolle, Poteau	Rush L. Wright, Poteau	
Lincoln	H. B. Jenkins, Tryon	Carl H. Bailey, Stroud	First Wednesday
Logan	William C. Miller, Guthrie	J. L. LeHew, Jr., Guthrie	Last Tuesday
Marshall	O. A. Cook, Madill	Philip G. Joseph, Madill	
Mayes	Ralph V. Smith, Pryor	Paul B. Cameron, Pryor	
McClain	B. W. Slover, Blanchard	R. L. Royster, Purcell	
McCurtain	A. W. Clarkson, Valliant	N. L. Barker, Broken Bow	Fourth Tuesday
McIntosh	James L. Wood, Eufaula	William A. Tolleson, Eufaula	First Thursday
Murray	P. V. Annadown, Sulphur	F. E. Sadler, Sulphur	Second Tuesday
Muskogee-Sequoyah-Wagoner	H. A. Scott, Muskogee	D. Evelyn Miller, Muskogee	First and Third Monday
Noble	C. H. Cooke, Perry	J. W. Francis, Perry	
Okfuskee	L. J. Spiekard, Okemah	M. L. Whitney, Okemah	Second Monday
Oklahoma	Walker Morledge, Oklahoma City	E. R. Musick, Oklahoma City	Fourth Tuesday
Okmulgee	A. R. Holmes, Henryetta	J. C. Matheney, Okmulgee	Second Monday
Osage	C. R. Weirich, Pawhuska	George K. Hemphill, Pawhuska	Second Monday
Ottawa	W. B. Sanger, Picher	Matt A. Connell, Picher	Third Thursday
Pawnee	E. T. Robinson, Cleveland	R. L. Browning, Pawnee	
Payne	L. A. Mitchell, Stillwater	C. W. Moore, Stillwater	Third Thursday
Pittsburg	John F. Park, McAlester	William H. Kaeiser, McAlester	Third Friday
Pontotoc	O. H. Miller, Ada	R. H. Mayes, Ada	First Wednesday
Pottawatomie	A. C. McFarling, Shawnee	Clinton Gallaher, Shawnee	First and Third Saturday
Pushmataha	John S. Lawson, Clayton	B. M. Huckabay, Antlers	
Rogers	C. W. Beson, Claremore	C. L. Caldwell, Chelsea	First Monday
Seminole	Max Van Sandt, Wewoka	Mack I. Shanholtz, Wewoka	Third Wednesday
Stephens	W. K. Walker, Marlow	Wallis S. Ivy, Duncan	
Texas	R. G. Obermiller, Texhoma	Morris Smith, Guymon	
Tillman	R. D. Robinson, Frederick	O. G. Bacon, Frederick	
Tulsa	James C. Peden, Tulsa	E. O. Johnson, Tulsa	Second and Fourth Monday
Washington-Nowata	J. G. Smith, Bartlesville	J. V. Athey, Bartlesville	Second Wednesday
Washita	A. S. Neal, Cordell	James F. McMurry, Sentinel	
Woods	C. A. Traverse, Alva	O. E. Templin, Alva	Last Tuesday Odd Months
Woodward	C. E. Williams, Woodward	C. W. Tedrowe, Woodward	Second Thursday

THE JOURNAL

OF THE

OKLAHOMA STATE MEDICAL ASSOCIATION

| VOLUME XXXVI | OKLAHOMA CITY, OKLAHOMA, JUNE, 1943 | NUMBER 6 |

The Medical Management of Diseases of the Gallbladder And Biliary Tract*

FRED C. REWERTS, M.D.

BARTLESVILLE, OKLAHOMA

Gallbladder disease as studied today presents difficulties not encountered in other of the common conditions. Correct diagnosis is often difficult and seldom early. The indications for medical or surgical treatment are variable, the morbidity and mortality are high, and the results of treatment are not uniformly good. Disease of the biliary tract, according to a survey recently made by Dean MacDonald, occurs twice as often as duodenal ulcer and ten times as often as gastric ulcer. It may be associated with either. Functional changes, or dyskinesias, which are just as real and more difficult of both diagnosis and treatment are not uncommon, and they present a problem which requires all the integrity, clinical acumen and judgment that one can call upon. It is so common that operations on the extra-hepatic system are, next to the appendix, the most common cause of operative interference in general practice. It seems rather strange that a condition so prevalent, and one whose operative treatment allows sufficient time for thorough study should have an average global mortality of from 12 per cent to 15 per cent. These facts would seem to warrant a more careful consideration of biliary tract disease and, wherever possible, to give these patients the advantages of the methods now in use for the study of the gallbladder, its functions and the basic changes which result in disease.

PHYSIOLOGY

Ivy states that the physiology of the gallbladder resembles in principle the general activities of the intestine; namely, absorp-

tion, secretion and motor activity. According to the classical concept, the viscus stores and concentrates much of the bile secreted by the liver during the interdigestive period in order to supply a store of concentrated bile at the beginning of the next digestive period and so to aid in the digestion and absorption of fatty foods in particular. This functional activity is made possible by the coordinated action of three types of primary activity mentioned above. The normal gallbladder concentrates the hepatic bile to a density of from four to ten times that of the original, principally by the absorption of water and inorganic salts so that the bile tends to come into osmotic equilibrium with the blood serum. In this process the bile is slightly acidified. The gallbladder proper forms only a small quantity of mucoid secretion, and in conditions of acute irritation it ceases to concentrate hepatic bile and instead, it pours out a secretion which may vary from normal bile. Because of these changes we find a great variation in the composition of bile in disease.

The gallbladder manifests two types of motor activity, one, a tonic contraction, produces a sustained rise in pressure for from five to 30 minutes. The other type might be called a tonus rhythm and is manifested by rhythmic contraction and relaxation occurring at the rate of from two to five times a minute. The actual evacuation of the gallbladder is the result of muscular contraction, and as has been demonstrated by Ivy, is brought about by this presence of fatty acids in the duodenum which form a hormone, cholecystokinin, the action of which is primarily to stimulate contraction and emptying of the gallbladder. Thus the importance of the sphincteric mechanism at the duo-

*Read before the Washington-Nowata County Medical Society, March 17, 1943.

denal end of the common duct is brought to mind. Pain may be brought about by contraction of the gallbladder concurrently with spastic obstruction in the intramural portion of the common duct. These observations made by Ivy, et. al., may explain the intolerance to fats which is a frequent complaint of patients with chronic cholecystitis. When one considers the several mechanisms and the precise integration of their action, which is necessary for normal function of the gallbladder and biliary tract, and the variety of influences which may affect one or the other, the existence of functional disorders of motility, the so-called biliary dyskinesias is not surpasing. The gallbladder and biliary tract seem to derive most of their inervation from the sympathetic chain, being derived from the motor cells of the semilunar ganglion of the coeliac plexus. There also exist connector fibers with the thoracic nerves of the fifth to ninth segments. The spinal system reaches the region through the phrenic, and phrenico-abdominalis, and its afferent impulses are carried back to the third and fourth cervical segment of the cord through the right phrenic, and thus may produce reflex pain in the right shoulder. The nervous regulation of the gallbladder itself is probably through vagus fibers which have a motor function and the sympathetic fibers which act as inhibitors. Vagus stimulation, therefore, would result in discharge of bile into the duodenum, while splanchnic stimulation would inhibit rhythmic contraction of the gallbladder and bring about a contraction of the sphincter of Oddi. It is on this basis that Lyon established the non-surgical drainage of the gallbladder.

The above physiological review, it is felt, will serve to give a better understanding of the principles of treatment which follow. Little mention will be made of acute cholecystitis as the great majority of these are surgical. The pre-operative treatment, however, in acute cases is important as is the judgment used in selecting the time for operation. The entire outcome of a case may depend on these two things. The signs and symptoms in these acute cases will often subside after adequate treatment with fluids, rest and the relief of pain. Occasionally these cases can be prepared for surgery in five or six days. Of course, a great deal depends on the individual, as to whether the case can be classed as a good surgical risk and whether the case is progressing satisfactorily under conservative management. An a t t e m p t should be made to individualize the treatment of each patient in acute cases.

CHRONIC CHOLECYSTITIS

These cases, with or without stones, comprise a vast majority of all diseases of the gallbladder and biliary tract. It is also in these cases without stones that surgical treatment is so often a failure, or at least does not yield good results. In the very efficient gallbladder clinic of the New York Post Graduate Hospital headed by Carter and Twiss on surgery and medicine respectively, it is the opinion of clinic members that surgery offers valuable assistance in the medical care of gallbladder disease by the removal of specifically inflamed ɔladders and the stones when the gallbladder is irreparably damaged. It is also the opinion of the members of this clinic that cholecystectomy rarely removes the basic cause for bile stasis, and dilation of the gallbladder and bile ducts which was originally productive of symptoms, and probably the cause of gall stones. Furthermore, that in spite of surgery in these patients, the need for specific medical therepy persists in the vast majority of cases after the removal of the gallbladder or stones in any stage of the disease. On the basis of this understanding of the problem, the surgeon is not held responsible for the failure to relieve symptoms after cholecystectomy for so-called chronic cholecystitis.

A majority of cases with indefinite pain in the right upper quadrant belong to the internist more often than the surgeon who can do little to relieve functional disturbances. Kraemer believes that the stoneless, diseased gallbladder is a medical problem and that these patients should be kept under observation for life. He warns against surgery in these cases except where the gallbladder becomes and remains functionless as evidenced by cholecystography. Gallbladders which will not empty usually have a strictured cystic duct and are surgical cases. Patients often get along more comfortably with adhesions about the gallbladder than they do following its surgical removal for attempted relief. The indications for medical treatment are (1) functional changes, (2) absence of stones, (3) neuresthenic temperaments associated with vague symptoms, and (4) poor risk patients.

TREATMENT: GENERAL CONSIDERATIONS:

The patients should be gotten into as good condition as possible. Regularity of meals, sleep, muscular and breathing exercises, bowel movements, sunshine, fresh air, etc., are most necessary. Over-eating and rapid eating, exhaustion and worry are to be avoided. Plenty of water and plenty of fruit juice are beneficial. Weight s h o u l d be brought to as near normal as possible, but care should be used to avoid rapid loss of weight, the safe rate of reduction should not exceed four to six pounds per month. Due attention should be given all foci of infection and their removal wherever possible. The benefits resulting from the discipline and relaxation of a well regulated and followed regime are great. Aside from general consideration mentioned above, special considerations must be given to diet. This is of paramount importance in medical treatment alone or pre-operatively and post-operatively.

DIETS

Diets often require individualization and are often determined on a trail and error basis. Atonic and hypertonic bladders do not respond to the same stimulus, and often such stimulation will produce pain in one instance and not in the other. In general, however, diets should be bland to prevent reflex symptoms and should contain sufficient bulk. Frequent feedings are often beneficial. The judicious use of fatty, but not greasy foods, at intervals will promote natural evacuation of the biliary tract. Egg yolk, olive oil and cream are good examples. Vitamin therapy should be adequate and the normal mineral requirements should not be disregarded. In general, low lipid diets may consist of two types; namely, (1) low cholesterol, low fat, low caloric, and (2) low cholesterol, low fat and high caloric. The indications for these are the same and are fat intolerance, cystic, duct obstruction, infection of the gallbladder or ducts, hypercholestermia, cholelithiasis and post-operative cholecystectomy. The only difference in these two diets lies in their calorific value—one being used in obesity and the second in cases of malnutrition, loss of weight and hepatitis. Bland hyperacidity diets are indicated in gastric hyperacidity, pylorospasm, duodenitis and functional disturbances of the biliary tract with colic. High lipid diets are indicated in functionally impaired or atonic gallbladders with biliary stasis, and where there is no obstruction of the cystic duct; no fat intollerance, infection of the biliary tract, cholelithiasis or obesity. High carbohydrate, low fat, low protein diets are indicated in all types of jaundice except hemolytic. These are important in pre-operative patients with dehydration or malnutrition.

Foods prohibited in all diets are: fried foods, fats, pork, shellfish, thickened gravies; all rich and highly seasoned foods; condiments, spiced and pickled foods, salad dressings; heavy cheeses, nuts, olives; pies, pastries, chocolate; alcohol and carbonated drinks; roughage, as cabbage, cauliflower, corn, brussels sprouts, cucumbers; bran and whole wheat products.

Meals should be small in amount and taken at the same time each day. Large meals are detrimental. Food should be chewed thoroughly. Rest of one-half hour after the noon and evening meal allows food to be more readily assimilated. The bowels should move every day after breakfast. Exercise such as walking and deep breathing stimulate the action of the gallbladder and liver. Except for those who are over-weight, eight glasses of water should be taken daily upon arising and between meals rather than with meals. Time does not permit mention of the specific foods represented in the above diets but these are readily found in any text book on treatment by diets.

DRUGS

These have as their chief value relief of spasm of the duct, duodenum or intestine, the prevention of non-mechanical stasis and, more rarely, sterilization of the tract. To date there is no satisfactory treatment for sterilization of the gallbladder or biliary tract, although the sulfonamide group of drugs, analine dyes, hexamine and vaccines may occasionally give a measure of relief and improvement. In most cases their value is doubtful. The most satisfactory results are obtained in the group of antispasmodic drugs, and their use in functional dyskinesias. Bellergal and belladenal tablets can, in most cases, be relied upon to give good results, and should be given about one-half hour before meals. Trasentin is often benificial. It should be remembered here that morphine, dilaudid, pantopon, codeine and hydrochloric acid cause an increase in the resistance of the spincter of Oddi. Morphine and its derivatives overcome the pain of spasms of the sphincter only through their sedative action on the central nervous system, as their local action is one of contraction. Intestinal and biliary stasis must be thoroughly treated and these are the most likely to respond to treatment. The more important correctable causes of biliary stasis are duodenal irritation, and the absence of normal stimulus, functional spasms and inactivity of the gallbladder. Occasionally the correction of colon stasis will result in the appearance of a shadow which was not previously visible before. It must not be forgotten that stasis usually precedes infection and reflex symptoms. For colon dysfunction equal parts of sodium phosphate, sodium sulfate and sodium bicarbonate will give excellent results given in doses of one teaspoonful, or more if required, before breakfast. If the hydrochloric acid of the stomach is deficient, as it often is, adequate doses of dilute hydrochloric acid given 15 minutes before each meal will frequently relieve the dyspepsia which is present in these cases.

Important also is the fact that other disturbances may co-exist, such as metabolic and glandular dysfunction. Thyroid gland is often of benefit and this with or without estrogens may often relieve the dyspepsia associated with the menapause.

Duodenal drainage prevents stasis by emptying the biliary tract, but is probably of more importance in diagnosis. Drainage into the duodenum is more successfully accomplished by the use of other methods such as dehydrocholic acid, egg yolk, cream, etc., and is much less trouble.

The patients with the more severe types of gallbladder disease are not always relieved satisfactorily by the above-mentioned measures. These often comprise those with severe persistent symptoms following cholecystectomy. If surgery were a cure all attended with no mortality, there would be no need for medical treatment. Surgery does not attack the problem at its root but only removes the end result. However, it is often indispensible and frequently brilliant in its result, so no quarrel is intended with surgery. However, it has been clearly demonstrated during the last few years that early recognition and proper medical care will, in the majority of cases obviate surgical procedures, by attacking and eliminating the factors which lead to the dead gallbladder and gall stones. There is no question in my mind that many needless deaths have occurred because of injudicious surgery on the gallbladder. It has often been done either to avoid the trouble of complete investigation or because of lack of available facilities for such investigation. Neither is excusable in my opinion. It is also just as readily admitted that conservative treatment based on unsound clinical judgment has often led to disasterous results.

SUMMARY

(1) The physiology and inervation of the gallbladder and biliary tract is reviewed briefly in order to give a better understanding of the principles of treatment.

(2) General and special consideration is given in regard to habits, exercise and diets. Dietary treatment is given in some detail but an attempt is made to avoid confusion. A few important drugs are mentioned together with their indications and pharmacological action.

(3) Advances in medical treatment in the past few years indicate that early recognition and proper treatment will, in a majority of cases prevent injury and death of the gallbladder, together with its attendant suffering and uncertainty.

CONCLUSION

In conclusion, it is not contended that medical treatment is on a satisfactory basis, but rather that more caution should be exercised in selecting cases for surgery, and that it is better to worry along, even if not so lucrative, with a troublesome case if surgery is not likely to prove beneficial. A plea is made for more active cooperation between the physician and surgeon, and the importance of thorough investigation of each patient as an individual is stressed. Shortcuts to diagnosis, never more tempting than they are today because of the war, must be avoided as much as possible in order to give these patients the benefits of the newer discoveries and methods now used in the modern treatment of biliary tract disease.

BIBLIOGRAPHY

1. Dean McDonald: The Canadian Medical Assoc. Journal. 45: 29-36. 1941.
2. Richard E. Ching, M.D.: Memphis Medical Journal. March, 1940.
3. Carter, Greene & Twiss: Diagnosis and Management of Diseases of the Biliary Tract. 1939.
4. Manfred Kraemer, M.D.: Journal of the Medical Society of New Jersey. 270-273. May, 1939.

A Simplified Treatment for Impetigo Neonatorum

CHARLES ED. WHITE, M.D.

MUSKOGEE, OKLAHOMA

In a recent outbreak of impetigo neonatorum in the nursery of one of our hospitals we were able to control the infection with the following regime, much better than any other method previously used.

The treatment of impetigo with the sulfathiazole drug is not particularly new. There are various methods of application such as ointment and crystals applied directly to the lesion. We found that by rupturing each new pustule that appeared on the infant with cotton saturated with green soap and then immediately dusting on powdered salfathiazole the infection was controlled in two or three days.

This treatment is not as efficacious if the crystals are used and it is important that the powder be applied before the green soap dries. The rupturing of the pustule with cotton saturated in green soap acts as a mild antiseptic which prevents the spread of the impetigo to the healthy tissue. We were very liberal in the application of the powder to these lesions and on some of the infants the skin was almost denuded in the folds of the neck, arms and buttocks.

There has been some question about the absorption of the sulfathiazole drugs when used as a topical application. No attempt was made to determine the amount or rate as there were no apparent side affects as far as we were able to observe. However in a recent application to a seven month premature of 2.2 pounds in weight the infant became very cyanotic. At first we attributed this to respiratory failure but a week later sulfathiazole was applied and it again became cyanotic. On removal of the drug the color cleared up. Therefore it is probably advisable to watch for absorption of sulfathiazole in prematures if the lesions are very extensive.

CONCLUSION

The use of powdered sulfathiazole and green soap was found to be the most effective means of controlling impetigo neonatorum. Its application should be watched for absorption in extensive lesions in prematures.

Treatment of Burn Cases Off The U.S.S. Wasp

R. G. JACOBS, M.D.*

ENID, OKLAHOMA

There have been many discussions and plans of procedure for the treatment of burns in the combat area, but unfortunately no definite type of therapy has been agreed upon. So it was with our medical company when we first set up our field hospital in the advanced base area in the New Hebrides. Prior to this we decided to treat all burn cases with 5 per cent sulfathiazole ointment made up by using lanolin and petrolatum as a base. We at least had a plan of attack.

Our organization on this Sunday was treating the many ailments of the Marines and doing all kinds of elective surgery, when suddenly we were ordered to prepare for an unknown number of severe burn cases from the U.S.S. Wasp. The first of the cases arrived at 17:00 and continued far into the night. Approximately 65 per cent were burns of the 1st and 2nd degree covering from 40 per cent to 70 per cent of the body surface.

The initial treatment used on the destroyers was tannic acid covered with gauze or cotton dressings. The latter was extremely difficult to remove.

As each case arrived a team of corpsmen and a medical officer rapidly but carefully removed the original bandage. The loose skin was removed and the denuded area was covered with a dressing composed of a 5 per cent sulfathiazole ointment. There was considerable loss of time in opening our sterile gauze strips and then applying the ointment much after the matter of spreading butter.

As these weeping wounds attracted clouds of large flies, the dressings were changed daily. Mosquito netting contributed greatly to the comfort of the patients. During the change of dressings two men were busy keeping away the flies.

Since speed in changing dressings was essential in the interest of the patient and because of the flies, a new method was devised in making the ointment dressings. Full length strips of three inch ordinary bandage rolls saturated in the ointment were placed layer upon layer in a small surgical tray. The ointment was smeared by hand in the cloth so as to saturate it. Tier upon tier of these layers were made until the tray was full. Two mounds of ointment dressings were placed in one tray and the space between the mounds was filled with free ointment to prevent drying out during sterilization. (Fig. 1). A mental cover was made from the top of a five gallon gasoline can, then covered with cloth and placed in a pressure sterilizer. This was autoclaved for ten to fifteen minutes under two hundred and twenty pounds of pressure.

It is a simple and fast maneuver using sterile forceps and straight scissors to cut off the desired length of ointment dressing and lay it on the burned area. Having learned that, in the war zone, patients come in large numbers and at the wrong time, we now have two large trays ready for emergency.

*Doctor Jacobs is now a Lieutenant Commander in the Navy and is presently stationed at U. S. Marine Corps, c/o Postmaster, San Francisco, California.

The black tannic acid protein crust was likewise covered with the ointment dressing and this prevented infection on the borders. The crusts were removed when no longer adherent. The face burns were covered with the free ointment several times each day.

Commander French R. Moore, MC, U.S. Navy, introduced and demonstrated the use of the femoral vein as the intravenous route

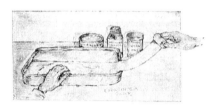

to give plasma. The other superficial veins in the severe burns were not available. Apparently the sailor's shorts and trousers give excellent protection in this area. The abdomen and thighs would be denuded but never that little triangle of skin in the inner groin.

A convalescent patient in each ward was detailed as "water boy" whose duty it was to force fluids every hour of the day and night. A free output of urine was thus assured.

Morphine was the great pain reliever. At first we give sulfa drugs by mouth, but this was discontinued because of the nausea and vomiting. We decided that it was more important that the fluid intake not be disturbed. Apparently the local sulfathiazole ointment was adequate, as there were no secondary infections.

The great value of plasma was clearly demonstrated in our series of cases. The severe cases were selected and they received from 1000 to 1750 cc daily for the first five days. At the onset all the medical officers individually made estimates on the probable mortality and the average figure arrived at was 16 per cent. We were extremely fortunate in having no deaths and we attribute this largely to the use of plasma.

We have found this simple method of preparing burn dressings efficient, time saving, and practical. The cooling effect of the ointment was comfortable and there were no infections. This excellent dressing is recommended to medical officers on destroyers and cruisers because they see these cases first, and because the great volume of war burns occur at sea.

The statements contained in this article are based upon the author's personal observations and do not reflect the views of the Navy Department.

NOTE: The author is indebted to B. M. Edwards, PhM1c, USN for the accompanying illustration and to E. E. Vanover, PhM1c, USN for typing.

A Consideration of the Kenny Treatment of Infantile Paralysis

D. H. O'DONOGHUE, M.D.

OKLAHOMA CITY, OKLAHOMA

The phrase "Sister Kenny" has much the same effect on a large group of our medical profession as the slogan "Erin go Brach" has on natives of the Emerald Isle. At one of our large national orthopedic meetings recently, we were treated to a debate on the Kenny method by well known and capable men, which progressed f r o m discussion through argument and dispute to actual recrimination and finally degenerated into expostulation, strangely reminiscent of the "tis—taint" of our boyhood days. What is it about this innovation that has such a volcanic effect upon ordinary sane and reasonable men of science? It is my opinion that the *method* of presentation has been greatly at

fault on the part of the proponents of the Kenny method, rather than the material presented. Certainly we should cultivate a healthy skepticism, but not the downright antagonism so often manifested by those opposing the Kenny method.

Let us analyze that statement for a moment and see if it cannot be clarified. The Kenny method was developed by Sister Kenny (the word Sister not designating any religious order, but rather representing a courtesy title given to an Australian bush nurse). Justifiably so, or not, Sister Kenny has antagonized a large group of the medical profession by a "chip-on-the-shoulder" attitude which refuses all accolades save the final one, and she has the utmost contempt for any previous method of treatment. She is a poor teacher, and completely intolerant of any opion save her own. Though her imperious attitude invites antagonism, it is my opinion, after considerable study and a minimum of observation, that the Kenny method offers a definite improvement in the management of infantile paralysis.

Sister Kenny insists that her method and the so-called orthodox method are as different as night and day, both as to concept of disease and as to treatment. In her mind, her idea is *revolutionary;* namely, casting aside everything which has gone before. To me, it is *evolutionary* and presents just another step foward in the comparatively short history of progress in the treatment of infantile paralysis.

To intelligently evaluate this treatment, we must have some idea as to the difference in concept of the disease between orthodox and Kenny. To over-simplify, let us list the comparative features of the two ideas:

Orthodox	Kenny
1. Virus disease	1. Virus disease
2. Cord affected	2. Cord affected
	a. Local involvement of muscle
3. Symptomatology	3. Symptomatology
a. General symptoms	a. General symptoms
—same	—same
b. Flaccid paralysis	b. Flaccid paralysis
c. Tender muscles	c. *Spasm*
d. Incoordination	d. *Incoordination*
e. Temporary and pseudo-paralysis	e. *Mental Alienation*

As can be seen from a glance at this outline, the three essential factors of the Kenny idea of infantile paralysis are *muscle spasm, incoordination,* and *mental alienation.* Thus, we find no essential difference in the cause, some difference in the primary pathology, but decided difference in the interpretation of symptoms. The Kenny idea does explain certain features that we have been all too glib about in the past. We have long known that soreness of muscles is one of the earliest symptoms in the disease, but have been vague as to its cause. Kenny predicates an actual involvement of the neuro-muscular end plate within the muscle, itself. This causes spasm

of the individual muscle fibers, not synchronously, but individually, with all of the fatigue phenomena attendant upon it. The result is not a muscle in contraction, but is an inelastic muscle not capable of useful contraction as a whole which is unable to shorten itself and, thus, cause functional motion of a joint. Sometimes there will be actual fibrillation of the muscle which can be demonstrated clinically.

"Mental alienation" is the term used to describe the well known phenomena that the stimulus of an hypertonic muscle will relax its opponent, thus, if the calf stays hypertonic long enough, the pathway to the dorsiflexor of the foot is lost and it cannot contract, thus, being alienated, or temporarily paralyzed. If continued long enough, this alienation becomes permanent and we have an apparently paralyzed muscle which is not, in itself, directly involved. We used to explain this by a theory that certain anterior horn cells were compressed enough to lose their function but not long enough to completely die. This theory was not proven pathologically and is not too tenable clinically. In the Kenny concept, the major involvement is in the muscle, itself, and the muscle is spastic and not flaccid; that is, the individual fibers are spastic. This is not the same as a contracted, or spastic muscle. Thus, the foot drop so commonly seen is due to calf muscle contracture and alienated dorsiflexors, rather than paralyzed dorsiflexors with the calf muscle shortening because it has no resistance from its opponent. The dorsiflexor muscle, itself, is normal. Its nerve pathway is is physiologically blocked but anatomically intact. So, too often, we have directed attention to the normal muscle, and ignored the involved muscle which is in spasm. Thus, we are able to account for the contracture deformity which is so common in infantile paralysis. The contracture is not a normal strong muscle overpulling a weak paralyzed one, but rather is a diseased muscle in spasm, shortening up and encountering no resistance from its alienated opponent.

As previously mentioned, incoordination has been long recognized and, indeed, often encouraged in some of its phases. It must not be confused with simple substitution in which a strong muscle takes over the job of a weak one voluntarily; thus, in substitution, the paralyzed hip may be flexed by voluntarily rotating the thigh externally and flexing it with the adductors. This is only one phase of incoordination. Much more often the incoordinate muscle is one that contracts, not rhythmically and smoothly, but jerkily, often attempting to carry out a motion for which it is not primarily intended. For example, flexing of the thigh by the rectus femoris muscle which actually should be an extensor of the knee. Under the Kenny concept, the "paralyzed muscle" is actually not paralyzed, but alienated; that is, the block is physiological and due to a sidetracking of impulses away from the alienated muscle. If this is true, it is obvious that substitution, or incoordination of function would add to alienation, since to overcome alienation, the normal rhythmic coordination between opposing muscles is a "sine qua non." For the hip flexor to contract smoothly, the extensor must relax. The contracting adductor muscle does not relax the extensor muscle. Therefore it makes a poor flexor since the synergistic action of the two muscles is lost.

Before we hasten on to consideration of treatment, let us again make a chart at the risk of a too gross simplification of the problem:

TREATMENT

Orthodox	Kenny
1. General care	1. General care
2. Rest	2. Rest
a. Bed	a. Bed
b. Splints	b. Foot board
c. Casts	
3. No local treatments	3. *Hot Packs*
4. Muscle training	4. *Muscle re-education*
5. Braces	5. *No braces*
6. Surgery	6. Surgery
7. Respirator	7. No respirator

The real essential difference here is the replacements of early support by hot packs which is based upon a different concept of the disease. Assuming local muscle pathology with muscle spasm, the alternate use of heating and cooling is certainly more rational management than is fixation. The Kenny concept does not deny flaccid paralysis, but it does assert that this is not the major involvement and even goes so far as to say that it is actually rare. The common condition, the one uniformly present, is direct involvement of the muscle, itself, with corresponding muscle spasm; whereas, the so-called paralyzed muscle is simply alienated. The application of support, therefore, not only prevents local treatment, but actually increases the muscle spasm by constantly irritating a hypersensitive muscle, since it is well known that

to keep tension on a muscle that is irritable or in spasm simply tends to increase its spasm (vide-ankle clonus). Local heat relaxes the spasm and prevents deformity.

Muscle re-education is a procedure that has been used in most clinics. The major change here is method, rather than concept. Sister Kenny is meticulous and wonderfully adept and patient with these children and the degree of difference between orthodox and Kenny muscle re-education will depend upon the degree of excellence of the physical theraphy previously practiced in each individual institution. Certain it is that the true Kenny method is painstaking and highly refined and will require highly trained personnel. The results will depend largely upon the extent to which each institution can approach the prefection of Sister Kenny's technique. Obviously, there will be various results in different places, since some technicians will be good and some bad. To my mind, the Achille's heel of the method is the necessity for depending upon inadequately trained, or uninterested personnel. Already, we have experienced this in cases supposedly treated by the Kenny method who had treatment only vaguely resembling the original Kenny technique.

Sister Kenny states categorically that the orthodox treatment is entirely wrong and that it does more harm. I believe sincerely that the Kenny method presents an outstanding advance in management of infantile paralysis. I am, however, equally convinced that with improper facilities and untrained personnel, the Kenny method will do more harm than good and that without appreciation of this fact by the physician, the method will rapidly fall into disrepute. "That which is worth doing at all is worth doing well." Given understanding and cooperation between physician, nurse, and physical therapist, the method seems ideal and, I believe, can be adapted to most situations. It behooves us to give this method a thorough trial with an open mind and with complete elimination of the personal factor.

Let there be no misconception, Sister Kenney has not presented us with a panacea. Her treatment, after all, is symptomatic and does not attack the cause. She has, however, given us a fresh viewpoint of certain features of the disease and above all, has stimulated thought along new lines which may ultimately permit us to approach the solution of this disease, as we have so many others, through its source. Until that goal is reached, the problem of infantile paralysis has not been solved.

In no profession does culture count for so much as in medicine, and no man needs it more than the general practitioner.—OSLER.

The Private Practitioner and the War Industry*

DONALD H. MACRAE, M.D., C.M.

OKLAHOMA ORDANCE WORKS

CLAREMORE, OKLAHOMA

Strickly speaking, this paper is not confined to a medical subject. It contains no gems of medical thought, nor does it set forth any astute observations resulting from meticulous research. Rather, it is a brief general discussion of some of the causes of Absenteeism in our War Industry. By War Industry, we mean collectively, the many types of industrial activity directly or indirectly essential to the war effort. As loyal Americans, you are interested in every cause of Absenteeism. As private practitioners of medicine, you are directly concerned with the medical aspects of Absenteeism, for it is here that you can play a vital role.

It might be said that in this war there are two armies: those on the fighting front and· those on the home front. A fighting army superbly equipped but ridden with disease is an ineffective army. Likewise, an industrial army crippled by illness or voluntary absence will produce little of the so-called sinews of war. The health of the armed forces is adequately protected by the several Medical· Corps. The health of the production army rests in large measure in the hands of private practitioners. You are part of the Medical Corps for the home army.

Modern warfare is waged with modern weapons, fabricated in modern factories and assembled on modern assembly lines. The armaments of yesterday, even of World War I, have given way to more complicated types of tanks, planes, munitions, surface and undersea craft and a multitude of intricate precision instruments. Our failure to produce these weapons of war, literally means death to thousands of our soldiers, sailors and marines and can bring defeat instead of victory. Absent workers do not produce.

Failure of the industrial army to remain on the job, is quite as serious as would be the refusal of our armed forces to face the enemy. The term Absenteeism signifies the collective absence of workers from the indus-

*Read before the Section on General Medicine, Annual Session, Oklahoma State Medical Association, May 12, 1943.

trial front, and includes justifiable as well as unjustifiable absence. It is sometimes called "The National Malady." Others call it "Desertion," an ugly word, but the slaughter of our troops or their incarceration in the prison camps of the enemy is also an ugly thing; utterly reprehensible if those deaths or imprisonment are a result of "Too Little and Too Late." In modern war, victory is not won by raw courage alone. It is won by courage plus the planes, tanks, guns and munitions which arrive in sufficient quantity and on time. Our enemy too has courage. To win we must out-produce him in death-dealing devices.

It is agreed by those who have made a thorough study of the subject that a normal absentee rate is 2.5 per cent of the working force, which can perhaps be considered the irreducible minimum. Compare this with an absentee rate of 20 per cent now being reported from some of our shipyards. Think of it! At a time when our nation is struggling for its very life, 20 out of every hundred workers are failing to report for work in some of our war industries. In reference to the shipyards· is it any wonder that the submarine packs of the enemy are causing the gravest concern in our highest military and governmental circles? Absentee rates in other war plants are somewhat better. The lost man hours flee never to be regained. Those badly needed tanks, guns, planes and ships which could have been produced are not. No victory can be won by ghosts or blueprints.

Let me cite for your consideration a few of the reasons, other than personal illness, given by chronic Absentees for their failure to stay on the job. These excuses are common to most plants and are not confined to one. Before I quote, it might be well to keep in mind a common finding—that the best attendance record is on payday and the worst the day following.

Here are a few of the non-illness excuses: "The hunting season has just opened, so I went hunting. I like to get out into the open."

"I earn more money now in four days than I ever earned in a week before. I can't buy a new car, so I took a trip."

"Transportation is pretty bad so I decided I wouldn't come to work for a few days."

"The tires on my car are bad, and I'm afraid to drive."

"I just had to get some shopping done."

"I went to the dentist."

"I don't like my foreman so I don't care whether I work or not."

"We have so many in our gang that I'm never missed so I stay at home to rest up."

"I had to see my rationing board."

"I guess I drank a little too much last night."

In all fairness to the workers, it is admitted that many war plants are located in areas where transportation is inadequate. Often the worker does need tires and his rationing board may be slow in granting him them or the tire quota for that month is used up. Housing facilities near many plant sites are grossly inadequate with landlords gouging the worker at high rents. In desperation, a worker takes a few days off in the faint hope of finding some suitable dwelling.

Nevertheless, most of the reasons cited above are due to poor morale on somebody's part. The hunter might well delay his hunting till after the war. The man who is making more money than he knows what to do with could siphon off his excess by purchasing War Bonds. The tire rationing board should make a special effort to provide the war worker with necessary tires. The transportation authorities might well attempt to provide more adequate facilities. The drinker should adjust his activities to these times which will not interfere with his work.

And so it goes. No one factor can be blamed nor can any one group of people be censured categorically. We, as physicians, from the specialized nature of our work, can do little to influence this side of Absenteeism, but we can do our bit in trying to bolster the general morale whenever the opportunity arises. In doing so we must look to our own personal morale. The worker must be convinced of the great importance of his job if this war is to be won with a minimum of delay.

Let us now consider the medical aspect of

Absenteeism. Recent surveys of war plants show that illness accounts for less than 50 per cent of Abenteeism; however, even less than 50 per cent of the lost time represents millions of lost man hours. Most of the illness is non-occupational, thus, as private practitioners you are the key man to the situation. The War Industry looks to you and needs your help in the treatment of non-plant-connected illness and injuries. In many plant-connected illnesses, too, the private practitioner is also called upon. It is interesting to note that accidents off the plant cause more lost-time than do plant injuries. At least this is the finding of one large insurance company whose accident percentages for 1943 are as follows:

Automobiles .... 16.68 per cent
At Home—Inside .... 25.26 per cent
At Home—Outside .... 15.81 per cent
Pedestrians .... 13.33 per cent
Sports and Recreation .... 20.85 per cent
Travel .... 2.79 per cent
Miscellaneous .... 5.28 per cent

In the miscellaneous group are included the lost-time injuries occurring in some of the largest war plants in the country for which this particular company is the carrier. Non-plant illness and off-the-plant accidents thus account for an overwhelming majority of Absenteeism due to illness. Therefore, these workers will be placed under the care of the private practitioner. Despite all of the health and safety programs fostered by the various industries always a certain number of workers will be ill. This is especially true when it is recognized that many oldsters and many physically handicapped persons are now being employed in war plants due to the loss of the best physical specimens to the Armed Forces.

Respiratory infection is the illness which causes the most lost time. Barring complications, the duration is usually limited to a few days. Perhaps you will be called to see the patient on but one occasion after which you lose contact. In such cases, assuming that you will see the patient but once, the golden opportunity for planting in his mind the desire to get back on the production line as quickly as possible should be grasped on the first visit. This can also be used as an argument for the patient's following your treatment orders explicitly which under ordinary circumstances many of them will not do. Naturally, if the patient is so ill that your fight talk would be disturbing to him, the probability is that you will visit the patient at a later date and can wield your influence during convalescence. Conversely, in the case of a patient who desires to return to work before he is well and whose too-early return would be conductive to a prolongation or exacerbation of his illness, it is in order to advise his remaining under treatment for a longer period.

Many of the war plants have a follow-up service by their Medical Departments. A physician or a nurse visits the employees who are absent because of illness. This investigation by the plant Medical Department in no way interferes with the function of the private practioner.

In reality it is a service designed to cooperate with the patient's physician and to help influence the patient to follow his physician's orders so that a speedy recovery may result. In our particular plant, a definite effort is made to discuss causes with the physician by phone, letter or personally. By pooling our information, plant Medical is in a better position to assist the private physician, and he, us. This is especially important in the case of a patient who has a tendency to be resistant to medical advice.

Inability to see a physician at night is another standard excuse for absence. Often it is the case of a worker who may have a non-incapacitating but annoying condition. He states that the reason he was absent on the day shift was because he was unable to locate a physician who kept night office hours, therefore, he took a day off to see one. In other cases, the employee was not ill himself but wished to accompany a sick wife or child to the doctor's office.

Consider another type of worker—the extremely conscientious one. He hates to lose time from work realizing that he is needed on the job. His condition is not disabling at the onset. Being on straight day shift his only free time is at night. Unable to find a physician he neglects his illness and finally may become incapacitated for a greater or lesser period because of the lack of simple, early care.

With most physicians overworked at present, it is desirable and indeed necessary that they obtain as much rest as possible because it is quite as important to keep the physician in good health as it is the worker in the factory. The provision of medical services in the evenings could, however, eliminate one excuse for absenteeism. To lighten the strain on physician, would it not be feasible for each County Medical Society to arrange for groups of its members to take night calls on certain nights. The number of physicians on call at any time, of course, would vary with the size of the community and the number of physicians available. A list of physicians who will be on duty on specified nights could be given to all war plants in the immediate vicinity for ready references. For the lone physician in an isolated community, there would appear to be no relief.

Another cause of lost time is the unnecessary prolongation of convalescence following certain surgical procedures. There is a case on record of an employee's leaving work without notifying his foreman or the Medical Department that he was ill. He could not be reached at his local address and none of his fellow workers would admit that they knew his whereabouts. A month after his first day of absence he wrote requesting sick benefits. He was in his home state several hundreds of miles away and had undergone an appendectomy. His disability, being certified by a licensed physician, entitled him to sick benefit payments. Another week or two passed, but the employee did not return. Several letters were sent to his surgeon asking for information and particularly whether there had been any complicating factors which would necessitate such a lengthy absence. Finally, one of the letters of inquiry was returned, and at the bottom, apparently written by the office girl, was the following, "It is my custom, following appendectomy, to allow the patient to return to office work only after eight weeks and to do physical labor only after three months." To say the least, that is rather a long convalescence from a simple appendectomy.

Another case that we heard about was that of a technical worker who was injured in an automobile accident. The injury was painful but no fracture or other evidence of severe injury was found. A rest period of a week seemed indicated and the worker was so instructed. During the week absence, a letter was received from this worker stating that his physician flatly ordered him to remain away from work for ten weeks. Although entitled to full salary, plus extra accident insurance, the employee wrote that he knew he could do his work and would return the following Monday. He did so without further disability. Nine unnecessary weeks of losttime of a critically-needed war worker were saved.

These last two cases are extreme, I must admit, and fortunately in the minority. They serve a purpose, however, by giving you a better idea of some of the diverse problems encountered by the war plants in relation to Absenteeism.

The classical three months of convalescence for simple hernia repair, without complications, which some surgeons still feel is necessary, has been proven in many cases to be unwarranted. We have seen a great number of these cases return to work six weeks from date of operation. Following an initial period of a few days of rather light work, the worker has been able to do even the heaviest type of labor. We have followed several such cases for over a year and feel that the results have been excellent.

If you have a patient whose health you think is being affected by his work, feel free to discuss the case with the plant Medical Supervisor. Many workers wittingly or unwittingly give their private physician an erroneous idea in regard to the hazards of their jobs. A phone call or a letter to the plant Medical Superintendent will usually clear up a misunderstanding. Conversely, if a patient has not reported to plant Medical and does have an occupational condition, we would be more than grateful for your information. The causative condition can frequently be eliminated or controlled for the benefit of all workers in that area.

Briefly, I have tried to bring to your attention the subject of Absenteeism, its adverse effect on war production, and the opportunity of the private practitioner to play a specific part. You and I know that organized medicine has always given fully of its time and skills in the hour of emergency as well as during the less spectacular times of peace. We have been sorely and unwarrantedly criticized in certain quarters. Let us give our critics no opportunity to say that we are not doing our duty, in this, the hour of our country's greatest peril.

DISCUSSION
PAUL B. RICE, M.D.
OKLAHOMA CITY, OKLAHOMA

Dr. McCrae has discovered the problem of absenteeism in War Plants very fully. I think that the average practitioner needs only to understand these problems in order to cooperate fully.

The war has changed all rules and, in some measure, we are deprived of the greatest of all therapeutic agents, rest. We are now keeping employees on the job who would be put to bed in normal times. For example: a few weeks ago at our own plant, we had an employee who sustained a fracture of the middle one third of both bones of the forearm. This man was sent to an orthopedic specialist for reduction and cast. He was back on the job the next day, losing a total of six hours working time. Again, we have in injury common to airplane plants where there is contusion to the end of a finger with laceration through the nail and a compound comminuted fracture of the distal phalanx. Such an injury is repaired and the employee sent back to work in a couple of hours.

All this is new to both the patient and the private physician. We will appreciate your cooperation, and we will assure you that when rest is really necessary your patients will be encouraged to take it.

We keep repeating to our employees that "they are in a war," and in spite of "Hell and high water," production must roll. We are employing a new class of people, many of whom have never worked before and they find the strain terrific. We see more neurotics than we do injuries and our difficulties will be repeated in your private practice. Our difficulties are increased by the fact that our workers are frozen on the job, and they must get a release in order to take a new job. They have found that about the only way to do this is to convince the Personnel Department that their employment is affecting their health. We are all hearing weird tales about nervousness, loss of weight, etc., from employees who are dissatisfied or restless. The pressure is even stronger on private physicians than on those in industry. I think a united front of the medical profession is necessary to stamp out this evil. When your patient comes in with a statement from you that his work is affecting his health, we cannot do much else but release him. I suggest that it might be better to set down y o u r physical findings and let the plant physician draw what conclusions are necessary.

Finally, I think that we should all remember that war plant workers have Rhinitis and Pharyngitis from colds as well as from plant dust; that some may have had skin eruptions even before they started working in war plants; and that they do develop Lumbago and Sciatica as well as Industrial Back Sprain. A chance word from his physician may plant a phobia in a worker's mind that can never be eradicated.

The informed cooperative influence of private physicians can be of enormous value to the efficient operation of our war plants.

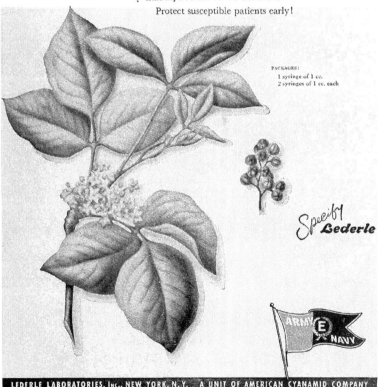

· THE PRESIDENT'S PAGE ·

For obvious reasons, it seemed best to appoint no physicians serving in the armed forces on Committees of the Oklahoma State Medical Association this year except on the Military Affairs Committee. This has thrown an additional burden on our members at home. I am deeply grateful to the many of you who have cheerfully accepted another responsibility.

Several of us attended the recent American Medical Association meeting in Chicago as interested spectators. A determined effort was made by a number of Delegates, including those from Oklahoma, to establish an Office of Information in Washington, D. C. similar to those now maintained there by the American Dental and the American Hospital Associations.

The Committee of the House of Delegates to which was referred the above proposal, at an open meeting, listened to the arguments presented in favor of the plan, but proposed a substitute which was adopted by the House of Delegates. This substitute sets up a new Council on Medical Service and Public Relations. It is hoped that this new council will be aggressive in the field of public relation, as well as in its study of the economic, social and other aspects of medical care for all the people.

Being held in conjunction with the House of Delegates, was the second meeting of the Council on Prepaid Medical and Surgical plans that has been established by State and Territorial Medical Associations.

This meeting brought together, for discussion of their mutual problems, the directors of these plans, and the information gained from the meeting was of exceptional interest in two major instances. One being that the plans succeeded in direct ratio to the interest and support of the medical profession and secondly that enrollment procedures could not be based upon any set rules but could be made adaptable to any condition when there was cooperation between the employer, employee and the plan. It was also pointed out that, mainly, the greatest problems were attendant to medical plans rather than surgical.

Certainly the plan to be inaugurated in Oklahoma by our own Association can profit from the experiences of these pioneer plans.

Sincerely yours,

James Stevenson

President.

The JOURNAL Of The
OKLAHOMA STATE MEDICAL ASSOCIATION

EDITORIAL BOARD

L. J. MOORMAN, Oklahoma City, Editor-in-Chief

E. EUGENE RICE, Shawnee

NED R. SMITH, Tulsa

MR. R. H. GRAHAM, Oklahoma City, Business Manager

EDITORIALS

THE DEVELOPMENT OF PUBLIC HEALTH

The basic principles of public health were developed in the first half of the nineteenth century. Their origin and evolution resulted from many converging influences. A careful analysis of these influences leads to the conclusion that some of them were selfish and some were wholly unselfish. It may be said that necessity, the prolific mother of invention, initiated national and international health regulations. Asiatic cholera invading Europe and America in the eighteen thirties served as the first great motivating calamity. Heinrich Heine described its catastrophic course in Paris with lurid effect, and observed the ever recurring obstacle in the way of public health progress; viz., "The dread of disturbing private business."

This great awakening came on the eve of a great mechanistic and industrial movement which, with steam transportation, brought about rapid urbanization. The latter soon called attention to the evils of poverty plus over-crowding, bad housing, poor sanitation and inadequate nutrition. The obvious rise in morbidity and mortality rates caused public concern, which, in turn, led to the creation of government agencies committed to the task of bringing about better social and hygienic conditions in the home, in the community and in industry. This was a laborious undertaking because of the diffidence and ignorance of the people and the opposition of industry.

The need for education of both the low and the high was obvious. In this connection, Fielding H. Garrison[1], after referring to other spiritual and educational influences, makes this significant statement "Through the efforts of such great writers as Charles Dickens, Charles Reade, Thomas Carlyle, Goethe (Mignon) and Victor Hugo (Cosette), it began presently to be perceived that the real wealth of a nation is its population, as Johann Peter Frank had originally maintained."

But it required persistent educational efforts on the part of the medical profession to show that the preservation of the population is dependent upon private and public medicine. No doubt the most powerful initial factor and the most effective influence in the marvelous development of the public health program came through interested members of the medical profession. It may be said that this unselfish contribution of the medical profession began with Tuke, Pinel, Riel and Benjamin Rush, who plead for more humane treatment of the insane. In fact, the whole public health program has been leargely motivated by the dominating spirit of medicine which is based upon "the primal sympathy of man for man."

In private practice and in the field of public health, doctors have put the patient and the public above their own private interests. Garrison[2] has said "It is to the credit of modern medicine that, in spite of intense competition, thousands of physicians have continued to practice their profession along the old honorable lines, giving largely and nobly of their time to the poor, although, in the crowded streets of finance, a man whose heart is better than his head is a fool by definition. The most enlightened physicians of today are advancing preventive medicine, which tends to do away with a great deal of the medical practice." Supplementing this, we quote the following from J. B. Nichols[3]: "Certainly men who regularly render a large part of their services gratuitously and are constantly striving to eradicate their own means of livelihood cannot be convicted of being altogether mercenary."

BIBLIOGRAPHY

1. Garrison, Fielding H.: An Introduction to the History of Medicine. 1924. Page 798.
2. Garrison, Fielding H.: An Introduction to the History of Medicine. 1924. Page 772.
3. Nichols, J. B.: "Medical Sectarianism," Wash. Med. Ann., 1918, xii, 12.

UNITED STATES OR APPALACHIAN

Just as we had bound our hands in charity's bonds, the Chamber of Commerce of the United States created its National Health Advisory Council for the consideration of the nation's health in connection with the war program. Twelve noteworthy physicians were named as members of the council. Ten of them hail from the Appalachians, one from Mississippi and one from Minnesota. When we think of the great middlewest, the southwest and the far west, and when we consider the relative importance of these sections of the country in the production of raw materials, food supplies, the training of our army and navy personnel, the production of the implements of warfare and our responsibility with reference to the health of our men in training, our civilian population and our natural exposure to all the tropical and oriental health problems, the quality of charity is so strained that we free our hands in behalf of just demands.

On the principle of no cooperation without representation, the Chamber of Commerce of the United States would find its operations limited to the eight states represented on its council and the District of Columbia. Doctors are so prone to spurn personal and political preferment that they will participate in the program without hampering prejudicies, but there is a clinging sense of unjust discrimination and our consciousness of the Chamber's lack of vision. The Chamber of the United States, designated to deal with less generous groups and less humane problems than those having to do with medicine, will never gather all her chicks unless she learns to spread her administrative wings westward.

If we, in the west, should withhold our cooperation and our commerce, the Chamber's chances for more stately mansions would be sadly shattered. If our natural resources were blatted out, our training camps closed, our war industries discontinued, the war program would suffer a serious setback. Finally, if it were not for our fair weather, our far flung horizons and our blue sky, how would our American youth ever learn to fly?

ONE WORLD*

When one travels around the world with Wendell L. Wilkie, he realizes that through improved intercommunications and transportation, both speeded by present emergencies, world dimensions rapidly dwindle. But, the load on the shoulders of Atlas has not been correspondingly lightened and unless we find some way to steady the rocking old sphere, we may experience a tremendous crash.

Mr. Wilkie's observations on the spiritual, political and economical trends in the various countries visited are most interesting. They are important to the medical profession because they take into account the value of modern medicine, including sanitation and public health. In addition, the author calls attention to the value of medical education abroad, sponsored by American agencies, and the influence of medical missionaries as emissaries of good will. The references in regard to health conditions encountered by Mr. Wilkie and his party definitely imply recognition of the superior medical service, sanitation and public health which they have become accustomed to in the United States.

Of far greater interest to the medical profession is the fact that his panacea for a sick world represents a formula which is largely composed of the principles laid down in the Hippocratic oath. This leads Mr. Wilkie to recommend international relationships similar to those prevailing between patient and doctor in all countries where personal freedom still lives. In other words, the author stresses the art, as well as the science of government.

*ONE WORLD. By Wendell L. Wilkie. Simon and Shuster, New York. 1943.

No one can accurately plan a post-war international program, but speculative dreaming based upon the privilege of individual thought and the freedom of personal initiative, is most hopeful.

THE LURE OF OVERTIME

The inconsistency of the forty-eight hour rule for seasoned laborors and the optional, unlimited overtime, especially for the novice, is not consistant with the government's concern about so-called better medical service for all the people.

Many ambitious workers in war industries are developing tuberculosis and other disabling conditions through the physical and mental strain resulting from excessive overtime and holiday work in order to draw time-and-one-half and double pay.

The highest type of medical service is the prevention of disease. In connection with the government's attitude toward the medical profession, many difficult questions arise. But there is one which the man in the street can answer with assurance. It may be stated as follows: Compared with the members of the medical profession, what does the bureaucrat know about the cause, prevention and cure of disease?

THE GOOD PHYSICIAN

"It is not my purpose, however, to go into a discussion of the methods of treating functional disturbances, and I have dwelt on the subject only because these cases illustrate so clearly the vital importance of the personal relationship between physician and patient in the practice of medicine. In all your patients whose symptoms are of functional origin, the whole problem of diagnosis and treatment depends on your insight into the patient's character and personal life, and in every case of organic disease there are complex interactions between the pathologic processes and the intellectual processes which you must appreciate and consider if you would be a wise clinician. There are moments, of course, in cases of serious illness when you will think solely of the disease and its treatment; but when the corner is turned and the immediate crisis is passed, you must give your attention to the patient. Disease in man is never exactly the same as disease in an experimental animal, for in man the disease at once affects and is affected by what we call the emotional life. Thus, the physician who attempts to take care of a patient while he neglects this factor is as unscientific as the investigator who neglects to controll all the conditions that may affect his experiment. The good physician knows his patients through and through, and his knowledge is bought dearly. Time, sympathy, and understanding must be lavishly dispensed, but the reward is to be found in that personal bond which forms the greatest satisfaction of the practice of medicine. One of the essential qualities of the clinician is interest in humanity, for the secret of the care of the patient is in caring for the patient."—Doctor and Patient by Francis W. Peabody, M.D.

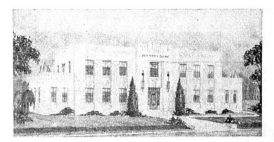

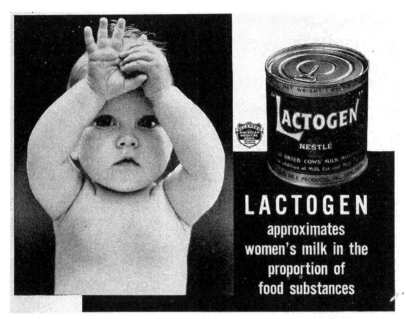

LACTOGEN
approximates
women's milk in the
proportion of
food substances

The cow's milk used for Lactogen is scientifically modified for infant feeding. This modification is effected by the addition of milk fat and milk sugar in definite proportions. When Lactogen is properly diluted with water it results in a formula containing the food substances—fat, carbohydrate, protein, and ash—in approximately the same proportion as they exist in woman's milk.

No advertising or feeding directions, except to physicians. For feeding directions and prescription blanks, send your professional b l a n k to "Lactogen Dept." Nestle's Milk Products, Inc., 155 East 44th St., New York.

> "My own belief is, as already stated, that the average well baby thrives best on artificial foods in which the relations of the fat, sugar, and protein in the mixture are similar to those in human milk."
>
> John Lovett Morse, A. M., M. D.
> Clinical Pediatrics, p. 156.

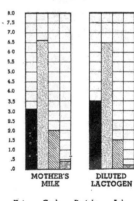

MOTHER'S MILK   DILUTED LACTOGEN

Fat   Carb.   Protein   Ash

ASSOCIATION ACTIVITIES

Official Proceedings of House of Delegates
Oklahoma State Medical Association
May 10-11, 1943, Oklahoma City

MINUTES OF FIRST SESSION
Monday, May 10, 1943

The 51st Annual Meeting of the Oklahoma State Medical Association was officially opened Monday, May 10, 1943, at 8:30 p.m., with a meeting of the House of Delegates in the Crystal Room, Skirvin Hotel, Oklahoma City. The House of Delegates was called to order by the Speaker of the House, Dr. George H. Garrison, Oklahoma City, and the roll call showed a majority of delegates present.

On *motion* by Dr. James Stevenson, Tulsa, seconded by Dr. Claude S. Chambers, Seminole, and *carried*, the minutes of the meetings of the House of Delegates held on April 22 and 23, 1942, were *approved* as published.

Following the adoption of the above motion, the Speaker, in compliance with the provisions of Chapter III, Section 4, Subsection (a), of the By-Laws, appointed the following Reference Committees: *Resolutions Committee*—Dr. W. A. Showman, Tulsa, Chairman; Dr. L. E. Woods, Chickasha, and Dr. W. M. Gallaher, Shawnee. *Sergeant-at-Arms*—Dr. Claude S. Chambers, Seminole, Chairman, and Dr. J. T. Phelps, El Reno. *Tellers and Judges of Elections*—Dr. R. E. Cowling, Ada, Chairman; Dr. Virginia Olson Curtin, Watonga, and Dr. M. A. Connell, Picher.

Following the appointment of the above committees, the following guests were introduced who, in turn, acknowledged their introduction by expressing appreciation for the privilege of being present. Mr. C.P. Loranz, Secretary-Manager of the Southern Medical Association, Birmingham, Alabama; Mr. N. D. Helland, Executive Director of Group Hospital Service in Oklahoma, Tulsa, and Mr. Jack Spears, Executive Secretary of the Tulsa County Medical Society.

At this time, the Speaker, in compliance with the provisions of Chapter VII, Section 3, of the By-Laws of the Association, called for the reports of Officers.

Upon request of the President of the Association, Dr. J. D. Osborn, Frederick, Mr. R. H. Graham, Executive Secretary, read the Report of the Council.

Report of the Council

Since the last report of the Council to the House of Delegates, the medical profession has gone to war. A war that, from the health standpoint, must be fought on two major fronts—the home and military, and both of equal importance.

Records of the Procurement and Assignment Service and those of the Association show 491 Oklahoma physicians in the armed forces with 332 being members of the Association. To these men the council pays homage, with a sincere appreciation of the sacrifices they are making and charges every member of the Association with the individual responsibilty of protecting the practices of these men to the end that they may return to as normal a life as humanely possible. It pledges its activities to that end without equivocation.

The activities of the Association, during the past year, are reflected in the reports of its committees that have been published in the April Journal and those that will be made during the sessions of the House of Delegates. For this reason, the Report of the Council will be limited to a report and recommendations of the finances of the Association and future activities.

The finances are in satisfactory condition. There is an operating reserve fund in the membership account of $4,058.09, which is an increase of $1,827.52 over that of 1942. The Journal account also shows an increase in operating reserve of $487.21 in excess of the reserve on hand at the end of last year. In addition to these cash balances, the Association owns unencumbered $1,235.78 in U. S. Treasury Bonds payable to the membership account and $8,163.10 in Treasury and Defense Bonds payable to the medical defense account, the latter cannot be used in the operation of Association activities. With this condition existing, the Council recommends that the dues for 1944 remain the same as 1943 ($12.00), and that no dues be charged members of the armed forces. For a detailed analysis of the finances of the Association, the Delegates are referred to the Audit published in the April Journal.

The budget of the Association for the coming year, as prepared by the Secretary-Treasurer, has been approved by the Council, and no increases have been recommended for any one expenditure with the exception of the salaries of the Editor in the amount of $600.00 and Miss Betche for the same amount. The raise in salary for Miss Betche is due to her additional activities with the Procurement and Assignment Service, and will be paid in the majority by that service. Decreases have been made in the majority of other items of expense.

Concerning the operation of the medical defense account, which is maintained by the placing of $1.00 of each member's dues to the account, the Council recommends that the account be stabilized in the amount of bonds now on hand plus an operating cash reserve of $500.00. This recommendation is made on the basis that, during the last five years, there has never been a single year when the fund has expended in excess of $300.00. This recommendation, in no way, limits the amount which may be paid out in excess of the $500.00 as, should this condition present itself, the cash operating fund would be augmented from moneys in the membership account. The Council also recommends that this action be retroactive to January 1, 1943.

Future programs to be undertaken by the Association during the war, in the opinion of the Council, should be limited to those that will directly contribute to the war effort and economic problems confronting the profession. These efforts will naturally be divided between the home and war fronts.

The Council recommends that the Executive Office of the Association and the appropriate committees continue to give full and complete cooperation to the American Medical Association and the Procurement and Assignment Service with reference to physicians entering the military forces. It is further recommended that the House of Delegates go on record as approving the appointment of a special committee by the President to study and prepare for the return of the physicians now serving in the military forces—this committee to consider the problems of locations and postgraduate education as part of its study. The latter recommendation to be correlated with the Postgraduate Medical Teaching Committee, which has a full-time director and office assistant.

Activities of the Association, through its county societies, must be broadened to cover the problems of pub-

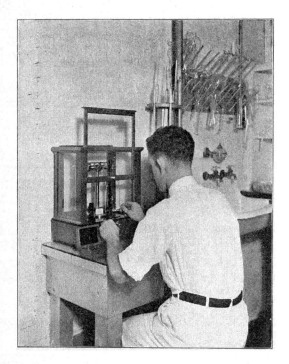

lic health whether political, economic or scientific. Aggressive leadership is imperative and should extend from the individual physician through the County, State and American Medical Association. The House of Delegates is admonished that the true effect of the Association in the protection of the health of the public is in direct ratio to the activities of the county societies.

Your Council, this year, in making its annual report, has changed its past procedure concerning recommendations of further activities, and will this year offer them as resolutions in order that the House of Delegates will give greater consideration and discussion to them.

The following resolutions are herewith submitted to the Resolutions Committee without recommendation unless otherwise stated in the resolution. The Council does, however, request that the Resolution Committee announce a place and time of meeting in order that any member of the Association may appear to speak on any resolution. (Resolutions recommended by the Council are listed here by title and may be found in complete form in the proceedings of Tuesday morning, May 11: American Medical Association Journal, Activities of the American Medical Association, Amendment to Constitution American Medical Association, Medical Education, Commonwealth Fund, Institute on Industrial Health, Public Health Department, Continuation of Postgraduate Course, Expression of Appreciation and Civilian Medical Care.)

In concluding its report, the Council urges that the Delegates give special consideration to the reports of the following committees: Prepaid Medical and Surgical Service, Malpractice Insurance and Public Health, as these committee reports, if accepted, will establish certain principles which will be binding upon the Council and Officers of the Association.

It is the considered opinion of the Council that as many Officers of the Association as possible, who feel that they can, attend the House of Delegates of the American Medical Association being held in Chicago, June 7-9, in order that they may acquaint themselves with the war program to be participated in by the profession.

The Council desires to compliment and commend the individual committees for their work during the past year. Had it not been for this cooperation, the work of the Association would have been seriously hampered.

The House of Delegates may be assured that, in the year to come, your Council will render service to the Association to the best of its ability constantly keeping in mind its obligation and heritage.

Upon completion of the reading of the Council Report by Mr. Graham, the Chairman called for approval of the report not in resolution form.

On *motion* by Dr. A. S. Risser, Blackwell, duly seconded by Dr. F. W. Boadway, Ardmore, and *carried*, the Report of the Council was *accepted*.

At this time, the Chairman stated that he would entertain a motion for the acceptance of the Councilor Reports of Districts No. 1, 8, and 9, as published in the April issue of the Journal, if there were no objections to the contrary.

On *motion* by Dr. H. K. Speed, Sayre, seconded by Dr. V. C. Tisdal, Elk City, and *carried*, it was moved that the three above-named reports be *accepted* as printed in the Journal.

Following this action, Dr. Garrison asked for the report of Councilor District No. 2, and Dr. V. C Tisdal, Elk City, was recognized and presented his report.

Annual Report District No. 2

Officers and Members of the House of Delegates
Of the Oklahoma State Medical Association
Gentlemen:

District No. 2, which consists of nine counties, brings you the following report of the state of conditions existing among the county societies and doctors.

We are pleased to report that the county societies are functioning with a stable degree of enthusiasm and a desire for medical advancement in the way of knowledge of both state and national affairs pertaining to medicine, and has been materially advanced since our district meeting which was so well attended by the officers of the State Medical Association, our President, Dr. J. D. Osborn, and President-Elect, Dr. James Stevenson. We were honored by the presence of a number of our men in the service who gave us encouraging reports of the work being done by the medical personnel in our armed forces.

There is a progressive and patriotic atmosphere demonstrated in all of our meetings, and the harmony in our district is worthy of imitation in any district in the state. With few exceptions, the doctors are sufficient to care for the actual work that is demanded of them.

Only a few years ago, the Oklahoma State Medical Association realized the importance of having the services of an executive secretary. We are unable to measure the results and achievements accomplished by this advanced step in our state Association. After a rather extensive survey of the membership of District No. 2, we feel, that under the stress of the time, we should have a like representation in our national capital—that a permanent office should be established there. We feel that, with the information brought to us by our President during our district meeting, it is only fair to our national government and to the doctors at home that we are due representation by the strongest individual that it is possible to secure.

We know that the American Dental Association, the American Hospital Association and every other organization that is serving suffering humanity and is a public necessity has representation that can give Congress the proper information in Washington. Such a service to our national Congress has been advocated by some of our senators and representatives, advocating a well-informed physician or a shrewd lawyer. We have been told that the A. M. A. leadership, still jittery about the defeat that was given them at the hands of the Supreme Court, absolutely refused to be involved. We are of the opinion that one defeat in battle or six defeats in battle should not deter us from having such a representation on a high and ethical plane disseminating information we can offer that will be a service to the masses.

Therefore, it is our sincere belief since our State Medical Association is made up of men who have pioneered in the fields of development and have achieved the degree of success that is visible to our nation that we, as a body, recommend to the Delegates to the American Medical Association that they demand a foward step sponsored by the American Medical Association or an association recommended by said body and that immediately have proper representation in our national capital for the following reasons:

1. There is so much of vital concern to the physicians that is taking place in our national capitol these days that we need representation on the spot to supply reliable information to our Congressmen and to our doctors at home.

2. Such representation might also play an important part in influencing the decisions affecting medicine.

3. That our National Congress is desirous of serving the medical profession to the best interest of the public.

4. That experience in our own state has proved the feasibility of having a public relations committee in our law making body.

It is our recommendation that in case the A. M. A. sponsorship is impossible that they, the Delegates to the American Medical Association, could consider the endorsement of the National Committee on Medical Service or the National Physicians Committee or a specially created association led by the legislative committeemen of state and county medical societies. In any event, the office would be financed by the U. S. doctors in gen-

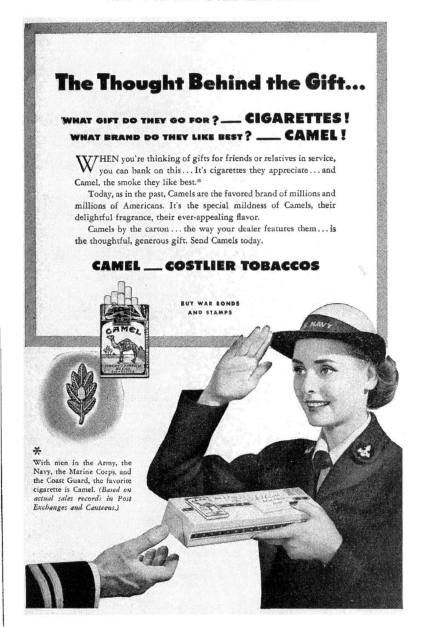

eral, either through voluntary contributions or by increases in medical society dues.

> Respectfully submitted,
> V. S. Tisdal, M. D.,
> Councilor, District No. 2

On *motion* by Dr. H. K. Speed, seconded by Dr. J. M. Bonham, Hobart, and *carried*, it was moved that the Report of Councilor District No. 2 be *adopted*.

The Councilor of District No. 3, Dr. C. W. Arrendell, Ponca City, was next granted the privilege of the floor and made his report.

Annual Report District No. 3

To the President and House of Delegates
Oklahoma State Medical Association
Gentlemen:

The Third Councilor District wishes to report satisfactory progress during the past year. Garfield, Payne and Kay Counties have seen almost one-third of their membership go into military service, and this naturally meant longer, harder hours for those remaining at home. However, this has not prevented their regular and enthusiastic attendance at monthly meetings. The quality of their programs has been excellent and stimulating. The Garfield County Medical Society is doing an especially commendable thing in publishing a monthly bulletin. The doctors who realize the value of this project and give their time to its preparation and editing deserve unstinted praise.

The roster of members in the other four counties of the district; namely, Grant, Noble, Major and Pawnee counties, is so small that it is impractical to maintain active societies. However it might be suggested that the doctors in these counties, individually and/or collectively, join in the activities of their neighboring societies. The county medical society is the unit of organized medicine, and it, therefore, follows that organized medicine will be only as strong as its weaker units. Doctors working as individuals have little influence in shaping the course of things to come; however, when the voice of the majority becomes the voice of the whole membership, then and then only will the members of this profession feel the security of their position in this turbulent world.

> Respectfully submitted,
> C. W. Arrendell, M. D.,
> Councilor, District No. 3.

On *motion* by Dr. R. E. Cowling, Ada, seconded by Dr. G. S. Baxter, Shawnee, and *carried*, the Report of Councilor District No. 3 was *accepted*.

Following the report of Dr. Arrendell, the Speaker called for the Report of Dr. Tom Lowery, Oklahoma City, Councilor of District No. 4. The Executive Secretary read the report of Dr. Lowry.

Annual Report District No. 4

Members of the House of Delegates
Oklahoma State Medical Association
Gentlemen:

The Councilor for the Fourth District reports that the component County Societies of this District are in good condition. Due to illness, the Councilor was able to attend only a few of the county meetings in his district; however, he was kept informed of the proceedings of these societies through the office of the Executive Secretary, and is glad to report progress.

> Respectfully submitted,
> Tom Lowry, M. D.,
> Councilor, District No. 4.

On *motion* by Dr. Claude S. Chambers, seconded by Dr. Clinton Gallaher, Shawnee, and *carried*, the Report of Councilor No. 4 was *approved*.

The Speaker next asked for the report of the Councilor from District No. 5, and Dr. J. I. Hollingsworth, Waurika, was granted the floor.

Annual Report District No. 5

Members of the House Of Delegates
Oklahoma State Medical Association
Gentlemen:

The Fifth District is rather behind in its activities.

Outside of visiting a county society or two and a Tri-county Meeting in Waurika in February, consisting of Cotton, Stephens and Jefferson counties, the Fifth District has lain practically dormant. When one puts on a big feed, free mind you, and can't get over 12 including the guest speakers in three counties to attend, things are getting a little low in enthusiasm.

As Councilor, I had planned at least three district meetings this year, one at Lawton, one at Chickasha and one at Ardmore, but met with such poor encouragement that the idea was abandoned, especially after the Tri-county failure.

Most doctors have really been busy in my District, and I don't think the majority of them are too enthusiastic about meetings at this time.

For the past six weeks, we have been having lectures in several cities in District No. 5 by Dr. L. W. Hunt of Chicago on Internal Medicine. They have been interesting as well as enlighting. Dr. Hunt is an able speaker and we are to be congratulated on having him.

I am making no promises for next year, but we are going to have a District meeting if none goes but the Councilor of the Fifth District.

> Respectfully submitted,
> J. I. Hollingsworth, M. D.,
> Councilor, District No. 5.

On *motion* by Dr. W. S. Larrabee, Tulsa, duly seconded by Dr. Galvin L. Johnson, Pauls Valley, and *carried*, the Report of Councilor District No. 5 was *accepted*.

At this time, the Chair called for the report of the Councilor from District No. 6, and privilege of the floor was granted to Dr. J. V. Athey, Bartlesville, who presented his report.

Annual Report District No. 6

Officers and Members of House of Delegates
Of Oklahoma State Medical Association
Gentlemen:

I am glad to report that the societies in District No. 6 seem to have carried on according to schedule, in spite of handicaps brought about by the war time dislocations. Your Councilor has visited all of the counties and has met with all the societies except one. This exception was due to a conflict in, and unforeseen change in, dates.

No report has come to me of lack of harmony. The various meetings have been held regularly, and interesting and instructive papers have been presented. Following is a report of the individual county societies:

Osage

In addition to regular meetings through the year with most of the speakers from outside the county, this Society initiated experimental tri-county meetings for the societies of Kay, Osage and Washington-Nowata. These three meetings were held in February, March and April, at Pawhuska, Ponca City and Bartlesville, with mostly out-of-state speakers. While the attendance was somewhat cut down by reason of gasoline and rubber restrictions, the meetings were generally held to have been successful. With three members of the Society in uniform and away, this Society's record of 65 per cent attendance is very high.

Rogers

This Society also has a splendid attendance record of about 68 per cent of total membership, with four members in the armed forces. Fewer meetings have been held than in some of the other societies, but good papers have been presented.

Creek

It is regrettable from the standpoint of attendance that members in this Society are scattered in three centers, quite a distance from each other. Meetings have been alternated between Sapulpa and Bristow and the attendance has been less than 50 per cent of the membership. The members are alert and have a very definite interest in organized medicine. The Sapulpa men have established and are maintaining a plasma bank. Four members of the society are in the armed forcse.

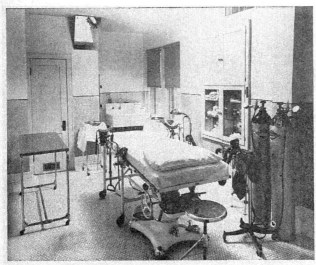

Tulsa

The Tulsa Society is fortunate in having many advantages (large membership, adequate hospitals, location in every active business and industrial centers, etc.), which enables it to accomplish things in a big way, where smaller societies must be content to attempt less and do less.

Outstanding among the many activities of this Society are the maintenance of a Medical Credit Bureau, which has been of great help to the members in the collection of accounts, the building and maintenance of a fine Medical Library with a full-time librarian, and the continuation of the Tulsa County Clinic, saving the taxpayers of the county thousands of dollars—this in the face of strong political opposition. Forty-eight members, approximately one-fourth of the total membership, are serving in the armed forces. Regular meetings have been held, with an average attendance of about 30 per cent. The members of this Society are very generous with their time and talents, helping weaker societies in this area with programs.

Washington-Nowata

This claims to be the banner Society in the state as to attendance at regular meetings. For years the average attendance has been 70 per cent or more of the membership. Good scientific papers have been presented at all meetings. Two $25.00 War Savings Bonds have been purchased. The Nowata County members have been very faithful in their attendance and committee work. Four members of this Society are in the armed service.

All Societies in the District report their finances in good condition, comfortable working balances being carried over into the present year.

It has been gratifying to hear from every Society in the District favorable comments on the postgraduate lectures delivered by Dr. L. W. Hunt on Internal Medicine. A very large proportion of the membership in each county attended these lectures, and hope that the course will be repeated next year, with a different group of topics.

Respectfully submitted,
J. V. Athey, M. D.,
Councilor, District No. 6.

On *motion* by Dr. Clinton Gallaher, seconded by Dr. Claude S. Chambers, and *carried*, Dr. Athey's report was *accepted*.

Following the report of Dr. Athey, Dr. Garrison called for the Report of the Councilor from District No. 7, Dr. Clinton Gallaher, Shawnee. Dr. Gallaher made the following remarks:

Annual Report District No. 7

Officers and Members of the House of Delegates
Of the Oklahoma State Medical Association
Gentlemen:

The Seventh District is in good order and good shape. Of the eight counties in my district, at least five are well organized and are definitely active. In some counties from two to five meetings are held each and every month and are well attended. It is my opinion that at least 80 per cent of the doctors in my District attended the postgraduate course in Internal Medicine recently conducted by Dr. L. W. Hunt.

One Society in the District maintains a monthly Bulletin and, regardless of the fact that it is my home county, it is a good one.

I have observed that it is important that each and every physician participate in the programs and activities of the society in order that he will be interested. In the District as a whole and in Pottawatomie County in particular, we have insisted that within the meetings there be established and maintained the precedent that the members of the society shall prepare and present the programs themselves. It is well and good to import speakers for special occasions, such as, fall and spring clinics, but this practice should not be followed for all meetings. A procedure of this type will develop the individuals in the society and make for the active par-

ticipation of each member. The extent to which a society is able to gain this cooperation is valuable to the development of the members.

Respectfully submitted,
Clinton Gallaher, M. D.,
Councilor, District No. 7.

On *motion* by Dr. Claude S. Chambers, seconded by Dr. Sam A. McKeel, Ada, and *carried*, the report of Councilor District No. 7 was *approved*.

The Speaker next called for the report of Councilor District No. 10, and inasmuch as it was impossible for Dr. J. S. Fulton, Atoka, to be present because of excessive rains, no report was given.

At this time, the Speaker stated the next order of business would be the report of the Standing Committees.

The first Committee to report was the Annual Session Committee, and Dr. J. D. Osborn, Frederick, as Chairman, made the following remarks:

Report of Annual Session Committee

There is not much of a report for my Committee to make other than it is our duty to decide where the Annual Meeting is to be held. The remainder of the plans are turned over to the Executive Secretary who, in turn, makes proper arrangements with the doctors in the host city.

On *motion* by Dr. O. E. Templin, Alva, seconded by Dr. J. M. Bonham, and *carried* the report was *approved*.

The Speaker next requested the report of the Scientific Work Committee and, in the absence of the Chairman, Dr. Ben H. Nicholson, the Chair called upon the Executive Secretary for remarks. Very briefly, Mr. Graham stated that the report of the committee was the program to be presented the following two days and that the committee appreciated the cooperativeness of those who had offered their assistance in the preparation of it. He further observed that no outside speakers had been secured other than those pertaining to the military services.

On *motion* by Dr. W. S. Larrabee, duly seconded by Dr. Claude S. Chambers, and *carried*, the report of the Scientific Work Committee was *approved*.

At this time, the Speaker requested the pleasure of the House concerning the disposition of the reports of the Public Policy Committee, the Committee on Medical Education and Hospitals and the Committee on Judicial and Professional Relations, which reports had appeared in the April issue of the Journal.

On *motion* By Dr. O. E. Templin, seconded by Dr. R. E. Cowling, and *carried*, the reports of the three committees were *approved*.

In order, the Speaker requested the report of the Committee on Publicity, and in the absence of the Chairman, Dr. L. J. Starry, Oklahoma City, Mr. Graham made several observations concerning the request of the Daily Oklahoman and Times, Oklahoma City, that they be given scientific assistance from the medical profession of the state with regard to the preparation of a series of articles on public health to be presented in the newspapers. Mr. Graham stated that a special committee had been apppointed by the President and that details were being worked out to the satisfaction of all concerned. He further remarked that editors had heard of the project that had been suggested by the Oklahoman and Times and that they were also clamoring for permission to run the same articles in their particular editions. Mr. Graham concluded his remarks by saying that the profession would not be called upon to write the articles since someone from the Oklahoman office would do this with the advice and counsel of the special committee appointed for this purpose, and no articles would be published that did not have committee approval. Credit will be given to the State Medical Association.

On *motion* by Dr. Galvin L. Johnson, duly seconded by Dr. Clinton Gallaher, and *carried*, the report of the Publicity Committee was *accepted*.

In order, the Speaker announced that this completed

The
Menninger Sanitarium

For the Diagnosis and Treatment
of Nervous and Mental Illness.

The
Southard School

For the Education and Psychiatric
Treatment of Children of Average
and Superior Intelligence.

Boarding Home Facilities.

Topeka, Kansas

the Reports of the Standing Committees and that the next order of business would be that of the presentation of Reports of Special Committee. Further, the Speaker stated that the following reports of Standing Committees had appeared in the April issue of the Journal: Benevolent Fund, Medical Economics, Medical Testimony, Postgraduate Medical Teaching, Study and Control of Cancer, Study and Control of Tuberculosis and Study and Control of Venereal Diseases.

On *motion* by Dr. Claude S. Chambers, duly seconded by Dr. Clinton Gallaher, and *carried*, the above-mentioned reports were *accepted*.

Following this action, the privilege of the floor was granted to Dr. Clinton Gallaher, who stated that the report of the Committee on Medical Testimony of which he was Chairman had been published but that he wished to *move* that the House dismiss the Committee since it had accepted the report. The motion was seconded by Dr. W. S. Larrabee, and *carried*.

The speaker stated that the next report to be presented would be that of the Committee on Conservation of Vision and Hearing. The Chairman, Dr. F. Maxey Cooper, Oklahoma City, was not in attendance, consequently, no report was given.

At this time, the Speaker called for the report from the Crippled Children's Committee, and Dr. D. H. O'Donoghue, Oklahoma City, Chairman, presented the following report:

Report of Crippled Children's Committee

The Crippled Children's Committee has no formal report to make at this time, however, the Committee has been active in cooperation with the Oklahoma Society for Crippled Children and has carried on investigations with regard to infantile paralysis, and it is hoped that your Committee will be able to submit a formal report for your approval next year.

On *motion* by Dr. Galvin L. Johnson, duly seconded by Dr. W. S. Larrabee, and *carried*, the report of the Crippled Children's Committee was *approved.*

Next, the Speaker called for the report of the Committee in Industrial and Traumatic Surgery. The Chairman, Dr. H. C. Weber, Bartlesville, made the following remarks:

Report of Committee on Industrial and Traumatic Surgery

The Committee on Industrial and Traumatic Surgery in cooperation with the Committee on Postgraduate Medical Education and the State Health Department held two Institutes on Wartime Industrial Health during the past year—in Tulsa on March 18 and in Oklahoma City on March 19, with a number of outstanding speakers for the occasion. Due to its vast importance, like programs on Industrial Health should be conducted throughout the coming year.

On *motion* by Dr. J. M. Bonham, duly seconded by Dr. D. H. O'Donoghue, and *carried*, the report of Dr. Weber was *approved.*

The Speaker next called for the report of the Committee on Malpractice Insurance, and Dr. V. K. Allen, Tulsa, Chairman, presented the report of his committee, *(Report of committee published in May issue of Journal.)*

Following the reading of the report, Dr. V. C. Tisdal, *moved* the adoption of the report, and the motion was seconded by Dr. W. S. Larrabee. At this time, discussion followed concerning the importance of the securing of more policies under the group master policy of the association in order that the premium might be reduced to the minimum. In order that this might be accomplished, Dr. Allen urged that the Delegates cooperate in their individual counties by giving the information to their members. Following discussion, the motion was *carried.*

The Speaker next called for the Report of the Committee on Maternity and Infancy, and in the absence of the Chairman, Dr. Charles Ed White, Muskogee, Dr. J. B. Eskridge, Oklahoma City, a member of the Committee, presented the report.

(Report of committee published in May issue of Journal.)

On *motion* by Dr. Galvin L. Johnson, seconded by Dr. F. W. Boadway, and *carried*, the report was *approved.*

At this time, Dr. Garrison asked that Mr. Graham, the Executive Secretary, read the report of the Committee on Public Health as published in the April Journal since there were several things in the report that should be thoroughly understoood before the report was acted upon.

Following the reading of the report and after discussion, it was *moved* by Dr. W. S. Larrabee, seconded by Dr. F. W. Boadway, and *carried* that the report be *received* at this time.

Next, the Speaker called for the report of the Committee on Prepaid Medical and Surgical Service, and Dr. John F. Burton, Chairman, Oklahoma City, presented the report.

(Report of committee published in May issue of Journal.)

Upon completion of the report, it was *moved* by Dr. J. M. Bonham, and seconded by Dr. H. K. Speed, that the report be received and action *deferred* until the next session of the House of Delegates.

Immediately following this motion, Dr. Philip C. Risser, Blackwell, moved that the motion be amended to read that the report be brought up for consideration the following morning at the second meeting of the House of Delegates. This *amendment* was accepted by Dr. Bonham, seconded by Dr. C. W. Arrendell, and *carried.*

At this time, Dr. C. M. Hodgson, Kingfisher, requested that if in order to move that the report of Dr. Burton be turned to the Council for action. The Speaker stated that the report had received Council approval in a previous meeting.

Following this, the original motion was voted upon and carried.

At this time, Dr. C. R. Rountree, Oklahoma City, requested permission of the floor and moved that Mr. N. D. Helland, Executive Director of Group Hospital Service in Oklahoma, be granted audience. The motion was seconded by Dr. A.S. Risser, and carried. Mr. Helland made pertinent observations to the House concerning the importance of such a plan as provided for in the report as presented by Dr. Burton.

Next, the Speaker called for the report of the Medical Advisory Committee to the Public Welfare Department, and the floor was granted to the Chairman, Dr. C. R. Rountree.

On *motion* by Dr. C. R. Rountree, seconded by Dr. J. B. Hollis, Mangum, and *carried*, it was moved that the report not be read on the floor of the House of Delegates and that it be published in the Journal.

(Report of committee published in May issue of Journal.)

In order, the Speaker stated that the last report to be presented was that of the Necrology Committee, and in the absence of the Chairman, Dr. J. M. Byrum, Shawnee, Mr. Graham read the following report:

Report of Committee on Necrology

To the officers and members of the Oklahoma State Medical Association, assembled in its Fifty-first Annual Session, Oklahoma City, Oklahoma, May 11-12, 1943:

Your Committee on Necrology takes cognizance of the membership records of the current year ending with this meeting, and observes with sincere regrets that the following members have passed to the Great Beyond since we last met in annual meeting one year ago. To wit:

William C. Sain—Ardmore........................March 7, 1942
Samuel N. Stone—Edmond..........................April 16, 1942
Albert H. Taylor—Anadarko...
Henry J. Daily—Oklahoma City...................April 26, 1942
Henry C. Childs—Tulsa................................May 7, 1942
Francis C. Myers—Tulsa.............................June 7, 1942
Jesse C. Bushyhead—Claremore...................July 11, 1942

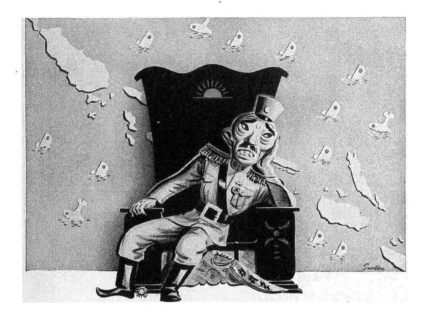

IPRAL WILL PUT JAPS TO SLEEP

IPRAL* will induce a sound restful sleep closely resembling the normal. It can, of course, put the Japanese war lords to sleep —but . . .

Since Ipral is usually free from untoward, after-effects when given in the customary therapeutic dosage and . . .

Since Ipral is readily absorbed and rapidly eliminated and . . .

Since the subject awakens generally calm and refreshed . . .

We suggest that Ipral—generally free from

undesirable cumulative effects—be used to allay the sleeplessness of your own patients and that you purchase War Bonds to help our government buy toxic and fatal "knock-out drops" for use on the Axis powers.

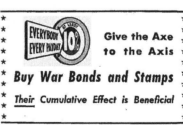

Give the Axe
to the Axis

Buy War Bonds and Stamps

Their Cumulative Effect is Beneficial

* "Ipral" is a trade-mark of E. R. Squibb & Sons. Supplied as Ipral Calcium (calcium ethylisopropylbarbiturate) in ¾- and 2-gr. tablets and Ipral Sodium (sodium ethylisopropylbarbiturate) in 4-gr. tablets.

Member of American Drug Manufacturers Association

Robert M. Anderson—Shawnee........................July 16, 1942
William G. Ramsay—McAlester........................July 25, 1942
J. M. Denby—Carter..August 22, 1942
Thomas T. Norris—Krebs........................September 6, 1942
James C. Smith—Ardmore....................September 9, 1942
George S. Barger—Purcell....................September 15, 1942
William D. Baird, Jr.—Oklahoma City-September 19, 1942
H. Dale Collins—Oklahoma City...........October 12, 1942
Fred H. Clark—Calumet...
John M. McFarling—Shawnee................October 27, 1942
*John C. Duncan—Forgan...................November 25, 1942
*J. E. Cullum—Earlsboro......................December 6, 1942
W. M. Browning—Waurika.....................February 5, 1943
Francis E. Rosenberger—Oklahoma City-February 8, 1943
Arthur D. Bunn—Savanna
Francis A. DeMand—Oklahoma City..February 11, 1943
Louis Bagby—Vinita...........................February 15, 1943
Ora O. Dawson—Wayne.............................April 20, 1943
F. C. Brown—Sparks..................................April 27, 1943
J. S. Meredith—Duke..

* Honorary

It is observed that some of these members, deceased, were in the early years of their professional life and were already achieving marked success. Others had served long and well in the ranks of the profession and had arrived at the top of the ladder of success in professional life and in the honors of the State Association.

The chairman of this very committee, one year ago, is numbered now among the absent. Since we live, we must die, and as we live, we surely die.

Those remaining on the roster of membership bow in humble and painful submission to the inexorable laws of nature, but resolve to carry on where our deceased members left off.

THEREFORE, BE IT RESOLVED, That this report be spread on the minutes of the 1943 Annual Meeting and that a copy be published in the Journal of the State Medical Association.

On *motion* by Dr. C. W. Arrendell, seconded by Dr. W. M. Gallaher, Shawnee, and *carried*, the report was *adopted.*

Following the adoption of the motion, the Speaker requested that the members of the house stand in a moment's silence in reverence to the memory of the deceased members.

At this time, the Speaker called for presentation of amendments to the Constitution and By-Laws from the floor.

Dr. D. H. O'Donoghue was granted permission of the floor and presented an amendment to the By-Laws in behalf of the Oklahoma County Society. (The amendment appears in the proceedings of Tuesday morning, May 11.) There being no more amendments presented by the members of the House from the floor, the Speaker stated that final consideration would be given to the amendments to the By-Laws and Constitution the following morning.

Dr. W. S. Larrabee was next recognized by the Chair: "It is with pleasure that I, as Chairman of the Tulsa County Delegation, extend to the members of the Oklahoma State Medical Association an invitation to be guests of the Tulsa County Medical Society for the 1944 Annual Meeting." Following this invitation, Dr. Larrabee read two letters—one from the Tulsa County Medical Society and one from the Chamber of Commerce—extending invitations that the 52nd Annual Meeting be held in Tulsa.

On *motion* by Dr. L. C. McHenry, Oklahoma City, seconded by Dr. F. W. Boadway, and *carried*, the invitation was *accepted.*

Following this action, the Speaker recognized Dr. W. A. Showman, Tulsa, Chairman of the Resolutions Committee, who requested that an advisory committee be appointed to meet with them immediately following adjournment. The Speaker appointed the following: Dr. J. D. Osborn, Frederick: Dr. James Stevenson, Tulsa, and Dr. Ellis Lamb, Clinton.

The next order pertained to the introduction of new business, and the Speaker recognized the Executive Secretary, who read the Offical Call to the Officers, Fellows and Members of the American Medical Association signed by the President, Dr. Fred W. Rankin; the Speaker of the House of Delegates, Dr. H. H. Shoulders, and the Secretary, Dr. Olin West, that had been received in the office of the Association.

At this time, Dr. Garrison asked if there were additional resolutions to be submitted to the Resolutions Committee other than those already in the possession of Dr. Showman,· and Dr. W. S. Larrabee submitted one in behalf of the Tulsa County Medical Society. (The resolutions appear in full in the proceedings of Tuesday morning, May 11.)

The Speaker stated that the next order of business to be considered would be the election of Honorary Members to the Association. Mr. Graham was recognized and stated that, in accordance with the provisions of Chapter I, Section 3, Subsection (b), of the By-Laws, the three following names had been submitted to the office of the Association for election to Honorary Membership: L. W. Cotton, Enid; R. W. Holbrook, Perkins, and J. T. Frizzell, Clinton.

On *motion* by Dr. D. H. O'Donoghue, seconded by Dr. J. M. Bonham, and *carried*, it was moved that these physicians be *elected* to Honorary Membership.

Following this approval, the Executive Secretary was again recognized by the Speaker and stated that in compliance with the amendment to By-Laws, Chapter I, Section 3, Subsection (d), as of 1942, the following names, as published in the March issue of the Journal, had been submitted for election to Associate Membership: Dr. David W. Gillick, Shawnee; Dr. Louis A. Turley, Oklahoma City, and Dr. S. G. Mollica, Muskogee. In addition, Mr Graham stated that the name of Mr. Fred Hansen, Assistant Attorney General, had been submitted.

On *motion* by Dr. Finis W. Ewing, Muskogee, seconded by Dr. C. R. Rountree, and *carried*, the above mentioned names were *approved* for Associate Membership.

On *motion* by Dr. R. E. Cowling, duly seconded by Dr. D. H. O'Donoghue, and *supported*, the House adjourned to recess until 8:30 A. M., Tuesday Morning.

MINUTES OF SECOND SESSION
Tuesday, May 11, 1943

The second and final session of the 51st Annual Meeting of the House of Delegates was called to order by the Speaker, Dr. George H. Garrison, at 8:30 A. M., Tuesday, May 11, Crystal Room, Skirvin Hotel, Oklahoma City.

Following roll call by the Credentials Committee, the Committee announced a quorum present, and upon motion duly seconded, the report was adopted.

The Speaker opened the morning session by stating that unfinished business of the preceding session would first be considered. At this time, he called for the report of the Committee on Prepaid Medical and Surgical Service.

Dr. John F. Burton, Chairman of the Committee, was extended the privilege of the floor and after introductory remarks to the effect that his committee was asking that this plan be tried as an experiment rather than a plan immediately available for the entire population, read the report of his committee.

Discussion in behalf of the adoption of the report followed by Dr. Philip C. Risser, Blackwell: Dr. C. R. Rountree, Oklahoma City: Dr. McLain Rogers, Clinton, and Dr. A. S. Risser, Blackwell. Dr. H. K. Speed, Sayre, spoke against its adoption. Following discussion by the above, Dr. J. M. Bonham, Hobart, requested that Mr. N. D. Helland, Executive Director of Group Hospital Service in Oklahoma, be accorded the privilege of the floor to explain what is being done in other states in regard to prepaid medical and surgical care. In his discussion, Mr. Helland emphasized salient points with regard to the benefit derived from such a plan.

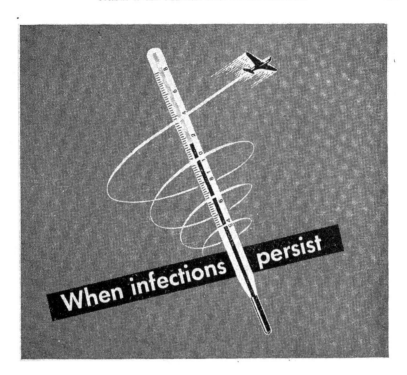

When infections persist, careful study for symptoms of adrenal cortical insufficiency should be undertaken. The patient may show unusual asthenia and pronounced hypotension, in addition to low resistance to exposure and strain. ADRENAL CORTEX EXTRACT (UPJOHN) is a potent specific therapy now available for increasing resistance, muscle tone and capacity for work in adrenal cortical insufficiency.

Adrenal Cortex Extract (Upjohn)

Sterile solution in 10 cc. rubber-capped vials for subcutaneous, intramuscular and intravenous therapy

On *motion* by Dr. A. S. Risser, duly seconded by Dr. C. R. Rountree, and *carried*, the report of the Committee on Prepaid Medical and Surgical Service was *adopted*.

The Speaker next recognized Dr. Carroll M. Pounders, Oklahoma City, Chairman of the Committee on Public Health, who moved that action be taken on the report of his committee which report had only been received in the proceeding session and no disposition made. The motion was seconded by Dr. Dewey Mathews, Tonkawa, and carried.

After a brief discussion, on *motion* by Dr. R. E. Cowling, Ada, duly seconded by Dr. J. D. Osborn, Frederick, and *carried*, the report of Dr. Pounders' committee was *adopted*.

The next order of business was the reading of resolutions which had been referred to the Resolutions Committee at the preceding session. The Speaker recognized the Executive Secretary, who read the resolutions, and final disposition follows each resolution. They are as follows:

Amendment to Constitution
American Medical Association
Article 6, Section 3

WHEREAS, The American Medical Association is composed of the 48 constituent state and territorial Medical Associations, and

WHEREAS, 22 of these State Associations lay west of the Mississippi River and are considered more or less rural states where the problems of medicine and public health are different from those of the industrial states

NOW, THEREFORE, BE IT RESOLVED, That the House of Delegates of the Oklahoma State Medical Association instruct its Delegates to introduce the following amendment to the Constitution of the American Medical Association.

Amendment

Amend Article 6, Section 3, by adding the following language:

"After the adoption of this amendment, the House of Delegates shall elect at the earliest possible time at least three Trustees from the states west of the Mississippi River, and all appointments to fill unexpired terms of those Trustees shall be from states west of the Mississippi River and that this ratio of members shall at all times be retained."

On *motion* by Dr. J. D. Osborn, seconded by Dr. Finis W. Ewing, Muskogee, and *carried*, the resolution was *adopted*.

American Medical Association Journal

WHEREAS, The Journal of the American Medical Association is accepted as the leading publication of its kind in America and in all probability the world, and

WHEREAS, The publication of this Journal calls for a physician of outstanding attainment as is embodied in the present Editor, and

WHEREAS, The Editor of any Journal of such a specialized nature should devote his full time to the editing and publishing of the Journal

NOW, THEREFORE, BE IT RESOLVED, That the Delegates from the Oklahoma State Medical Association to the House of Delegates of the American Medical Association be instructed to introduce the following resolution before that body.

Resolution

That the Board of Trustees of the American Medical Association be instructed by the House of Delegates to limit the duties of the Editor of the Journal to the necessary activities attendant to its publication and all other outside activities, in which the Editor shall participate as Editor of the Journal and spokesman for the American Medical Association, shall be limited to appearances pertaining solely to scientific medicine.

On *motion* by Dr. W. A. Howard, Chelsea, duly seconded by Dr. Finis W. Ewing, and *carried*, the resolution was *adopted*.

Activities of American Medical Association

WHEREAS, The American Medical Association is

the parent organization of all State Medical Associations and is therefore looked to for leadership by the public in matters pertaining to health and welfare, and

WHEREAS, The office of the American Medical Association and its executive officers are located in Chicago, Illinois, and therefore not easily accessible to the Congress of the United States and other departments of the Federal Government dealing with matters of health for the people

NOW, THEREFORE, BE IT RESOLVED by the House of Delegates of the Oklahoma State Medical Association that its Delegates be instructed to either introduce or support a resolution such as proposed by the National Conference on Medical Service and the Federated Medical Boards of Examiners which will establish an office of information of the American Medical Association in Washington, D. C., with full-time personnel in attendance in order that the Congress and Bureaus of Federal Government may have the advice and guidance of the American Medical Association on health legislation at all times. It is further resolved that the Delegates of the Oklahoma State Medical Association to the American Medical Association be instructed to work to the end that any committee, council, bureau or board appointed by the Board of Trustees of the American Medical Association, to act in an advisory capacity to a Bureau of Information in Washington, D. C., be of sufficient size to have representation on it of physicians taken from geographic localities of the United States and that these physicians be in the majority to any other physicians appointed to a committee, council, bureau or board, and it is still further resolved that any appointments to any committee, council, bureau or board by the Board of Trustees be made upon the recommendations of the Delegates from the States represented in the different geographic divisions.

In explanation, Mr. Graham stated that this resolution had been presented by the Council, and that the Resolutions Committee had recommended that the following wording be inserted in the third paragraph as an amendment: "such as proposed by the National Conference on Medical Service and the Federated Medical Boards of Examiners."

On *motion* by Dr. C. W. Arrendell, Ponca City, duly seconded by Dr. Finis W. Ewing, and *carried*, the amendment was *adopted*.

This action was followed by a *motion* by Dr. Finis W. Ewing, seconded by Dr. James Stevenson, Tulsa, and *carried*, that the resolution as amended be *adopted*.

Civilian Medical Care

WHEREAS, The medical profession has an obligation to give adequate medical care to the civilian population, and

WHEREAS, The present war has withdrawn many physicians from communities in Oklahoma to a place where medical care is reaching a minimum

NOW, THEREFORE, BE IT RESOLVED, That the House of Delegates of the Oklahoma State Medical Association urges every county medical society to assume the obligation of providing adequate care to these communities with the aid and assistance of established civilian agencies, such as, the State War Council, and it is further resolved that the need for community cooperation is paramount for the successful operation of plans for medical care and that the sole responsibility cannot be placed on the medical profession.

On *motion* by Dr. A. S. Risser, duly seconded by Dr. J. D. Osborn, and *carried*, the resolution was *adopted*. Following this adoption, a series of four resolutions were presented prior to any action.

Institute on Industrial Health

The House of Delegates of the 51st Annual Session of the Oklahoma State Medical Association wishes to express its appreciation and thanks to Dr. Grady F. Mathews, Commissioner, Oklahoma State Health Department, and his staff, for the wholehearted cooperation and financial assistance given the Oklahoma State Medical Association in sponsoring the Institute on Wartime Industrial Health

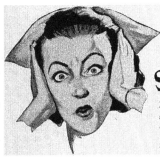

Such language!

My boss used to be as grumpy as a bear. He'd growl and bang around and his wife said: "Poor George, he's working too hard. It's wearing him down to a frazzle!"

So, I told her a few plain facts:

... how I'd discovered the most amazing thing ... that physicians who prescribe S-M-A* actually have more time for other things ... because it isn't necessary to change the formula throughout the entire feeding period. (She sat up at that.)

... how S-M-A eliminates many unnecessary questions that mothers usually ask about other modified milk formulas.

When I had finished, she said she would certainly speak to George about using S-M-A as a routine formula.

* * *

Just because my boss turned over a new leaf ... he wants everybody to pat him on the back for it. But he's not fooling us ... we know how he got to be such a nice man.

BUSY DOCTORS TODAY — PRESCRIBE S-M-A!

With the exception of Vitamin C ... S-M-A is nutritionally complete. Vitamins B_1, D and A are included in adequate proportion ... ready to feed. Their presence in S-M-A prevents the development of subclinical vitamin deficiencies ... because the infant gets all the necessary vitamins right from the start.

S-M-A has still another highly important advantage not found in other modified milk formulas. It contains a special fat that resembles breast milk fat ... resembles it chemically and physically—according to impartial laboratory tests. S-M-A fat is more readily digested and tolerated by most infants than cow's milk fat.

S-M-A IS EASIER TO PREPARE. ONE MEASURE OF POWDER TO EACH OUNCE OF WARM, BOILED WATER, COMPLETES THE FORMULA ... TWENTY CALORIES TO THE OUNCE

The infant food that is nutritionally complete

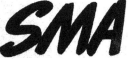

*REG. U. S. PAT. OFF.

S. M. A. Corporation
8100 McCormick Boulevard
Chicago, Illinois

S-M-A, a trade-mark of S.M.A. Corporation, for its brand of food especially prepared for infant feeding—derived from tuberculin-tested cow's milk, the fat of which is replaced by animal and vegetable fats, including biologically tested cod liver oil; with the addition of milk sugar and potassium chloride; altogether forming an antirachitic food. When diluted according to directions, it is essentially similar to human milk in percentages of protein, fat, carbohydrate and ash, in chemical constants of the fat and physical properties.

in Tulsa and Oklahoma City, and particularly wishes to commend the fine spirit and effort made by Dr. V. C. Myers, who handled many of the details, by adoption of the following resolution:

WHEREAS, The Industrial Health program in the war effort is of inestimable value in the protection of the industrial worker, and

THEREFORE, BE IT RESOLVED by the House of Delegates of the Oklahoma State Medical Association that the Oklahoma State Health Department, its Commissioner, Dr. Grady F. Mathews, and Dr. V. C. Myers, Industrial Hygiene Physician, are hereby commended for the financial assistance of the department and their individual efforts in sponsoring this outstanding program.

IT IS FURTHER RESOLVED that a copy of this resolution be sent to the Oklahoma State Health Department.

Postgraduate Education

The House of Delegates of the 51st Annual Session of the Oklahoma State Medical Association wishes to express its appreciation and thanks to the Oklahoma State Health Department and the U. S. Public Health Service of Washington, D. C., for their financial support in making possible the postgraduate program in internal medicine in the state of Oklahoma by the adoption of the following resolution:

WHEREAS, Postgraduate medical education in the war effort is of inestimable value in the protection of the public health, and

WHEREAS, The course in internal medicine of the Oklahoma State Medical Association has received substantial financial support from the Oklahoma State Health Department and the U. S. Public Health Service.

NOW, THEREFORE, BE IT RESOLVED by the House of Delegates of the Oklahoma State Medical Association that the Oklahoma State Health Department and Dr. Grady F. Mathews, personally, the Commissioner, and the U. S. Public Health Service be advised that the Association appreciates this cooperation and pledges its entire facilities to the end that the people of Oklahoma will at all times receive the best medical care.

IT IS FURTHER RESOLVED that a copy of this resolution be sent to the Oklahoma State Health Department and the U. S. Public Health Service of Washington, D. C.

Commonwealth Fund

The House of Delegates of the 51st Annual Session of the Oklahoma State Medical Association wishes to express its appreciation and thanks to The Commonwealth Fund of New York for their financial support in making possible the postgraduate program in internal medicine in the state of Oklahoma by the adoption of the following resolution:

WHEREAS, Postgraduate medical education in the war effort is of inestimable value in the protection of the public health, and

WHEREAS, The course in internal medicine of the Oklahoma State Medical Association has received substantial financial support from The Commonwealth Fund of New York

NOW, THEREFORE, BE IT RESOLVED by the House of Delegates of the Oklahoma State Medical Association that The Commonwealth Fund be advised that the Association appreciates this cooperation and pledges its entire facilities to the end that the people of Oklahoma will at all times receive the best of medical care.

IT IS FURTHER RESOLVED that a copy of this resolution be sent to The Commonwealth Fund of New York.

Continuation of Postgraduate Course

Since the response to questionnaires about the extension program of postgraduate medical education indicates a definite desire on the part of members of the Oklahoma State Medical Association for a course in surgical diagnosis beginning in February, 1944, the House of Delegates approves participation of the Oklahoma State Medical Association in such a course and the appropriation of $2,000.00 per annum for such a participation, and requests the Postgraduate Committee to arrange financial assistance from outside agencies as in the past courses.

On *motion* by Dr. J. D. Osborn, seconded by Dr. A. S. Risser, and *carried*, the above resolutions were *adopted*.

Expression of Appreciation

It has come to the attention of the House of Delegates of the Oklahoma State Medical Association that because of his pioneer efforts, expenditure of personal time and funds, for travel to New York and other points, for assembly of finances and solicitation of instructors, brings to the career of Dr. Henry H. Turner the distinction of being the "Father of Postgraduate Medical Education" under the present sponsorship of the State Association in Oklahoma, and further that the Oklahoma program has repeatedly attracted national attention and interest, resulting in his present chairmanship of the National Associated State Postgraduate Committees,

NOW, THEREFORE, BE IT RESOLVED, That because Doctor Turner has advised the Council that he must resign the Chairmanship of the Postgraduate Committee, the Oklahoma State Medical Association does herewith express its thanks and appreciation to Doctor Turner for his untiring efforts, efficient promotion and chairmanship of many courses in extension medical teaching in Oklahoma since the year 1928.

On *motion* by Dr. A. S. Risser, seconded by Dr. F. W. Boadway, Ardmore, and *carried*, the resolution was *adopted*.

Amendment to Constitution

WHEREAS, An amendment to the Constitution will be up for consideration by the House of Delegates concerning the taking of office of newly-elected Delegates which would, in effect, make a "lame duck" of the defeated Delegate and seriously hamper his effectiveness,

NOW, THEREFORE, BE IT RESOLVED, That the Council of the Association recommends that in its considered judgment this ammendment should not be accepted.

After the reading of the resolution proper, the following interpretation not as an amendment but as an explanation of this action was read:

The Resolutions Committee in consideration of the above amendment, after a complete and thorough discussion of extengencies existing with reference to the amendment, desires to add its approval to the Council that this amendment should not be adopted. The Committee in further substantiation of its action submits the following information received from Dr. W. C. Woodward as contained in a letter to the Speaker of the House of Delegates which is hereby quoted:

"It would certainly be unreasonable for the Association to elect a delegate in May of one year, effective on January 1 of the next year, but by reason of the circumstances of the case, unable to perform any of his official duties until June of the second year, at the time of the regular session of the House of Delegates of the American Medical Association. Such a rule would delay a delegate in the discharge of his duties for more than a year and would allow an annual meeting of the House of Delegates of the association that he represents and an annual meeting of the House of Delegates of the American Medical Association to intervene between his election and the beginning of the actual discharge of his duties, which annual meeting might even be made up of delegates out of sympathy with him, possibly antagonistic, and without confidence in his ability to represent the association properly. It was to correct such a condition, in much less aggravated form, that it was thought necessary to amend the Constitution of the United States so as to permit the Presidents, Senators, and Representatives elected in November to take office in the following January, rather than in the following March, as had been the custom for more than a century, the purpose being to keep the elected officers and representatives of the people at all times in immediate sympathy of the people by whom they were elected."

On *motion* by Dr. C. W. Arrendell, duly seconded by Dr. J. M. Bonham, and *carried*, the above resolution pertaining to the amendment to the Constitution was *adopted*.

Medical Education

WHEREAS, It appears that in the prosecution of the war to a successful conclusion that it now becomes necessary for the armed services to enter into certain contracts with the approved medical schools of the United States, and

WHEREAS, The purpose of the present medical training program is being chiefly directed toward providing physicians for military service, and

WHEREAS, The present tendency in medical education has thus far taken no serious cognizance of urgent need for civilian medical replacements

NOW, THEREFORE, BE IT RESOLVED, That the House of Delegates of the Oklahoma State Medical Association do hereby call attention to the fact that it will become increasingly difficult to maintain medical services which are essential to the health, welfare and safety of the civilian population, unless a provision is made for replacement of physicians for civilian medical care. It is further resolved that unless adequate attention is given the problem of civilian medical care, it is inevitable that a breakdown of even minimal medical attention may result. In any event, this tendency has already proved a serious embarrassment to the war effort in major congested war areas and deserves serious consideration by the proper military authorities.

It was moved by Dr. R. E. Cowling, Ada, and seconded by Dr. J. D. Osborn that the resolution be adopted. Prior to final disposition, discussion followed by Dr. Tom Lowry, Dean of the Medical School, who was of the opinion that the resolution should be forwarded to the Council on Medical Education and Hospitals of the American Medical Association. Dr. L. J. Moorman, Oklahoma City, offered the following amendment to the original motion: ''I move that we amend the resolution to word it so that the resolution will be sent to the Council on Medical Education and Hospitals of the American Medical Association rather than to proper military authorities.'' The amendment was seconded by Dr. C. R. Rountree, and adopted.

On *motion* by Dr. C. R. Rountree, seconded by Dr. G. I. Walker, Hominy, and *carried*, the resolution as amended was *adopted*.

Annual Registration Act

WHEREAS, The members of the Tulsa County Medical Society as duly licensed medical practitioners of the State of Oklahoma have complied with the terms of the Laws of Oklahoma, 1941, Title 59, Chapter II, popularly known as the Annual Registration Act, by payment of an annual registration fee of $3.00 each, and

WHEREAS, This legislative act specifically provides that a portion of the proceeds so derived shall be used in the employment of an attorney to investigate flagrant violations of the Medical Practice Act of Oklahoma, and/or to assist state and county officers in the prosecution of such offenders, and

WHEREAS, It has come to the attention of the membership of the Tulsa County Medical Society that certain persons residing within the limits of Tulsa County, State of Oklahoma, are violating the terms of the Medical Practice Act of Oklahoma,

NOW THEREFORE, BE IT RESOLVED, That the House of Delegates of the Oklahoma State Medical Association join the Tulsa County Medical Society in requesting the Board of Medical Examiners to supply an attorney to investigate and call to the attention of the local civil authorities violations of the Medical Practice Act and, if these local authorities refuse to take action, that the Medical Board be requested to ask of the Governor that a special prosecutor of the Attorney General's office be assigned to the case to assist the Fraudulent Practice Committee of the Tulsa County Medical Society in the protection of the public health by an enforcement of the Medical Practice Act.

On *motion* by Dr. H. C. Weber, Bartlesville, seconded by Dr. H. K. Speed, and *carried*, it was moved that action on the resolution be *delayed*.

Physicians in Service

WHEREAS, 332 members of the Oklahoma State Medical Association are now serving in the armed forces at a great personal sacrifice,

NOW, THEREFORE, BE IT RESOLVED, That the House of Delegates recognizes the sacrifices being made by these physicians and sincerely pledges its full facilities to the end that they may be accorded the entire facilities of the Association and its members to the end that their practices shall be protected to the greatest ability of every member of the Association.

On *motion* by Dr. R. E. Cowling, seconded by Dr. V. C. Tisdal, Elk City, and *carried*, the resolution was *adopted*.

Procurement and Assignment Service

WHEREAS, The Procurement and Assignment Service has been created by executive order of the President of the United States, and

WHEREAS, This Service has secured 135 per cent of its quota of Oklahoma physicians for 1942 under the direction of the present Chairman, Dr. W. W. Rucks of Oklahoma City,

NOW, THEREFORE, BE IT RESOLVED, That the House of Delegates of the Oklahoma State Medical Association commends this committee of the War Manpower Commission for the efficient and fair administration of the function of the Procurement and Assignment Service, and

IT IS FURTHER RESOLVED, That the Association pledges its cooperation when requested for a furtherance of the war effort.

On *motion* by Dr. Finis W. Ewing, seconded by Dr. Dewey Mathews, and *carried*, the resolution was *adopted*.

Governor Robert S. Kerr

WHEREAS, The Honorable Robert S. Kerr, Governor of Oklahoma, has during the Nineteenth Session of the Oklahoma Legislature demonstrated a broad understanding of the problems of medicine, public health and the general welfare of the people,

NOW, THEREFORE, BE IT RESOLVED, That the House of Delegates of the Oklahoma State Medical Association does hereby commend Governor Kerr for his conservative and progressive attitude toward problems affecting the health of the people and urges Governor Kerr in the approximate two years that will intervene between now and the Twentieth Session of the Legislature to give careful and deliberate consideration to the recommendations of the Public Health Committee of the Association which has been adopted by the House of Delegates with reference to the establishment of a Public Health Commission for the State of Oklahoma and the passage of a state immunization law.

BE IT FURTHER RESOLVED, That the entire resources of the Association are hereby offered to Governor Kerr for a study of this important health project.

On *motion* by Dr. Finis W. Ewing, seconded by Dr. R. E. Cowling, and *carried*, the resolution was *adopted*.

Oklahoma State Health Department

WHEREAS, The present war has developed problems in the public health field, foreign and unusual to the normal activities of Public Health Departments,

NOW, THEREFORE, BE IT RESOLVED, That the House of Delegates of the Oklahoma State Medical Association does hereby commend and compliment the Public Health Department of the State of Oklahoma under the leadership of Governor Robert S. Kerr and the directorship of Dr. Grady F. Mathews, Commissioner, for its energetic and efficient handling of these war conditions, and

BE IT FURTHER RESOLVED, That the House of Delegates recognizes that, for the first time in the history of Oklahoma, the director of the Department of Public Health has been retained for a period longer than his original appointment which, in the opinion of the

House of Delegates, indicates the desire of Governor Kerr to place the health of Oklahoma on as high a plane as possible and is the paramount need for the continued operation of an efficient health department.

On *motion* by Dr. Finis W. Ewing, seconded by Dr. A. J. Weedn, Duncan, and *carried*, the resolution was *adopted*.

Following the disposition of resolutions, Dr. C. M. Hodgson, Kingfisher, *moved* that the House of Delegates authorize the Editor of the Journal, if the procedure be legal, to offer the pages of the Journal for an annual financial statement of the State Board of Medical Examiners for the benefit of the profession of Oklahoma. The motion was seconded by Dr. Sam A. McKeel, Ada, and *adopted*.

In order, the Speaker stated that final consideration would be given to amendments to the By-Laws and Constitution that had been submitted. The Executive Secretary was recognized, and presented the following:

Article VIII, Section 4
Re: Vacancy of the Speaker of the House

That Article VIII, Section 4, of the Constitution, be amended as follows in order that the existing conflict with Chapter VI, Section 4, of the By-Laws, will be eliminated:

"Vacancies created by the death, resignation or removal of the above-named officers shall be filled by temporary appointment by the Council, such appointment being effective until the next annual meeting of the House of Delegates, which shall elect a successor to complete the unexpired term, if any, except the President, whose place shall be filled by the Vice-President, and the Speaker of the House of Delegates, whose unexpired term shall be filled by the Vice-Speaker."

On *motion* by Dr. Finis W. Ewing, seconded by Dr. Philip C. Risser, and *carried*, the amendment was *adopted*.

Article VIII, Section 3
Re: Term of A. M. A. Delegate

Article VIII, Section 3, of the Constitution, be amended as follows:

"All of the above officers shall assume the duties of their respective offices immediately upon the close of the annual session at which they were elected to serve and shall serve until their successors have been elected and installed with the exception of Delegate to the American Medical Association who shall take office the first of January succeeding his election."

On *motion* by Dr. Finis W. Ewing, seconded by Dr. W. A. Howard, and *carried*, it was moved that the amendment *be not adopted*.

Chapter V, Section 4
Re: Term of A. M. A. Delegate

That Chapter V, Section 4, of the By-Laws, be amended as follows:

"*Installation.* All officers elected at the final session of the House of Delegates shall assume office at the close of the annual session, except the President-Elect who shall assume the duties of President at the close of the next annual session and Delegate to the American Medical Association who shall assume office the first of January succeeding his election. The terms of office shall be as herein provided or until their successors have been elected and qualified."

Chapter III, Section 1
Re: House of Delegates Representation

Chapter III, Section 1, of the By-Laws, to be amended as follows:

Delete the word "corresponding" in line four and thirteen.

On *motion* by Dr. D. H. O'Donoghue, Oklahoma City, seconded by Dr. V. C. Tisdal, and *carried*, the amendment was *adopted*.

Following this action, Mr. Graham was accorded the privilege of the floor at which time he expressed his appreciation to the members of the Association for the assistance and cooperation they had rendered the office of the Executive Secretary during the past four and a half years.

The next order was the election of officers.

The Speaker announced that the first election would be that of President-Elect and recognized Dr. H. C. Weber, Bartlesville, who made the following remarks: "Mr. Chairman and Members of the House of Delegates: At this time, I should like to place in nomination for President-Elect of this Association a man who is active in the Society and who is known locally as well as state wide. He has practiced medicine in the state for 15 years. There can be no unkind words said of him. At this time, I should like to present Dr. Charles R. Rountree of Oklahoma City." The motion was seconded by Dr. Galvin L. Johnson, Pauls Valley.

Dr. F. W. Boadway, Ardmore: "I move that the nominations cease and that Dr. Rountree be elected by acclamation." The motion was seconded by Dr. V. C. Tisdal, Elk City, and carried.

Following his election, Dr. Rountree made the following remarks to the Delegates: "Mr. Speaker and Members of the House: I hardly know what to say. As I look over the crowd, I realize there are many who could do better than I; however, I shall promise to carry forth the work of this Association as it has been carried out in the past. I have never received an honor that I appreciate more deeply than this."

Following the election of President-Elect, nominations were in order for Vice-President. Dr. J. C. Matheney, Okmulgee, was recognized, by the Speaker: "Mr. Speaker and Gentlemen: For the office of Vice-President, I have in mind a gentleman, a doctor and a member of this House of Delegates. He was born in the state of South Carolina and graduated from the University of Tennessee 35 years ago. For the past 29 years, he has enjoyed a large and respectable practice of medicine in this state. May I present for consideration Dr. J. G. Edwards of Okmulgee."

Dr. Finis W. Ewing, Muskogee: "I desire to second the nomination of Dr. Matheney."

Dr Sam A. McKeel, Ada: "I move that the nominations cease and that Dr. Edwards be elected Vice-President by acclamation." The motion was seconded by Dr. V. C. Tisdal, and carried.

After his election, Dr. Edwards made the following remarks: "Gentlemen: After Dr. Matheney's oratory, I believe it is not necessary for me to say anything. I am very proud and shall do everything I can in my humble way to assist organized medicine."

Next, the Speaker stated nominations were open for the office of Secretary-Treasurer.

Dr. Finis W. Ewing: "I would like to place in nomination Dr. L. J. Moorman of Oklahoma City to succeed himself as Secretary-Treasurer." The motion was seconded by Dr. J. D. Osborn.

Dr. V. C. Tisdal: "I move that the nominations cease and that Dr. Moorman be elected by acclamation." The motion was seconded by Dr. C. W. Arrendell, Ponca City, and carried.

The Speaker next called for nominations for that of Delegate to the American Medical Association to serve for 1943-1944. Dr. Carroll M. Pounders, Oklahoma City, was recognized: "Members of the House of Delegates: It is my desire to remind you that this in an important position. We need to be very careful in the selection of a man for this office. I believe we have had a man in this office for the past two years who is competent to fill the office, who is aquainted with the situation and who knows how to perform the duties that are expected of him. At this time, may I present the name of Dr. A. S. Risser of Blackwell to succeed himself." The nomination was seconded by Dr. O. E. Templin, Alva.

Dr. Harper Wright, Oklahoma City: "I move that the nominations cease and that Dr. Risser be elected by acclamation." The motion was duly seconded by Dr. H. C. Weber, and carried.

Following the election of Dr. Risser as Delegate to the American Medical Association, Dr. Garrison observed that nominations were in order for Alternate Delegate to the American Medical Association. Dr. Galvin L.

Johnson was recognized by the Speaker and moved that Dr. J. D. Osborn, Frederick, be elected to this position. It was moved by Dr. F. W. Boadway, and seconded by Dr. Finis W. Ewing, and carried, that the nominations cease and that Dr. Osborn be elected by acclamation.

At this time, the Speaker stated that the Delegates from District No. 3, District No. 6 and District No. 9 might retire in order to prepare their nominations for Councilors from their respective districts.

Following recess, the Speaker called the House to order and requested nominations for Councilor from District No. 3. Dr. Dewey Mathews, Tonkawa, nominated Dr. C. W. Arrendell of Ponca City. On motion by Dr. O. E. Templin, seconded by Dr. J. G. Edwards, and carried, Dr. Arrendell was elected by acclamation.

n order, Dr. W. S. Larrabee, Tulsa, moved that Dr. J. V. Athey, Bartlesville, be re-elected Councilor of District No. 6 by acclamation. The motion was seconded by Dr. D. H. O'Donoghue, and carried.

Because of flood conditions, there were no Delegates present from Councilor District No. 9. In the presence of this situation, the Speaker stated that no election would be held for this District and that Dr. L. C. Kuyrkendall, McAlester, in compliance with Chapter V, Section 4, of the By-Laws, would serve in this capacity until his successor had been duly elected and qualified.

At this time, Dr. Garrison announced that the desk of the Speaker was cleared and unless there was other business to be transacted, a motion for adjournment was in order.

On *motion* by Dr. W. S. Larrabee, seconded by Dr. D. H. O'Donoghue, and *carried*, a motion for adjournment was *adopted*.

For the physician there is only one rule: Put yourself in the patient's place.—LORD LISTER.

One pound of learning requires ten pounds of common sense to apply it.—Persian Proverb.

DR. GRIDER PENICK WINS GOLF TOURNAMENT

The Annual Golf Tournament of the Association, held in conjunction with the Annual Meeting, was played this year over the exacting course of the Oklahoma City Golf and Country Club. Thirteen physicians competed for the trophies with the following results: Dr. Grinder Penick, Oklahoma City, was the winner of the Lev Prichard Low Medal Award, having an eighty-three for first place.

Dr. Roy Emanual, Chickasha, was the runner-up and recipient of the A. F. Buckley Trophy.

Dr. Max Van Sandt, Wewoka, received the Nestle Milk Cup as winner in the Handicap Flight, having a score, counting his handicap, of sixty-five.

Dr. J. J. Caviness, Oklahoma City, was runner-up and winner of the Industrial Printing Company Trophy.

Reports from the tournament officials indicate that there will be revisions of the handicaps for next year. Anyone shooting the style of golf as displayed by Dr. Van Sandt should be a scratch player.

Dr. Hugh Jeter, Oklahoma City, as Chairman of the local Committee, again was responsible for a fine tournament. It is suggested that the golfers let Dr. Jeter win a trophy sometime—he has earned it!

According to statistics submitted by the various state health departments, 59,173 persons died of tuberculosis in the United States during the past years, and there have been 105,714 new cases reported thus far.

The average human heart beats more than two and a quarter billion times in a lifetime of sixty years.—The Pathfinder.

Give me health and a day and I will make the pomp of emperors ridiculous.—Ralph Waldo Emerson.

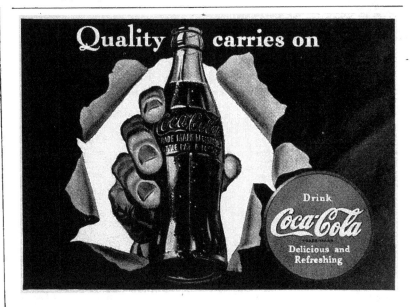

WOMEN'S AUXILIARY NEWS

Report of the Annual Meeting of Auxiliary

OKLAHOMA CITY, OKLAHOMA
May 11-12, 1943

**Officers
1943-1944**

President..............Mrs. F. Maxey Cooper, Oklahoma City
President-Elect..........Mrs. Clarence C. Young, Shawnee
Vice-President..........Mrs. Warren T. Mayfield, Norman
Secretary..........Mrs. Charles R. Rountree, Oklahoma City
Treasurer..............Mrs. C. P. Bondurant, Oklahoma City
Historian..................Mrs. Alfred R. Sugg, Ada
Parliamentarian..................Mrs. Frank L. Flack, Tulsa

Committee Chairman

Public Relations..................Mrs. S. J. Bradfield, Tulsa
Program..................Mrs. Gerald Rogers, Oklahoma City
Hygeia..................Mrs. Clarence C. Young, Shawnee
Press and Publicity..Mrs. L. Chester McHenry, Okla. City
Convention..................Mrs. J. W. Rogers, Tulsa
Legislative..............Mrs. George Garrison, Oklahoma City
Tray Award..................Mrs. Hugh Perry, Tulsa
Printing..............Mrs. W. Floyd Keller, Oklahoma City
Organization..................Mrs. Warren T. Mayfield, Norman

The Women's Auxiliary to the Oklahoma State Medical Association met in Oklahoma City May 11 and 12, with headquarters at the Skirvin Hotel. Mrs. Neil Woodward, registration chairman, reported 110 registered. Forty out-of-the-city women and 70 local women were present at the meetings. Two guests came from out of the state, one from Amarillo, Texas, and one from Casey, Illinois. Mrs. Henry H. Turner, Convention Chairman, Mrs. W. Floyd Keller, Oklahoma County President, and Mrs. Gerald Rogers, Entertainment Chairman, were in charge of arrangements.

The Pre-Executive Board Meeting was held in the home of Mrs. F. Maxey Cooper, president-elect, on Tuesday afternoon, May 11. The business meeting was preceded by tea and a social hour. The meeting was called to order by the president, Mrs. Frank L. Flack, Tulsa. Roll call showed the following counties represented: Cleveland, Pottawatomie, Tulsa and Oklahoma. After a discussion of matters of interest to the Auxiliary, the Nominating, Finance and Tray Award Committees were appointed. The meeting adjourned to permit these committees to meet.

The out-of-city doctors' wives were guests of the Oklahoma County Medical Association at a dinner given Tuesday evening at 7:00 o'clock in the Rainbow Room of the Beacon Club. Seventy-eight were present. The evening was spent in visiting in the club lounge.

The general meeting of the Auxiliary was held in the Venetian Room of the Y. W. C. A., May 12, at 10:00 o'clock. Mrs. Frank L. Flack, President, presided. The invocation was given by Mrs. W. K. West of Oklahoma City, a member of the National Board. Mrs. Henry H. Turner, Convention Chairman, extended a welcome to the delegates and guests. Mrs. John C. Perry, Tulsa, gave the response. The Memorial Service for Mrs. S. E. Frierson, Oklahoma City, was conducted by Mrs. J. M. Alford, Oklahoma City. Special guest speakers at the meeting were Dr. James Stevenson, President-Elect of the State Medical Association, and Lieutenant Elizabeth Hartman of the Army Nurse Corps. Mrs. Joseph Kelso, Oklahoma City, gave a report of the National Auxiliary meeting last June, stating that Tulsa's exibit at the Convention was outstanding.

Officers' reports were given as follows: Recording Secretary, Mrs. James Stevenson, Tulsa; Treasurer, Mrs. H. Lee Farris, Tulsa, read by Mrs. Stevenson and Historian, Mrs. Clinton Gallaher, Shawnee.

Reports of Committee Chairman were given as follows: Public Relations and War Activities, Mrs. S. J. Bradfield, Tulsa read by Mrs. Carl Hotz, Tulsa; Hygeia, Mrs. F. Maxey Cooper, Oklahoma City; Press and Publicity, Mrs. Carl Hotz, Tulsa; Organization, Mrs. Jim Haddock, Norman, and Legislation, Mrs. George Garrison, Oklahoma City.

Reports of the County Presidents were given by: Mrs. W. T. Mayfield, Cleveland; Mrs. W. Floyd Keller, Oklahoma; Pontotoc report read by Mrs. Flack; Mrs. W. Powell, Pittsburg; Mrs. Clinton Gallaher, Pottowatomie, and Mrs J. W. Childs, Tulsa.

The Tray Committee awarded the Tray to the Oklahoma County Society.

Mrs. James Stevenson, Tulsa, was elected delegate to the meeting of the National Auxiliary in Chicago, June 7-9.

The meeting adjourned for a special hour over "coffee" served by the local Auxiliary. The Post-Executive Board Meeting was held immediately following with Mrs. F. Maxey Cooper, Oklahoma City, presiding.

The dinner-dance of the Association, held Wednesday evening at the Skirvin Hotel, concluded the entertainment of the Convention.

"Something New Has Been Added"

The Doctors' Aide Corps is the newest defense organization, the first of its kind in America. This service may be just what your Auxiliary has been needing. Further information about this wartime service for doctors' wives only will be published in the Auxiliary News of the August Journal of the Oklahoma State Medical Association.

Classified Advertisements

OKLAHOMA DOCTORS ATTEND NEW ORLEANS MEETING

The following Oklahoma doctors attended The New Orleans Graduate Medical Assembly meeting, held from March 15 to March 18 in New Orleans, Louisiana; Charles E. Barker, George N. Barry, F. Maxey Cooper, Edward N. Smith, Oklahoma City; Ian Mackenzie, Tulsa; Finis W. Ewing, J. H. White, Muskogee; Turner Bynum, Chickasha; J. Holland Howe, Ponca City; Russell L. Kurtz, Nowata; Emmett C. Lindley, Duncan; Emmett O. Martin, Cushing; L. A. Mitchell, Stillwater, and J. C. Rumley, Stigler.

FIGHTIN' TALK

Special Article

MILK

(*Editor's Note: Each month the Journal office receives many notices of change of address of our members in Service, letters from the men themselves, and bits of news about them. We feel that all of these would be of great interest to our readers, and thus we are initiating a new monthly column, "Fightin' Talk." We strongly urge all members in Service to send us any news, for we on the home front are vitally interested in where you are, and what you are doing.*)

Major James O. Hood, Norman, advises that his new address is now A. P. O. No. 45, c/o Postmaster, New York.

Major John W. Records, formerly of Oklahoma City, reports that he is now an instructor at the Medical Field Service School at Carlisle Barracks, Pennsylvania.

Major Cole D. Pittman, formerly stationed at Bolling Field, Washington, D. C., is now stationed at Rosecrans Field, St. Joseph, Missouri.

Major Orville H. Tackett of Oklahoma City is home for his first visit in 17 months. Major Tackett has been stationed in the Caribbean defense area.

Lt. Comdr. R. B. Ford of Tulsa and Lt. John A. Cunningham of Oklahoma City report the following address: Fleet Post Office, San Francisco, California.

The following communication concerning the activity of Colonel Lee R. Wilhite, who was in charge of the Medical Recruiting Board in Oklahoma last year, has been received in the office:

1ST HQ., SPECIAL TROOPS
SECOND ARMY
FORT BRAGG, N. C.

201.22

Subject: Commendation

TO: Colonel Lee R. Wilhite, M. C., 134th Medical Regiment, Fort Bragg, N. C.

1. Colonel John H. Carruth, C. E., Captain of Inspection Team No. 1 for the period April 15, 1943, has advised me that your Regiment deserves credit for excellent training and classes in "Dog Surgery."

2. Your training programs have received only the most favorable comments from all observers. Only through training can we attain our ultimate objective—"Success in Battle."

3. It gives me great pleasure and satisfaction to commend you and your staff on this training.

/s/ H. B. Crea
H. B. Crea
Colonel, Infantry
Commanding

(Extracted 134th Med Regt)
1st Ind.

To: All Officers, 134th Medical Regiment.

I do not consider the above as a personal commendation, because it was obtained only through your wholehearted cooperation and attention to training details. I wish to commend you for this fine work.

LEE R. WILHITE
Colonel, M. C.
Commanding

John O. Bradshaw, M.D., formerly of Welch, is now Major Bradshaw, Surgeon of the Station Hospital, Camp Monticello, Ark.

Milk is one of the most important foods, therefore, it must be produced and handled with utmost care. It is the only food derived from animals which is consumed in the raw state. No other article of food so nearly contains all the elements of a well balanced diet. It is the perfect food for infants, and should be consumed in liberal quantities by older children and adults. No single article of food is exposed to so many sources of contamination, and it is probable that milk is the source of more diseases than all other articles of food combined.

Milk is an especially good culture media for the growth of bacteria, and under favorable conditions a few bacteria in milk will increase to millions in a very few hours. In the production of milk there is a constant danger of contamination through the handling to which it is subjected. Infected milk has caused numerous and, at times, extensive epidemics. No other food, except water, has been responsible for so much food-borne disease.

The principal ways in which milk may convey infection are:

1. The animal from which milk is obtained, usually the cow, may be infected with certain diseases which are transmitted through milk.

2. Persons handling the milk or milk utensils who are infected with certain diseases or who have been infected and remain carriers.

3. Indirectly from one of the above sources through contaminated water, flies, or dust.

The objectives of the milk sanitation program of the State Health Department are primarily, protection of Public Health and secondarily, economic. The Public Health objectives are:

1. To protect the health of the consumer from diseases transmitted by milk. The most common of such diseases are: tuberculosis, typhoid, and para-typhoid fevers, streptococcus infections (scarlet fever and septic sore throat), undulant fever, enteritis and diarrheas of children, food poisoning, and diphtheria.

2. To improve the taste, flavor, and keeping quality through sanitary handling and production methods, and through improved feeding of the cattle.

3. To increase the consumption of milk and milk products through education of the public to the superior food value of milk and through increased confidence in its safety.

The economic objectives are:

1. To reward the dairyman who complies with the regulations, by requiring all dairies to properly label their milk as to grade.

2. To protect the public from fraud by prohibiting the use of adulterants or the addition of preservatives.

3. To encourage the development of the dairy industry by sponsoring programs which will increase the market for dairy products.

To attain these objectives, the Oklahoma State Health Department recommends to the cities and towns of the state, the adoption of the U. S. Public Health Service Standard Milk Ordinance, and the employment of competent enforcement officers. This ordinance sets out the minimum requirements for the production, handling, and processing of good, clean, wholesome milk, to be labeled Grade A. It provides for frequent visits by the Health Officer or Milk Sanitarian, to the farm dairies and pasteurization plants, to aid and educate the dairymen in making the necessary improvements. It also provides for adequate laboratory analysis of milk samples as the final check on the wholesomeness and safety of the milk supply.

The consuming public and city officials must also be educated as to the need of this program. This can be done best by the medical profession and members of the public health department. We need more interest and better planning, more concerted effort and team work by every person connected with the milk program, if we are to realize the full benefits of an adequate, safe milk supply.

NEWS FROM THE COUNTY SOCIETIES

On Wednesday, May 5, an interesting program on syphilis was presented to the members and guests of the Pontotoc County Medical Society by Colonel Udo J. Wile, professor of Dermatology and Syphilogy from the University of Michigan, and Major John Cowan, Director of Venereal Disease Division of the Oklahoma State Health Department.

Colonel Wile, one of the most important syphilologists in the United States, has been loaned to the United States Public Health Service for the duration of the war. It was the good fortune of the Oklahoma State Health Department to obtain, during the month of May, the services of Colonel Wile for addresses on the management and control of syphilis.

Fifty members attended the meeting of the Tulsa County Medical Society on May 24 at the Mayo Hotel. The subject for discussion was ''Laryngeal Obstructions in Children—A Symposium.'' Speakers included Dr. Maurice J. Seale, Dr. George R. Russell and Dr. Donald L. Mishler.

The Society will adjourn for the summer months and will resume meetings on September 13 in Tulsa.

The Garvin County Medical Society met on May 19 for a report on the State Meeting at Oklahoma City. Reports were given by Dr. G. L. Johnson and Dr. M. E. Robberson, Jr., who were delegates. There was a general discussion by the members present.

It has been the custom of the Okmulgee-Okfuskee County Medical Society to discontinue regular meetings during the months of June, July and August. Unless there is a specific need for a call meeting, there will be no further meeting until the second Monday in September.

Dr. Dewey Mathews gave a report on the State Meeting at the regular meeting of the Kay County Medical Society on May 20 in the City Hall at Blackwell.

''Differentiation between Peptic Ulcer and Gall Bladder Disease'' was discussed by Dr. A. S. Risser, and Dr. Thomas McElroy spoke to the members on various phases of surgery.

Due to the State Meeting, no regular meeting of the Custer County Medical Society was held in May. The members will meet with the Western Oklahoma Society in June.

No regular meetings will be held by the Washington-Nowata Society until September. The last meeting was held on May 5 in Bartlesville. Dr. L. D. Hudson of Dewey was the speaker and his subject was ''Habitual Abortion.''

Dr. Clinton Gallaher delivered a paper on the ''Local Use of Sulfonamides in Treatment of Upper Respiratory Tract Infections'' at the meeting of the Pottawatomie Society on May 15 in Shawnee. A report on the annual meeting was given by the delegates.

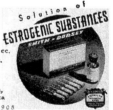

Blue Cross Reports

Every day 3,000 patients leave the hospital with their bills paid by the Blue Cross.

These hospital service plans, 77 in number, sponsored by the American Hospital Association now place hospital care in the family budget for 11,000,000 workers and family dependents and have paid American hospitals $160,000,000.00 since their establishment.

The voluntary Blue Cross Hospital Service plan movement sponsored by the American Hospital Association had enrolled scarcely 1,000,000 suscribers five years ago. Now Blue Cross protection is available in 36 states which contain 90 per cent of the population of the United States, and employees are protected through the cooperation of 150,000 employers, large and small, throughout the nation.

The movement continues to grow with more than 6,000 additional participants becoming eligible for benefits every day. They make regular payments, equal to a few cents a day per family, into a common fund which is used to pay the hospital bills for those people requiring such care. The basis of the Blue Cross movement is a guarantee of service by more than 2,500 member hospitals wich maintain contracts with their local plans.

Impressive as the past attainment of Blue Cross plans has been, they must be measured by the unfinished task of the future. What is good for 11,000,000 Americans is still better for 110,000,000. The popularity of non-profit Blue-Cross protection has led to the offering of indemnity benefits for hospital insurance by many commercial companies in the United States, many of which are entirely reputable organizations. But the more significant development of the past year has been the suggestion that hospitalization protection be added to the present social security program with each employed person and his dependents entitled to a number of days of hospitalization or an indemnity for expense incurred during a period of hospitalized illness. It has been estimated such a program would cost the American people approximately one per cent of all payrolls up to $3,000.00 per year and would provide from $3.00 to $6.00 per day for a period of 30 to 60 days per year for each individual eligible for benefits.

Hospitalization is a personal experience and hospitalization protection is most satisfactory when its benefits are available in service, not in cash. For no one can tell exactly what his hospital experience will cost. It is important that he be assured of necessary hospital services rather than cash indemnification which may pay only a portion of the expenses involved.

Money is not the only consideration in the receipt of hospital care. Many people forego hospital service because of ignorance or fear. But regular subscription to a convenient and economical Blue Cross plan would soon remove the ignorance and fear which comes from lack of contacts with or understanding of hospital service.

The future of the voluntary hospital system is dependent upon the development and continuance of a voluntary method of financing hospital care. The people of America wish to be assured of necessary hospitalization, and have welcomed an opportunity to place hospital care in the family budget along with other necessities. Administrators and trustees of Blue Cross plans and voluntary hospitals are hopeful that the Blue Cross plan will reach an even more substantial portion of the population within the immediate future.

Blue Cross plans are non-profit organizations established primarily to bring good hospital care to the American people on a convenient and economical basis, with a quality of service which assures the maximum protection against the hazards of unforeseen sickness costs. But if Blue Cross plans hope to make a compulsory hospital insurance program unnecessary, the tempo of enrollment must be increased. The addition of 2,000,000 participants each year is a great achievement, but the membership growth must be accelerated if we are to achieve the objectives claimed for a compulsory hospital insurance plan.

• OBITUARIES •

U. S. Cordell, M.D.
1868-1943

Dr. U. S. Cordell died at his home in Macomb, Oklahoma, on May 28 following a two months' illness caused by a heart ailment.

He was born in Valley Head, Alabama, on December 16, 1868. In 1880 the family moved to Colbert in Indian Territory where Dr. Cordell began studying and reading medicine under the preceptorship of Dr. Howell. He was graduated from the Medical College at Chattanooga, Tennessee and in 1902 moved to Romulus, Oklahoma, where he practiced until 1918, moving then to Macomb where, except for a few years of practice in Tecumseh, he continued to practice until the time of his death. Dr. Cordell was a pioneer physician of this county and was a typical "horse and buggy doctor." His passing will be a great loss to his many friends and patients.

He is a member of the Pottawatomie County, the the Oklahoma State, and the American Medical Associations, a member of the Masonic and Odd Fellows lodge in Romulus, Oklahoma.

He is survived by seven children, two sons, Wille and Eugene Cordell, and five daughters, Miss Beulah Cordell, Mrs. Lester Wilson, Mrs. Beatriz Hellman, Mrs. W. R. Muncey and Mrs. Farris Willingham. Four of his daughters, following his training, became nurses. His wife died in 1936.

Services were held in Tecumseh at the First Christian Church with Dr. W. F. Reynolds of the Presbyterian Church of Pauls Valley officiating. The body was cremated.

F. C. Brown, M.D.
1872-1943

Dr. Fredrick Charles Brown died at his home in Sparks, April 27, 1943, following a long illness.

He had practiced medicine in Sparks since the opening of that community in 1902. Born near St. Mary's, Ontario, Canada, August 5, 1872, he received his precollege education in that country. He came to Chicago, Illinois, and entered Rush Medical College, graduating in 1900. After spending a year in Alaska with an exploration organization he came to Oklahoma in 1901 and to Lincoln County in 1902.

In 1918 Dr. Brown was assigned to overseas service in World War No. 1. After the signing of the Armistice, he took a postgraduate course at Dijon, France. He remained overseas sixteen months, returning in August 1919.

Dr. Brown was an active member of the State and Medical Societies and the American Legion. He was also very active in civic and political circles.

Funeral services were held at the Methodist Church of Sparks on April 29, with Reverend E. T. Cooprider, pastor of the Chandler Methodist Church, and Manford Cox, of the American Legion officiating.

He is survived by his widow and five sisters.

MEDICAL ABSTRACTS

"SOME ANOMALOUS FORMS OF AMAUROTIC IDI-
OCY AND THEIR BEARING ON THE RELATIONSHIP
OF THE VARIOUS TYPES." Mason R. Wyburn. The
British Journal of Ophthalmology. (London). Vol. 27,
pp. 145-173, April, 1943.

In 1881, Tay described a familial disease of infants
in which, within the first year of life, there appears at
the maculæ of both retinæ a cherry-red spot surrounded
by a fairly well-defined white area. The child becomes
weak, unable to hold up his head or move his limbs and
finally completely paralyzed and progressively demented.
Blindness develops, the disc becoming white and atrophic.
Hyperacusis is often present. The child usually dies before the age of two years.

Sachs, in 1887, described autopsy findings and called
the condition amaurotic idiocy. In 1901, Higier suggested the name Tay-Sach's disease. It was first thought
to be confined to Jews, but although, occurring predominantly in Jews, occasional non-Jewish cases have
been reported from all parts of the world, including
Japan. Slome, in 1933, found it to be inherited as a
recessive character, as 111 cases occured in 69 families
containing two or more members and consanguinity of
the parents was present in over 50 per cent of the cases.

At autopsy, a brain of firm rubbery consistency is
found, usually smaller than normal, with widened sulci.
Microscopically the nerve cells, dendrites and axis cylinders show generalized swelling with diffuse gliosis.
Fat stains show the granules in the cells to be formed
of prelipoid lecithin-like material. The changes are present throughout the central nervous system including the
cerebellum. The ganglion cells of the retina are heavily
affected leading to an enlargement of the normal small
red area present at the macula and allowing more of
the choroidal coat to show through, while the lipoid in
the ganglion cells produces the opaque whitish appearance of the surrounding zone. Lipoid degeneration of
ganglion cells may occur, however, without giving rise
to a cherry-red spot. The periphery of the fundus is
generally normal, though pigmentary changes have been
described. In the early stages the discs are normal,
but later are atrophic. The final stage consists of
a gradual spreading of the white area to involve the
whole retina which atrophies with pigmentary changes.
The red spot disappears and is replaced by a reticulated,
white and circular area and the disc becomes dead
white. The author mentions several cases, some of them
atypical, observed in Jewish and non-Jewish infants.

In some of the cases various peculiar reflex phenomena
were observed. One of the infants has been having
thirty curious attacks a day in which her hands clenched,
her legs flexed, her eyes rolled and she seemed to be
trying to raise herself up. In addition, there was marked
hyperacusis, the child being easily startled at the slightest sound and screaming as if nervous and frightened.

In 1903, Batten drew attention to the occurrence of
cerebral degeneration with symmetrical changes in the
maculæ in two members of a family. One patient developed symptoms at the age of six and his sister at
the age of five. The retinæ showed generalized peppered
pigmentary changes and at each macula there was an irregular reddish-black spot, the region immediately surrounding the spot being paler than the rest of the
fundus and more atrophic looking. Cerebral degeneration was manifest by mental changes, feeble knee jerks,
and extensor plantar responses. Shortly afterwards, Mayou
and also Vogt, demonstrated further multiple cases in

familes, and the latter tried to establish the condition as a
variant of Tay-Sach's disease. Spielmeyer later described
similar cases in which the fundus appearances resembled
retinitis pigmentosa. Sjogren established the condition
as an heredodegeneration of a simple recessive type and
showed that there is a great frequency of consanguinity
amoung the parents, but in contrast to Tay-Sachs' disease there is no racial predilection for Jews.

The patient develops normally until the age of five
to eight years and then the first signs of the disease
usually manifest themselves by failure of vision, the
patient in most cases becoming blind within two years.
Later, epileptic attacks occur followed by mental degeneration, disturbance of speech, ataxia, spastic weakness of the legs, and incontinence, all of which progress,
the patient finally dying between 14 and 18 years of age,
occasionally reaching the age of 25 or more.

In retina, fine pigmentary changes at the macula are
probably the first signs. Gradually the whole retina
atrophies sometimes with pigmentary degeneration like
that of retinitis pigmentosa, but differing in that the
central areas are affected as well as the periphery. Later
optic atrophy and narrowing of the vessels appears and
irregular nystagmus is almost constant in the terminal
stages. Microscopically the degenerative changes in the
retina are less extensive in the ganglion cells than in
the infantile type and rod and cone layer, which is little
affected in the latter type, is completely destroyed.

In the brain the changes found are essentially those
present in the infantile type of the disease, but the cerebellum, basal ganglia and medulla may be only slightly
affected. The staining reactions of the lipoid cells give
different results. In the infantile type the prelipoid
lecithin-like material is present, whereas in the juvenile
type, the lipoids are of a simpler form approaching the
constitution of neutral fats. The author reports a number
of examples of this condition occurring in 10 families
and affecting 15 persons.—M. D. H., M. D.

"THE COMBINED OPERATION IN LOW BACK AND
SCIATIC PAIN." R. K. Ghormley, J. Grafton Love, and
H. Herman Young. The Jour. of A.M.A., CXX, 1171,
Dec. 12, 1942.

The combined operation is a combination of exploration of the spinal canal and bone grafting to bridge the
affected parts in patients suffering from low back pain.
The number of combined operations has been steadily increasing at the Mayo Clinic, rising from one per cent
in 1937 to 14 per cent in 1940. The reason for this is
that the orthopedic consulatants see all patients suspected of having an intraspinal lesion of the intervertebral-
disc type before operation is done.

A careful history is taken to evaluate the early symptoms for evidence of the static type of back pain relieved
by rest, and superimposed evidence of protruded disc
is made. Evidence for or against fusion is not determined
solely by roentenographic findings. In a group of 77 patients in whom results of myelographic examination were
positive, spinograms were positive in 49 cases, and in
five cases the protruded discs were found with radiopaque oil, making a total of 54 of the 77 patients.

In a group of 62 patients for whom results of exploration were negative, results of spinograms were positive in 20 cases, and in one case results of examination
with radiopaque oil were positive. This discrepancy between the results of the spinogram and the results of
surgical exploration was due to the interpretation of

hypertrophied ligamentum flavum as protrusion of the intervertebral disc in cases in which the results of exploration had been negative.

Tibial grafts were used in closing the laminectomy defects, as well as for stabilizing the low back, as it was felt that these were superior to chip grafts, and also because they could be obtained from the tibia at the time the neurosurgeons were doing the laminectomy. Plaster fixation was not employed postoperatively, and a normal schedule was generally reached by the end of three or four months after operation.

In the tabulation of end results, 64 per cent of the patients had good results, 25 per cent fair, and 11 per cent poor results. In an analysis of some of the fair and poor results, three cases were found in which the graft was unsatisfactory; one case of infected graft and questionable fusion; one of psychoneurosis, and one on whom compensation had not been settled. It is felt that laminectomy plus fusion need not limit a patient's career as far as his work is concerned. Protruded discs, as far as the authors were able to ascertain, have not recurred after fusion.

An interesting abstract of discussion follows this well-written article.—E. D. M., M. D.

"SOLITARY UNICAMERAL BONE CYST WITH EMPHASIS ON THE ROENTGEN PICTURE, THE PATHOLOGIC APPEARANCE AND THE PATHOGENESIS." Henry L. Jaffe and Louis Lichtenstein. Archives of Surgery. XLIV. 1004. 1942.

Solitary unicameral bone cyst occurs as a rare, but distinct, entity in childhood and adolescence. The lesion consists of a fairly large, fluid-filled, unicameral cavity, located in the interior of the affected bone shaft, and delimited by a more or less thinned and expanded cortex of the shaft, the inner surface of which is lined by a rather thin membrane of connective tissue from which little material can usually be curetted. The cyst may attain a large size before its presence is discovered, and a pathological fracture may be the first evidence of the condition. The disease is readily amenable to cure by surgical intervention, and occasionally even heals spontaneously after pathological fracture.

The lesion usually begins its development in the shaft, at or near an epiphyseal cartilage plate, of some one of a few predilected long tubular bones. The upper portion of the shaft of the humerus or femur are particularly prone to involvement.

On microscopic examination the contents of the cyst consist of fibrin clots undergoing organization, and even calcification and ossification. In an occasional case, it also contains some cholesterol crystals, with or without nests of multinuclear giant cells, and phagocytes containing lipoid and hemosiderin.

As to pathogenesis, the authors favor the view of Mickuliez that the lesion has its basis as a local disorder of development and bone growth. The cyst has an active growth as long as it remains abutting on the epiphyseal cartilage plate, but following a spontaneous fracture it assumes a latent or static phase, moving farther away from the epiphyseal plate as the longitudinal growth of the bone progresses.

Whether in the growing or in the static stage, solitary unicameral bone cysts are amenable to operative cure by curettage and filling the cavity with autogenous bone chips. Radiation therapy by itself never leads to healing of the type of cyst in question, and even seems to be contraindicated as an adjuvant to surgical intervention.—E. D. M., M.D.

KEY TO ABSTRACTORS

E. D. M. ....Earl D. McBride, M.D.
M. D. H. ....Marvin D. Henley, M.D.

BOOK REVIEWS

"The chief glory of every people arises from its authors."—Dr. Samuel Johnson.

STEDMAN'S MEDICAL DICTIONARY—ILLUS-TRATED. Fifteenth Revised Edition. Stanley Thomas Garber, B. S., M. D. The Williams and Wilkins Companies, Baltimore, Maryland. 1942 Price $7.50.

Stedman's Medical Dictionary, with a record of thirty years of service, is now in its fifteenth edition. It has been thoroughly revised to meet the changing nomenclature in medicine and other scientific fields. It comes from the press in compact, usable form with flexible binding. The editor is Dr. Stanley Thomas Garber, who collaborated with Dr. Stedman in the preparation of the proceeding edition. Consequently, the volume embodies the accumulated knowledge and experience of Stedman, plus the current contributions of Dr. Garber.

In addition to 1,234 pages devoted to the pronunciation and definition of indispensable words and medical terms, there is an appendix containing valuable data, including symbols and abbreviations. Also, there are valuable comparative tables and the new nomenclature in Latin and English adopted by the National Society of Great Britian and England with the Basle anatomical nomenclature equivalent.

We can heartily recommend this volume to all students of medicine and the allied sciences.—Lewis J. Moorman, M. D.

TABLES OF FOOD VALUES. Alice V. Bradley, M. S., Associate Professor of Nutrition and Health Education, State College, Santa Barbara, California. Completely Revised and Enlarged. The Manual Arts Press, Peoria, Illinois. 1942. 224 pages. Cloth. Price $3.50.

This book, which has very recently been completely revised and enlarged having been brought thoroughly up-to-date, is outstanding and valuable as an authority on the subject of nutrition.

Chapter 1 is a brief discussion of dietary componets, including the energy foods, tissue builders and body regulators, while Chapter II is devoted to diet calculation and menu planning.

The remainder of this book is divided into two parts. The complete nutritive value, raw or cooked, of a food all in one table in both average servings and in 100-gram portions is listed. Part I lists the average servings and is accompanied by recipes in order that the ingredients used in each is readily accessible. Part II gives the 100-gram portions of commonly used foods. Each part covers 27 classifications of foods and at the same time lists the commonly known foods of each classification. Another convenient arrangement is that of listing the name of the food at the end of each line thereby avoiding much confusion.

This book is a tabulation that is a necessary part of the equipment of every physician, as well as other interested persons, desiring detailed information with regard to the composition of food and the nutritive value of specific diets.—Anne Betche.

BABIES ARE FUN. Jean Littejohn. Aaberg William Penn Publishing Corporation, 220 Fifth Avenue, New York, New York. Price $1.00.

"Babies Are Fun" would be a very helpful addition to the usual variety of prescribed reading for young mothers and mothers-to-be. The valuable but stereotyped information found in these books too often leaves the inexperienced mother feeling as though she were blessed with a rather bleak scientific accomplishment and psychological problem instead of an enchanting little human that could be more fun than anything in the world.

In this day of the harassed and over-worked war time physician and the many young mothers far away from the comforting reassurance of their family doctors, a copy of "Babies Are Fun" should be stressed as a first article of the layette. Many a frantic telephone call could be avoided and many an anxious parent calmed.

The author has managed to answer all of the perplexing small questions that are too often taken for granted as a matter of female instinct. She has dealt humorously and accurately with each aspect of everyday infant care from the correct method of folding a diaper to the small problems of behaviorism. Although she has stressed the importance of each routine task, it is all made to sound like an exciting adventure thereby helping the young mother to retain her sense of balance and her sense of humor no matter what Junior may think of next.—Betty S. Moorman.

SURGICAL PATHOLOGY. (Fifth edition thoroughly revised.) William Boyd, M. D. 502 illustrations and 16 colored plates. W. B. Saunders Company, Philadelphia and London. 1942. Price $10.00.

It is a most worthy addition to the reference library of every surgeon, internist and pathologist. The pathology of surgical conditions is placed before both student and practitioner, from a practical standpoint, Dr. William Boyd has had wide experience in the pathological department of the Winnepeg General Hospital and as professor of pathology at the University of Toronto, and writes in a clear style with excellent description and illustration.

The chapter on the thyroid gland is one of the best in literature. The diseases of the vermiform appendix are excellently portrayed. The chapter on the cranium and its contents, gives a practical approach to the difficult terminology of brain tumors. The diseases of the bones are covered in a manner which thoroughly deals with the underlying pathology.—Major W. A. Howard, M. C.

FULL TIME INTENSIVE COURSE IN ELECTROCARDIOGRAPHY

From August 16 to August 28, 1943, an intensive graduate course in Electrocardiography will be offered to physicians at the Michael Reese Hospital by Dr. Louis N. Katz, Director of Cardiovascular Research.

There will be practice on several electrocardiographic machines and discussion of the principals of their construction and use. Sessions will be held on interpretations of electrocardiograms illustrated by lantern slides, and practice by the student with unknown records. Emphasis will be placed on chest leads and on importance of the electrocardiogram in coronary sclerosis and myocardial infraction. The mechanism and interpretation of heart irregularities will be developed.

As group and individual instruction will be given, the course is open to both the beginning and advanced student in Electrocardiography. It is planned to individualize the course so that at the end of the period each student will be capable of taking and properly interpreting routine electrocardiograms. In order to accomplish this purpose, the class will be limited in number. It is imperative, therefore, that reservations be made early.

For further information address Michael Reese Hospital, Cardiovascular Department, 29th and Ellis Avenue, Chicago Illinois.

DISCOVERING THE OBVIOUS

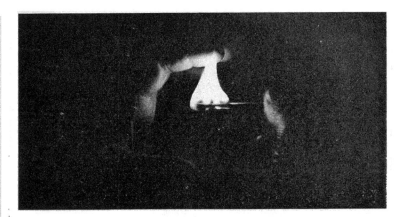

OFFICERS OF COUNTY SOCIETIES, 1943

★

COUNTY	PRESIDENT	SECRETARY	MEETING TIME
Alfalfa	H. E. Huston, Cherokee	L. T. Lancaster, Cherokee	Last Tues. each Second Month
Atoka-Coal	J. B. Clark, Coalgate	J. S. Fulton, Atoka	
Beckham	H. K. Speed, Sayre	E. S. Kilpatrick, Elk City	Second Tuesday
Blaine	Virginia Olson Curtin, Watonga	W. F. Griffin, Watonga	
Bryan	J. T. Colwick, Durant	W. K. Haynie, Durant	Second Tuesday
Caddo	F. L. Patterson, Carnegie	C. B. Sullivan, Carnegie	
Canadian	P. F. Herod, El Reno	A. L. Johnson, El Reno	Subject to call
Carter	Walter Hardy, Ardmore	H. A. Higgins, Ardmore	
Cherokee	P. H. Medearis, Tahlequah	James K. Gray, Tahlequah	First Tuesday
Choctaw	C. H. Hale, Boswell	E. A. Johnson, Hugo	
Cleveland	J. A. Rieger, Norman	Curtis Berry, Norman	Thursday nights
Comanche	George S. Barber, Lawton	W. F. Lewis, Lawton	
Cotton	A. B. Holstead, Temple	Mollie F. Scism, Walters	Third Friday
Craig	F. M. Adams, Vinita	J. M. McMillan, Vinita	
Creek	H. R. Haas, Sapulpa	C. G. Oakes, Sapulpa	
Custer	F. R. Vieregg, Clinton	C. J. Alexander, Clinton	Third Thursday
Garfield	Paul B. Champlin, Enid	John R. Walker, Enid	Fourth Thursday
Garvin	T. F. Gross, Lindsay	John R. Callaway, Pauls Valley	Wednesday before Third Thursday
Grady	Walter J. Baze, Chickasha	Roy E. Emanuel, Chickasha	Third Thursday
Grant	I. V. Hardy, Medford	E. E. Lawson, Medford	
Greer	G. P. Cherry, Mangum	J. B. Hollis, Mangum	
Harmon	W. G. Husband, Hollis	L. E. Hollis, Hollis	First Wednesday
Haskell	William Carson, Keota	N. K. Williams, McCurtain	
Hughes	Wm. L. Taylor, Holdenville	Imogene Mayfield, Holdenville	First Friday
Jackson	E. S. Crow, Olustee	E. W. Mabry, Altus	Last Monday
Jefferson	F. M. Edwards, Ringling	L. L. Wade, Ryan	Second Monday
Kay	Philip C. Risser, Blackwell	J. Holland Howe, Ponca City	Third Thursday
Kingfisher	C. M. Hodgson, Kingfisher	H. Violet Sturgeon, Hennessey	
Kiowa	B. H. Watkins, Hobart	J. William Finch, Hobart	
LeFlore	Neeson Rolle, Poteau	Rush L. Wright, Poteau	
Lincoln	H. B. Jenkins, Tryon	Carl H. Bailey, Stroud	First Wednesday
Logan	William C. Miller, Guthrie	J. L. LeHew, Jr., Guthrie	Last Tuesday
Marshall	O. A. Cook, Madill	Philip G. Joseph, Madill	
Mayes	Ralph V. Smith, Pryor	Paul B. Cameron, Pryor	
McClain	B. W. Slover, Blanchard	R. L. Royster, Purcell	
McCurtain	A. W. Clarkson, Valliant	N. L. Barker, Broken Bow	Fourth Tuesday
McIntosh	James L. Wood, Eufaula	William A. Tolleson, Eufaula	First Thursday
Murray	P. V. Annadown, Sulphur	F. E. Sadler, Sulphur	Second Tuesday
Muskogee-Sequoyah-Wagoner	H. A. Scott, Muskogee	D. Evelyn Miller, Muskogee	First Monday
Noble	C. H. Cooke, Perry	J. W. Francis, Perry	
Okfuskee	L. J. Spickard, Okemah	M. L. Whitney, Okemah	Second Monday
Oklahoma	Walker Morledge, Oklahoma City	E. R. Musick, Oklahoma City	Fourth Tuesday
Okmulgee	A. R. Holmes, Henryetta	J. C. Matheney, Okmulgee	Second Monday
Osage	C. R. Weirich, Pawhuska	George K. Hemphill, Pawhuska	Second Monday
Ottawa	W. B. Sanger, Picher	Matt A. Connell, Picher	Third Thursday
Pawnee	E. T. Robinson, Cleveland	R. L. Browning, Pawnee	
Payne	L. A. Mitchell, Stillwater	C. W. Moore, Stillwater	Third Thursday
Pittsburg	John F. Park, McAlester	William H. Kaeiser, McAlester	Third Friday
Pontotoc	O. H. Miller, Ada	R. H. Mayes, Ada	First Wednesday
Pottawatomie	A. C. McFarling, Shawnee	Clinton Gallaher, Shawnee	First and Third Saturday
Pushmataha	John S. Lawson, Clayton	B. M. Huckabay, Antlers	
Rogers	C. W. Beson, Claremore	C. L. Caldwell, Chelsea	First Monday
Seminole	Max Van Sandt, Wewoka	Mack I. Shanholtz, Wewoka	Third Wednesday
Stephens	W. K. Walker, Marlow	Wallis S. Ivy, Duncan	
Texas	R. G. Obermiller, Texhoma	Morris Smith, Guymon	
Tillman	R. D. Robinson, Frederick	O. G. Bacon, Frederick	
Tulsa	James C. Peden, Tulsa	E. O. Johnson, Tulsa	Second and Fourth Monday
Washington-Nowata	J. G. Smith, Bartlesville	J. V. Athey, Bartlesville	Second Wednesday
Washita	A. S. Neal, Cordell	James F. McMurry, Sentinel	
Woods	C. A. Traverse, Alva	O. E. Templin, Alva	Last Tuesday Odd Months
Woodward	C. E. Williams, Woodward	C. W. Tedrowe, Woodward	Second Thursday

THE JOURNAL
OF THE
OKLAHOMA STATE MEDICAL ASSOCIATION

| VOLUME XXXVI | OKLAHOMA CITY, OKLAHOMA, JULY, 1943 | NUMBER 7 |

Spontaneous Pneumothorax in Apparently Healthy Young Adults

J. Floyd Moorman, M.D.

OKLAHOMA CITY, OKLAHOMA

Usually spontaneous pneumothorax has been considered due to tuberculosis until proved otherwise. If a tubercle should be located beneath the visceral pleura, it is possible that rupture through the pleura could occur and produce pneumothorax. On the other hand, if a tuberculous lesion develops at the periphery of the lung, adhesions are prone to occur rather early in a large percentage of cases. Laennec (1819) first recognized pneumothorax in the living patient by ausculation. Louis (1825) showed that it was a common complication of pulmonary tuberculosis. During the past few years, I have observed six cases of spontaneous pneumothorax in young adults, all of whom had apparently been in good health prior to the accident. It is now being recognized that pneumothorax occurs in apparently healthy persons, and accumulated data reveals rather conclusively that the condition is often entirely unrelated to clinical tuberculosis. Many names have been applied to this type of pneumothorax, such as "pneumothorax in the apparently healthy," "benign spontaneous pneumothorax" and "pneumothorax simplex." Perhaps the best name suggested is "idiopathic spontaneous pneumothorax." This condition not only occurs in the apparently healthy, but is usually manifested by an afebrile benign course with recovery in a few weeks.

Exertion is not a necessary precipitating factor. Laughing, coughing, sneezing, straining at stool, coitus and running have been reported as the immediate cause, but many cases occur while the patient is resting in bed or in a chair.

Etiology of spontaneous pneumothorax as recorded by Phillips and Kneopp:[1]

1. Exogenous
   (a) accidental
   (b) operative
2. Endogenous.
   (a) adhesions
   (b) blebs
   (c) necrosis
   (d) tuberculosis
   (e) carcinoma
   (f) cystic disease
   (g) other inflammations

Blebs are of two types (1) the scar-tissue variety which predominate at the apex, and (2) the emphysematous type which occur on the lung border.

Because of the benign nature of this type of pneumothorax, very few opportunities have ever occurred to study its pathologic basis. A number of cases have been reported in which subpleural emphysematous blebs have been found at autopsy, and five cases have been reported in which autopsy demonstrated congenital lung cysts as the cause of the spontaneous pneumothorax. Kjaergaard,[2] who has made a rather extensive study of the problem of etiology believes that subpleural vesicles may form and eventually rupture on any of three pathological bases: (1) congenital valve vesicles (2) emphysematous valve vesicles, and (3) scar tissue vesicles.

Whether the original lesion be a congenital subpleural cyst, localized and valvular emphysema, or a subpleural scar from any cause, the mechanism of the actual rupture is apparently the same. Air enters a subpleural space more readily than it can leave it, consequently, a positive pressure is built by respiration, the pleura becomes progressively thinner, and finally, with or without any slight strain such as a cough, sneeze, or laugh, the difference in pressures between the interior of the vesicle and the potential pleural space becomes too great for the tensile strength of the attentuated and avascular pleura, which tears, allowing air to enter the pleural space until the pressures are equalized. This accident is most frequent in early adult life because the intrapleural pressure is most negative at that age. Moreover, such valve vesicles are situated most commonly at the apex of the lung, where, according to Parodi,[3] the difference between intrapulmonary and intrapleural pressure is the greatest due to the effects of gravity and of the concentration of forces on that area.

The presence of valve vesicles explains the marked tendency of spontaneous pneumothorax to recur. Also, since such vesicles are apt to be found in the apices of both lungs if present in one, it explains the occurrence of bilateral, simultaneous, or successive pneumothoraces.

The preponderance of males in the cases reported and observed is an unexplained phenomenon. If it has been solely due to the more strenuous pursuits of young men, one would expect to hear of an increased number of such accidents among the young women who today exercise as vigorously as their brothers. An hereditary tendency is suggested by Atwood,[4] and his cases were in father and son. However, physical differences between the two sexes may suffice to explain the susceptibility of the male to pneumothorax. Between the end of the growth period and the loss of pulmonary elasticity accompanying the later decades of life, the lungs are at the greatest stretch. The predominately diaphragmatic type of breathing and the low position of the diaphram in the tall lean type of young man concentrate the tension at the lung apices favoring both vesicle formation and rupture.

The symptoms and physical findings will depend upon the extent of the collapse, this depending upon the size of the rent in the visceral pleura. The onset is usually sudden and the first symptom is usually pain in the chest, most often on the affected side. The pain may be referred to the shoulder or abdomen and the symptoms may sometimes simulate or be mistaken for some abdominal emergency. Dyspnea is complained of by most patients, the intensity of this symptom will depend upon the extent of the collapse and displacement of the mediastinum. Cough is present and usually unproductive. Absence of fever is the rule and the pulse rate is usually normal. Accumulation of fluid in the pleural cavity may result in elevation of temperature and this is usually accompanied by

soreness in the chest. Many cases have been diagnosed pleurisy, intercostal neuralgia, muscle strain or something else.

The physical signs of pneumothorax (absence of tactile fremitus, and diminution or absence of voice and breath sounds) are said to be present in all cases. In the ordinary routine examination of the chest these findings may often be overlooked, particularly in those patients where a thin layer of air is present. Lagging of the affected side can usually be detected by careful observation. Displacement of the mediastinal structures will be evident in some left sided cases and when collapse is complete. The coin test is usually negative and amphoric breath sound or rales are seldom found.

Fluoroscopic examination alone is not reliable, small pneumothoraces without thickening of the pleura may not be visible by fluoroscopy. An x-ray film is the most reliable method of diagnosis and any patient who presents himself with the complaint of pain in the chest should have an x-ray. Oftentimes spontaneous pneumothorax had not been suspected until the roentgenogram revealed its presence.

Routine laboratory examinations are usually negative. The tuberculin test is important, in that a patient presenting a positive test might offer a clue as to the etiology. A positive test does not mean clinical tuberculosis but a negative one virtually excludes this etiology. No acid fast organisms were found in the sputum of any of our cases. If productive cough is present, a diligent and persistent search should be made for tubercle bacilli, because if the etiology should prove to be tuberculous, the treatment would be different.

TREATMENT

Most observers recommend nothing more than several weeks of rest in bed. Rest is the first requisite. All but one of our cases have been converted into artificial pneumothorax which is contrary to the recommendations of other observers. My reasons for this method of treatment are: (1) when I first observed this condition, I was of the opinion that tuberculosis was the etiology, (2) all patients were relieved of pain in the chest, and dyspnea. Frequent floroscopic examinations revealed the fact that after the introduction of air into the pleural cavity re-expansion of the lung was hastened permitting a more accurate opinion as to the presence or absence of pulmonary pathology which might have been obscured by the collapse. The intrapleural pressure is usually negative and changing this to a more neutral pressure seems to be the most logical explanation for the relief of symptoms. Naturally, if collapse were complete, air would have to be removed.

In some of the idiopathic cases collapse might recur. In one of our patients, this happened three times, the lung would apparently re-expand completely and then at a later date manifest recurrence of symptoms (pain in the chest and dyspnea) and examination and x-ray would reveal a partial collapse of the lung. This case was then converted into an artificial pneumothorax and maintained for approximately twelve months after which there was no recurrence. At one time it was felt that the pneumothorax should be obliterated as quickly as possible by the introduction of cauterizing solutions and frequently an open operation was recommended. Experience has shown that such procedures are unnecessary and not without danger.

If, after a few weeks observation, the physician can feel reasonably sure that tuberculosis does not exist, the lung may be permitted to re-expand. If the artificial pneumothorax is maintained for several months, re-expansion usually results in the development of adhesive pleuritis, obliterating the normal pleural cavity, which is the attainment desired in cases of idiopathic spontaneous pneumothorax.

A certain number of these patients will develop fluid which is usually in small amounts and is most always absorbed. Exploratory thoracentesis in an Oklahoma University student with a spontaneous pneumothorax revealed the presence of blood in the pleural cavity. He had no fever, and pain in the chest and dyspnea were the only symptoms. He was kept in bed for one week after which the lung re-expanded.

Recurrent pneumothorax is not uncommon. In one of our cases it occurred three times. One of Wilson's[5] cases had three attacks, another two. Sale[6] reported a case with eleven attacks of p n e u m o t h o r a x. Hawes[7] reported a case with at least twelve attacks. Wilson[5] states that the incidence of recurrence is about 20 per cent of all cases. Wood[8] found 21 per cent recurrent in reporting a series of 71 cases from the Mayo Clinic. Bilateral pneumothorax may occur, the second lung seeming to rupture under the stress of compensating for the collapse of the first. This condition naturally carries with it a much more serious immediate prognosis than the unilateral form. In cases of repeatedly recurrent spontaneous pneumothorax, conversion into an artificial pneumothorax is the safest and most effective treatment. Maintaining this for several months, then permitting the lung to re-expand, results in obliteration of the pleural space. Injecting various substances into the pleural sac, such as the patient's own blood, 30 per cent glucose and 0.5 per cent solution of silver nitrate has been recommended for the recurrent cases.

Bilateral pneumothorax calls for emergency aspiration of air. In this type of case, one should not hesitate to use continuous suction to re-expand one lung until the other perforation can close. Oxygen therapy is valuable in this type.

CASE REPORTS

B. L. M., white female, age 17, highschool student. First examined February 10, 1934. Chief complants: pain in the right chest, fatigue, dry cough. Family history negative. Past history negative except an operation for cleft palate when three years of age. Present illness: On January 27, 1934, she developed pain in the right chest that was aggravated by deep breathing. She was out of school for one week. The pain was relieved by rest and application of heat. The pain persisted, but was not constant and was often referred to the right shoulder. Examination: weight 95, temperature 98.8, pulse 112, respiration 20, blood pressure 118/80. Limited expansion and diminished breath sounds right chest. X-ray revealed approximately 75 per cent

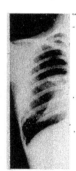
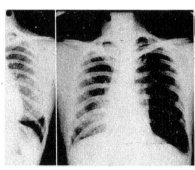
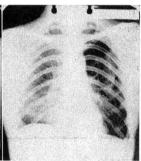

Fig. 1   Fig. 2   Fig. 3

collapse of the right lung. (Fig. 1). Air, 200-350 cc, was introduced into the right pleural cavity February 23, March 2 and 9, 1934, then discontinued. On March 30, 1934, fluoroscopy showed the right lung completely re-expanded. She has had no further trouble and is now a student in the University of Oklahoma.

O. S. J. white male, age 28, postoffice clerk. First examined March 8, 1938. Chief complaints: Shortness of breath, cough, pain in the left shoulder. Family history unimportant. Past history unimportant. Present illness: began in February 1938, with a pain in left chest and shoulder, followed later by unproductive cough and shortness of breath. This was a recurring spontaneous pneumothorax as the roentgenologist who referred him to me had observed him from February 11 to March 8. The lung had collapsed and re-expanded twice during this time. (Fig. 2)

chest, dry cough. Present illness: On January 6, 1940, while sitting in an automobile after having been hunting he noticed a dull pain in the lower left chest which gradually increased in severity. By the time he got home the pain was very severe, "cutting off" his breath and making talking difficult. His family physician was called who attributed the pain to an abscessed gum where a tooth had been extracted several days previously. The pain became less severe during the night, but shortness of breath and soreness in the left chest have persisted. Change of position aggravates the symptoms. Examination: Weight 127½, temperature 98.6, pulse 96, respiration 22, blood pressure 105/80. Limited expansion of the left chest, distant breath sounds and displacement of the mediastinal structures to the right. Fluoroscopic examination revealed approximately 80 per cent collapse of the left lung with displacement of

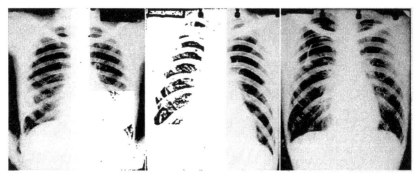

Fig. 4   Fig. 5   Fig. 6

Examination revealed a well developed and well nourished male. Weight 154, temperature 98.4, pulse 80, blood pressure 118/80. Expansion of left chest was restricted, the percussion note was hyperresonant and breath sounds were distant over the left side. Fluoroscopic examination showed approximately 75 per cent collapse of the left lung. This case was converted into an artificial pneumothorax which was maintained until March, 1939. During the course of treatment he continued to work as a clerk in a postoffice, his general condition was excellent and at the time of the last examination July 7, 1939, the left lung had completely re-expanded, there was no evidence of thickening of the visceral pleura and the left hemidiaphragm moved normally during respiration.

W. J. J., white male, age 32, baker. First examined January 11, 1940. Chief complaints: shortness of breath, soreness in left

the heart to the right and fluid in the costophrenic angle. X-ray confirmed these findings. (Fig. 3). This case was converted into an artificial pneumothorax and collapse was maintained for six months, the last refill being given June 29, 1940. On July 29, 1940, fluoroscopy showed the lung completely re-expanded. He is now in good condition and continuing his occupation as a baker.

T. H., white female, age 27, housewife. First examined April 22, 1941. Chief complaints: fatigue, cough, loss of weight, dyspnea, pain in right chest. Family history: maternal grandmother, mother, an aunt and two cousins died of tuberculosis, father has pulmonary tuberculosis. Close contact with mother, father and two cousins. Examination revealed a fairly well nourshed white woman. Temperature 98.8, pulse 66, respiration 24, blood pressure 118/80, weight 109. There was diminution of breath sounds over the right chest. Otherwise negative. X-ray revealed approximately 50 per cent collapse of the right lung and slight displacement of the mediastinal structures to the left. (Fig. 4). Three sputum tests were negative for tubercle bacilli. Four refills, 150-300 cc, air was given at weekly intervals and then discontinued because she had mild reactions (fever, pain in chest and malaise) following refills. She was last examined September 16, 1941. No rales were heard and fluoroscopic examination showed complete re-expansion of the lung.

D. L., white male, age 27, student at University of Oklahoma. First examined April 3, 1941. Chief complaints: pain in the right chest, shortness of breath. Family and past history negative. Present illness: on April 2, 1941, while walking to class he was seized with a severe pain in the right chest and dyspnea. The day before he had pain in the right shoulder which was relieved to some extent by heat. He entered the University Infirmary and an x-ray revealed collapse of right lung. (Fig. 5). Examination: weight 169¼, temperature 98.2, pulse 84, respiration 22, blood pressure 112/80. Breath sounds were distant over the right chest. Fluoroscopic examination showed approximately 40 per cent collapse of the right lung with small amount of fluid in the pleural cavity. Diagnosis: Hydropneumothorax (right).

On April 5, 1941, fluoroscopic examination showed less collapse of the right lung with a small amount of fluid still present. An exploratory thoracentesis was done and 5cc. of dark blood was aspirated. The diagnosis was hemopneumothorax. He was advised to rest as much as possible and was seen again November 11, 1941. Temperature 98.6, weight 167, pulse 96. No constant rales were heard. No pneumothorax space was visible by fluoroscopy, a small amount of fluid filled the right costophrenic angle.

G. M., white male, age 23, student at University of Oklahoma. First examined March 28, 1941. Chief complaints: pain in the right chest, shortness of breath, cough, sore throat. He gave a history of having had pleurisy, left side, in 1936. Present illness: on March 22, 1941, while sitting in a chair he felt a sudden sharp pain in the right chest which was aggravated by movement or a deep breath. March 24, 1941, he was examined at the University Infirmary. An x-ray revealed a spontaneous pneumothorax and a small amount of fluid. (Fig. 6). An intracutaneous tuberculin test was 3 plus. Examination: weight 141½, temperature 98.4, pulse 80, respiration 20, blood pressure 100/66. Expansion of the right chest was limited and breath sounds were distant over this side. Hospitalization was advised, and he entered the Farm Sanatorium March 31, 1941. The

spontaneous pneumothorax was converted into an artificial pneumothorax. After four weeks in the sanatorium, he was permitted to resume his studies at the University. During his stay in the sanatorium his temperature never exceeded 99.4 and was usually normal. Repeated sputum tests were negative for tubercle bacilli. Artificial pneumothorax was discontinued September 20, 1941. At that time his weight was 158 and he had no symptoms. He is a senior in the University of Oklahoma. Collapse was maintained for several months because the x-ray showed some infiltration and fibrosis in the second right interspace which was suggestive of tuberculous infiltration.

SUMMARY

Six cases of spontaneous pneumothorax have been presented, four males and two females between the ages of 17 and 32 years. There were four right-sided and two left-sided cases. With the exception of the case of hemopneumothorax, all were converted into artificial pneumothoraces because past experience had shown that this procedure relieved symptoms and because we were not absolutely convinced that tuberculosis was not an etiological factor. Only one of the six patients had a tuberculin test but this should never be neglected even though a positive tuberculin test does not warrant a diagnosis of tuberculosis without other confirmatory evidence. Particulary in cases of recurring spontaneous pneumothorax conversion into an artificial pneumothorax would seem to be the treatment of choice and this would also apply to cases in which there is any suspicion of tuberculosis as revealed either by the history, physical or x-ray examination.

Although this is a small series, it confirms the opinion of many investigators that exertion is not a necessary precipitating factor.

BIBLIOGRAPHY

1. Phillips, J. R. and Knoepp, L. F.: Diseases of the Chest VI: 243-247, (August) 1940.
2. Kjaergaard, H.: Acta Med. Scandinav., 43 (Suppl.) 1, 1932.
3. Parodi, J.: "La Mechanique Pulmonaire," Masson et Cie, Paris, 1933.
4. Atwood, A. W.: Boston M. & S. J., 195: 1287, 1926.
5. Wilson, J. L.: Spontaneous Pneumothorax, Internat. Clin. 1: 157-175, (March) 1937.
6. Sale, J. C.: Lancet 1: 1572, 1907.
7. Hawes, J. B.: Boston M. & S. J. 186: 528, 1922.
8. Wood, H. G.: Minnesota Med., 14: 550, 1931 (cited by Leggett et al).

Decreased Rate of Tubercular Deaths

In a recent announcement, the National Tuberculosis Association with headquarters in New York City has disclosed the fact that in 1941 the death rate resulting from tuberculosis had decreased from 44 per 100,000 population as compared to 46 for every 100,000 population in 1940. The association further warned that, due to wartime conditions, the disease would probably show an increase for the year 1942.

Rocky Mountain Spotted Fever*

PAUL SIZEMORE, M.D.

DURANT, OKLAHOMA

It is my object in this paper to bring out a fairly well generalized knowledge I learned in dealing with seven cases of Rocky Mountain Spotted Fever. This experience dates to August and September 1941, and all relates to the same locality, in fact, all but one being in the same family. There is a distinct possibility that an eighth case could be mentioned in this discussion.

These cases occurred in Bryan County which is located in the south central section of Oklahoma. The town of Armstrong, where these cases occurred, is in the northwest part of the county, some five miles north of Durant. This section is semi-prairie with sandy loam soil. A small river runs about one-eighth mile away. Both a railway and a national highway pass through the town. Many trees are seen along the river banks but only a few are scattered throughout the village. A heavy growth of grass and weeds predominate throughout the locality. Numerous gopher mounds are seen, especially surrounding the house where cases occurred. Since this is a typical farming region there is the usual number of cattle, horses and dogs in evidence.

The family had lived in the described vicinity for several years but had been on a visit to Texas, some hundred miles away, two weeks previous to the onset of the first case of fever. Upon their return from Texas they moved into a new, unpainted, green lumber house only a short distance from their previous home. As far as I was able to learn there had been no cases in the part of Texas where the family had visited.

On August 27, 1941 I was asked by Dr. Allen Flythe, a former Durant physician, to accompany him on a call to Armstrong. The first patient seen, Mrs. M. Q., was a well developed white female, aged 37. She was acutely ill. The history of the onset was as follows, which by the way, was quite typical of the other cases: fourteen days previous to this visit the patient developed fever, anorexia, headache, photophobia, chilly sensations, generalized aching accompanied by muscular tenderness. In three or four days

*Read at the Annual Meeting of the Oklahoma State Medical Association, May 12, at Oklahoma City, Oklahoma.

a macular rash appeared on ankles and wrists which gradually spread over her entire body. Restlessness and insomnia became prominent and distressing symptoms. Please note that I first saw this patient several days after she became sick.

Physical and laboratory findings were as follows: a generalized petechial rash was seen over the body, including soles of feet, palms of hands and buccal mucosa. In scattered areas over the body surface, the skin presented a bluish, mottled appearance. The sclera and conjunctiva were injected. Generalized muscular tenderness was present, this being more marked in the lower extremities and lumbar region. Examination of the abdomen revealed some tympanites and a slightly enlarged spleen. The temperature by mouth was 102 F., pulse 118, respiration 30, and blood pressure 130/84. Records showed that the temperature had varied from 101 F. to 104 F. since onset. The leucocyte count was 10,000. Urinalysis was negative for pus, sugar and albumin. Widal and stool examinations were negative for typhoid fever. No laboratory examinations had been made for typhus or Rocky Mountain Spotted Fever. Blood serology was negative for syphilis.

May. I say that, in an adjoining room, two small sons of the patient described had been sick a few days with a strikingly similar condition. The smaller of the two, a three year old child, had gotten sick seven days after onset of the mother's illness. A similar rash appeared three days after fever developed. During the course of the disease the child's temperature ranged from 102 F. to 106 F. rectally, and during the height of the fever, convulsions were not uncommon. The leucocyte count ranged as high as 20,000. Insomnia, muscular tenderness, photophobia and headache were marked. The other child, a five year old boy, developed fever, headache, anorexia, etc., four days before this visit. A macular rash which disappeared on pressure, was present on wrists and ankles and in three or four days it spread over the body and had become slightly raised and petechial in character. This case differs somewhat from the other two in that constipation was more marked. Temperature varied from 101 F. to 103.6 F. rectally, with a leucocyte count of 13,000. Although this patient was delirious at times, no convulsions occurred.

The remainder of the household examined on this first visit consisted of Mrs Q.'s husband, daughter, and mother. On questioning, the husband was found to have a slight elevation of temperature. He complained of dull headache, chilly sensations, anorexia, generalized aching and was noticeably apprehensive. The next day he had a severe headache, photophobia, temperature of 101 F., and pulse rate of 115. Two days later he developed a macular rash, first on wrists and ankles, which later spread over abdomen, back, face, and buccal mucosa. His condition became gradually worse and on the seventh day he developed bronchial pneumonia. This cleared up and he was able to be up and about on the 25th day.

Naturally, investigations were begun on the first visit as to what we were dealing with. Typhus fever was suspected but further questioning brought out the fact that all members of the household had been bitten repeatedly, since moving to this house, by ticks which infested the yard. The family stressed the fact there were numerous ticks on the premises. These statements put a new angle in the picture. Rocky Mountain Spotted Fever was suspected. Blood samples were sent to the State Laboratories for examination. The diagnosis of Rocky Mountain Spotted Fever was later confirmed at the Rocky Mountain Laboratories, Hamilton, Montana.

On September 1, or about three weeks after the first member of this group became sick, Mrs. M. Q.'s mother, aged 67, developed Rocky Mountain Spotted Fever. On the fifth day bronchopneumonia complicated the tick fever and she died three days later.

On September 12, or one month after the onset of the first patient's illness, her eight year old daughter developed the disease. The course was uneventful and recovery was complete within 2 weeks.

The attending physician, Doctor Allen Flythe, age 44, became sick September 13. He gave a history of having found a tick under his right axilla 12 days previous to onset of fever. This case was fulminating in character. The onset was with a chill, fever,

severe headache, generalized muscular tenderness and aching, then photophobia, extreme restlessness and insomnia which seemed to be aggravated by a feeling of apprehension. By the end of the fourth day the rash was well generalized. Large petechia became numerous and produced a generalized bluish mottling of the skin. Early in the course of the disease the leucocyte count was 9,000 but later it reached 14,000. The temperature (oral) ranged from 102 F. to 105 F. and pulse 118 to 140 per minute. He went into a coma several hours before death. During this period his temperature reached 106 F., and pulse became thready, irregular and very rapid. The use of opiates was resorted to, to help control the nervousness, headache, and insomnia. The toxic condition of the patient became worse and he died early the seventh day.

Another person that was probably infected was a white male, aged 47, who stayed at the Q. home while the first three members of the family were sick. At the end of the first week he became ill and returned to his home. His family said that he developed a rash a few days later and died on the eighth day of his illness. It so happened that the same embalmer who took care of the other Spotted Fever fatalities also saw this one. He said the appearance of the skin in all three cases was the same. From this evidence I am inclined to think that this was also a case of Spotted Fever.

The eight year old girl received 1 c.c. of Rocky Mountain Spotted Fever vaccine 7 days previous to onset of fever. Dr. Flythe was given 1 c.c. of vaccine 5 days before onset of fever or seven days after having been bitten by the tick, and another 1 c.c. injection at onset of the disease. No other members of this group were given any vaccine.

The treatment of all cases was symptomatic and supportive, i.e., bland diet, forced fluids, intravenous glucose, sedatives, tepid sponges, enemas as needed, and opiates when necessary. Sulfonamide therapy was tried but was of no proven value.

Prophylaxis or preventive measures consists in destruction of ticks, especially in areas where the disease exists or has existed. This of course, is a difficult undertaking. In the Armstrong area, where above cases occurred, the gopher proved to be the ticks'

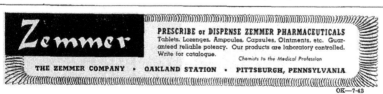

host, consequently many have since been destroyed.

Secondly, the use of vaccine in infested areas each year is indicated. This is best given in late winter or early spring. Recommended dosage by the United States Public Health Service for adults is two injections of 2 c.c.'s each or three injections of 1 c.c. each, five to ten days apart. An additional injection is desirable in areas of high case fatality. For children ten years of age or over, the adult dosage may be given. Children under 10 years may be given one half the adult dosage. The vaccination should be completed at least ten days before the first expected exposure. The vaccine is not recommended for therapeutic use. It certainly did not help in the case of Dr. Flythe.

The diagnosis consists chiefly in history of tick bite, character and distribution of the rash and laboratory examination of blood and serum. These consist of the agglutination test, guinea pig inoculation and lastly, the protection or virus neutralization test. When collecting blood to be sent to the laboratory at least 10 c.c.'s should be obtained.

Rocky Mountain Spotted Fever must be differentiated from typhus fever, typhoid fever, measles, and meningitis. History is very important. However, laboratory

In case of doubt a spinal puncture should be resorted to.

In conclusion it may be said that in Oklahoma, Rocky Mountain Spotted Fever is not a rare disease. I wish to say it is not only probable but highly possible that in several cases Spotted Fever has either been mis-diagnosed or not diagnosed at all. This probably accounts for the fact that such a disease was not suspected. Besides the seven cases mentioned in this paper several others have been reported from various sections over the state during the past two or three years and in general the mortality rate has not been low.

DISCUSSION

LEA A. RIELY, M.D.

OKLAHOMA CITY, OKLAHOMA

Dr. Sizemore has done a distinct service to the profession in so ably and minutely giving the clinical details of these seven cases which he personally observed.

The Board of Health has a record of one case in 1936, one in 1937, and one in 1938, three in 1939, ten in 1940, fourteen in 1941, and twelve in 1942, males being three times as frequent as females. Ages range from eighteen months to sixty-eight years, no negroes being reported throughout. The mortality is about 30 per cent. These cases are

SUMMARY OF CASES

	Sex	Age	Onset	Duration	Complications	Outcome
1.	Female	37	8-13-41	19 days	None	Recovery
2.	Male	37	8-29-41	24 days	Broncho-pneumonia	Recovery
3.	Male	3	8-20-41	21 days	None	Recovery
4.	Male	5	8-23-41	20 days	None	Recovery
5.	Female	67	9-1-41	8 days	Broncho-pneumonia	Died
6.	Female	8	9-12-41	12 days	None	Recovery
7.	Male	44	9-13-41	7 days		Died

methods may have to be resorted to, in order to distinguish Rocky Mountain Spotted Fever from typhus. In typhoid the prodromal symptoms are longer, the rash is different, diarrhea is usually present whereas in Rocky Mountain Spotted Fever constipation is the rule. Laboratory procedures can also be resorted to. Measles at its height may present some difficulty, as the rash may resemble the early rash of Spotted Fever. In fact, at the onset Mrs. Q. was thought to have measles. The history of slower onset, coryza symptoms, the absence of severe muscular pain and tenderness, and the character and distribution of the rash serve to differentiate between the two. In epidemic meningitis the onset is more sudden and nervous symptoms with rigidity of the neck appear early.

reported from the counties of southern, eastern and central portions of this State.

Rickettsia infections are a public health problem through the whole of the United States. In the Bitter Root Valley of Montana the mortality reaches 90 per cent, while only 15 per cent in eastern Montana, and 3 per cent in the Eastern states. Brills disease was only one per cent. Some think the variance of mortality is due to the different vectors and their modification of the pathogenicity of the germ.

The rural districts are the ones infected, and the vector is the tick. The Dermacenter Andersoni in the West and the Dermacenter Variabilis in the east. Animals, including rodents, may act as reservoirs of these vectors. Rats are the animal reservoir and fleas are the vectors in Typhus, also caused by the Rickettesia. When anyone is infected with ticks, they should use forceps to remove them, either from themselves or their dogs, as the unbroken skin will be pervious to the bacilli harbored in the excrement of these ticks. These infected ticks are found only in about one per cent of the ticks examined in the regions where the disease prevails, and only laboratory measures can tell the infected ones.

Those working in these regions such as farmers, hunters, and those in the many vocations of the petroleum industry should be especially careful about these ticks. I have seen many with ticks clinging to them. Dogs are prone to harbour them and their owners should have the same care in deticking them with forceps as they do themselves. These ticks are not infectious until they have been adherent to the body one hour or two, so early deticking is urgent. Kolmer says "that Spencer-Parker Vaccine is of value, capable of preventing the disease or reducing the severity and mortality. Duration of acquired immunity about one year. Wholesale immunity is not practical. Advisable in endemic areas for those particularly exposed to wood ticks."

Rocky Mountain Spotted Fever is not contagious, despite the fact that Dr. Sizemore found several cases in one family, hence isolation and quarantine are not advisable. It does not spread from man to man as in typhus fever. It occurs only from May to September, as the ticks are dormant during the colder period. The incubation period is from four to twelve days. The onset is sudden with headache, chills and rising temperature. Temperature may fluctuate, reaching 105 to 106 degrees, and continue from 15 to 22 days or until death, going down by lysis as contrasted with crisis in typhus. Macular rash and later possibly a papular rash beginning on the wrist and ankles after three to five days, and later becoming generalized and varying from rose red to petechial or hemorrhagic spots and may even be confluant.

Delerium, hyperesthesia and tremors noted. Peripheral vascular system has definite residual trouble, sometimes simulating thrombo-angitis abliterans. Like typhoid it has a splenomegaly and after the second week agglutination may or may not occur, which agglutinate proteus x19 in many cases, some even to 1-10,000. Cross immunity or neutralization tests in guinea pigs are used in differential diagnosis. Immunity is established in each case when recovered.

Rabbit immune seras are effective in the treatment of experimental infections of guinea pigs and monkeys. This has not been stabilized in the treatment of human beings. Five cases were treated by serum in this state in 1942 with one death. Sulfa group are found ineffective in the treatment of Richettesial group. Vaccine is of no value in the treatment.

BIBLIOGRAPHY:

1. Kolmer-Tuft: Clinical Immunology, Biotheraphy and Chemotheraphy. 1941.
2. Christian, H. A.: Osler's Principles and Practice of Medicine. Fourteenth Edition. 1892-1942.

The Plasma Bank

A. RAY WILEY, M.D.

TULSA, OKLAHOMA

This is the first of a series of articles on plasma, its place in our armamentarium, items of interest to the active clinician, as well as those engaged in the setting up and supervising a plasma bank. While technical detail will not be eliminated, emphasis will be upon the practical use for the clinician. Since all practical phases of the study of plasma cannot be suitably condensed in one article, others will follow in succeeding months.
—A.R.W.

During very recent years plasma has taken such a definite place in the armamentarium of the doctor, that it is necessary that each one of us gather as much knowledge on the subject as possible, and because the public has become so "plasma conscious" since the beginning of the war, we will be asked many questions by the laity. Be prepared to answer them. If the present Red Cross program is fulfilled, between three and four million Americans will volunteer as blood doners in 1943. The American doctors or their assistants will bleed these donors. The conduct of these doctors, their "Esprit de Corps", their ready knowledge of all facts about the blood banks, will greatly aid the morale of the public and enhance that traditional respect the public bears to the profession. There are certain requirements made of the donors which will at times necessitate considerable tact and finesse. This will be discussed further in the chapter on the transmission of diseases by transfusion.

I shall point out the uses and abuses of whole blood transfusions, plasma transfusions and crystalloid infusions. I believe these are very important and some points not as well understood as they should be. The use of plasma in various diseases and abnormal conditions such as shock, burns, infections, intestinal obstruction, nephrosis, certain heart diseases, etc., has been recognized. These conditions render the patients' blood deficient in blood protein by the loss of the plasma content of the blood, or in some conditions, such as shock, both a loss of tissue protein and blood stream plasma.[1] The physiological mechanism of plasma protein therapy needs considerable emphasis.

SHOCK

To properly appreciate the use of plasma in shock a better understanding of the pathology of shock is necessary. The condition that we know as shock still stands as a major surgical problem. While it has received exhaustive study, especially in recent years, there is a wide difference of opinion of its mechanism. No less than 22 theories are current in present medical literature. There are many types of shock by various causes and physical conditions and no one definition will cover all. The following was given by this author in 1939 and is as practical as any today. "Shock is the end result of certain efferent sympathetic nerve impulses, induced by a definite agent (toxic, trauma, etc.,) producing an abnormal capillary permeability." While many students in this work will not subscribe to the "leak-loss Theory," certainly there is a definite change in the osmotic pressure between the capillary and the tissue cells. The capillary endothelium loses its ability to retain the plasma protein within the capillary. The following quotation from the Military Surgical Manual[2] is of interest. "Increased capillary permeability as the ultimate cause of the progressive loss of volume of circulating blood, is probably the most accurate criterion of shock." The graphic illustration by Gamble,[3] clearly shows the interchange of body fluids, blood plasma and crystalloid solutions between the blood stream and the body tissue. Quoting Gibbons and Smith,[3] "the composition of blood plasma is simular to that of the inter-

stitial fluid, with the exception that the latter fluid contains a negligible amount of protein while the blood contains an important and significant amount. The plasma and the interstitial fluid with the exception of their proteins interchange freely with one another through the wall of the capillaries. The pressure of the protein in the plasma is essential to the retention of water and salts in the blood vessel, the osmotic pressure of the plasma proteins being equal, roughly, to the blood pressure in the capillaries.

The restoration or maintenance of blood volume has long been recognized as essential to the treatment of shock. No entirely satisfactory method for the accurate estimation of blood volume is known. This is especially true in small hospitals with limited equipment. Since it has been shown that restoration and maintenance of the blood protein is essential to the production of blood volume, it follows that the accurate determination of the plasma protein of the patient must be the criteria to plasma dosage or, in other words, the amount required from the plasma bank in each individual case.

In 1926 Barbour and Hamilton introduced the falling drop method of determining the specific gravity of body fluids, including total plasma protein. With a developed formula and improved instruments, the protein determination is now fairly simple. Every hospital using a blood bank should be equipped to make plasma protein determination by the falling drop method. The estimation of cell volume by the hematocrit method, though long known, was studied by Hedin in 1891. This interest in cell volume led to its use in determining changes in fluid losses. An increase in cell volume is the result of plasma loss from the blood vessels, whether the loss is the result of burns, trauma, shock, vomiting, or abnormal kidney action. The protein determination and estimation of cell volume by the hematocrit are used to determine the protein needs of the blood. Of course the exception to the use of the hematocrit is in marked cell loss as well as plasma loss in specific conditions, particularly hemorrhage. The use of the hematocrit in estimating plasma dosage will be further discussed in a chapter on burns. This data should be kept in mind for further articles on this subject, particularly in estimating plasma dosage. A normal person weighing 154 pounds (70 kilograms) has 5500 cc of whole blood or about 3000 cc of plasma. The normal plasma protein ranges from 5.9 gm. o/o to 7.9 gm. o/o with 6.5 to 7.5 being the usual range. Normal blood contains, roughly, 55 o/o plasma and 45 o/o cells.

In summarizing the treatment of shock, the most important and practical concept of shock is the loss of plasma protein, with its important and vita' onstituents. In order that this plasma may be replaced quickly and sufficiently, a blood specimen should be obtained just before administration of the

plasma, provided this causes no delay in giving the plasma, and further determinations should be made frequently, even every few hours, depending upon the clinical condition of the patient. As we shall see later, our ideas and dosage have changed, now knowing that much larger amounts of plasma are needed than was first thought.

BIBLIOGRAPHY

1. Culbertson: Lancet. Vol. 1, pp. 433. April 11, 1943.
2. Military Surgical Manuel. Vol. 5. 1943.
3. Gibbons, J. H. and Smith, Harold: Blood Chemical Aids to Surgical Therapy. Surgical Clinics of North America. Vol. 19, pp 1585. December, 1939.

Neuropsychiatric Problems Arising in the Civilian Population

JAMES ASA WILLIE, M.D.

OKLAHOMA CITY, OKLAHOMA

War is not a direct but more of a precipitating cause for an increased number of nervous and mental breakdowns in predisposed individuals. Probably no American can escape the emotional stresses of this present conflict. Many persons, for instance, are now suffering from a sense of insecurity, apprehension or frustration relative to increased work and responsibilities, changing family life, altered finances, difficulties with priorities or rationing, the departure or possible loss of loved ones, etc. The combination of such disturbing forces will undoubtedly undermine the vital nervous reserve of many persons and will throw them into a state in which nervous and mental breakdowns will more readily flourish.

One group of emotional problems is arising in some Selective Service Registrants just prior to induction. The fellow who is expecting to be called for induction may suffer an emotional crisis, because mobilization into the armed forces means a complete disorganization of the individual's peacetime design of living. Certain men have emotional conflicts which are likely to be intensified by a military set-up. I think here, for example, of a patient of mine who has been aware of strong, passive homosexual tendencies since five years of age, but who has successfully repressed them since the age of 15. He has just received notice to appear for examination by his Local Board and now he comes to the Psychiatrist all upset because he knows that close association with large numbers of men is likely to again stimulate his homosex-

ual tendencies and lead to homosexual acts again. Or worse still, if he tries to defend himself against the wish to perform such acts, he feels that it would drive him into a psychosis. An explanatory letter to his Local Board solved the situation.

Another set of civilian problems arises in those unstable fellows who have somehow slipped through the various screening-outs set up by Selective Service and whose misfitness soon became apparent to the military authorities and led to dismissal. These discharged men feel shame, class themselves as social inferiors and think that other people regard them as slackers. One such example was discharged from the Army after one month's service due to a severe compulsive-obsessive neurosis. He then felt strange because he was no longer in the Army. He thought that he had disgraced himself, that people would look down on him and that his Army discharge was a stigma. He developed various hypochondriacal complaints and later slipped into mental confusion and deep depression. The Red Cross, by the way, is doing a very commendable work in establishing follow-ups on all such discharged individuals and is helping to rehabilitate them.

Certain employers sometimes refuse to take on or to re-employ those who have been rejected for nervous or mental defects. The employer's attitude is: "If you are not good enough for the Army then you are not good enough for me!" This is true despite the fact that many of these men have a long standing, excellent employment record. I recall at this point a fine young man rejected by the Army because of latent homosexual inclinations which, however, had not bothered him for years. He was accepted by a local defense plant, only to be dismissed when they learned the cause of his Army rejection. The same thing happened at another defense plant, despite the fact that the discharged individual possessed much needed technical skill.

The parents and other dependents of those in the service are also showing various types of emotional response. I remember an Italian who has been accustomed to having his children always live close by. One son was inducted six months ago. The father became mildly depressed, and lost weight, appetite and sleep, however, when a second son was inducted two months ago, the father became very deeply depressed and suicidal.

Some of the wives of service men are reacting badly, especially those who follow their husbands around over the country. They have too little to occupy their minds and too much time to worry about such things as the possibility of the husband being sent across, killed, etc. I am observing two such wives at present, one in a severe depression and the other a severe Schizophrenic. Furthermore, many so-called "service marriages" are being hastily performed, where children are born with the father away and the mother has no knowledge of child-care. Or we have the postponement of marriages until the war is over which also causes many unhealthy problems.

Defense plant workers and their families are also a fruitful source of emotional problems. Where incompatibility between the parents preceded the war, the increased pay given by defense plants offers a greater opportunity for divorce, which causes more broken homes. This in turn leads to more delinquents. In addition, too little effort and study are being given to the problem of fitting the right personality to the right job. For instance, certain personality types cannot stand the responsibility of executive positions. I have in mind, for example, an engineer who had little formal education but who had worked successfully under others for years. For two years now he has been employed by a local defense plant. Two months ago he was given the foremanship of a large building at the defense plant. He soon began to worry and said that he lacked the education and that he was not smart enough to be a foreman. His superiors did not agree with this idea. He was torn between his feelings of inadequacy and a patriotic duty to do as he was told. Two weeks ago he attempted to commit suicide. He recovered from his depression quickly following a few metrazol shocks and it was recom-mended that he avoid such executive positions.

Finally we must not ignore the impact of this war upon our young children and adolescents. It is impossible to measure the psychological damage done to the small child by this war. The mental state of the child is of great importance to its own present and future; also it reacts to the anxieties and tensions produced in its parents by the war. In addition, extra loads are being placed upon teachers at the worse possible time and upon already overworked social agencies by an increased number of emotional problems that are cropping up in children. Strangely enough we are finding that children, instead of being shocked by war, are becoming hardened by it.

But the adolescent reacts more to war than the younger child. Because of the serious drain on man-and-woman-power, the adolescent is being called upon to assume added responsibilities. In return he expects and demands more freedom. The 14 and 16 year old boy is resenting parental guidance and scholastic obligations. He is more independent and cares less what his parents think about how he spends his leisure time. In other words, he is trying to go through the period of emancipation from his parents two or three years too early. He is demanding the privileges and responsibilities of adulthood without having gone through that two or three years' period of additional experience and training which is necessary to fit him for adulthood. The adolescent also is not mature enough yet to tolerate much frustration. War calls for more frustration and less gratification. The result is that the adolescent wants to live fully and dangerously. His attitude is that it may be too late to live tomorrow for then he may be killed. Many adolescent marriages are being contracted even by fifteen year old boys! One such immature youth recently even tried in a local court to force his mother's consent to his marriage to a worthless girl. Similar attitudes abound in adolescent girls also. There has been an alarming increase in sexual escapades by girls who rationalize their misbehaviour on the grounds that it is the patriotic thing to do. Many adolescent girls are hastily marrying because they resent parental guidance. They get annulments of the marriage quickly when their premature taste of marriage sours them on it and proves their lack of sufficient maturity to make a go of it. As one author recently put it, "We are heading for a wave of juvenile delinquency the like of which we have never seen!"

Such, in brief, are a few neuropsychiatric problems now arising in our civilian population.

Special Article

Recommendations for a Venereal Disease Control Program in Industry

Report of the
Advisory Committee on the Control of Venereal Diseases

Otis L. Anderson, Chairman

In order to assemble current authoritative information and to formulate basic principles applicable to a program of venereal disease control in industry, the Surgeon General has appointed an Advisory Committee to the United States Public Health Service. This Committee has outlined the objectives of such a program as:

A. Medical and Public Health:
1. To find and refer for proper medical management all cases of venereal diseases among workers in industry.
2. To establish equitable policies for the employment of applicants and continuation of services of employees who have venereal diseases.
3. To coordinate the community and industrial venereal disease control programs.

B. Employee:
1. To improve the physical condition of employees.
2. To reduce the number of workers lost through illness or injury.
3. To provide job placement.
4. To prolong and increase the earning power of employees.

C. Employer:
1. To reduce compensation costs.
2. To lessen work interruptions and labor turnover.
3. To enhance production by increasing the efficiency of workers.
4. To minimize personnel problems.

In order to assure agreement on all phases of fundamental policy, the committee recommends that the following agencies be consulted in carrying out this program: the State Labor Department, Industrial Commission, or similar department of State Government, the appropriate committee of the State Medical Society, the association representing employers, the labor organizations, appropriate voluntary health and welfare associations.

Responsibility for the administration of the program should be shared by the industrial hygiene and venereal disease divisions of the State Health Department. The program should not be inaugurated without a complete educational program. The employee should be convinced that adequate treatment protects both his health and his ability to earn a living, and the employer, that not all cases of venereal disease are infectious, through an educational program before venereal disease control measures are introduced.

In order that the control program may be effective, pre-employment examinations should be mandatory for all workers. Laboratory tests for syphilis and gonorrhea should be made a part of the periodic, re-employment or "return from illness" physical examinations which are the policy of the industry. The interval between examinations should under no circumstances be more than three years.

It is of utmost importance that the results of the medical examination be considered confidential between the worker and the medical staff. Information should be furnished to others only with the consent of the individual concerned or, failing this, on legal advice. The medical staff should make proper recommendations to the management as to the physical fitness of the employee for work. When the usual clinical record is kept in an open file, venereal disease forms should be filed in the medical departments for the use of the medical staff only.

There is no reason for denying employment to an applicant or for discharging an employee because an examination has revealed evidence of syphilis or gonorrhea, provided:
1. That the employee agrees to place himself under competent medical management.
2. That, if the disease is in the infectious stage, employment should be delayed or interrupted until such time as a noninfectious state is established through treatment and open lesions are healed.
3. That when syphilis exists in a latent stage, employment should not be delayed nor interrupted.
4. That employment may be deferred or denied when the individual is an industrial hazard.
5. That occupational readjustments of employees be made of individuals developing disabling manifestations.
6. That workers with syphilis in any of its stages be excluded from areas where there is exposure to chemicals which may produce toxic reactions, and those having cardiovascular syphilis or neurosyphilis should not be exposed to physiologic stresses.
7. That workers with gonorrhea should be allowed to work only under special medical observation during the administration of sulfonamide drugs.

The applicant or the employee whose examination reveals evidence of a venereal disease should be called to the industrial physician's office for a conference. He should be instructed as to the nature of the disease which he has in order that he may cooperate intelligently with the requirements of the program. He should be referred to a reputable source for medical attention and be furnished with a letter directed to his physician stating the results of the examination and what is expected of the employee as to regularity of treatment if he is to be employed. The industrial physician should receive a record of treatment at about monthly intervals. The names of individuals who have neglected or refused treatment should be turned over to the health department for appropriate action in bringing them back to treatment.

The plant physician, making a tentative diagnosis of communicable syphilis or gonorrhea, should, without delay, acquaint the appropriate health authority with the facts.

· THE PRESIDENT'S PAGE ·

OUR ADVERTISING FRIENDS

Advertising is the life of any publication. Only through the income from advertising is it possible for your Journal to exist. The Executive Secretary and the Editorial Board are constantly faced with the necessity of turning down lucrative offers from unethical, unknown and unscrupulous merchants who would pay well to take advantage of the Journal's endorsement of their product.

Primarily, our advertisers desire to create a market for the product or service offered, but with many of them we sense also a friendly interest and support for our publication and what it stands for. Let us reciprocate with this spirit of giving as well as seeking support. Let us use a little of our reading time to keep acquainted with our advertising friends. They are in sympathy with the aims and ideals of the profession in this state. They are loyal to us—they ask our friendship as well as our business. Let's give it.

James Stevenson

President.

The JOURNAL Of The
OKLAHOMA STATE MEDICAL ASSOCIATION

EDITORIAL BOARD

L. J. MOORMAN, Oklahoma City, Editor-in-Chief

E. EUGENE RICE, Shawnee

NED R. SMITH, Tulsa

MR. R. H. GRAHAM, Oklahoma City, Business Manager

CONTRIBUTIONS: Articles accepted by this Journal for publication including those read at the annual meetings of the State Association are the sole property of this Journal.

The Editorial Department is not responsible for the opinions expressed in the original articles of contributors.

Manuscripts may be withdrawn by authors for publication elsewhere only upon the approval of the Editorial Board.

MANUSCRIPTS: Manuscripts should be typewritten, double-spaced, on white paper 8½ x 11 inches. The original copy, not the carbon copy, should be submitted.

Footnotes, bibliographies and legends for cuts should be typed on separate sheets in double space. Bibliography listing should follow this order: Name of author, title of article, name of periodical with volume, page and date of publication.

Manuscripts are accepted subject to the usual editorial revisions and with the understanding that they have not been published elsewhere.

NEWS: Local news of interest to the medical profession, changes of address, births, deaths and weddings will be gratefully received.

ADVERTISING: Advertising of articles, drugs or compounds unapproved by the Council on Pharmacy of the A.M.A. will not be accepted. Advertising rates will be supplied on application.

It is suggested that members of the State Association patronize our advertisers in preference to others.

SUBSCRIPTIONS: Failure to receive The Journal should call for immediate notification.

REPRINTS: Reprints of original articles will be supplied at actual cost provided request for them is attached to manuscripts or made in sufficient time before publication. Checks for reprints should be made payable to Industrial Printing Company, Oklahoma City.

Address all communications to THE JOURNAL OF THE OKLAHOMA STATE MEDICAL ASSOCIATION, 210 Plaza Court, Oklahoma City. (3)

OFFICIAL PUBLICATION OF THE OKLAHOMA STATE MEDICAL ASSOCIATION

Copyrighted July, 1943

EDITORIALS

ACUTE POLIOMYELITIS

Unfortunately we are now facing a treacherous enemy on the home front. Anxious mothers are guarding their children against unnecessary contacts hoping to avert the vague, invisible virus of a dreadful disease which even the doctors do not wholly understand.

In behalf of these mothers and their children, it is every doctor's duty to be on the alert in order that each new case of acute poliomyelitis may have an early diagnosis and immediate isolation. It is not easy to make an early diagnosis, consequently it is the purpose of this editorial to sound the warning and to call attention to the fact that the incubation period probably is three to ten days; that the initial period of general infection may last from a few hours to three to four days.

In 61 cases at this date under observation at the Crippled Children's Hospital, with a few exceptions, the onset has been characterized by fever, headache, nausea and vomiting. The temperature runs approximately seven days, reaching a maximum of 103 on the third or fourth day.

Any illness, especially in a child, with onset and progression as described above, calls for a spinal puncture and isolation while awaiting the laboratory report on the spinal fluid. The symptoms of meningeal irritation should immediately arouse suspicion and hasten the diagnostic procedure. It should be remembered that the meningitis and paralytic stages come later. For the protection of the patient and the public, the diagnosis should not await these shocking developments.

"FROM BISMARCK TO BEVERIDGE" PLUS WAGNER AND MURRAY

What a headache for the unsuspecting American people who truly represent pioneering stock. A people who ran away from unwarranted political domination only a few generations ago cannot accept such a total resubmission, with the sacrifice of many personal liberties, without a sense of distinct loss. Our citizenry should know that Social Security Legislation, including compulsory health insurance, had its origin in Germany where the common people have never seen the light of liberty, therefore, never happy without regimentation.

With the vision of a poet and the education of a doctor, Frederich Schiller cried out against the injustice of government control and military discipline. His stinging tragedy "The Robbers" tells the story of his rebellion and his "William Tell" depicts his love of liberty as portrayed in a true democracy. Duke Charles could force upon the uninterested Schiller the study of law, later he could selfishly approve the less objectionable study of medicine, he could temporarily silence the freedom of speech but never the freedom of thought, neither could he stay the secret record of Schillers restless pen which proved a powerful vehicle against the evils of a merciless discipline. In this connection, we cannot refrain from quoting Karl Moser who at the moment of bitterness, said, of his own nation, "Germany is a great, but despised people . . . my heart trembles at the sight of our chains." The same author, in an attempt to ascribe to every nation a governing principle, says, "In England it is liberty; in Holland, truth; in France, the honor of the king; while in Germany, it is obedience."

All this for the purpose of calling attention to the fact that it was in this national atmosphere that modern, socialized medicine was born. Bismark, with the sagacity of a true politician, rather than the clear vision of a poet, seized his opportunity and as the real spokesman through the mouth of the Emperor, sent his plan for accident insurance to the Reichstag as a message from the throne. This was in November, 1881. In the spring of 1882, Bismarck had two bills before the Reichstag; the Accident Insurance Act and the Sickness Insurance Act. The debate upon this proposed legislation was tempestuous. Bismarck was accused of being a socialist and charged with a desire to destroy individualism. This opposition, however, came from the conservatives and represented the vain periscopic view of those not yet hopelessly submerged. Next in succession came the Old Age and Health Insurance and, finally, the Unemployment Insurance. In justification of the accusation that Bismarck was politically sagacious, it should be remarked that he argued that the best way to secure and maintain existing political policies was to place the people under obligation through paternalistic practices. In the Fourteenth Edition of the Encyclopedia Britannica, Erich Brandenburg, lecturer in Philosophy and History at The Prussian Akademie der Wissenschaften, Berlin, says, "The people was and remained in his eyes purely a thing to be governed, unfit, in his opinion to influence the conduct of its own affairs in any large degree."

Unfortunately, England has already slipped into the whirling vortex and is now being urged to feed the last vestiges of professional freedom into the political shredder. Those who may question this statement should read the Beveridge Report, the Report of the Planning Commission of the British Medical Association and, finally, the Report of the Medical Research.

The United States is likewise slipping. Bismarck's wildest dreams never surpassed the provisions of the Wagner Bill, S. 1161, which is now before the Congress of the United States. Time and space will not permit an analysis of this proposed legislation, but every doctor is urged to secure a copy* at once in order that he may study its contents and point out to his patrons the undemocratic provisions which virtually will destroy the time honored patient and doctor relationship so vital to a free people. Contemplation of this bill is not only confusing but depressing. If it becomes law many members of the medical profession may find themselves sitting in the sad twilight of their freedom, looking upon the mangled torso of their humanitarian dreams. The proposed administration of this bill provides for a board containing a majority of laymen. But this is not surprising, with few exceptions, experience shows that in a bureaucratic government, slave driving is the prerogative of laymen arriving at the port of bureaucratic authority without justifiable portfolio.

*A copy may be obtained from the Clerk of the Senate, Senate Office Bldg, Washington, D. C.

"COGITO EGO SUM"

It was Descartes who said "I think, therefore, I am." Upon the spur of the moment it may seem that the father of philosophy was careless not to add "what I am" rather than to leave us speculating and doubting. Spinoza was disturbed by Descartes' philosophy, he discarded the rabinical teachings which had dominated his early life and accepted the Cartesian philosophy. However, Spinoza's most lucid concepts of the intellect leave us still wondering what we are. John Locke supplemented philosophy with his knowledge of medicine. His reasoning on the development of knowledge and the building of personality anticipated the Freudian theory by more than 200 years. Locke was not the first to apply medical knowledge in the solution of psychological problems. A certain degree of psychoanalysis was practiced by Hippocrates and Galen. Hippocrates recognized the influence of dreams and the stabilizing effect of the normal sex life. The notable work of Pinel and Benjamin Rush in behalf of the insane was not without significant effect.

The so-called "Freudian Epoch" was to some extent dependent upon the above evolutionary influences which converged to provide favorable manifest destiny for Freud.

It should be remembered that Breuer, who collaborated with Freud, was the first to employ mental and emotional catharsis, e.g., free vent to otherwise repressed thought. He reported having used this method with good effect in a case of hysteria. Breuer collaborated with Freud until professional and popular criticism caused him to withdraw in favor of his accustomed private practice. If Breuer had not accidentally discovered the value of mental catharsis, in all probability there would be no "Freudian Epoch." Breuer and Freud originally employed hypnotism in connection with mental catharsis, but Freud later discarded the former as being unsatisfactory. Thus Freud's psychoanalytical method is based upon the cathartic theory which requires the patient to give up all conscious reflection and to relinquish all inhibitions with frank expression of all spontaneous thought. The accumulation and careful interpretation of the resulting data constitutes our present concept of psychoanalysis. Certainly, Freud has given us a better understanding of sex, and his method has thrown new light upon the diagnosis and management of the neuroses and phychoses. But for those who have sufficient equanimity to keep them near the imaginary line between sanity and insanity, we recommend psychoanalytical abstinence. After all, there is not much comfort in finding out that the stuff we are made of is the summation of sex and dreams. Those who have faith should cling to their prayers with the assumption that we are made of common clay, but not *too common* for the potter. Descartes, if not consciously wise, was at least merciful in withholding the full truth.

Arthritis Now Linked to Rheumatic Fever

Evidence that chronic infectious arthritis in adults may have resulted from rheumatic fever in childhood was given the American Association of Pathologists and Bacteriologists by Dr. Archie H. Baggenstoss and Dr. Edward F. Rosenberg of the Mayo Clinic.

The two Mayo physicians felt that arthritis involves more than disease of the joints; that it involves the vital organs, the crippled joints being merely one expression of the malady.

They examined the organs of thirty patients who had had chronic infectious arthritis and found evidence of disease in the heart, kidneys, liver and other organs. There was damage to the heart in twenty-four cases and in sixteen of these the injury was indistinguishable from that caused by rheumatic fever. Also significant was the pathologic condition discovered in the kidneys. It was felt that heart and kidney damage was due to some underlying set of causes.

Drs. Baggenstoss and Rosenberg concluded there may be a relationship between chronic infectious arthritis and rheumatic fever, typically a disease of childhood.—Science News Letter.

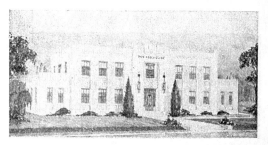

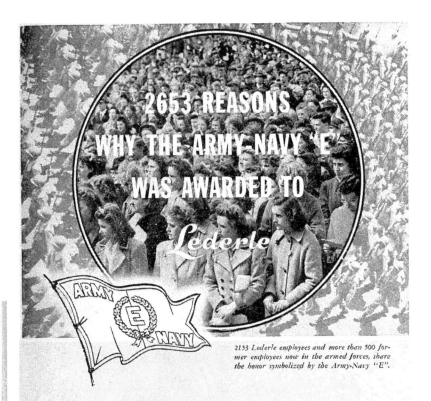

ROSTER
Oklahoma State Medical Associatian
1943

(*Members are listed according to the county of their residence*).

(*Indicates the member is serving in the armed forces*).

ALFALFA

*BEATY, C. SAM ....*Cherokee*
DOUGAN, A. L. ....*Carmen*
   (*member Woods Co. Medical Society*)
*DUNNINGTON, W. G. ....*Cherokee*
HALE, FORREST ....*Cherokee*
HARRIS, G. G. ....*Helena*
HUSTON, H. E. ....*Cherokee*
LANCASTER, L. T. ....*Cherokee*
STEPHENSON, WALTER L. ....*Aline*
   (*member Woods Co. Medical Society*)
WEBER, A. G. ....*Goltry*

ATOKA

BRIGGS, T. H. ....*Atoka*
*COTTON, W. W. ....*Atoka*
DALE, CHARLES D. ....*Atoka*
FULTON, J. S. ....*Atoka*
HUNTLEY, H. C. ....*Atoka*

BEAVER

BENJEGERDES, THEODORE D. ....*Beaver*
   (*member Woods Co. Medical Society*)
McGREW, EDWIN A. ....*Beaver*
   (*member Woods Co. Medical Society*)

BECKHAM

BAKER, L. V. ....*Elk City*
*DEVANNEY, P. J. ....*Sayre*
KILPATRICK, E. S. ....*Elk City*
*LEVICK, J. E. ....*Elk City*
McCREERY, R. C. ....*Erick*
McGRATH, T. J. ....*Sayre*
MURRAY, F. L. ....*Elk City*
PHILLIPS, G. W. ....*Sayre*
*SLABAUGH, R. M. ....*Sayre*
SPEED, H. K. ....*Sayre*
SPENCE, W. P. ....*Sayre*
STAGNER, G. H. ....*Erick*
STANDIFER, O. C. ....*Elk City*
TISDAL, V. C. ....*Elk City*

BLAINE

ANDERSON, H. R. ....*Watonga*
BOHLMANN, W. F. ....*Watonga*
**BUCHANAN, F. R. ....*Canton*
COX, A. K. ....*Watonga*
CURTIN, VIRGINIA OLSON ....*Watonga*
GRIFFIN, W. F. ....*Watonga*
HARP, ROBERT F. ....*Okeene*
   (*member Greer Co. Medical Society*)
HARTSHORNE, WILLIAM O. (*Indian Ser.*) ....*Geary*
   (*member Seminole Co. Medical Society*)
KIRBY, L. R. ....*Okeene*
MILLIGAN, E. F. ....*Geary*
STOUGH, D. F., JR. ....*Geary*
STOUGH, D. F., SR., (*honorary*) ....*Geary*
   (*member Canadian Co. Medical Society*)
**Deceased, June 4, 1943.*

BRYAN

BLOUNT, W. T. ....*Durant*
BOLINGER, E. W. ....*Achille*
CAIN, P. L. (*honorary*) ....*Albany*
COCHRAN, R. L. ....*Caddo*
COLWICK, J. T. ....*Durant*
COLWICK, O. J. ....*Durant*
HAYNIE, JOHN A. ....*Durant*
HAYNIE, W. KEILLER ....*Durant*
HYDE, W. A. ....*Durant*

McCALIB, D. C. ....*Colbert*
MOORE, CHARLES F. ....*Durant*
MOORE, W. L. ....*Bokchito*
PRICE, CHARLES G. ....*Durant*
RUSHING, G. M. ....*Durant*
RUTHERFORD, J. P. ....*Bennington*
SAWYER, R. E. ....*Durant*
SIZEMORE, PAUL ....*Durant*
TONEY, S. M. ....*Bennington*
WANN, C. E. (*honorary*) ....*Albany*
WEBB, JAMES P. ....*Durant*
WELLS, A. J. ....*Colera*
WHARTON, J. T. ....*Durant*

CADDO

BENWARD, JOHN H. ....*Doernbecker Hospital*
                                 Portland, Ore.
DIXON, W. L. ....*Cement*
HASLAM, G. E. ....*Anadarko*
HAWKINS, E. W. ....*McGregor, Tex.*
HENKE, J. R. ....*Hydro*
JOHNSTON, R. E. ....*Anadarko*
KERLEY, W. W. ....*Anadarko*
McMILLAN, C. B. ....*Gracemont*
PATTERSON, FRED L. ....*Carnegie*
PUTNAM, W. B. ....*Carnegie*
ROGERS, F. W. ....*Carnegie*
SULLIVAN, CLARENCE B. ....*Carnegie*
WILLIAMS, R. W. ....*Anadarko*
WRIGHT, PRESTON ....*Anadarko*

CANADIAN

ADERHOLD, THOMAS M. (*honorary*) ....*El Reno*
BROWN, HADLEY C. ....*El Reno*
CATTO, W. B. ....*El Reno*
DEVER, HARVEY K. ....*El Reno*
GOODMAN, GEORGE L. ....*Yukon*
HEROD, PHILIP F. ....*El Reno*
JOHNSON, ALPHA L. ....*El Reno*
LAWTON, W. P. ....*El Reno*
MILLER, W. R. ....*Cowgill, Mo.*
MYERS, PIRL B. ....*El Reno*
NEUMANN, MILTON A. ....*Okarche*
PHELPS, JOSEPH T. ....*El Reno*
PHELPS, MALCOM E. ....*El Reno*
RICHARDSON, D. P. ....*Union City*
RILEY, JAMES T. ....*El Reno*
WARREN, R. C. ....*Yukon*

CARTER

BARKER, E. R. ....*Healdton*
BOADWAY, F. W. ....*Ardmore*
CANADA, J. C. ....*Ardmore*
*CANTRELL, D. E., JR. ....*Healdton*
CANTRELL, D. E., SR. ....*Healdton*
CANTRELL, EMMA JEAN ....*Healdton*
COX, J. L. ....*Ardmore*
GILLESPIE, L. D. ....*Ardmore*
HARDY, WALTER ....*Ardmore*
HATHAWAY, W. G. ....*Lone Grove*
HIGGINS, H. A. ....*Ardmore*
JACKSON, T. J. ....*Ardmore*
JOHNSON, G. E. ....*Ardmore*
JOHNSON, WALTER ....*Ardmore*
KETCHERSID, J. W. ....*Ardmore*
MOTE, W. R. ....*Ardmore*

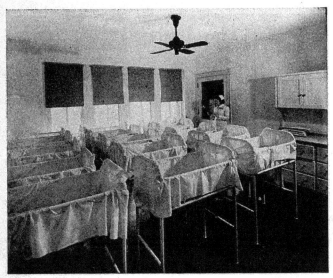

POLLOCK, JOHN R. _____Ardmore
REID, ROGER _____Ardmore
SULLIVAN, R. C. _____Ardmore
VEAZEY, J. HOBSON _____Ardmore
*VEAZEY, LYMAN C. _____Ardmore

CHEROKEE

ALLISON, J. S. _____Tahlequah
BAINES, SWARTZ _____Tahlequah
*GRAY, JAMES K. _____Tahlequah
HINES, S. J. T. _____Tahlequah
MASTERS, H. A. _____Tahlequah
MEDEARIS, P. H. _____Tahlequah
WOOD, W. M. _____Tahlequah

CHOCTAW

BOYER, H. L. _____Fort Towson
GEE, ROBERT L. _____Hugo
GREGG, O. R. _____Hugo
HALE, C. H. _____Boswell
JOHNSON, E. A. _____Hugo

CIMARRON

HALL, HARRY B. _____Boise City

CLEVELAND

ATKINS, W. H. _____Norman
BERRY, CURTIS _____Norman
BRAKE, CHARLES A. _____Norman
*BUFFINGTON, F. C. _____Norman
CARROLL, W. B. _____Norman
FOWLER, W. A. _____Norman
GASTINEAU, F. T. _____Norman
GRIFFIN, D. W. _____Norman
HADDOCK, J. L. _____Norman
*HADDOCK, PHIL _____Norman
HOWELL, O. E. _____Norman
MAYFIELD, W. T. _____Norman
MERRITT, IVA S. _____Norman
NIELSEN, GERTRUDE _____Norman
*PROSSER, MOORMAN P. _____Norman
*RAYBURN, CHARLES R. _____Norman
RIEGER, J. A. _____Norman
SCHMIDT, ELEONORA L. _____Norman
STEEN, C. T. _____Norman
STEPHENS, E. F. _____Norman
WICKHAM, M. M. _____Norman
*WILLARD, D. G. _____Norman
WOODSON, O. M. _____Norman

COAL

CLARK, J. B. _____Coalgate
CODY, ROBERT D. _____Centrahoma
HENRY, R. C. _____Coalgate
HIPES, J. J. _____Coalgate

COMANCHE

ANGUS, DONALD A. _____Lawton
ANGUS, H. A. _____Lawton
ANGUS, HOWARD _____Lawton
ANTONY, JOSEPH T. _____Lawton
BARBER, GEORGE S. _____Lawton
BERRY, G. L. _____Lawton
DOWNING, GERALD G. _____Lawton
DUNLAP, ERNEST B. _____Lawton
FERGUSON, LAWRENCE W. _____Lawton
FOX, FRED T. _____Lawton
GOOCH, L. T. _____Lawton
HAMMOND, FRED W. _____Lawton
HATHAWAY, EUEL P. _____Lawton
JOYCE, CHARLES W. _____Fletcher
KNEE, LOREN C. _____Lawton
LEWIS, W. F. _____Lawton
MARTIN, CHESLEY M. _____Elgin
PARSONS, O. L. _____Lawton

COTTON

BAKER, G. W. _____Walters
CALVERT, HOWARD A. _____Walters
HOLSTED, A. B. _____Temple
JONES, M. A. _____Walters
SCISM, MOLLIE F. _____Walters
TALLANT, GEORGE A. _____Walters

CRAIG

ADAMS, F. M. _____Vinita
*BRADSHAW, J. O. _____Welch
CHUMLEY, C. P. _____Vinita
    (member Woodward Co. Medical Society)
*DARROUGH, J. R. _____Vinita
FAUST, HUGH H. _____Vinita
HAYS, P. L. _____Vinita
HERRON, A. W. _____Vinita
LEHMER, ELIZABETH E. _____Vinita
MARKS, W. R. _____Vinita
McMILLAN, J. M. _____Vinita
McPIKE, LLOYD H. _____Vinita
SANGER, PAUL G. _____Vinita

CREEK

BISBEE, W. G. _____Bristow
COPPEDGE, O. C. _____Bristow
COPPEDGE, O. N. _____7100 Walnut St.,
                                    Philadelphia, Pa.
COPPEDGE, O. S. _____Depew
*COWART, O. H. _____Bristow
CROSTON, GEORGE C. _____Sapulpa
*CURRY, J. F. _____Sapulpa
HAAS, H. R. _____Sapulpa
HOLLIS, J. E. _____Bristow
KING, E. W. _____Bristow
LAMPTON, J. B. _____Sapulpa
LEWIS, P. K. _____Sapulpa
LONGMIRE, W. P., JR. ___Johns Hopkins Hospital,
                                    Baltimore, Md.
LONGMIRE, W. P., SR. _____Sapulpa
McDONALD, C. R. _____Mannford
*MOTE, PAUL _____Sapulpa
OAKES, CHARLES G. _____Sapulpa
*PICKARDT, W. L. _____Sapulpa
REESE, C. B. _____Sapulpa
REYNOLDS, S. W. _____Drumright
SCHRADER, CHARLES T. _____Bristow
SHRYOCK, LELAND F. _____Sapulpa
SISLER, FRANK H. _____Bristow
*SISLER, FRANK H., JR. _____Bristow
STARR, O. W. _____Drumright
WHARTON, J. L. _____Depew

CUSTER

ALEXANDER, C. J. _____Clinton
ASHER, JAMES O. _____Clinton
    (member Oklahoma Co. Medical Society)
BLACK, THOMAS C. _____Montgomery, Ala.
BOYD, T. A. _____Weatherford
BRUNDAGE, BERT T. _____Thomas
*BULLOCK, BERNARD _____Clinton
CUNNINGHAM, C. B. _____Clinton
*CUSHMAN, H. R. _____Clinton
DEPUTY, ROSS _____Clinton
DOLER, C. _____Clinton
FRIZZELL, J. T. (honorary) _____Clinton
GAEDE, D. _____Weatherford
GOSSOM, K. D. _____Clinton
*HINSHAW, J. R. _____Butler
*KENNEDY, LOUIS _____Clinton
LAMB, ELLIS _____Clinton
*LINGENFELTER, PAUL B. _____Clinton
McBURNEY, C. H. _____Clinton
*PAULSON, ALVIN W. _____Clinton
ROGERS, McLAIN _____Clinton
RUHL, N. E. _____Weatherford
SMITH, WILLARD H. _____Clinton
STOLL, A. A. _____Clinton
*TISDAL, WILLIAM C. _____Clinton
VIEREGG, F. R. _____Clinton
*WILLIAMS, GORDON _____Weatherford
*WOOD, J. GUILD _____Weaterford

DELAWARE

WALKER, C. F. _____Grove
    (member Craig Co. Medical Society)

DEWEY

LOYD, E. M. _____Taloga
    (member Custer Co. Medical Society)

MABRY, W. L. ....Leedey
   (member Beckham Co. Medical Society)
SEBA, W. E. ....Leedey
   (member Beckham Co. Medical Society)

ELLIS

BEAM, J. P. ....Arnett
   (member Woodward Co. Medical Society)
*DUBE, PAUL H. ....Shattuck
   (member Woodward Co. Medical Society)
*NEWMAN, FLOYD ....Shattuck
   (member Woodward Co. Medical Society)
NEWMAN, M. HASKELL ....Shattuck
   (member Woodward Co. Medical Society)
NEWMAN, O. C. ....Shattuck
   (member Woodward Co. Medical Society)
NEWMAN, ROY ....Shattuck
   (member Woodward Co. Medical Society)

GARFIELD

*BAKER, R. C. ....Enid
BITTING, B. T. ....Enid
BONHAM, KENNETH W. ....Enid
CHAMPLIN, PAUL B. ....Enid
*CORDONNIER, BYRON J. ....Enid
COTTON, LEE W. (honorary) ....Enid
DUFFY, FRANCIS M. ....Enid
FEILD, JULIAN ....Enid
FRANCISCO, GLENN ....Enid
HAMBLE, V. R. ....Enid
HARRIS, D. S. ....Drummond
*HINSON, BRUCE R. ....Enid
HOPKINS, P. W. ....Enid
HUDSON, F. A. ....Enid
HUDSON, HARRY H. ....Enid
*JACOBS, RAYMOND C. ....Enid
McEVOY, S. H. ....Enid
*MERCER, WENDELL J. ....Enid
METSCHER, ALFRED J. ....Enid
*NEILSON, W. P. ....Enid

*NEWELL, W. B., JR. ....Enid
NEWELL, W. B., SR. ....Enid
REMPEL, PAUL H. ....Enid
RHODES, W. H. ....Enid
*ROBERTS, C. J. ....Enid
ROBERTS, D. D. ....Enid
*ROSS, GEORGE ....Enid
ROSS, HOPE ....Enid
SHANNON, H. R. ....Enid
SHEETS, MARION E. ....Enid
*TALLEY, EVANS E. ....Enid
VANDEVER, H. F. ....Enid
WALKER, JOHN R. ....Enid
WATSON, JOHN M. ....Enid
WIGNER, R. H. ....Enid
   (member Noble Co. Medical Society)
WILKINS, A. E. ....Covington
WILSON, GEORGE S. ....Enid

GARVIN

ALEXANDER, ROBERT M. ....Paoli
CALLAWAY, JOHN R. ....Pauls Valley
GREENING, WILLIAM P. ....Pauls Valley
GROSS, T. F. ....Lindsay
JOHNSON, GALVIN L. ....Pauls Valley
*LINDSEY, RAY H. ....Pauls Valley
MONROE, HUGH H. ....Pauls Valley
ROBBERSON, MARVIN E. ....Wynnewood
ROBBERSON, MORTON E. ....Wynnewood
SHI, AUGUSTIN H. ....Stratford
SHIRLEY, EDWARD T. ....Pauls Valley
SULLIVAN, CLEVE L. ....Elmore City
WILSON, H. P. (honorary) ....Wynnewood

GRADY

BAZE, WALTER J. ....Chickasha
BONNELL, W. L. ....Chickasha
BOON, U. C. ....Chickasha
BYNUM, W. TURNER ....Chickasha
COOK, W. H. ....Chickasha

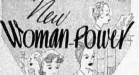

DOWNEY, D. S. ....*Chickasha*
EMANUEL, LEWIS E. ....*Chickasha*
EMANUEL, ROY E. ....*Chickasha*
HENNING, A. E. ....*Tuttle*
*JOYCE, FRANK T. ....*Chickasha*
LEEDS, A. B. ....*Chickasha*
LITTLE, AARON C. ....*Minco*
LIVERMORE, W. H. (*honorary*) ....*Chickasha*
MASON, REBECCA H. ....*Chickasha*
McCLURE, H. M. ....*Chickasha*
MITCHELL, C. P. ....*Chickasha*
PYLE, OSCAR S. ....*Chickasha*
RENEGAR, J. F. ....*Tuttle*
WOODS, LEWIS E. ....*Chickasha*

GRANT

HARDY, I. V. ....*Medford*
KEELER, E. T. ....*Lamont*
LAWSON, E. E. ....*Medford*

GREER

CHERRY, G. P. (*honorary*) ....*Mangum*
HOLLIS, J. B. ....*Mangum*
LANSDEN, J. B. ....*Granite*
LEWIS, R. W. ....*Granite*
LOWE, J. T. ....*Mangum*
PEARSON, LEB. E. ....*Mangum*
POER, E. M. ....*Mangum*
*RUDE, JOE C. ....*Mangum*

HARMON

HUSBAND, W. G. ....*Hollis*
LYNCH, R. H. ....*Hollis*
RAY, W. T. (*honorary*) ....*Gould*
STREET, O. J. ....*Gould*
YEARGAN, W. M. ....*Hollis*

HARPER

CAMP, EARL (*honorary*) ....*Buffalo*
   (*member Woodward Co. Medical Society*)
HILL, H. K. ....*Laverne*
   (*member Woodward Co. Medical Society*)
*PIERSON, DWIGHT ....*Buffalo*
   (*member Woodward Co. Medical Society*)
WALKER, HARDIN ....*Buffalo*
   (*member Woodward Co. Medical Society*)
WINCHELL, F. Z. ....*Buffalo*
   (*member Woodward Co. Medical Society*)

HASKELL

CARSON, WILLIAM S. ....*Keota*
RUMLEY, J. C. ....*Stigler*
THOMPSON, W. A. ....*Stigler*
WILLIAMS, N. K. ....*McCurtain*

HUGHES

DAVENPORT, A. L. ....*Holdenville*
FLOYD, W. E. ....*Holdenville*
GEORGE, L. J. ....*Stuart*
   (*member Pittsburg Co. Medical Society*)
HAMILTON, S. H. ....*Non*
HICKS, C. A. ....*Holdenville*
HOWELL, H. A. ....*Holdenville*
KERNEK, PAUL ....*Holdenville*
MAYFIELD, IMOGENE ....*Holdenville*
MORRIS, C. H. ....*Wetumka*
PRYOR, V. W. ....*Holdenville*
TAYLOR, W. L. ....*Holdenville*
WALLACE, C. S. ....*Holdenville*

JACKSON

BERRY, THOMAS M. ....*El Dorado*
CROW, E. S. ....*Olustee*
MABRY, E. W. ....*Altus*
McCONNELL, L. H. ....*Altus*
McFADIN, J. S. ....*Altus*
**MEREDITH, J. S. ....*Duke*
   (*member Greer Co. Medical Society*)
REID, JOHN R. ....*Altus*
SPEARS, C. G. ....*Altus*
STULTS, J. S. (*honorary*) ....*Altus*
TAYLOR, R. Z. ....*Blair*
**Deceased.

JEFFERSON

ANDRESKOWSKI, W. T. ....*Ryan*
BOBBITT, F. S. ....*Mojave, Calif.*
**BROWNING, W. M. ....*Waurika*

COLLINS, D. B. ....*Waurika*
DERR, J. I. ....*Waurika*
EDWARDS, F. M. ....*Ringling*
HOLLINGSWORTH, J. I. ....*Waurika*
MAUPIN, C. M. ....*Waurika*
WADE, L. L. ....*Ryan*
YEATS, H. WESLEY ....*Ringling*
**Deceased February 5, 1943.

JOHNSTON

RAINES, S. W. ....*Wapanucka*
   (*member Bryan Co. Medical Society*)

KAY

ARMSTRONG, W. O. ....*Ponca City*
ARRENDELL, C. W. ....*Ponca City*
BEATTY, J. H. ....*Tonkawa*
BECKER, L. H. ....*Blackwell*
CLIFT, MERL ....*Blackwell*
*CURRY, JOHN R. ....*Blackwell*
GARDNER, C. C. ....*Ponca City*
GHORMLEY, J. G. ....*Blackwell*
GIBSON, R. B. ....*Ponca City*
*GORDON, D. M. ....*Ponca City*
GOWEY, H. O. ....*Newkirk*
*HARMS, EDWIN M. ....*Blackwell*
HOWE, J. HOLLAND ....*Ponca City*
*KENNEDY, VIRGIL ....*Newkirk*
KINSINGER, R. R. ....*Blackwell*
*KREGER, G. S. ....*Tonkawa*
MALL, W. W. ....*Ponca City*
MATHEWS, DEWEY ....*Tonkawa*
McELROY, THOMAS ....*Ponca City*
MILLER, D. W. ....*Blackwell*
*MOHLER, ELDON C. ....*Ponca City*
MOORE, G. C. ....*Ponca City*
*MORGAN, L. S. ....*Ponca City*
*NEAL, L. G. ....*Ponca City*
NIEMANN, G. H. ....*Ponca City*
NORTHCUTT, C. E. ....*Ponca City*
NUCKOLS, A. S. ....*Ponca City*
RISSER, A. S. ....*Blackwell*
RISSER, PHILIP C. ....*Blackwell*
VANCE, L. C. ....*Ponca City*
WAGGONER, E. E. ....*Tonkawa*
WAGNER, J. C. ....*Ponca City*
WALKER, I. D. ....*Tonkawa*
*WHITE, M. S. ....*Blackwell*
*WRIGHT, L. I. ....*Blackwell*
YEARY, G. H. ....*Newkirk*

KINGFISHER

ANGLIN, J. E. ....*Dover*
DIXON, A. ....*Hennessey*
GOSE, C. O. ....*Hennessey*
HODGSON, C. M. ....*Kingfisher*
MEREDITH, A. O. ....*Kingfisher*
STURGEON, H. VIOLET ....*Hennessey*
TOWNSEND, B. I. ....*Hennessey*

KIOWA

BONHAM, J. M. ....*Hobart*
BRAUN, J. P. ....*Hobart*
FINCH, J. WILLIAM ....*Hobart*
HATHAWAY, A. H. ....*Mountain View*
MOORE, J. H. ....*Hobart*
WALKER, F. E. ....*Lone Wolf*
WATKINS, B. H. ....*Hobart*

LATIMER

HARRIS, J. M. ....*Wilburton*
   (*member Pittsburg Co. Medical Society*)

LE FLORE

BAKER, F. P. ....*Talihina*
BEVILL, S. D. ....*Poteau*
BOOTH, G. R. ....*LeFlore*
COLLINS, E. L. ....*Panama*
DEAN, S. C. ....*Howe*
DORROUGH, J. ....*Monroe*
FAIR, E. N. ....*Heavener*
GILLIAM, WILLIAM C. ....*Spiro*
MIXON, A. M. ....*Spiro*
ROLLE, NEESON ....*Poteau*

WOODSON, E. M. ....*Poteau*
WRIGHT, R. L. ....*Poteau*

LINCOLN

ADAMS, J. W. ....*Chandler*
BAILEY, CARL H. ....*Stroud*
**BROWN, F. C. ....*Sparks*
BROWN, R. A. ....*Prague*
  (*member Pottawatomie Co. Medical Society*)
BURLESON, NED ....*Prague*
DAVIS, W. B. ....*Stroud*
ERWIN, PARA ....*Wellston*
HURLBUT, E. F. ....*Meeker*
JENKINS, H. B. ....*Tryon*
MARSHALL, A. M. ....*Chandler*
NICKELL, U. E. ....*Davenport*
NORWOOD, F. H. ....*Prague*
ROBERTSON, C. W. ....*Chandler*
ROLLINS, J. S. ....*Prague*
**Deceased April 27, 1943.

LOGAN

BARKER, PAULINE ....*Guthrie*
BUSSEY, H. N. ....*Mulhall*
CORNWELL, N. L. ....*Coyle*
GARDNER, P. B. ....*Guthrie*
GRAY, DAN ....*Guthrie*
HAHN, L. A. ....*Guthrie*
HILL, C. B. ....*Guthrie*
LeHEW, J. LESLIE, JR. ....*Guthrie*
MILLER, W. C. ....*Guthrie*
PETTY, C. S. ....*Guthrie*
*PETTY, JAMES S. ....*Guthrie*
REDING, ANTHONY C. ....*Coyle*
RINGROSE, R. F. ....*Guthrie*
*RITZHAUPT, LOUIS H. ....*Guthrie*
ROGERS, C. L. ....*Marshall*
SOUTER, J. E. ....*Guthrie*

LOVE

LOONEY, M. D. ....*Marietta*
  (*member Carter Co. Medical Society*)

MAJOR

McCROSKIE, M. R. ....*Fairview*
  (*member Garfield Co. Medical Society*)
RYAN, ROBERT O. ....*Fairview*
  (*member Garfield Co. Medical Society*)
SPECHT, ELSIE ....*Fairview*
  (*member Garfield Co. Medical Society*)

MARSHALL

COOK, ODIS A. ....*Madill*
HOLLAND, JOHN LEE ....*Madill*
JOSEPH, PHILIP G. ....*Madill*
YORK, JOSEPH F. ....*Madill*

MAYES

CAMERON, PAUL B. ....*Pryor*
HERRINGTON, V. D. ....*Pryor*
MORROW, B. L. ....*Salina*
RUTHERFORD, S. C. ....*Locust Grove*
SMITH, R. V. ....*Pryor*
WERLING, E. H. ....*Pryor*
WHITAKER, W. J. ....*4657 Arts St.*
  New Orleans, La.
WHITE, L. C. ....*Adair*

McCLAIN

COCHRANE, J. E. ....*Byars*
DAVIS, S. C. ....*Blanchard*
**DAWSON, O. O. ....*Wayne*
KOLB, I. N. ....*Blanchard*
McCURDY, W. C., JR. ....*Purcell*
McCURDY, W. C., SR. ....*Purcell*
ROYSTER, R. L. ....*Purcell*
SLOVER, BENJAMIN W. ....*Blanchard*
**Deceased April 20, 1943.

McCURTAIN

BARKER, N. L. ....*Broken Bow*
CLARKSON, A. W. ....*Valliant*
HAMILTON, J. G. ....*Clebit*
KELLEAM, E. A. ....*Wright City*
  (*member LeFlore Co. Medical Society*)
McBRAYER, WILLIAM H. ....*Haworth*
MORELAND, J. T. ....*Idabel*
MORELAND, W. A. ....*Idabel*

OLIVER, R. B. ....*Idabel*
SHERRILL, R. H. ....*Broken Bow*
WILLIAMS, R. D. ....*Idabel*
WILLIAMS, W. W. ....*Idabel*

McINTOSH

BAKER, J. HOWARD ....*Eufaula*
FIRST, F. R. ....*Checotah*
JACOBS, LUSTER I. ....*Hanna*
LITTLE, DANIEL E. ....*Eufaula*
*STONER, RAYMOND W. ....*Checotah*
TOLLESON, WILLIAM A. ....*Eufaula*
WOOD, JAMES L. ....*Eufaula*

MURRAY

ANNADOWN, P. V. ....*Sulphur*
DeLAY, W. D. ....*Sulphur*
SADLER, F. E. ....*Sulphur*
SLOVER, GEORGE W. ....*Sulphur*

MUSKOGEE

BALLANTINE, H. T. ....*Muskogee*
BRUTON, L. D. ....*Muskogee*
COACHMAN, E. H. ....*Muskogee*
*DORWART, F. G. ....*Muskogee*
*DOYLE, W. H. ....*Muskogee*
EARNEST, A. N. ....*Muskogee*
*ELKINS, MARVIN ....*Muskogee*
EWING, FINIS W. ....*Muskogee*
FITE, E. HALSELL ....*Muskogee*
FITE, W. PAT ....*Muskogee*
FULLENWIDER, C. M. ....*Muskogee*
HAMM, SILAS G. ....*Haskell*
*HOLCOMBE, R. N. ....*Muskogee*
KLASS, O. C. ....*Muskogee*
KUPKA, JOHN F. ....*Haskell*
McALISTER, L. S. ....*Muskogee*
MILLER, D. EVELYN ....*Muskogee*
MOBLEY, A. L. ....*Aubuquerque, N. M.*
*NEELY, SHADE D. ....*Muskogee*
NICHOLS, J. T. ....*Muskogee*
OLDHAM, I. B. ....*Muskogee*
RAFTER, JAMES G. ....*Muskogee*
RAFTER, JOHN R. ....*Muskogee*
REYNOLDS, JOHN ....*Muskogee*
*REYNOLDS, JOHN H. ....*Muskogee*
ROGERS, ISAAC W. ....*Muskogee*
*SCHNOEBELEN, RENE E. ....*Muskogee*
SCOTT, H. A. ....*Muskogee*
STARK, W. W. ....*Muskogee*
  (*member Okmulgee Co. Medical Society*)
THOMPSON, M. K. ....*Muskogee*
WALKER, JOHN H. ....*Muskogee*
WARTERFIELD, F. E. ....*Muskogee*
*WEAVER, W. N. ....*Muskogee*
WHITE, CHARLES ED ....*Muskogee*
WHITE, J. HUTCHINGS ....*Muskogee*
*WOLFE, I. C. ....*Muskogee*
*WOODBURN, J. TINDER ....*Muskogee*

NOBLE

COLDIRON, D. F. ....*Perry*
COOKE, C. H. ....*Perry*
DRIVER, JESSE W. ....*Perry*
FRANCIS, J. W. ....*Perry*
HEISS, J. E. ....*Perry*
RENFROW, T. F. ....*Billings*

NOWATA

DAVIS, KIEFFER D. ....*Nowata*
KURTZ, R. L. ....*Nowata*
LANG, S. A. ....*Nowata*
ROBERTS, S. P. ....*Nowata*
SCOTT, M. B. ....*Delaware*

OKFUSKEE

BOMBARGER, C. C. ....*Paden*
BRICE, M. O. ....*Okemah*
COCHRAN, C. M. ....*Okemah*
JENKINS, W. P. ....*Okemah*
LUCAS, A. C. ....*Castle*
MELTON, A. S. ....*Okemah*
PEMBERTON, J. M. ....*Okemah*
PRESTON, J. R. ....*Weleetka*
SPICKARD, L. J. ....*Okemah*
WHITNEY, M. L. ....*Okemah*

OKLAHOMA

ABSHIER, A. BROOKS ....1200 *N. Walker*
ADAMS, ROBERT H. ....515 *N. W. 11th St.*
AKIN, ROBERT H. ....400 *N. W. 10th St.*
ALFORD, J. M. ....*Medical Arts Bldg.*
ALLEN, E. P. ....1200 *N. Walker*
*ALLEN, GEORGE T. ....1200 *N. Walker*
ANDREWS, LEILA E. ....1200 *N. Walker*
*APPLETON, M. M. ....400 *N. W. 10th St.*
AYCOCK, BYRON W. ....301 *N. W. 12th St.*
BAILEY, F. M. ....1219 *N. W. 21st St.*
*BAILEY, W. H. ....301 *N. W. 12th St.*
BAKER, MARGUERITE M. ......1104 *N. E. 63rd St.*
BALYEAT, RAY M. ....1200 *N. Walker*
*BARB, T. J. ....318 *S. W. 25th St.*
BARKER, C. E. ....1200 *N. Walker*
BARRY, GEORGE N. ....*Medical Arts Bldg.*
*BATCHELOR, JOHN J. ....*Medical Arts Bldg.*
*BATTENFIELD, JOHN Y. ....*State Health Dept.*
BAUM, E. ELDON ....*Perrine Bldg.*
*BEDNAR, GERALD ....*Medical Arts Bldg.*
*BELL, AUSTIN H. ....301 *N. W. 12th St.*
BELL, J. T. ....*State Health Dept.*
BERRY, CHARLES N. ....*Medical Arts Bldg.*
BINDER, HAROLD J. ....628 *N. W. 21st St.*
BINKLEY, J. G. ....*Medical Arts Bldg.*
*BIRGE, JACK P. ....204 *N. Robinson St.*
BLACHLY, CHARLES D. ....2752 *N. W. 18th St.*
BLACHLY, LUCILE SPIRE ....605 *N. W. 10th St.*
BOATRIGHT, LLOYD C. ....*Perrine Bldg.*
BOGGS, NATHAN ....*Perrine Bldg.*
*BOLEND, REX ....*Medical Arts Bldg.*
BONDURANT, C. P. ....*Medical Arts Bldg.*
BONHAM, WILLIAM L. ....*Medical Arts Bldg.*
*BORDER, CLINTON L. ....*American Natl. Bldg.*
*BORECKY, GEORGE L. ....204 *N. Robinson St.*
BRADLEY, H. C. ....*Perrine Bldg.*
*BRANHAM, D. W. ....*Medical Arts Bldg.*
BREWER, A. M. ....*Perrine Bldg.*
*BROWN, GERSTER W. ....*Medical Arts Bldg.*
BRUNDAGE, C. L. ....1200 *N. Walker*
BURKE, R. M. ....*Medical Arts Bldg.*
BURTON, JOHN F. ....1200 *N. Walker*
BUTLER, H. W. ....1200 *N. Walker*
CAILEY, LEO F. ....*Medical Arts Bldg.*
CAMPBELL, COYNE H. ....131 *N. E. 4th St.*
CAMPBELL, J. MOORE, III ......*Medical Arts Bldg.*
CANNON, J. M. ....210½ *W. Commerce St.*
CAPPS, J. F. ....*Tinker Field*
(member Seminole Co. Medical Society)
CATES, ALBERT M. (*honorary*) ....2733 *N. E. 20th St.*
CAVINESS, J. J. ....*Medical Arts Bldg.*
*CHAFFIN, ZALE ....*Municipal Bldg.*
*CHARNEY, L. H. ....*Medical Arts Bldg.*
(member Seminole Co. Medical Society)
CLARK, ANSON L. ....*Medical Arts Bldg.*
*CLARK, JOHN V. ....1706 *S. E. 29th St.*
CLARK, LeMON ....*Medical Arts Bldg.*
CLARK, RALPH O. ....1706 *S. E. 29th St.*
CLOUDMAN, H. H. ....*Medical Arts Bldg.*
CLYMER, C. E. ....*Medical Arts Bldg.*
COLE, W. C. ....1200 *N. Walker*
COLEY, A. J. (*honorary*) ....*Hightower Bldg.*
*COLEY, JOE H. ....105 *N. Hudson St.*
COOPER, F. MAXEY ....*Medical Arts Bldg.*
COSTON, TULLOS O. ....*Medical Arts Bldg.*
COTTEN, DAISY V. H. ....807 *N. W. 23rd St.*
CRICK, L. E. ....*Britton*
DANIELS, HARRY A. ....610 *N. W. 9th St.*
DERSCH, WALTER H. ....*Medical Arts Bldg.*
DEUPREE, HARRY L. ....*Medical Arts Bldg.*
*DEVANNEY, LOUIS R. ....1200 *N. Walker*
DICKSON, GREEN K. ....1200 *N. Walker*
*DILL, FRANCIS E. ....*Medical Arts Bldg.*
DOUDNA, HUBERT E. ....800 *N. E. 13th St.*
DOWDY, THOMAS W. ....*Medical Arts Bldg.*
*DRUMMOND, N. ROBERT ....*Medical Arts Bldg.*
EARLY, RALPH O. ....*Medical Arts Bldg.*
EASTLAND, WILLIAM F. ....*Medical Arts Bldg.*
ELEY, N. PRICE ....400 *N. W. 10th St.*
*EMENHISER, LEE K. ....*Medical Arts Bldg.*

EPLEY, C. O. ....1200 *N. Walker*
ERWIN, FRANTZ B. ....*Medical Arts Bldg.*
ESKRIDGE, J. B., JR. ....1200 *N. Walker*
FAGIN, HERMAN ....*Natl. Aid Life Bldg.*
FARIS, BRUNEL D. ....*Medical Arts Bldg.*
FARNAM, LARRY M. ....1200 *N. Walker*
FELTS, GEORGE R. ....625 *N. W. 10th St.*
FERGUSON, E. GORDON ....*Medical Arts Bldg.*
FISHMAN, C. J. ....132 *N. W. 4th St.*
FLEETWOOD, D. H. ....*Edmond*
FLESHER, THOMAS H. ....*Edmond*
*FOERSTER, HERVEY A. ....*Medical Arts Bldg.*
*FORD, HARRY C. ....*Medical Arts Bldg.*
FRIERSON, S. E. ....*Medical Arts Bldg.*
*FRYER, SAM R. ....119 *N. W. 5th St.*
*FULTON, C. C. ....*Medical Arts Bldg.*
FULTON, GEORGE ....*American Natl. Bldg.*
GALBRAITH, HUGH M. ....*First Natl. Bldg.*
GALLAGHER, C. A. ....610 *N. W. 9th St.*
GARRISON, GEORGE H. ....1200 *N. Walker*
GEE, O. J. ....*Medical Arts Bldg.*
*GIBBS, ALLEN G. ....*Apco Tower*
*GINGLES, R. H. ....*State Health Dept.*
GLISMANN, M. B. ....1021 *N. Lee*
GLOMSET, JOHN L. ....1200 *N. Walker*
GOLDFAIN, E. ....228 *N. W. 13th St.*
GOODWIN, R. Q. ....*Medical Arts Bldg.*
GRAENING, P. K. ....605 *N. W. 10th St.*
GRAHAM, A. T. ....26 *S. W. 25th St.*
GRAY, FLOYD ....1200 *N. Walker*
HACKLER, JOHN F. ....*State Health Dept.*
HALL, CLARK H. ....*Medical Arts Bldg.*
HAMMONDS, O. O. ....623 *N. E. 18th St.*
HARBISON, FRANK ....510 *N. W. 12th St.*
HARBISON, J. E. ....510 *N. W. 12th St.*
HARRIS, HENRY W. ....1200 *N. Walker*
HASKETT, PAUL E. ....*Hales Bldg.*
HASSLER, GRACE C. ....*Medical Arts Bldg.*
HAYES, BASIL A. ....625 *N. W. 10th St.*
*HAZEL, ONIS G. ....1200 *N. Walker*
HEATLEY, JOHN E. ....*Medical Arts Bldg.*
*HERRMANN, JESS D. ....*Medical Arts Bldg.*
HETHERINGTON, A. J. ....2014 *Gatewood*
HICKS, FRED B. ....*Medical Arts Bldg.*
HIGHLAND, J. E. ....634 *N. E. 13th St.*
HIRSHFIELD, A. C. ....*Medical Arts Bldg.*
*HOLLINGSWORTH, C. E. ....*Medical Arts Bldg.*
HOLLIS, LYNN E. ....*Tinker Field*
(member Harmon Co. Medical Society)
*HOOD, F. REDDING ....1200 *N. Walker*
*HOWARD, ROBERT B. ....1200 *N. Walker*
HOWARD, R. M. ....1200 *N. Walker*
HUFF, RHEBA L. ....1200 *N. Walker*
*HUGGINS, J. R. ....2225 *Exchange Ave.*
HULL, WAYNE M. ....1200 *N. Walker*
HUNTER, GEORGE ....*County Court House*
*HYROOP, GILBERT L. ....*Medical Arts Bldg.*
HYROOP, MURIEL ....131 *N. E. 4th St.*
*ISHMAEL, WILLIAM K. ....605 *N. W. 10th St.*
JACKSON, A. R. ....25284½ *S. Robinson*
JACOBS, MINARD F. ....*Medical Arts Bldg.*
JANCO, LEON ....10 *W. Park*
JETER, HUGH ....1200 *N. Walker*
JOBE, VIRGIL R. ....400 *N. W. 10th St.*
JONES, HUGH ....*Medical Arts Bldg.*
JONES, RALPH E. ....*Tinker Field*
(member Pawnee Co. Medical Society)
KELLER, W. FLOYD ....*Medical Arts Bldg.*
KELSO, JOSEPH W. ....*Medical Arts Bldg.*
KELTZ, BERT F. ....*Medical Arts Bldg.*
KERNODLE, STRATTON E. ....*First Natl. Bldg.*
*KIMBALL, GEORGE H. ....*Medical Arts Bldg.*
*KUHN, JOHN F. ....*Medical Arts Bldg.*
*KURZNER, MEYER ....1200 *N. Walker*
LACHMAN, ERNEST ....801 *N. E. 13th St.*
LAIN, E. S. ....*Medical Arts Bldg.*
LAMB, JOHN H. ....*Medical Arts Bldg.*
LAMBKE, PHIL M. ....105 *N. W. 23rd St.*
LaMOTTE, GEORGE A. ....*Colcord Bldg.*
LANGSTON, WANN ....*Medical Arts Bldg.*

*LEMON, CECIL W. ....Medical Arts Bldg.
LENEY, FANNIE LOU ....1200 N. Walker
LEONARD, C. E. ....131 N. E. 4th St.
LEVY, BERTHA M. ....1200 N. Walker
LEWIS, A. R. ....Hightower Bldg.
*LINDSTROM, W. C. ....Medical Arts Bldg.
LINGENFELTER, F. M. ....1200 N. Walker
*LITTLE, JOHN R. ....Apco Tower
LONG, LeROY D. ....Medical Arts Bldg.
LONG, WENDELL ....Medical Arts Bldg.
LOVE, R. S. ....Perrine Bldg.
LOWRY, TOM ....1200 N. Walker
LOY, C. F. ....400 N. W. 10th St.
LUTON, JAMES P. ....Medical Arts Bldg.
LYON, JAMES I. ....Edmond
MACDONALD, J. C. ....301 N. W. 12th St.
MARGO, ELIAS ....605 N. W. 10th St.
*MARIL, JOSEPH J. ....Medical Arts Bldg.
*MARTIN, HOWARD C. ....204 N. Robinson St.
MARTIN, J. T. ....1200 N. Walker
MASTERSON, MAUDE M. ....Medical Arts Bldg.
MATHEWS, GRADY F. ....State Health Dept.
    (member Cherokee Co. Medical Society)
*MATTHEWS, SANFORD ....400 N. W. 10th St.
McBRIDE, EARL D. ....605 N. W. 10th St.
*McCLURE, WILLIAM C. ....1200 N. Walker
McGEE, J. P. ....1200 N. Walker
McHENRY, L. C. ....Medical Arts Bldg.
McKINNEY, MILAM F. ....Medical Arts Bldg.
McLAUCHLIN, J. R. ....Plaza Court Bldg.
McNEILL, P. M. ....Medical Arts Bldg.
MECHLING, GEORGE S. ....1200 N. Walker
*MELVIN, JAMES H. ....First Natl. Bank
MESSENBAUGH, J. F. ....Medical Arts Bldg.
*MESSINGER, R. P. ....807 N. W. 23rd St.
*MILES, W. H. ....1200 N. Walker
*MILLER, NESBITT L. ....Medical Arts Bldg.
MILLS, R. C. ....Hightower Bldg.
MOOR, H. D. ....800 N. E. 13th St.
MOORE, B. H. ....Perrine Bldg.
MOORE, C. D. ....Perrine Bldg.
MOORE, ELLIS ....Medical Arts Bldg.
MOORMAN, FLOYD ....1200 N. Walker
MOORMAN, LEWIS J. ....1200 N. Walker
MORGAN, C. A. ....First Natl. Bank
MORLEDGE, WALKER ....1200 N. Walker
MORRISON, H. C. ....807 N. W. 23rd St.
MOTH, M. V. ....American Natl. Bldg.
*MULVEY, BERT E. ....Medical Arts Bldg.
MURDOCH, L. H. ....Medical Arts Bldg.
    (member Blaine Co. Medical Society)
*MURDOCH, RAYMOND L. ....Medical Arts Bldg.
MUSICK, E. R. ....Medical Arts Bldg.
MUSICK, V. H. ....Medical Arts Bldg.
MUSSIL, W. M. ....Medical Arts Bldg.
MYERS, RALPH E. ....1200 N. Walker
*NAGLE, PATRICK S. ....1021 N. Lee
*NEEL, ROY L. ....Medical Arts Bldg.
*NEFF, EVERETT B. ....1200 N. Walker
NICHOLSON, BEN H. ....301 N. W. 12th St.
*NOELL, ROBERT L. ....Medical Arts Bldg.
O'DONOGHUE, D. H. ....Medical Arts Bldg.
O'LEARY, CHARLES M. ....Medical Arts Bldg.
PARRISH, J. M., JR. ....1200 N. Walker
PAULUS, D. D. ....301 N. W. 12th St.
PAYTE, J. I. ....2429 Aurora Court
PENICK, GRIDER ....Colcord Bldg.
PHELPS, A. S. ....Medical Arts Bldg.
PINE, JOHN S. ....Medical Arts Bldg.
POINTS, THOMAS C. ....1200 N. Walker
POSTELLE, J. M. ....Medical Arts Bldg.
POUNDERS, CARROLL M. ....1200 N. Walker
PRATT, CHARLES M. ....1449 Westwood
    (member Garvin Co. Medical Society)
PRICE, JOEL S. ....1200 N. Walker
PUCKETT, CARL ....22 West 6th St.
    (member Mayes Co. Medical Society)
RANDEL, HARVEY O. ....Medical Arts Bldg.
RECK, JOHN A. ....Colcord Bldg.
*RECORDS, JOHN W. ....301 N. W. 12th St.

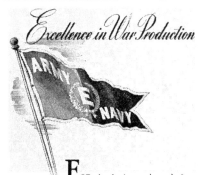

FOR developing and producing Sterile Shaker Packages of Crystalline Sulfanilamide especially designed to meet military needs, for supplying Mercurochrome and other drugs, diagnostic solutions and testing equipment required by the Armed Forces, and for completing deliveries ahead of contract schedule—these are the reasons for the Army-Navy "E" Award to our organization.

Until recently our total output of Sterile Shaker Packages of Crystalline Sulfanilamide was needed for military purposes. As a result of increased production, however, we can now supply these packages for civilian medical use. The package is available only by or on the prescription of a physician.

Supplied in cartons of one dozen Shaker Packages each containing 5 grams of Sterile Crystalline Sulfanilamide, 30-80 mesh.

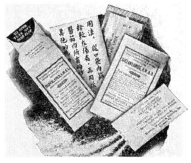

REED, HORACE ....1200 N. Walker
REED, JAMES R. ....Medical Arts Bldg.
REEVES, C. L. ....400 N. W. 10th St.
REICHMANN, RUTH S. ....124 N. W. 15th St.
*RICKS, J. R. ....1200 N. Walker
RIELY, LEA A. ....Medical Arts Bldg.
RILEY, J. W. ....118 N. W. 5th St.
ROBINSON, J. H. ....301 N. W. 12th St.
RODDY, JOHN A. ....Apco Tower
ROGERS, GERALD ....1200 N. Walker
ROUNTREE, C. R. ....1200 N. Walker
*ROYCE, OWEN, JR. ....890 N. E. 13th St.
*RUCKS, W. W., JR. ....301 N. W. 12th St.
RUCKS, W. W., SR. ....301 N. W. 12th St.
*SADLER, LeROY H. ....1200 N. Walker
SALOMON, A. L. ....1200 N. Walker
*SANGER, F. A. ....Key Bldg.
SANGER, F. M. ....Perrine Bldg.
SANGER, WINNIE M. ....Perrine Bldg.
*SANGER, W. W. ....301 N. W. 12th St.
*SEBA, CHESTER R. ....1200 N. Walker
SEBRING, MILTON H. ....807 N. W. 23rd St.
SELL, L. STANLEY ....Medical Arts Bldg.
SERWER, MILTON J. ....1200 N. Walker
*SEWELL, DAN R. ....400 N. W. 10th St.
SHACKELFORD, JOHN W. ....State Health Dept.
SHELTON, J. W. ....Hightower Bldg.
SHEPPARD, MARY S. ....1200 N. Walker
*SHIRCLIFF, E. E., JR. ....128 N. W. 14th St.
*SHORBE, HOWARD B. ....605 N. W. 10th St.
*SMITH, CHARLES A. ....717 N. Robinson St.
SMITH, DELBERT G. ....First Natl. Bldg.
SMITH, EDWARD N. ....400 N. W. 10th St.
SMITH, L. L. ....229 S. W. 29th St.
SMITH, RALPH A. ....4434½ N. W. 23rd St.
*SNOW, J. B. ....1200 N. Walker
STANBRO, GREGORY E. ....Medical Arts Bldg.
STARRY, L. J. ....1200 N. Walker
STILLWELL, R. J. ....American Natl. Bldg.
STOUT, MARVIN E. ....209 N. W. 13th St.
*STRADER, S. E. ....105 N. Hudson St.
*STRECKER, WILLIAM E. ....Medical Arts Bldg.
SULLIVAN, ELIJAH E. ....Medical Arts Bldg.
TABOR, GEORGE R. (honorary) ....First Natl. Bldg.
TAYLOR, CHARLES B. ....Medical Arts Bldg.
*TAYLOR, JIM M. ....Medical Arts Bldg.
TAYLOR, WILLIAM M. ....625 N. W. 10th St.
THOMPSON, WAYMAN J. ....1200 N. Walker
*TOOL, DONOVAN ....Edmond
TOWNSEND, CARY W. ....Medical Arts Bldg.
TRENT, ROBERT I. ....Medical Arts Bldg.
TURNER, HENRY H. ....1200 N. Walker
*VAHLBERG, E. R. ....First Natl. Bldg.
VON WEDEL, CURT ....610 N. W. 9th St.
WAILS, T. G. ....Medical Arts Bldg.
*WAINWRIGHT, TOM L. ....Medical Arts Bldg.
*WATSON, I. NEWTON ....Edmond
WATSON, O. ALTON ....1200 N. Walker
WATSON, R. D. ....Britton
WEIR, MARSHALL W. ....Apco Tower
WELLS, EVA ....Medical Arts Bldg.
WELLS, LOIS LYON ....1200 N. Walker
WELLS, W. W. ....Medical Arts Bldg.
WEST, W. K. ....1200 N. Walker
WESTFALL, L. M. ....Medical Arts Bldg.
WHITE, ARTHUR W. ....Medical Arts Bldg.
WHITE, OSCAR ....1200 N. Walker
WHITE, PHIL E. ....Perrine Bldg.
*WILDMAN, S. F. ....Medical Arts Bldg.
WILKINS, HARRY ....Medical Arts Bldg.
WILLIAMS, LEONARD C. ....1200 N. Walker
WILLIAMSON, W. H. ....128 N. W. 14th St.
WILLIE, JAMES A. ....218 N. W. 7th St.
WILSON, KENNETH J. ....Medical Arts Bldg.
*WITTEN, HAROLD B. ....Harrah
*WOLFF, JOHN POWERS ....1200 N. Walker
WOODWARD, NEIL W. ....1200 N. Walker
WRIGHT, HARPER ....318 S. W. 25th St.
YOUNG, A. M., III ....Medical Arts Bldg.

OKMULGEE

ALEXANDER, LIN ....Okmulgee
*ALEXANDER, R. L. ....Okmulgee
BOLLINGER, I. W. ....Henryetta
BOSWELL, H. D. ....Henryetta
CARLOSS, T. C. ....Morris
CARNELL, M. D. ....Okmulgee
*COTTERAL, J. R. ....Henryetta
EDWARDS, J. G. ....Okmulgee
HAYNES, W. M. ....Henryetta
HOLMES, A. R. ....Henryetta
HUDSON, W. S. ....Okmulgee
KILPATRICK, G. A. ....Henryetta
LESLIE, S. B. ....Okmulgee
MABEN, CHARLES S. ....Okmulgee
MATHENEY, J. C. ....Okmulgee
McKINNEY, G. Y. ....Henryetta
MING, C. M. ....Okmulgee
MITCHENER, W. C. ....Okmulgee
PETER, M. L. ....Okmulgee
RAINS, HUGH L. ....Okmulgee
RODDA, E. D. ....Okmulgee
SIMPSON, N. N. ....Henryetta
*SMITH, C. E. ....Henryetta
TRACEWELL, GEORGE L. ....Okmulgee
VERNON, W. C. ....Okmulgee
WATSON, F. S. ....Okmulgee

OSAGE

AARON, WILLIAM H. ....Pawhuska
ALEXANDER, E. T. ....Barnsdall
DOZIER, BARCLAY E. ....Shidler
GUILD, CARL H. ....Shidler
HEMPHILL, GEORGE K. ....Pawhuska
*HEMPHILL, PAUL H. ....Pawhuska
KARASEK, MATTHEW ....Shidler
KEYES, E. C. ....Hominy
LIPE, EVERETT N. ....Fairfax
SULLIVAN, B. F. ....Barnsdall
WALKER, G. I. ....Hominy
WALKER, ROSCOE ....Pawhuska
WEIRICH, COLIN REID ....Pawhuska
WILLIAMS, CLAUDE W. ....Pawhuska
WORTEN, DIVONIS ....Pawhuska

OTTAWA

*AISENSTADT, E. ALBERT ....Picher
BARRY, J. R. ....Picher
*BISHOP, CALMES ....Picher
BUTLER, V. V. ....Picher
CANNON, R. F. ....Miami
*CHESNUT, W. G. ....Miami
COLVERT, GEORGE W. ....Miami
CONNELL, M. A. ....Picher
CRAIG, J. W. ....Miami
CUNNINGHAM, P. J. ....Miami
DeARMANN, M. M. ....Miami
DeTAR, GEORGE A. ....Miami
HAMPTON, J. B. ....Commerce
HETHERINGTON, L. P. ....Miami
HUGHES, A. R. ....Miami
JACOBY, J. SHERWOOD ....Commerce
KERR, WALTER C. H. ....Picher
McNAUGHTON, G. P. ....Miami
MURRY, A. V. ....Picher
PRATT, T. W. ....Miami
RALSTON, BENJAMIN W. ....Commerce
RUSSELL, RICHARD ....Picher
SANGER, W. B. ....Picher
*SAYLES, W. JACKSON ....Miami
SHELTON, B. WRIGHT ....Miami
SIEVER, CHARLES W. ....Picher
STAPLES, J. H. L. ....Afton
WORMINGTON, F. L. ....Miami

PAWNEE

BROWNING, R. L. ....Pawnee
HADDOX, CHARLES H. ....Pawnee
LeHEW, J. L. ....Pawnee
ROBINSON, E. T. ....Cleveland
SADDORIS, M. L. ....Cleveland
SPAULDING, H. B. ....Ralston

PAYNE

*BASSETT, CLIFFORD M. ....*Cushing*
CLEVERDON, L. A. ....*Stillwater*
*DAVIDSON, W. N. ....*Cushing*
DAVIS, BENJAMIN ....*Cushing*
FRIEDMANN, PAUL W. ....*Stillwater*
*FRY, POWELL E. ....*Stillwater*
HOLBROOK, R. W. (*honorary*) ....*Perkins*
LEATHEROCK, R. E. ....*Cushing*
MANNING, H. C. ....*Cushing*
MARTIN, E. O. ....*Cushing*
*MARTIN, JAMES D. ....*Cushing*
MARTIN, JOHN F. ....*Stillwater*
MARTIN, JOHN W. ....*Cushing*
MITCHELL, L. A. ....*Stillwater*
MOORE, CLIFFORD W. ....*Stillwater*
OEHLSCHLAGER, F. KEITH ....*Yale*
*PUCKETT, HOWARD L. ....*Stillwater*
RICHARDSON, P. M. ....*Cushing*
*ROBERTS, R. E. ....*Stillwater*
SEXTON, C. E. (*honorary*) ....*Stillwater*
SILVERTHORN, LOUIS E. ....*Stillwater*
SMITH, A. B. ....*Stillwater*
SMITH, HASKELL ....*Stillwater*
WAGGONER, ROY E. ....*Stillwater*
WEBER, ROXIE A. ....*Stillwater*
*WILHITE, L. R. ....*Perkins*

PITTSBURG

BALL, ERNEST ....*McAlester*
*BARTHELD, FLOYD T. ....*McAlester*
BAUM, FRANK J. ....*McAlester*
DAKIL, LOUIS N. ....*McAlester*
DORROUGH, JOE ....*Haileyville*
*GREENBERGER, EDWARD D. ....*McAlester*
KAEISER, WILLIAM H. ....*McAlester*
*KLOTZ, WILLIAM ....*McAlester*
KUYRKENDALL, L. C. ....*McAlester*
*LEVINE, JULIUS ....*McAlester*
*LIVELY, C. E. ....*McAlester*
McCARLEY, T. H. ....*McAlester*
MILLER, FRANK A. ....*Hartshorne*
MUNN, JESSE A. ....*McAlester*
PACKARD, LOUIS A. ....*McAlester*
PARK, JOHN F. ....*McAlester*
PEMBERTON, R. K. ....*McAlester*
POWELL, PAUL T. ....*McAlester*
RICE, O. W. ....*McAlester*
SAMES, W. W. ....*Hartshorne*
SHULLER, E. H. ....*McAlester*
SPRINKLE, D. L. ....*McAlester*
STOUGH, A. R. ....*McAlester*
WAIT, WILLIAM C. ....*McAlester*
WILLIAMS, C. O. ....*McAlester*
WILLOUR, L. S. ....*McAlester*
WILSON, HERBERT A. ....*McAlester*

PONTOTOC

*BIGLER, IVAN ....*Ada*
BRECO, J. G. ....*Ada*
BRYDIA, CATHERINE T. ....*Ada*
CANADA, ERNEST A. ....2549 *Howard Ave.*
                                                Memphis, Tenn.
*CHEATWOOD, W. R. ....*Ada*
COWLING, ROBERT E. ....*Ada*
*CUNNINGHAM, JOHN A. ....*Ada*
CUMMINGS, I. L. ....*Ada*
DEAN, W. F. ....*Ada*
GULLATT, ENNIS, M. ....*Ada*
LANE, WILSON H. ....*Ada*
LEWIS, E. F. ....*Ada*
LEWIS, M. L. ....*Ada*
MAYES, R. H. ....*Ada*
McBRIDE, OLLIE ....*Ada*
*McDONALD, GLEN ....*Ada*
McKEEL, SAM A. ....*Ada*
MILLER, O. H. ....*Ada*
*MOREY, J. B. ....*Ada*
MORRIS, R. D. ....*Allen*
    (*member Hughes Co. Medical Society*)
*MUNTZ, E. R. ....*Ada*

*MURRAY, E. C. ....*Ada*
NEEDHAM, C. F. ....*Ada*
*PADBERG, E. D. ....*Ada*
RICHEY, S. M. (*honorary*) ....*Ada*
    (*member Tulsa Co. Medical Society*)
ROSS, S. P. (*honorary*) ....*Ada*
SEABORN, T. L. ....*Ada*
SUGG, ALFRED R. ....*Ada*
*WEBSTER, HARRELL ....*Ada*
WEBSTER, M. M. ....*Ada*
WELBORN, O. E. ....*Ada*

POTTAWATOMIE

BAKER, M. A. ....*Shawnee*
BALL, W. A. ....*Wanette*
BAXTER, GEORGE S. ....*Shawnee*
BYRUM, J. M. ....*Shawnee*
CAMPBELL, H. G. ....*Tecumseh*
CARSON, F. L. ....*Shawnee*
CARSON, JOHN M. ....*Shawnee*
**CORDELL, U. S. ....*Macomb*
CULBERTSON, R. R. ....*Maud*
FORTSON, J. L. ....*Tecumseh*
GALLAHER, CLINTON ....*Shawnee*
*GALLAHER, PAUL ....*Shawnee*
GALLAHER, W. M. ....*Shawnee*
HAYGOOD, CHARLES W. ....*Shawnee*
HILL, R. M. C. (*honorary*) ....*McLoud*
*HUGHES, HORTON E. ....*Shawnee*
HUGHES, J. E. ....*Shawnee*
KAYLER, R. C. ....*McLoud*
KEEN, FRANK M. ....*Shawnee*
MATHEWS, W. F. ....*Tecumseh*
McFARLING, A. C. ....*Shawnee*
MULLINS, WILLIAM B. ....*Shawnee*
NEWLIN, FRANCES P. ....*Shawnee*
PARAMORE, C. F. ....*Shawnee*
RICE, E. EUGENE ....*Shawnee*
ROWLAND, T. D. ....*Shawnee*
WALKER, J. A. ....*Shawnee*
WILLIAMS, ALPHA McADAMS ....*Shawnee*
**YOUNG, C. C. ....*Shawnee*
**Deceased May 28, 1943.

PUSHMATAHA

CONNALLY, D. W. ....*Antlers*
HUCKABAY, B. M. ....*Antlers*
LAWSON, JOHN S. ....*Clayton*
PATTERSON, E. S. ....*Antlers*

ROGER MILLS

CARY, W. S. ....*Reydon*
    (*member Beckham Co. Medical Society*)
HENRY, J. WORRALL ....*Cheyenne*
    (*member Beckham Co. Medical Society*)

ROGERS

ANDERSON, F. A. ....*Claremore*
*ANDERSON, P. S. ....*Claremore*
*ANDERSON, W. D. ....*Claremore*
BESON, CLYDE W. ....*Claremore*
*BIGLER, E. E. ....*Claremore*
CALDWELL, C. L. ....*Chelsea*
COLLINS, B. F. ....*Claremore*
*HOWARD, W. A. ....*Chelsea*
JENNINGS, K. D. ....*Chelsea*
MACRAE, DONALD H. ....*Claremore*
MELINDER, ROY J. ....*Claremore*
MELOY, R. C. ....*Claremore*
WALLER, GEORGE D. ....*Claremore*

SEMINOLE

CHAMBERS, CLAUDE S. ....*Seminole*
GIESEN, A. F. ....*Radford, Va.*
GRIMES, JOHN P. ....*Wewoka*
HARBER, J. N. (*honorary*) ....*Phoenix, Ariz.*
HUDDLESTON, W. T. ....*Konawa*
McGOVERN, J. D. ....*Wewoka*
MOSHER, D. D. ....*Seminole*
PACE, L. R. ....*Seminole*
PRICE, J. T. ....*Seminole*
REEDER, H. M. ....*Konawa*
SHANHOLTZ, MACK I. ....*Wewoka*

STEPHENS, A. B. ....Seminole
TURLINGTON, M. M. ....Seminole
VAN SANDT, GUY B. ....Wewoka
VAN SANDT, MAX M. ....Wewoka
WALKER, A. A. ....Wewoka
WILLIAMS, J. CLAY ....Wewoka
WILLIAMSON, SAM H. ....Wewoka
   (member Oklahoma Co. Medical Society)
WRIGHT, H. L. ....Konawa

SEQUOYAH
NEWLIN, WILLIAM H. ....Sallisaw
   (member Cherokee Co. Medical Society)
MORROW, JOHN A. ....Sallisaw

STEPHENS
GARRETT, S. S. ....Duncan
IVY, WALLIS, S. ....Duncan
*KING, E. G. ....Duncan
McCLAIN, W. Z. ....Marlow
McMAHAN, A. M. ....Duncan
PATTERSON, J. L. ....Duncan
RICHARDSON, B. W. ....Duncan
TALLEY, C. N. ....Marlow
WALKER, W. K. ....Marlow
*WATERS, CLAUDE B. ....Duncan
WEEDN, ALTON J. ....Duncan

TEXAS
BLACKMER, L. G. ....Hooker
HAYES, R. B. ....Guymon
LEE, DANIEL S. ....Guymon
SMITH, MORRIS ....Guymon

TILLMAN
ALLEN, C. C. ....Frederick
ARRINGTON, J. E. ....Frederick
BACON, O. G. ....Frederick
*BOX, O. H., JR. ....Grandfield
CHILDERS, J. E. ....Tipton
COLLIER, E .K. ....Tipton
COMP, G. A. ....Manitou
*FISHER, ROY L. ....Frederick
FOSHEE, W. C. ....Grandfield
*FRY, F. P. ....Frederick
FUQUA, W. A. ....Grandfield
OSBORN, J. D. ....Frederick
ROBINSON, R. D. ....Frederick
SPURGEON, T. F. ....Frederick

TULSA
ADAMS, R. M. ....591 N. Boulder
*AKIN, J. O. ....Medical Arts Bldg.
ALLEN, V. K. ....Medical Arts Bldg.
ARMSTRONG, O. C. ....Medical Arts Bldg.
ATCHLEY, R. Q. ....507 S. Cincinnati
ATKINS, PAUL N. ....Medical Arts Bldg.
BARHAM, J. H. ....Daniels Bldg.
*BEST, RALPH L. ....Medical Arts Bldg.
BEYER, J. WALTER ....McBirney Bldg.
BILLINGTON, J. JEFF ....Medical Arts Bldg.
BIRNBAUM, WILLIAM ....915 S. Cincinnati
BLACK, HAROLD J. ....Medical Arts Bldg.
*BOONE, W. B. ....2112 W. 41st St.
BOWERS, JOSEPH S. ....2812 W. 40th St.
BRADFIELD, S. J. ....Medical Arts Bldg.
**BRADLEY, C. E. ....Medical Arts Bldg.
*BRANLEY, B. L. ....Medical Arts Bldg.
BRASWELL, JAMES C. ....Medical Arts Bldg.
*BROCKSMITH, H. A. ....Medical Arts Bldg.
BROGDEN, J. C. ....Medical Arts Bldg.
BROOKSHIRE, J. E. (honorary) ....409 S. Boulder
BROWNE, HENRY S. ....Medical Arts Bldg.
BRYAN, W. J., JR. ....Medical Arts Bldg.
CALHOUN, C. E. ....Sand Springs
CALHOUN, W. H. ....Medical Arts Bldg.
CARNEY, A. B. ....915 S. Cincinnati
CHALMERS, J. S. ....Sand Springs
CHILDS, D. B. ....1226 S. Boston Place
CHILDS, J. W. ....1226 S. Boston Place
CLINTON, FRED S. (honorary) 230 E. Woodward Blvd.
CLULOW, GEORGE H. ....1307 S. Main
COHENOUR, E. L. ....Medical Arts Bldg.
COOK, W. ALBERT ....Medical Arts Bldg.

COULTER, T. B. ....Medical Arts Bldg.
CRAWFORD, WILLIAM S. Natl. Bank of Tulsa Bldg.
CRONK, FRED Y. ....Medical Arts Bldg.
DAILY, R. E. ....Bixby
DAVIS, A. H. ....Medical Arts Bldg.
DAVIS, GEORGE M. ....Bixby
*DAVIS, T. H. ....Medical Arts Bldg.
DEAN, W. A. ....Medical Arts Bldg.
*DENNY, E. RANKIN ....Medical Arts Bldg.
DUNLAP, ROY W. ....Medical Arts Bldg.
*EADS, CHARLES H. ....Medical Arts Bldg.
*EDWARDS, D. L. ....Philcade Bldg.
*EDWARDS, JOHN ....Medical Arts Bldg.
ETHERTON, MONTE C. ....10-A S. Lewis
EVANS, HUGH J. ....Medical Arts Bldg.
*EWELL, WILLIAM C. ....1307 S. Main
FARRIS, H. LEE ....Medical Arts Bldg.
FLACK, F. L. ....Natl. Bank of Tulsa Bldg.
FLANAGAN, O. A. ....912 S. Boulder
FORD, H. W. ....915 S. Cincinnati
*FORD, RICHARD B. ....Braniff Bldg.
FORBY, W. W. ....Bixby
FRANKLIN, ONIS ....Broken Arrow
*FRANKLIN, S. E. ....Broken Arrow
FULCHER, JOSEPH ....Medical Arts Bldg.
FUNK, ROBERT E. ....Medical Arts Bldg.
GARRETT, D. L. ....Medical Arts Bldg.
GILBERT, J. B. ....Natl. Mutual Bldg.
GLASS, FRED A. ....Medical Arts Bldg.
GODDARD, R. K. ....Skiatook
GOODMAN, SAMUEL ....Medical Arts Bldg.
GORRELL, J. F. ....Medical Arts Bldg.
GRAHAM, HUGH C. ....1307 S. Main
*GREEN, HARRY ....Medical Arts Bldg.
GROSSHART, PAUL ....Medical Arts Bldg.
*HAMMOND, JAMES H. ....Medical Arts Bldg.
HARALSON, C. H. ....Medical Arts Bldg.
*HARDMAN, T. J. ....Medical Arts Bldg.
HARRIS, BUNN ....Jenks
HART, MABLE M. ....1228 S. Boulder
HART, M. O. ....1228 S. Boulder
HAYS, LUVERN ....Medical Arts Bldg.
HENDERSON, F. W. ....Medical Arts Bldg.
HENLEY, MARVIN D. ....Medical Arts Bldg.
*HENRY, G. H. ....Medical Arts Bldg.
HILL, O. L. ....915 S. Cincinnati
HOKE, C. C. ....Philtower Bldg.
*HOOVER, W. D. ....511 S. Boston
HOTZ, CARL J. ....Springer Clinic
HOUSER, M. A. ....McBirney Bldg.
HUBER, W. A. ....Medical Arts Bldg.
HUDSON, DAVID V. ....21 N. Cincinnati
HUDSON, MARGARET G. ....1759 S. Victor
HUMPHREY, B. H. ....Sperry
HUTCHISON, A. ....Bixby
HYATT, E. G. ....Springer Clinic
INGRAM, MARGARET A. ....915 S. Cincinnati
JOHNSON, E. O. ....Medical Arts Bldg.
JOHNSON, R. R. ....Sand Springs
JONES, ELLIS, ...Medical Arts Bldg.
   (member Creek Co. Medical Society)
JONES, WILLIAM M. ....915 S. Cincinnati
KEMMERLY, H. P. ....Medical Arts Bldg.
*KORNBLEE, A. T. ....1307 S. Main
KRAMER, ALLEN C. ....Medical Arts Bldg.
LARRABEE, W. S. ....Medical Arts Bldg.
LAYTON, O. E. ....Collinsville
*LEE, J. K. ....Medical Arts Bldg.
LeMASTER, D. W. ....Medical Arts Bldg.
LHEVINE, MORRIS B. ....Medical Arts Bldg.
LONEY, W. R. R. ....Medical Arts Bldg.
LOWE, J. O. ....915 S. Cincinnati
*LUSK, EARL M. ....915 S. Cincinnati
LYNCH, THOMAS J. ....Philcade Bldg.
MacDONALD, D. M. ....1739 S. Utica
MacKENZIE, IAN ....Medical Arts Bldg.
MARGOLIN, BERTHE ....2603 E. 14th St.
MARKLAND, J. D. ....Medical Arts Bldg.
*MATT, JOHN G. ....1304 E. 20th St.
MAYGINNES, P. H. ....Palace Bldg.

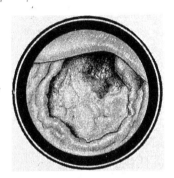

*McDONALD, J. E. ....Medical Arts Bldg.
McGILL, RALPH A. ....Medical Arts Bldg.
McKELLAR, MALCOLM M. ....Springer Clinic
McQUAKER, MOLLY ....1552 E. 17th Place
MILLER, GEORGE H. ....Atlas Life Bldg.
MINER, JAMES L. ....Medical Arts Bldg.
MISHLER, D. L. ....Springer Clinic
*MITCHELL, T. H. ....Natl. Bank of Tulsa Bldg.
MOHRMAN, S. S. ....Daniels Bldg.
*MUNDING, L. A. ....Medical Arts Bldg.
MURDOCK, H. D. ....Medical Arts Bldg.
MURRAY, P. G. ....Medical Arts Bldg.
MURRAY, SILAS ....Medical Arts Bldg.
NEAL, JAMES H. ....1944 N. Denver Place
NELSON, FRANK J. ....Medical Arts Bldg.
NELSON, F. L. ....Atlas Life Bldg.
NELSON, I. A. ....Medical Arts Bldg.
NELSON IRON H. ....Medical Arts Bldg.
NELSON, M. O. ....Medical Arts Bldg.
NESBITT, E. P. ....Medical Arts Bldg.
NESBITT, P. P. ....Medical Arts Bldg.
NORTHRUP, L. C. ....1307 S. Main
OSBORN, GEORGE R. ....Medical Arts Bldg.
PAVY, C. A. ....Medical Arts Bldg.
PEDEN, JAMES C. ....Medical Arts Bldg.
*PERRY, FRED J. ....Atlas Life Bldg.
PERRY, HUGH ....Atlas Life Bldg.
PERRY, JOHN C. ....Medical Arts Bldg.
PIATT, LOUIS M. ....Medical Arts Bldg.
PIGFORD, A. W. ....Medical Arts Bldg.
*PIGFORD, R. C. ....Medical Arts Bldg.
*PITTMAN, COLE D. ....Broken Arrow
*POLLOCK, SIMON ....Tulsa
*PORTER, H. H. ....Medical Arts Bldg.
PRESSON, L. C. ....1305 E. 15th St.
PRICE, H. P. ....Medical Arts Bldg.
*RAY, R. G. ....915 S. Cincinnati
REESE, K. C. ....Medical Arts Bldg.
REYNOLDS, E. W. ....915 S. Cincinnati
RHODES, R. E. L. ....Medical Arts Bldg.
ROBERTS, T. R. ....Wright Bldg.
ROBINSON, F. P. ....915 S. Cincinnati
      (member Grant Co. Medical Society)
ROGERS, J. W. ....Medical Arts Bldg.
ROTH, A. W. ....1616 S. Peoria Ave.
RUPRECHT, H. A. ....Springer Clinic
RUPRECHT, MARCELLA ....Springer Clinic
RUSHING, F. E. ....Medical Arts Bldg.
RUSSELL, G. R. ....Springer Clinic
SCHRECK, PHILIP M. ....Medical Arts Bldg.
*SCHWARTZ, H. N. ....Medical Arts Bldg.
SEARLE, M. J. ....Medical Arts Bldg.
SHAPIRO, DAVID ....Atlas Life Bldg.
SHEPARD, R. M. ....Medical Arts Bldg.
*SHEPARD, S. C. ....Medical Arts Bldg.
SHERWOOD, R. G. ....Wright Bldg.
*SHIPP, J. D. ....Medical Arts Bldg.
SHOWMAN, W. A. ....Medical Arts Bldg.
SIMPSON, CARL F. ....Medical Arts Bldg.
*SINCLAIR, F. D. ....Springer Clinic
SIPPEL, MARY EDNA ....1542 E. 15th St.
SISLER, WADE ....Mercy Hospital
SMITH, D. O. ....Springer Clinic
SMITH, NED R. ....Medical Arts Bldg.
*SMITH, ROY L. ....Medical Arts Bldg.
SMITH, RURIC N. ....Medical Arts Bldg.
SMITH, W. O. ....Stanolind Bldg.
*SPANN, LOGAN A. ....Braniff Bldg.
*SPOTTSWOOD, MAURICE D. ....Medical Arts Bldg.
SPRINGER, M. P. ....Springer Clinic
STALLINGS, T. W. ....724 S. Elgin St.
STANLEY, M. V. ....904 N. Denver
STEVENSON, JAMES ....Medical Arts Bldg.
STEWART, H. B. ....1932 S. Utica
*STUARD, C. G. ....Tulsa
*STUART, FRANK A. ....Natl. Mutual Bldg.
STUART, LEON H. ....Medical Arts Bldg.
SUMMERS, C. S. ....Daniels Bldg.
*SWANSON, K. F. ....Springer Clinic
THOMPSON, OLIVER H. ....615 W. 14th Place

TRAINOR, W. J. ....Medical Arts Bldg.
*TURNBOW, W. R. ....Medical Arts Bldg.
UNDERWOOD, DAVID J. ....Medical Arts Bldg.
UNDERWOOD, F. L. ....Medical Arts Bldg.
UNGERMAN, A. H. ....Medical Arts Bldg.
VENABLE, S. C. ....6th & Cheyenne
WALKER, WILLIAM A. ....Kennedy Bldg.
WALL, GREGORY A. (honorary) ....1159 N. Cheyenne
WALLACE, J. E. ....Medical Arts Bldg.
WARD, B. W. ....Wright Bldg.
WENDEL, WILLIAM E. ....915 S. Cincinnati
*WHITE, ERIC M. ....Medical Arts Bldg.
WHITE, N. S. ....Medical Arts Bldg.
WILEY, A. RAY ....Medical Arts Bldg.
WILLIAMS, THEO. S. ....Medical Arts Bldg.
WITCHER, R. B. ....Medical Arts Bldg.
*WOLFF, EUGENE G. ....St. John's Hospital
WOODSON, FRED E. ....Medical Arts Bldg.
*YANDELL, HAYS R. ....Medical Arts Bldg.
ZINK, ROY ....Daniels Bldg.
**Deceased July 6.

WAGONER

BATES, S. R. ....Wagoner
DIVINE, D. G. ....Wagoner
JOBLIN, W. R. ....Porter
PLUNKETT, J. H. ....Wagoner
RIDDLE, H. K. ....Coweta

WASHINGTON

ATHEY, J. B. ....Bartlesville
BEECHWOOD, E. E. ....Bartlesville
CHAMBERLIN, E. M. ....Bartlesville
CRAWFORD, HORACE G. ....Bartlesville
CRAWFORD, JOHN E. ....Bartlesville
DORSHEIMER, GEORGE V. ....Dewey
*ETTER, FORREST S. ....Bartlesville
*GENTRY, RAYMOND C. ....Bartlesville
GREEN, OTTO I. ....Bartlesville
HUDSON, LAWRENCE D. ....Dewey
KIMBALL, M. C. ....Box 391, Borger Texas
KINGMAN, W. H. (honorary) ....Bartlesville
LeBLANC, WILLIAM ....Ocheleta
PARKS, SETH M. ....Bartlesville
REWERTS, FRED C. ....Bartlesville
*RUCKER, RALPH W. ....Bartlesville
SHIPMAN, WILLIAM H. ....Bartlesville
SMITH, JOSEPH G. ....Bartlesville
SOMERVILLE, OKEY S. ....Bartlesville
STAVER, BENJAMIN F. ....Bartlesville
TORREY, JOHN P. ....Bartlesville
VANSANT, J. P. ....Dewey
WEBER, HENRY C. ....Bartlesville
WEBER, SHERWELL G. ....Bartlesville
WELLS, CEPHAS J. ....Bartlesville
WELLS, THOMAS ....Bartlesville
*WORD, LEE B. ....Bartlesville

WASHITA

ADAMS, ALLEN C. ....Cordell
BENNETT, D. W. ....Sentinel
BUNGARDT, A. H. ....Cordell
*DARNELL, E. E. ....Colony
FREEMAN, W. H. (honorary) ....Sentinel
      (member Kiowa Co. Medical Society)
HARMS, J. H. (honorary) ....Newton, Kansas
JONES, J. P. (honorary) ....Dill
*LIVINGSTON, L. G. ....Cordell
McMURRY, JAMES F. ....Sentinel
NEAL, A. S. ....Cordell
*STOWERS, AUBREY E. ....Sentinel
TRACY, C. M. ....Sentinel
WEAVER, E. S. ....Cordell
WEBER, A. ....Bessie

WOODS

CLAPPER, EBENEEZER, P. (honorary) ....Waynoka
ENSOR, DANIEL B. ....Hopeton
GRANTHAM, ELIZABETH (honorary) ......Alva
HALL, RAY L. ....Waynoka
HUNT, ISAAC S. (honorary) ....Freedom
LaFON, WILLIAM F. ....Waynoka
*ROYER, CHARLES A. ....Alva
*SIMON, JOHN F. ....Alva

SIMON, WILLIAM E. _____*Alva*
STEPHENSON, ISHMAEL F. _____*Alva*
TEMPLIN, OSCAR E. _____*Alva*

WOODWARD

DARWIN, D. W. _____*Woodward*
DAY, JOHN L. _____*Supply*
*DUER, JOE L. _____*Woodward*
*ENGLAND, MYRON _____*Woodward*
JOHNSON, H. L. _____*Supply*
*KING, FRANK M. _____*Woodward*
LEACHMAN, THAD C. _____*Woodward*
MITCHELL, CLARENCE _____*Supply*
ORRICK, GEORGE W. _____*Supply*
PIERSON, ORRA A. _____*Woodward*
*RUTHERFORD, V. M. _____*Woodward*
TEDROWE, C. W. _____*Woodward*
TRIPLETT, T. BURKE _____*Mooreland*
WILLIAMS, O. E. _____*Woodward*

ASSOCIATE MEMBERS

GILLICK, M.D., DAVID _____*Shawnee*
HANSEN, MR. FRED _____*Oklahoma City*
MOLLICA, M. D., S. G. _____*Muskogee*
TURLEY, PH. D., LOUIS A. _____*Oklahoma City*

• OBITUARIES •

F. R. Buchanan
1892-1943

Dr. F. R. Buchanan, born June 30, 1892 in Gallup, New Mexico, died June 4 at his home in Canton.

In 1895, Dr. Buchanan moved to Thomas where he resided until graduating from high school. He then attended the Arkansas University Department of Medicine transferring to the Chicago College of Medicine and Surgery in the Fall of 1912. He graduated in the Spring of 1914. From 1914 to 1915 Dr. Buchanan practiced in Thomas and then moved to Canton, where he practiced until the time of his death.

During the last War, Dr. Buchanan was with the U. S. Army Medical Corps and had eighteen months active duty. He was discharged in 1919 with the rank of Captain, immediately being promoted to the rank of Major in the inactive Reserve Corps. In 1928 he was discharged and at that time was appointed to the rank of Lieutenant Colonel.

Dr. Buchanan was Past Master of the A. F. and A. M. Lodge No. 418 of Canton and a member of the Lions Club. He was also a member of the Blaine County Medical Society and the Oklahoma State and Southern Medical Associations. He was medical examiner for the local draft board of Blaine and Dewey Counties.

Surviving relatives include his widow, two sons, H. Reuel and F. Randall and two daughters, Theresa M. Haigler and Carolee Abshire.

Classified Advertisements

COUNTY NEWS

The Payne County Medical Society met on June 17 at Stillwater. "Anaplasmosis" was discussed by H. E. Smith, V.N.D. of A. & M. College. Dr. Leatherock, Cushing, will make arrangements for the first program when meetings are resumed in September.

Members and visitors of the Pottawatomie Society met on June 6 for a report by the Public Relations Committee on a plan for Obstetric and Pediatric care for the families of the men in the armed forces.

Dr. C. C. Young was the speaker and chose as his subject "Leukorrhea."

The next meeting will be held July 17.

Meetings of the Southwest Oklahoma Medical Society will be resumed in September. The last meeting was held in Clinton on June 22 and Dr. F. R. Vieregg of Clinton spoke on "Use of local anesthetics in the Eye." Dr. Ellis Lamb, also of Clinton, selected "Hypertensive Heart Disease" as his topic for discussion. "Treatment of Functional Uterine Bleeding" was discussed by Dr. J. William Finch, Hobart.

Dr. J. L. Day, Superintendent of the Western Hospital gave an interesting talk to the Woodward County Medical Society on the history of Fort Supply from the start. Dr. Day displayed many souvenirs that had been dug up on the place. He has a nice collection for an historical museum.

The Newman Clinic will be host to the members when meetings are resumed in September.

A paper on "Thyroid Diseases" was read by Dr. E. T. Shirley and discussed by Dr. M. E. Robberson, Jr., at the meeting of the Garvin County Medical Society on June 16. Meetings will be resumed in September.

The Cleveland County Medical Society had as its guest speaker, Dr. E. S. Burge of the Naval Hospital. Dr. Burge presented a colored film on "Occiput Posterior" which he helped produce at Northwestern and Evanston Hospital. This was of great interest to the members and lengthy discussion followed the presentation.

A general business meeting followed the scientific period. It was decided that no further meetings would be held during the summer months. The program chairman and committee for the fall meetings were named.

AN OPPORTUNITY FOR PHYSICIANS TO STUDY WAR CASUALTIES

An opportunity to study Army and Navy treatment of casualties at two of the nation's leading military hospitals will be afforded physicians attending the annual convention of the Association of Military Surgeons of the United States in Philadelphia, Pennsylvania, October 21-23 inclusive.

Visits to the U. S. Naval Hospital, Philadelphia, and the U. S. Army Hospital at Valley Forge, where patients from war zones are under treatment, may be arranged for members of the Association during the three-day convention at the Bellevue-Stratford if they so wish.

Throughout the years Philadelphia has maintained its high place in medical circles and is also one of the historical centers of the United States. Within a short distance of convention headquarters are national shrines and other points that offer both interest and inspiration during these trying war days.

Cultivation is as necessary to the mind as food is to the body.—Cicero.

By gnawing through a dyke even a rat may drown a nation.—Edward Burke.

ASSOCIATION ACTIVITIES

ANNUAL MEETING
OF
AMERICAN MEDICAL ASSOCIATION

The annual meeting of the American Medical Association recently held in Chicago was highlighted by the refusal of the House of Delegates to definitely establish a Washington Bureau of Information to assist the Congress of the United States in the consideration of health problems. Resolutions introduced to this end were side tracked in the Reference Committee on Legislation and Public Relation by the substitution of a resolution resigned to accomplish a part of the suggested proposal through the establishment of a Council on Legal Medicine and Legislation in the headquarters of the American Medical Association in Chicago. It was significant to note that the officers and Board of Trustees of the American Medical Association were united in working for the adoption of the Reference Committee's report without allowing the House of Delegates to vote directly on the adoption of the original resolutions.

The report of the Reference Committee as adopted creates a Council on Legal Medicine and Legislation to be composed of six members of the American Medical Association geographically distributed over the United States, the President, the Secretary, the immediate Past President, and a member of the Board of Trustees. The six members of the American Medical Association for the first year shall be selected by the Board of Trustees and thereafter they shall be elected by the House of Delegates on a staggered term basis from nominations made by the Board of Trustees.

The duties of the Council as outlined in the Committee report are as follows: ''The duties of this Council shall be to make available all facts, data and medical opinions with respect to timely and adequate rendition of medical care to the American people and to keep informed the constituent state medical associations and component county medical societies of all proposed changes affecting medical care in the nation and also the activities of the Council. The present Bureau of Legal Medicine and Legislation shall be made a part of this Council, and the Board of Trustees shall provide adequate facilities for these activities.''

Regretable is the fact that the duties of the Council as outlined make no reference for assistance to be available in Washington for members of Congress on questions of health and medical care. It will also be interesting to watch for the information that will be transmitted to the State Association between now and the reconvening of Congress in September.

The Board of Trustees in a supplemental report to the House of Delegates made an exhaustive report on the principle involved with reference to Group Hospitalization and the practice of medicine, particularly as they pertained to the inclusion in the Hospital Plans of services in the fields of radiology, pathology and anesthesiology. This supplemental report should be read in full by every member of the profession and may be found in entirety on page 524 and 526 of the American Medical Journal, June 19, 1943.

The House of Delegates in adopting the complete report of the Reference Committee on Legislation and Public Relation, took a clear stand on a current topic, this being the present plan of the Federal Childrens Bureau of giving assistance to wives and children of Service Men. The Committee report supported a resolution introduced by the Oregon State Medical Association which proposed that the federal assistance be granted in aid to the families and in turn the families should select their own physicians and arrive at a mutually agreed fee.

Dr. A. S. Risser presented the resolutions adopted by the Oklahoma Association with reference to the establishment of a Washington Bureau of Information and the Amendment to the Constitution of the American Medical Association concerning the apportionment of membership on the Board of Trustees. The resolution on the Washington Bureau was referred to the Committee on Legislation and Public Policy along with similar resolutions from other State Associations but as previously stated, was not voted upon. The Amendment to the Constitution proposed by the Oklahoma Delegation must lie over one year before being acted upon.

Distinguished Service Award To Dr. Elliott P. Joslin

The Distinguished Service Award was voted to Dr. Elliott P. Joslin of Boston, Massachusetts. Dr. Joslin received the award on the basis of his contributions in the fields of diabetes research and education.

Dr. Herman L. Kretschmer President-Elect

Dr. Herman L. Kretschmer of Chicago whose resignation as Treasurer of the American Medical Association was accepted the first day of the Session, was duly elected President-Elect. Dr. Kretschmer had served for ten years as Treasurer and, as stated by Dr. Olin West, Secretary, upon announcing the resignation, his services have indeed been meritorious.

Other officers elected were Dr. John Amesse, Denver, Vice-President; Dr. Olin West, Chicago, Secretary; Dr. Josiah J. Moore, Chicago, Treasurer; Dr. Harrison H. Shoulders, Nashville, Speaker of the House; and Dr. Roy W. Fouts, Omaha, Vice-Speaker.

The two vacancies on the Board of Trustees were filled by the re-election of Dr. William F. Braasch, Rochester, and Dr. Ernest E. Irons, Chicago, to succeed themselves for five-year terms.

Nominations For Standing Committees

Dr. James E. Paullin, Atlanta, Georgia, who was installed as President, nominated for membership to Standing Committee, Dr. John H. O'Shea, Spokane, Washington to the Judicial Council for a term of five years and Dr. Edward L. Bortz, Philadelphia, to the Council on Scientific Assembly for a like term. Both Dr. O'Shea and Dr. Bortz were in turn elected by the House of Delegates. They succeed themselves on the two Councils.

The Board of Trustees likewise nominated Dr. Russell L. Hadden, Cleveland, Ohio, to serve another term on the Council on Medical Education and Hospitals and the nomination was approved by the House of Delegates.

Session To San Francisco in 1946

The House of Delegates in one of its final actions accepted the invitation extended by the California delegates to hold the 1946 meeting in San Francisco. This action by the House gave another opportunity for California to be hosts since the meeting for this year had previously been scheduled for that city but was transferred to Chicago due to transportation facilities.

Oklahoma Physicians Attending Meeting

Oklahoma physicians attending the Session in addition to Dr. A. S. Risser and Dr. W. A. Howard, were Dr. James Stevenson, Tulsa, Dr. C. R. Rountree, Oklahoma City; Dr. James D. Osborn, Frederick and Dr. Tom Lowry, Oklahoma City.

DR. J. D. OSBORN ELECTED TO NATIONAL BOARD OF EXAMINERS

Dr. J. D. Osborn who has recently been appointed by Governor Robert Kerr to his third consecutive term as a member of the State Board of Medical Examiners has been further honored in this same field by election to the National Board of Medical Examiners.

Dr. Osborn's name was one of three submitted by the Federated Boards of Medical Examiners to the National Board.

This election is the first ever bestowed upon a member of the Oklahoma Board and is not only a compliment to Dr. Osborn personally, but to the State of Oklahoma as well.

The election is for a term of six years.

PRESIDENT STEVENSON ANNOUNCES COMMITTEE APPOINTMENTS FOR 1943

Dr. James Stevenson, newly installed President of the Association announces in this issue of the Journal, his committee appointments for the coming year.. The committee appointments this year do not include any physicians serving in the military forces with the exception of the Committee of Military Affairs, an addition to the Special Committees. This procedure obviously was necessitated by the fact that committee work must be now delegated to those remaining on the home front. The response to appointments was 100 per cent.

The Special Committee, Prepaid Medical and Surgical Service, has been enlarged from four members to nine members since the Committee has been charged with the responsibility of doing the preliminary organizational work on the Prepaid Medical and Surgical Plan as initiated by the House of Delegates at the last Annual Meeting.

Those members appointed to Special Committees will serve concurrently with the term of the President. Appointments to Standing Committees are for a three year period.

NEW PAY-AS-YOU-GO TAX PROCEDURE

The following brief analysis of the new Pay-As-You-Go Tax Law has been prepared by the Association's auditors, H. E. Cole Company, 214 Plaza Court, Oklahoma City. The analysis covers only the provisions as they apply to employees. It is suggested that individual physicians, as well as those with employees, consult, whenever possible, competent tax authorities.

Provisions Concerning Deductions For Employees

Beginning July 1, 1943, the new Pay-As-You-Go Tax Plan becomes effective and each employer is required to deduct and withhold a tax from the wage or salary of every employee. The tax, which is 20 per cent ,applies only to the amount by which the wage or salary exceeds the amount of the withholding exemption. The tax which will be withheld from the wage or salary earned after July 1 will also include the Victory Tax, which has heretofore been deducted.

If the 1942 Income Tax is less than 1943, 75 per cent of the 1942 tax is forgiven. The payments which were made on March 15 and June 15 will be applied against the 1943 tax, and the remaining 25 per cent of the 1942 tax must be paid in 1944 and 1945. If the 1942 Income Tax exceeds the 1943 tax, then its treatment will be exactly the reverse of the procedure mentioned. Under certain conditions all of the 1942 tax is forgiven. Complete information will be provided those who make inquiry.

If the income exceeds the minimum specified in the income tax law, it is necessary that a return be filed with the Treasury Department on or before September 15, 1943, giving an estimate of the income in which will be included all income in excess of that earned from the employer, together with allowable deductions, and in the event that the estimated tax thereon exceeds the total of the March 15 and June 15 payments and the amount which the employer will withhold during the year, it will be required that all persons pay such additional amount of estimated tax—one-half on September 15 and the other half on December 15 of this year. All persons will file a final income tax return on March 15, 1944, which will reflect the actual tax liability and the amount of the underpayment or overpayment during 1943.

The law provides that the employer may elect to deduct exactly 20 per cent of the taxable income or may elect to apply the wage bracket withholding tables at his discretion.

If a person is married and husband or wife is receiving wages subject to withholding taxes, they must decide how much of the withholding exemption each will claim. The amount of exemption which each claims for the purpose of withholding does not affect the manner in which each may divide the married person's exemption in their income tax return. They may divide that as they wish. The withholding exemption for any dependent may be taken only by the person who furnishes the chief support for such dependent.

SUMMARY

As a summary, the following statements are reprinted from Circular WT issued by the Bureau of Internal Revenue of the U. S. Treasury Department:

"1. **Beginning July 1, 1943, employers are required to deduct and withhold a tax upon the wages of their employees. This is a tax of 20 per cent of the excess of each wage payment over the WITHHOLDING EXEMPTION allowable under the schedule shown in Specific Instruction 6.**

"Instead of making an exact computation, employers may elect to withhold specified amounts shown in the tables designated A-1 to A-5 which approximate the 20 per cent.

"It is the joint responsibility of the employer and the employee to see that "Employee's Withholding Exemption Certificate" (Form W-4) is made out by the employee and filed with the employer sufficiently in advance of July 1st.

"2. **It will be the duty of employers who withheld more than $100 during the month to pay the amounts withheld to a depositary authorized by the Secretary of the Treasury.**

"These payments are to be made within ten days after the close of each calendar month.

"Employers may get from any bank the name and address of authorized depositaries.

"3. **Employers must make quarterly returns on Form W-1 to their collectors of internal revenue ,showing the aggregate amount of taxes withheld during the quarter.**

"Returns must be made on or before the last day of the month following the close of each quarter.

"Each return must be accompanied by the payment of the full amount of the tax. It will be the duty of employers who withheld more than $100 during the month to make the payment of the tax in the following form: (1) depositary receipts for the full amount of the tax withheld, or (2) depositary receipts for the first two months of the quarterly period, together with a direct remittance for the amount withheld during the last month of the quarterly period.

"4. **With the final return for the calander year, employers must send to the collector on Form W-3 a reconciliation of "Quarterly Returns" (Form W-1) with "Statements" to employees of taxes withheld (Form W-2).**

"5. **Employers must provide each employee annually with a "Statement of Income Tax Withheld on Wages."**

"This is Form W-2 and must be delivered to employees on or before January 31 of the next year. For employment terminating during a calendar year, see Specific Instruction 14.

"6. **Employers may obtain all forms mentioned above from the collector of internal revenue for their district.**

"7. **Employers will discontinue the 5 per cent Victory Tax withholding when the 20 per cent withholding begins.**"

It is good to rub and polish our brain against that of others.—Montaigne.

No thoroughly occupied man was ever yet very miserable.—Landor.

★ *FIGHTIN' TALK* ★

Lt. Col. James H. Hammonds, formerly of Tulsa, who graduated from the Oklahoma University School of Medicine in 1937, has been assigned to Boling Field, Washington, D. C., where he will be in charge of the high altitude tests for the Army Air Forces.

Lt. Col. Charles Rayburn, Executive Officer of the Station Hospital at Hunter Army Air Field, Savannah, Georgia, has gone to San Antonio to take the Flight Surgeon's course.

Captain C. M. Bloss, Okemah, finished first in the class at Carlisle Barracks, Pa., Medical Field Service School and is now stationed at Camp Livingston, La.

Major Dan Sewell, Oklahoma City, base surgeon of the Station Hospital Army Air Base Flying School, Pecos, Texas, has been promoted to Lt. Colonel.

Col. Dwight M. Young, Kingfisher is now surgeon of the Air Forces in Alaska.

Lt. Frank Joyce, formerly of Chickasha, was on furlough in Chicago June 7-8, taking the American Board of Internal Medicine. Lt. Joyce was Secretary of the Grady County Medical Society at the time he left for the service.

Captain George Borecky, Oklahoma City, formerly stationed at Barksdale Field, Louisiana, has been assigned to the Avon Park Bombing Range, Avon Park, Florida as Venereal Disease Control Officer. Captain Borecky was the first doctor to be commissioned by the Medical Recruiting Board in Oklahoma City, May, 1942.

Major H. K. Speed, Jr., is now flight surgeon at De Ritter Army Air Field, De Ritter, Louisiana. Major Speed is the son of Dr. H. K. Speed, Sayre.

Major Rex Greer, Will Rogers Field, Oklahoma City, is being transferred to the Woodward Army Air Field as base surgeon.

Lt. W. W. Mead, U.S.N.R., formerly stationed at Orange, Texas, reports his new address as, c/o F.P.O., New York City, N. Y.

Lt. James K. Gray, of Carlisle Barracks, Pa., reports that he is ver ybusy and finds things most interesting, however, he will be glad to return to the familiar scenes of Oklahoma and Texas. Lt. Gray was formerly director of Health District No. 1 composed of four counties, Adair, Delaware, Cherokee and Sequoyah. He was also Secretary of the Cherokee County Medical Society before reporting for service.

Dr. John R. Taylor, who, prior to entering active service, practiced in Kingfisher, has recently been promoted to a Captain and is presently in charge of the Department of Medicine, Will Rogers Field, Oklahoma City. Captain Taylor's youngest brother Lloyd W., who entered the service immediately upon graduation, is a Captain in the Medical Corps and has participated in overseas duty for approximately a year. The other two brothers are also in active service — one is a sergeant in the marines on overseas duty and the other a private in the tank corps. The Taylors originally hail from Hugo.

Word has been received from *Major W. W. (Buck) Sanger*, formerly with the Oklahoma City Clinic, that he is the proud 'papa' of W. W. Jr., born April 6. Major Sanger reports that he pulled through and is now doing fine.

Lieutenant Roy Baze is also numbered among the new fathers, his son having been born after he left for overseas duty approximately two months ago.

The following interesting letter was received from *Captain William C. Tisdal*, Clinton, who is now station-

ed at the Station Hospital, Roswell Internment Camp at Roswell, New Mexico:

"We have here German prisoners of war and of course, we hear some very interesting stories. These Germans have recently been captured in the African campaign and they are mostly all from Rommel's Army. They seem to be rather happy to be here rather than fighting on the other side.

"One of the most interesting stories is the fact that they were very much surprised to see the Statue of Liberty still standing as well as to see that New York had not been completely flattened out by bombs. On seeing so many flying fortresses in the air they came to the conclusion that the United States and Japan were at war here in the United States.

"They cannot understand why we had so many bombers here at home. They state that all of their bombers are on the front lines fighting.

"These prisoners are altogether different from the type of prisoners that were captured a year and a half ago. Some of these boys do not look to be over thirteen or fourteen years of age. As a whole, their physical condition is about the same as that of our limited-service men here.

"I have enjoyed the bone work such as long-standing cases of osteomyelitis. Several of these cases have been operated two or three times in Station Hospitals in Africa. Evidently, they are short on the sulfa drugs. I have had a good fortune to try the closed method and the use of sulfathiazole. So far I have not had a failure.

"Another interesting thing from the medical point of view is the fact that ninety per cent of these boys have four small pox vaccination scars. The only explanation I am able to find is that they use the scratch and intradermal methods.

"It seems that the intradermal method gives the reaction each time. Some of them have as many as six and seven scars.

"It may be interesting to you to know the attitude these prisoners have toward our bombers. I have been told so many different stories by civilians as to how our bombers stack up with those of other countries. One boy I talked to who was in the anti-aircraft stated that our bombers were very strong and were very hard to shoot down.

"When asked how these bombers compared with the English bombers, he stated that our American bombers were much better. He was speaking more of the flying fortresses. He also said our bomber was superior to the German's. His choice of all planes seemed to be the flying fortresses and the P-38.

"This is a two-hundred bed Station Hospital which is well equipped and I am doing all types of surgical work. We have regular Tuesday afternoon staff meetings in which we give papers and present cases. On the whole, we are not losing sight of medicine at all.

"Colonel Murray Gibbons of Oklahoma City is Commanding Officer of this Camp, and Major Lorenzo D. Massey from Arkansas, is our Commanding Officer here in the Station Hospital. So you see, we have a very congenial group to work under.

"Thanking you again for the nice letter and hoping that these will continue in the future, I remain

Sincerely yours,
s/ William C. Tisdal
Captain, M.C."

Recently the Executive Office began assembling the photographs of the past presidents of the Association. In response to the request for pictures, the following letter was received from Col. David A. Myers, M.C., who was president in 1910-11, while a resident of Lawton.

No doubt many members of the Association will not only remember Dr. Myers but will be pleased to know he is still in the harness and going strong.

MEDICAL SECTION
Service Command Unit 1927
Station Dispensary
Office of the Commanding Officer
Presidio of San Francisco, California
June 7, 1943.

R. H. Graham, Executive Secretary,
The Oklahoma State Medical Association,
210 Plaza Court.
Oklahoma City, Oklahoma.
My dear Mr. Graham:

Your letter of June 1st is at hand. It is with pleasure that I respond to your request to forward a picture of myself for inclusion with the rest of the past presidents of the Oklahoma State Medical Association. It is impossible to provide a picture taken at the time I was President of the Association, therefore, I am forwarding one recently taken. There is also inclosed a second picture which I wish you would deliver to my old friend, Doctor Moorman.

It has been many years since I have been back to Oklahoma, but I still retain many pleasant memories of the old pioneer days, and of those up to the beginning of World War I.

I retired for statutory age (64) in June, 1940, and was recalled to active duty within a period of three months, and have been on continuous duty ever since. My entire service for twenty-five years was with the Air Corps as Flight Surgeon during which time I served as Chief Flight Surgeon for the United States Army Air Corps in Washington, D. C., for a period of four years. It pleased me very much to know that the Oklahoma Medical boys responded in such a wonderful manner to the Procurement and Assignment Service. This statement is made with considerable satisfaction as I had charge of Procurement and Assignment and Medical Personnel for the nine Western States for a period of two years, and I can assure you that there were many evasive answers received when physicians were desired for duty.

At the present time I am serving as Surgeon for the Post of Presidio, San Francisco, and Mrs. Myers and I are living in the city. Provided the war is ever over, we expect to adopt this as our future home. Please extend to any of the old timers who may remember me my best wishes, and with sincere thanks for remembering that I was once President of the Association, I remain

Sincerely yours,
DAVID A. MYERS
Colonel, Medical Corps
Surgeon.

Captain W. W. Rucks, Jr., and *Captain Everett Neff,* both of Oklahoma City, are on furlough and arrived home the last of June. Captain Rucks and Captain Neff are with the Evacuation Unit that was activated from the University School of Medicine approximately a year ago.

Captain William K. Ishmael, formerly associated with the McBride Clinic and Bone and Joint Hospital of Oklahoma City, now of Harding Field, Baton Rouge, Louisiana, reports:

"The Journal is being received. Enjoyed 'Fightin' Talk.' I have been fortunate in that I have been doing hospital work since in the army. Have had a very interesting service here. Virus infections outnumber all others in the contagious ward. There has been considerable amount of malarial fever. Rheumatic disease and G. I. disturbances make up the bulk of the metabolic diseases."

(Editor's Note: We wish to express our thanks and appreciation to the following for their most interesting and prompt contributions to our column "Fightin' Talk": Major E. Rankin Denny, Captain Floyd T. Bartheld, Colonel R. N.. Holcombe, Major Hervey A. Foerster, Major W. W. Sanger, Captain William K. Ishmael, Captain L. S. Morgan, Lt. Roy L. Smith and Captain William C. Tisdal).

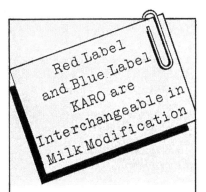

Red Label and Blue Label KARO are Interchangeable in Milk Modification

Both in chemical composition and in caloric value these two types of KARO are practically identical. There is only a difference in flavor.

Either is equally effective in milk modification. Your patients may safely use either type, if the other is temporarily unavailable at their grocers'.

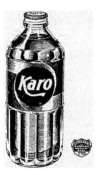

How much KARO for Infant Formulas?

The amount of KARO prescribed is 6 to 8% of the total quantity of milk used in the formula— one ounce of KARO in the newborn's formula is gradually increased to two ounces at six months.

CORN PRODUCTS REFINING CO.
17 Battery Place • New York, N. Y.

WOMAN'S AUXILIARY NEWS

A REPORT AND BRIEF HISTORY OF THE DOCTORS' AIDE CORPS

This plan of work was adopted by the Woman's Auxiliary to the Southern Medical Association at the annual convention held in Richmond, Virginia, November 10-12, 1942, and is recommended to State and County Auxiliaries represented in the Southern Medical Association. The Doctors' Aide Corps has been approved by the Advisory Committee of the Fulton County Medical Society, Atlanta, Georgia, and by the Advisory Committee of the Southern Medical Association. It is Atlanta's newest defense organization, the first of its kind in America, originating among the members of the Woman's Auxiliary of the Fulton County Medical Society, and was adopted as a special wartime service.

The organization of the Doctor's Aide Corps was the result of an earnest desire on the part of the president and the members of the Auxiliary to make a definite contribution to the war effort. The program is an ambitious one, the primary purpose being to release as many doctors and nurses as possible for vital war work. In normal times the doctor gives much of his time and effort to public health education. In wartime, when demands upon him are so greatly multiplied, some group must come to his aid in this important field. For this purpose, it was proposed that members of the Woman's Auxiliary who are willing to undergo training for this purpose, shall serve and be known as "Doctor's Aides."

Lecture Periods and Subjects Covered

1. Greetings and Purpose of Doctors' Aide Corps.
   a. Public Health Services.
      1. State Department of Health.
      2. County Health Department and its Services.
      3. Atlanta Health Department. Its Functions and Facilities.
2. Civic Housekeeping.
   a. Water Department and its Relation to Health.
   b. Sanitation as it Affects Health.
   c. Diseases—Insects and Rodents.
   d. Discussion on Milk Supply Problems.
3. Physical Fitness Program.
   a. Physical Disabilities Causing Army Rejections.
   b. Standard Requirements for School Cafeterias.
   c. Nutrition and National Defense.
   d. Physical Fitness of Adults Through Daily Exercise.
   e. Exercise and Supervised Play for the School Child.
4. Introduction of Departmental Chairmen.
   a. Information and Speakers' Bureau.
   b. Health Film Committee.
   c. Cooperative Service with Red Cross and other Volunteer Agencies.
   d. Blood Type Registry.

The instruction course consisted of 14 two-hour lectures on general health subjects and discussions of health problems, given over a two-weeks period by members of the local Medical Society, doctors in public health work and by experts in special fields. There was also two weeks' training in special activities necessary to the program in full. Special training classes were organized in public speaking for radio and organization work, in printing and filing and refresher courses for technicians and graduate nurses.. At the close of the Instruction Course, replies to questionnaires determined the volunteers for each type of work to be followed.

Induction Pledge

Because I believe that in the ideals and aims of the medical profession lie man's hope for future physical well-being, and because I wish to help in this service to humanity and my country, I, as a member of the Doctors' Aide Corps, pledge to you, the Doctors, my loyal and constant service. I will endeavor at all times to be faithful to the fulfillment of my pledged responsibilities; ethical in my every contact with the public; diligent in the acquiring of those skills and abilities which lead to larger spheres of usefulness; and unselfishly dedicated to the up-building of all those forces which promote universal health, safety, longevity and happiness.

Rules Governing Membership

1. The candidate must be a member in good standing of the Woman's Auxiliary to the County Medical Society, or wife of a physician, member of the American Medical Association, in service.
2. The candidate must subscribe to Hygeia Magazine.
3. The candidate must complete the four basic lecture periods as outlined for the Corps and approved by the Advisory Committee of the County Medical Society.
4. The candidate must take special training to equip herself for membership in the service groups.

Awards

1. The candidate will become a Doctors' Aide after she has taken the Pledge of Induction.
2. The Aide will receive and will be privileged to wear on the left sleeve of her uniform the insignia of the Corps.
3. The Aide, after each 100 hours of service, will be awarded a service stripe.

The Four Services of Doctors' Aide Corps

1. Information and Speakers' Bureau.
   a. Speakers on health subjects for radio and lay organizations.
   b. Speakers on Blood Type Registry.
   c. Filing and lending Bureau for the purpose of lending papers and books on health subjects, posters, charts and pamphlets.
   d. Health Education Centers at Academy of Medicine for the purpose of covering subjects of nutrition, tuberculosis, control of cancer and venereal diseases.
2. Health Films.
   a. Reviewing and showing health films.
   b. Showing films for the National Board of War Information.
   c. Showing films for the Office of Civilian Defense.
3. Cooperative Services with Other Volunteer Agencies.
   a. American Red Cross.
   b. Office of Civilian Defense.
   c. American Woman's Volunteer Service.
   d. Organization of classes in first aid, nutrition, home nursing and nurses' aides.
4. The Blood Type Registry.
   a. Receptionists.
   b. File Clerks.
   c. Typists.
   d. Technicians.
   e. Graduate Nurses.
5. (Service to be added).

A fifth service has been adopted by the Doctors' Aide Corps, which is now under consideration by the Advisory Committee. Many doctors are losing their office help on short notice as the secretary, technician and nurse is accepting work in munitions or bomber plants. Office routine need not be interrupted because of such absences. The doctor has only to call headquarters of the Academy of Medicine and a Doctors'

Aide will report to his office. This is a volunteer and temporary service arranged at the request of the doctors. A training class for this group will teach proper use of the telephone, duties of a receptionist, history taking, sterilization of instruments and draping a patient for examination.

Uniforms

The street uniform of the Doctors' Aide Corps consists of a two-piece coat suit of navy blue gabardine, with brass buttons, plain white blouse or slip over sweater with round neck, black shoes, beige hose, blue felt hat and a top coat of the same material as the suit. Insignia is worn on the left sleeve. In order that the Doctors' Aides will earn, through study and service, the right to wear the uniform and insignia of the Doctors' Aide Corps, permission to use the Medical caduceus as part of the insignia was granted by the local and Southern Medical organizations.

STUDENT NURSES NEEDED IMMEDIATELY

The Office of Civilian Defense in Washington, D. C. has issued an urgent appeal for 65,000 Student Nurses, needed immediately. Unless the nurse-power of the Nation is reinforced by the enrollment of 65,000 students in schools of nursing during 1943, America faces a real threat to civilian health. Nurses are absolutely vital in keeping civilians and soldiers alike healthy to carry on the war. A student nurse helps release a graduate nurse to serve in military or essential civilian positions.

The Health Committees of State Defense Councils should use the following procedure in order to help in securing these nurses:

1. Contact State Nursing Councils to work out specific steps and procedures for conducting the campaign throughout the State.
2. Stimulate Defense Councils to take part in this campaign through their local Health Committees and local Nursing Councils.

3. Emphasize to local Defense Councils the need for getting in touch with the local Nursing Councils for War Service or members of the nursing profession in the communities and working with and through them.
4. Secure from the State Nursing Council facts and figures on the shortage of and need for nurses.
5. Assist with publicity for nursing schools if they are on the accredited list (consult State Nursing Council for War Service).

The following organizations are taking an active part in the campaign by raising funds for scholarships; Federation of Women's Clubs, American Legion Auxiliary, Rotary, Kiwanis, Lions Club, Women of the Moose, American Hospital Association, American Association of University Women, Business and Professional Women, United Daughters of the Confederacy and others.

Our part in this campaign is definite. Every doctor should participate to the fullest extent in the program to secure Student Nurses. He has the ability to point out the history of nursing to the student and also the great service that can be rendered. It is imperative that every physician help in establishing the motto for the program—"Save His Life and Find Your Own—Become a Nurse."

Further information may be obtained from the National Nursing Council for War Service, 1790 Broadway, New York City or by contacting the Office of the Oklahoma State Board of Nurses Examiners, 531 Commerce Exchange Building, Oklahoma City, Oklahoma.

". . . books are the most important tools of our craft when assembled in mass in our great medical libraries: . . . books no less may be to the individual doctor his greatest source of relaxation, his greatest solace in times of trouble, when near to his hand on his own shelves."—Dr. Harvey Cushing.

The principal part of everything is the beginning.—Maxim.

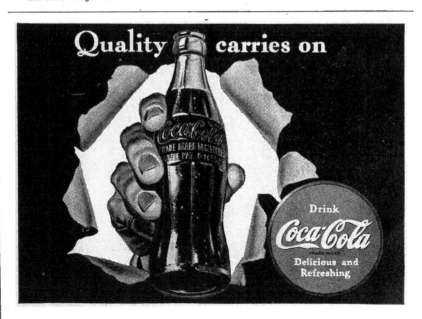

25 YEARS AGO

(Editor's Note: We feel that the column "25 Years Ago" will be of interest to our readers. Each month we will publish news items, editorials and personal news taken from the Journal of twenty-five years ago).

The following article, taken from the Journal of the Oklahoma State Medical Association published in 1918, shows that the Medical Corps of World War No. 1 very closely resembles the present day organization with the exceptions of the size and the speeding up of mobilization.

JOURNAL, 1918.

Present Condition of the Medical Reserve

Notwithstanding considerable misinformation to the contrary the Medical Reserve Corps of the Army is in splendid condition from the numerical standpoint. Late reports indicate that we now have more than 19,500 (*Editor's Note: As against approximately 45,000 today*) men engaged in the service and that figure does not include those in the Regular Army.

The men throughout the country are rapidly becoming familiar with military forms and usages and the especially difficult paper work so necessary in the handling of an immense work. Promotions are coming to many of the men and there is general satisfaction as a rule among them. The "Gasoline Board"—the title is unofficial of course, is busy in the camps and cantonments and when a man gets lazy or neglectful of his duties, he is soon sent home to ruminate again over the pleasures of civil life, where the 5:30 reville and "Taps" disturb him not. The special work given many of the officers is especially fine. They are sent to various medical centers for special training in that branch they feel most qualified to handle and as one officer very aptly puts it: "We get splendid postgraduate work with all the expenses paid." There is a growing idea, not confined to the physician, that the rank and corresponding pay of Medical Department should be raised. We have none, excepting the Surgeon General holding the rank of Brigadier General, yet there are scores of Brigadiers in other branches of the service, who have nothing like the responsibility placed on men of lower rank in the Medical Department.

A few men have not yet accepted the commissions sent them from the Surgeon General's office after completion of their examination, but as a rule this is due to altered circumstances of the applicant and not to a disposition to evade duty.

It is apparent that war time conditions in Tulsa were as serious on the housing problem twenty-five years ago as they are today. The following article shows an interesting comparison of the hotels and their rates with those of the present day.

JOURNAL, 1918

The Tulsa Meeting

This meeting will be held May 14, 15 and 16. Physicians contemplating attendance are warned now to make reservations for the meeting at a very early date. Ten days or two weeks notice will not do at all, as is the case with most conventions, but the reservation must be made far in advance. Tulsa is the most crowded city in the United States, all hotels and rooming houses, as well as apartments, are crowded to the utmost at all times and the local physicians are suggesting this warning at an early date in order that attendants may provide for themselves in time or otherwise be left without any accommodations.

Following is a list of the better hotels, but in addition to that there are others, which are good, not here listed; Alexander hotel, $1.00 and up; Tulsa Hotel, $2.00 up; Ketchum hotel, $2.00 up; Brady hotel, $1.00 up; Cordova hotel, $1.00 up; Detroit hotel, $1.00 up; Drexal, $1.00 up; Boswell, $1.00 up; Lee, $1.00 up; Lahoma, $1.00 up; Majestic, $1.00 up; Marquette, $2.00 up; Oxford, $1.00 up; Oklahoma, $1.50 up.

These are among the best in town. The Tulsa, Alexander, Ketchum, Marquette, Oklahoma and Brady. (*Note: The Mayo had not been built at this time*).

Personal News—JOURNAL, 1918

Dr. J. M. Bonham, Hobart, has been appointed a Captain in the Medical Reserve Corps.

Major R. M. Howard, M.R.C., paid his Oklahoma City friends a flying visit in December.

Dr. A. K. West, Oklahoma City, had his Ford Sedan appropriated by a thief while making a call.

Lieut. W. W. Rucks, M.R.C., formerly of Guthrie is recovering from an operation performed at Ft. Sam Houston.

Dr. Phil F. Herod, Lieutenant M.R.C., El Reno, has arrived safely in France.

Dr. W. P. Fite, Captain M.C.N.G., Muskogee, stationed at Camp Bowie, and Miss Maurine Mitchell of Fort Worth were married at Fort Worth June 1.

News From The State Health Department

During the recent flood when some 18 counties in the eastern part of the State were affected by high water, the State Health Department worked with other agencies in bringing relief to those who had lost their homes, crops and live stock. Full time departments which operated in seven of the affected counties immediately went into action and organized to meet the emergency of the disaster. One of the first steps in helping to prevent any kind of epidemic was the issuance of a bulletin, under the direction of the Engineering Department, again warning the people against the use of water which might have become contaminated either by surface water draining into the wells or by sub-surface contamination, and also giving simple directions for treating and purifying the domestic water supply.

Tours of inspection were conducted over the devastated area in order to obtain a clear picture of the immediate needs. Representatives of the State Health Department, together with those of the Red Cross, devised plans for the most effective means of distributing aid both to the individuals affected and to the area as a whole.

The State Health Department had, in years previously, conducted a wide-spread immunization program in this area and when the emergency arose, additional clinics were organized for giving immunization against typhoid fever to those who had not been reached. In Sallisaw on June 12, 700 people reported for innoculations. To date, due to the thoroughness of full time and part time health departments, more than 40,000 people have been immunized against typhoid and it is felt that this is something of a record. So far, only one case has been reported from any of the affected counties. Neither has there been any outbreak of dysentery, enteritis, or malaria. The fact that there has been no epidemics following this great castastrophe is proof that the work done previously and in the face of an emergency have been most effective.

The local authorities were assisted in the relief work by the American Red Cross, County Medical Societies, Emergency Medical Service of the State War Council, part time county health officers, and the State Health Department.

The way to cheerfulness is to keep our bodies in exercise and our minds at ease.—Steele.

University of Oklahoma School of Medicine

Army Specialized Training Unit No. 3805 has been activated at the University of Oklahoma School of Medicine with 161 medical students participating. The Unit is commanded by Captain Lyman F. Barry, Inf., assisted by 2nd Lt. Alfred L. Muse, Inf., Executive Officer. A staff of four non-commissioned officers will assist in the administration and training. Those students making up this Unit are now in uniform and form a part of the Army of the United States. The School of Medicine is operating as heretofore since these men are only assigned here to study medicine. All of them are the students regularly accepted and enrolled by the School of Medicine.

It is expected that the Naval Specialized Training Unit will be activated on or about July 1st. At least 59 medical students will compose this group.

Dr. H. A. Shoemaker, Acting Dean, will represent the University of Oklahoma School of Medicine at the Conference of Representatives of Institutions Participating in the Army Specialized Training Program, to be held in Dallas, Texas, June 21 and 22.

Miss Kathlyn Krammes, Superintendent of Nurses, University and Crippled Children's Hospitals, is attending the Meeting of the National League of Nursing Education in Chicago.

Dr. Arthur A. Hellbaum, Associate Professor of Physiology, will return to the medical school July 1, 1943, following a Sabbatical Leave of Absence for study at the University of Chicago School of Medicine.

Dr. John Walter Barnard has been appointed Research Fellow in Anatomy for the period October 1 to December 1, 1943. On January 1, 1944, he will occupy the position of Assistant Professor of Anatomy. Dr. Barnard holds the degree of Ph. D. in Neuro-Anatomy from the University of Michigan. He is a member of Sigma Xi and the American Society of Anatomists.

Dr. Kenneth M. Richter, who has been serving as Research Fellow in Pathology since 1939, was appointed to the Position of Assistant Professor of Histology and Embryology on June 1, 1943.

Dr. Jack Louis Valin, M.D., University of Cincinnati, has been appointed Assistant Professor of Anaesthesiology effective July 1, 1943. Dr. Valin served as Resident in Anaesthesia in the University and Crippled Children's Hospitals during the past year.

Dr. Peter E. Russo, M.D., St. Louis University School of Medicine, former Resident in Radiology. University and Crippled Children's Hospitals, will assume the position of Assistant in Roentgenology on July 1, 1943.

Dr. Samuel A. Corson, Assistant Professor of Physiology, has resigned his position effective July 15, 1943.

Miss Roberta Huff, former Secretary to the Dean, is now a member of the SPARS and is stationed at New Orleans, Louisiana. Miss Huff left the medical school on April 3, 1943. Mrs. Beverly Howard has been appointed Secretary to the Acting Dean since the departure of Miss Huff. Mrs. Howard formerly served in the capacity of Secretary to the Admissions Committee of the medical school.

Mrs. Mildred T. Gossett has been appointed Executive Secretary of the University of Oklahoma School of Medicine. Mrs. Gossett served six years as Secretary to Maj. Gen. Rob't. U. Patterson, former Dean of the Medical School, and has also served as Secretary to the Medical Director of the University and Crippled Children's Hospitals.

Miss J. Marie Helgaard, Director, Dietary Department, The University Hospitals, has announced the following dietetic staff for July 1: Administration Dietitian, Mrs. Ethel Sykes Guilford; Teaching Dietitian, Vera I. Parman; First Assistant Dietitian, Martha F. Spradlin; and Ward Dietitians, Ellen M. McMurray, University Hospital, and Florine E. Craig, Crippled Children's Hospital.

Miss Eloise Argo, Administrative Dietitian, The University Hospitals, and Dr. Maurice Gephardt, University of Oklahoma School of Medicine, Class of '43, were married on May 16th at Stroud, Oklahoma. They are living in Chicago where Dr. Gephardt is serving an internship in the Research Hospital.

Student Dietitians who will complete their course in July are: Florine E. Craig, Ellen M. McMurray, J. Paul, and Leona Whipple. The graduation exercises took place on June 25th at The University Hospital.

The following students will enter the Hospitals for their ten-month dietetic training course: Ramah Louise Gaston, Montana State University; Eileen Elizabeth Hazel, Iowa State College; Jeanne House Hutchinson, Oklahoma A. & M. College; and Mattie Lou Robertson, Texas State College for Women.

Opal Howard and Aley Goldsmith, Ward Dietitians, The University Hospitals, resigned in June to accept positions at the Norton Memorial Infirmary, Louisville, Kentucky, and the Mid-West Air Depot, Oklahoma City, respectively.

Medical Preparedness

"MEDICAL REPLACEMENT TRAINING CENTER, Camp Barkeley, Texas—June 15, 1943.

(SPECIAL)—Beginning with the class which reports for training on July 9, the Medical Administrative Corps Officer Candidate School is lengthening its training period to 16 weeks, four more than the present program calls for.

In announcing this scheduled compliance with a War Department directive, Col. George E. Armstrong, Medical Corps, assistant commandant of the Camp Barkeley school, also said, "The new schedules will involve no addition of material. it will merely mean a more intensive coverage of the work now included." All the departments of the school, training, administration, logistics, tactics, sanitation and chemical warfare will be allotted some of the extra hours added to the curriculum.

The present field work will be especially affected by the new schedules which have been submitted to the War Department training division. A continuous problem in medical support will be carried out during a six-day bivouac for each Camp Barkeley class, and the candidates will practice choosing aid station sites, evacuation routes, and other medical installations in simulated battle conditions.

The strength of the school, 12 companies, will remain the same, with the result that the output will be slightly decreased. It is felt that this decrease will be more than compensated by the extra time spent upon the subjects in the new curriculum.

Over 6,000 men have already received commissions as second lieutenants in the Medical Administrative Corps from the Camp Barkeley school, which is commanded by Brig. Gen. Roy O. Heflebower. Another large group was commissioned by the school at Carlisle Barracks, Pa., before the MAC school there closed this spring. The non-medical functions of this youngest of the army Medical Department's officer corps have proved invaluable in many fields."

MEDICAL ABSTRACTS

"A MEDICAL ECONOMIC SITUATION REGARDING LABORATORY DIAGNOSIS." Thomas L. Ramsey, M.D., C.P., Toledo, Ohio. Reprinted from The Toledo Academy of Medicine Bulletin. Vol. XIX No. 9, November, 1935.

The American Society of Clinical Pathologists has made a study of the economic situation regarding laboratory diagnosis and in this published report by one of its members, some of the pertinent facts are disclosed, as follows:

The Clinical Pathologist would be very glad to confine his work entirely to his specialty, and would become more proficient and better equipped in it, were is possible for him to do so. As matters now stand, some are forced to practice in other fields besides their own, and to the detriment of both.

There is a progressive decrease in laboratory work that is being sent to private clinical laboratories. Reasons for this are:

(a) Expense of medical care. Many physicians do not use the laboratory services of private laboratories in their endeavor to keep down the cost of medical care to the patient.

(b) The use of free laboratory services extended by the state and other municipal laboratories. The amount of this work has yearly been increasing. The expense of maintaining the state and city laboratories has proportionally increased. This is a vitally important wedge toward generalized state medicine.

(c) The increased use of hospital laboratories for outside laboratory work. This is partially to increase the profit of the hospital laboratory and partially to offer a laboratory service to the staff for their private outside cases at a reduced laboratory fee. The hospital laboratories are therefore entering into cut rate competition with the private clinical laboratories.

(d) Hospitalization of patients for diagnosis only, thereby procuring the maximum amount of laboratory work at a minimum laboratory fee.

(e) Laboratory work is being performed by assistants in doctors' offices and clinics. Some of these are not trained technicians and often have no supervision as to the efficiency of their work; even technicians of experience need some supervision in most of the more complicated laboratory procedures.

The results are as follows:

(a) Many men of experience in laboratory procedure have already left this field and taken up more profitable lines of medical endeavor.

(b) Very few, if any, young physicians are taking up laboratory work as a specialty.

(c) Hospitals throughout the country need competent, trained men in this line of work.

(d) The salaries paid are not enticing.

(e) It takes years of study to become a competent tissue diagnostician.

(f) The future of clinical pathology is at stake.

We must maintain a high standard of efficiency in laboratory procedures and it is time for the medical profession to realize these facts.

This has been discussed repeatedly with health officers and directors of the state and municipal laboratories and the same answer is always received; that as long as the physicians demand these activities it seems necessary for them to continue.

I have endeavored in this short paper to call to your attention certain practices that seem unfair to the Clinical Laboratory Physician.

Certainly hospital laboratories should not enter into cut rate competition with private laboratories and the medical staff taking laboratory work for their office patients to the hospitals should in all fairness see that the pathologist of the hospital receives the fee fo rthis type of work.

Hospitals do not, and probably cannot, pay adequate salaries to the pathologists. This should be at least partially adjusted by allowing the pathologist the fee for the outside work.

It is also clearly unfair for physicians to send work to Municipal and State laboratories from patients able to pay for these services, this not only pertains to Wassermann tests but for all other diagnostic reactions and test regardless of the communicability of the disease. Until a diagnosis is made it is not the business of the health officer to enter into the picture. After the diagnosis is made it is a different matter, for then the protection of the health of the community is concerned.

On patients unable to pay, I have called to your attention the fact that any of the laboratory physicians would gladly perform the charity work on deserving cases for physicians who send to them their pay cases.

It is entirely up to the medical profession and not the fault of the Municipal Laboratories. Medical men must awaken to the fact that this free service has been carried entirely too far and that even now other fields of medical endeavor are being invaded.

These points have been reapidly discussed. This paper is only additional plea to the profession who may have foregotten that private laboratories do exist and that that clinical laboratory diagnosis is really an important specialty that must be given support and consideration. —H. J., M. D.

"COLOR IN PROTECTIVE NIGHT LIGHT." C. E. Ferree and Rand G. Ferree. The British Journal of Ophthalmology, Vol. 27, pp. 173-183, April, 1943.

In the selection of a color for a protective night light, the eye factors as well as power to penetrate the external atmosphere should be taken into consideration; namely, the comparative sensitivity of the eye to colored lights at very low intensities, visual acuity at low intensity, and the adaptation factors. Because of the eye factors, deep red has recently been recommended as superior to the fomrely widely-accepted, dark-blue light. The problem is to select that color or composition of light that will be of the greatest use in the discrimination of detail in nearby objects and will have the least visibility at a distance.

The authors constructed a special illuminator, which is also made in the form of a lamp with the opening turned downwards or obliquely downwards. With its control of intensity by means of the rotatable shutter, the light can be varied in continuous change from full to extinction, thus making it possible, by using it as a night light, do obtain a complete blackout or as near a complete black-out as may be desired.

The authors point out the infeasibility of the ordinary blackout devices as an all-the-year round means of securing a complete blackout. In southern cities the thought of obtaining a complete blackout of a fully lighted room on a hot summer night for any considerable length of time by means of curtaining or similar devices alone, is untenable and intolerable. The kind of blackout that is used in England may not be suitable in summer in the southern portion of the United States. Climatic conditions make the blackout device of the authors very desirable.—M. D. H., M. D.

"TECHNIQUE FOR OBTAINING BACTERIOLOGICAL SPECIMENS FROM THE ANTRUM. Moffett, A. J. The Journal of Laryngology and Otology. Vol. 57, page 537, December, 1942.

Bacteriological examination of the contents of the antrum is not easy. There are two risks: (a) contamination by casual organisms in the nose or nasal vestibule, and (b) destruction of the organisms by the methods employed to extract them from the antrum. The author describes a new method by which the first difficulty is greatly reduced, and the second difficulty is completely overcome. In his technique, the culture medium is brought to the organism, instead of, as is usual, the organism to the medium.

The culture specimen should be taken from an antrum not previously punctured. All instruments used are sterilized, particular care being taken that they are free from alcohol or other chemical antiseptic. The patient is seated with the head upright and the inferior meatus is then cocainized in the manner usual for puncture of the antrum by that route. When cocainization is complete, the vestibule of the nose is cleansed with alcohol and all excess dried off with sterile cotton wool. The antrum is then punctured with a trocar and cannula, contact with the nasal mucous membrane being kept to a minimum. The trocar is withdrawn and the cannula pushed inwards until it touches the posterior wall of the antrum. It is then withdrawn one-fourth of an inch.

The head of the patient is next bent backwards and to the side under investigation and the cannula connected with a 10 cc. syringe containing 8-10 cc. of sterile broth. Having made certain that the cannula is in the antrum, 5 cc. of broth are gently run in. If possible, this is then sucked back into the syringe. If no broth returns, the remainder in the syringe is run in and the piston again withdrawn. With 10 cc. a specimen is nearly always obtained. This has been directly inoculated by the organisms in the antrum.

The syringe is then disconnected from the cannula, the contents put into a sterile tube for incubation and the antrum washed out with saline. If there is any reason to suspect that the end of the cannula is not free in the antrum cavity, this method should not be employed.—M.D.H., M.D.

"ELECTRO-SURGICAL EXCISION OF PTERYGIUM." Daniel B. Kirby, M.D. American Journal of Ophthalmology, Series 3, Vol. 26, No. 3, page 301.

The author starts his article with the definition of pterygium. He states, as everyone knows, that excision has not always proved entirely satisfactory due to the tendency of the vessels growing forward and the growth recurring. He has a technique which he has been using for five years and to him has proven satisfactory.

Local anesthesia is used. A cataract knife is used to cut the head from the cornea. The knife is slipped under the growth at the limbus, the growth thus being sliced cleanly off the cornea. He does not use a curette to remove any of the remaining fibres from the cornea but slices them off with the same cataract knife. The head of the pterygium is next picked up with toothed forceps and lifted from its bed on the sclera. If necessary, Stevens scissors are used. Linear sections of conjunctiva above and below adherent conjunctiva are made toward the semilunar fold and joined beyond adherent conjunctiva. The mass of the body is now freed by scissors. The base is severed with high frequency needles, coagulating the base. The vessels for a width of 1 mm. are destroyed. He closes the denuded area of the sclera by dissecting the conjunctiva above and below until there is sufficient free conjuntiva to allow suturing without tension, using interrupted sutures.—M.D.H., M.D.

KEY TO ABSTRACTORS

E. D. M. ....Earl D. McBride, M.D.
M. D. H. ....Marvin D. Henley, M.D
H. J. ....Hugh Jeter, M.D.

THE COYNE CAMPBELL SANITARIUM, INC.

For Psychiatric Disorders

Established 1939

Admissions

1939	157
1940	379
1941	639
1942	699

A GROWING INSTITUTION

Coyne H. Campbell, M.D., F.A.C.P.

Chas. E. Leonard, B.S., M.D.
Muriel Hyroop, M.D.
Chas. A. Smith, M.D.

Aleen Bates, R.N.
Jessie Bent, Occ. Ther.
Margaret Drake, Bus. Mgr.

Fourth Street at Walnut Avenue, Oklahoma City, Oklahoma

BOOK REVIEWS

"The chief glory of every people arises from its authors."—Dr. Samuel Johnson.

THE YEAR BOOK OF PEDIATRICS—1942. Isaac Abt, D. Sc., M. D. Illustrated. 500 pages. Price $3.00. Year Book Publishers, Chicago, 1943.

This volume contains abstracts of many articles of pediatric interest which appeared in the current literature, both foreign and domestic, for the year named. Also included are a number of interesting and unusual case reports. The abstracts are so grouped that the references on one subject can easily be reviewed.

Regardless of the number of journals available, this book is of great value for brief, but rather comprehensive review of recent developments in pediatrics.—Bertha Levy, M. D.

UROLOGY IN GENERAL PRACTICE. Nelse F. Ockerblad, M.D., Hjalmar E. Carlson, M.D. The Year Book Publishers. Price $4.00.

"One must remember that while it may be desirable and in the best interests of the patient for a specialist to be in attendance, it is nevertheless true that in most instances just a plain doctor sees the patient first. This manual was written to meet the need presented by that situation — to help the general physician do better those things that are within the limits beyond which the best interests of his patients require that he obtain the help of a specialist."

These words distinctly state the intent of the authors —two earnest students of science who have spent many years studying diseases of the urinary system. The book contains twenty-one chapters of intensely practical information with all the frills, philosophy, and speculation left out. One especially well-written chapter discusses infections of the kidney and lays down plain and simple rules for the management of each type of case up to the point of instrumental interference. Another chapter summarizes the important facts about nephritis and coordinates this subject into the picture of kidney infections in general. For this effort the writers are to be especially commended. The usual urological diseases such as urinary lithiasis, prostatism, infections of the bladder and urethra, and gonorrhea are well covered. The female urethra is discussed in a very practical manner, and the signs and symptoms of ureteral diseases are thoroughly described. Carcinoma of the prostate is discussed from the modern viewpoint of hormonal therapy, and such up-to-the-minute subjects as sterility and impotence and use of sulfonamides in urology are handled in a way that any intelligent practitioner may know just how far it is safe for him to go before calling in a specialist for counsel and advice.

This is good book. It is the most up-to-date book on urology now in print. It has no padding. Last but not least, its authors are safe and sensible men who stick to known facts and standard practices.—Basil A. Hayes, M.D.

THE CONDENSED CHEMICAL DICTIONARY. Third Edition. Completely revised and enlarged under supervision of Thomas C. Gregory, Editor. Reinhold Publishing Corporation. 1942. 756 pages. Price $12.00.

The Third Edition of this valuable book has come from the press at a time when medicine and industry are greatly in need of all available knowledge in the field of Chemistry.

The following descriptive paragraphs from the preface to The Third Edition will convey to the reader a fair impression of the importance of this work.

"The general arrangement, which was so successful in the Second Edition, remains the same. But, over 6,000 new items have been added. They comprise chemicals, drugs, pharmaceuticals, chemical specialties, metals, minerals, clay products, petroleum products, essential oils, perfumery chemicals, leather processing agents, mothproofing agents, insecticides, fungicides, hydrogenated products, flavoring materials, and many others. Also, many new encyclopedic-type definitions have been added. And finally, the old items carried over from the previous edition have been brought up-to-date.

"A very valuable feature is the large number of chemical specialties, sold under trade or brand names, included in the present edition. So many chemicals and chemical products are now being sold under trade or brand names that this trend must be recognized. The publisher ventures to say that nowhere between two covers of a book will this vast fund of information be found in as great detail and variety. That these products are very important is evidenced by the marketing of so many in these last few years by the leading chemical manufacturers."

This volume is worthy of a place in every doctor's library.—Lewis J. Moorman, M.D.

CHEMOTHERAPY OF GONOCOCCIC INFECTIONS. Russell D. Herrold, M.D. C. V. Mosby Co., St. Louis, 1943. Pp. 132. Price $3.00.

Dr. Herrold's opinions as one of the pioneers in sulfonamide therapy are certainly worthy of careful consideration, both by the general practitioner and the urologist. His chapter on differential diagnosis is very complete. He does not pay much attention to secondary sources of infection such as teeth, tonsils, etc., and in my experience these are probably very important in the etiology of the non-specific infections.

The author's ideas of sulfathiazole dosage are sound, i.e., four grams daily for five days, then if there is a favorable clinical response and no discharge, with both urines clear, he observes for one week. He then proceeds with the usual criteria of cure. If one course of a sulfonamide fails, he gives a second one, but believes that any more than two courses will not cure the patient and can only result in damage to his general condition. He believes that sulfadiazine is just as efficient as sulfathiazole and is less toxic.

In the failures in chemotherapy, the author recommends the usual local treatment and used fever therapy in a large number of cases. It is my opinion that fever therapy entails too great a risk for most patients unless some complication such as gonorrheal arthritis is present. After all, the mortality of gonorrhea is practically zero and that statement cannot be made of fever therapy. Those of us who have read and taken to heart the theories of Pelovze in regard to the treatment of gonorrhea, will be slow to advocate this merely because sulfonamides have failed.

The author does not particularly stress one of the most important factors in the treatment, namely drainage. The small urinary meatus should be looked for and if present, should be enlarged. This will be curative in a fairly large number of cases. In others we should employ the well known drugs that have proven their efficacy through the years, or cystourethroscopy in a search for urethral sinuses or fistulae.

Dr. Herrold's book is well worth the time required to read it and offers a great deal in the way of a rational approach to the sulfonamide therapy of gonorrhea.—Robert H. Akin, M.D.

Athlete's Foot

A mixture of carbolic acid and camphor has been found effective in the treatment of "athlete's foot," Edward Francis, M.D., Washington, D. C., states in J.A.M.A.

OFFICERS OF COUNTY SOCIETIES, 1943

★

COUNTY	PRESIDENT	SECRETARY	MEETING TIME
Alfalfa	H. E. Huston, Cherokee	L. T. Lancaster, Cherokee	Last Tues. each Second Month
Atoka-Coal	J. B. Clark, Coalgate	J. S. Fulton, Atoka	
Beckham	H. K. Speed, Sayre	E. S. Kilpatrick, Elk City	Second Tuesday
Blaine	Virginia Olson Curtin, Watonga	W. F. Griffin, Watonga	
Bryan	J. T. Colwick, Durant	W. K. Haynie, Durant	Second Tuesday
Caddo	F. L. Patterson, Carnegie	C. B. Sullivan, Carnegie	
Canadian	P. F. Herod, El Reno	A. L. Johnson, El Reno	Subject to call
Carter	Walter Hardy, Ardmore	H. A. Higgins, Ardmore	
Cherokee	P. H. Medearis, Tahlequah	James K. Gray, Tahlequah	First Tuesday
Choctaw	C. H. Hale, Boswell	E. A. Johnson, Hugo	
Cleveland	J. A. Rieger, Norman	Curtis Berry, Norman	Thursday nights
Comanche	George S. Barber, Lawton	W. F. Lewis, Lawton	
Cotton	A. B. Holstead, Temple	Mollie F. Seism, Walters	Third Friday
Craig	F. M. Adams, Vinita	J. M. McMillan, Vinita	
Creek	H. R. Haas. Sapulpa	C. G. Oakes, Sapulpa	
Custer	F. R. Vieregg, Clinton	C. J. Alexander, Clinton	Third Thursday
Garfield	Paul B. Champlin, Enid	John R. Walker, Enid	Fourth Thursday
Garvin	T. F. Gross, Lindsay	John R. Callaway, Pauls Valley	Wednesday before Third Thursday
Grady	Walter J. Baze, Chickasha	Roy E. Emanuel, Chickasha	Third Thursday
Grant	I. V. Hardy, Medford	E. E. Lawson, Medford	
Greer	G. P. Cherry, Mangum	J. B. Hollis, Mangum	
Harmon	W. G. Husband, Hollis	L. E. Hollis, Hollis	First Wednesday
Haskell	William Carson, Keota	N. K. Williams, McCurtain	
Hughes	Wm. L. Taylor, Holdenville	Imogene Mayfield, Holdenville	First Friday
Jackson	E. S. Crow, Olustee	E. W. Mabry, Altus	Last Monday
Jefferson	F. M. Edwards, Ringling	L. L. Wade, Ryan	Second Monday
Kay	Philip C. Risser, Blackwell	J. Holland Howe, Ponca City	Third Thursday
Kingfisher	C. M. Hodgson, Kingfisher	H. Violet Sturgeon, Hennessey	
Kiowa	B. H. Watkins, Hobart	J. William Finch, Hobart	
LeFlore	Neeson Rolle, Poteau	Rush L. Wright, Poteau	
Lincoln	H. B. Jenkins, Tryon	Carl H. Bailey, Stroud	First Wednesday
Logan	William C. Miller, Guthrie	J. L. LeHew, Jr., Guthrie	Last Tuesday
Marshall	O. A. Cook, Madill	Philip G. Joseph, Madill	
Mayes	Ralph V. Smith, Pryor	Paul B. Cameron, Pryor	
McClain	B. W. Slover, Blanchard	R. L. Royster, Purcell	
McCurtain	A. W. Clarkson, Valliant	N. L. Barker, Broken Bow	Fourth Tuesday
McIntosh	James L. Wood, Eufaula	William A. Tolleson, Eufaula	First Thursday
Murray	P. V. Annadown, Sulphur	F. E. Sadler, Sulphur	Second Tuesday
Muskogee-Sequoyah-Wagoner	H. A. Scott, Muskogee	D. Evelyn Miller, Muskogee	First Monday
Noble	C. H. Cooke, Perry	J. W. Francis, Perry	
Okfuskee	L. J. Spickard, Okemah	M. L. Whitney, Okemah	Second Monday
Oklahoma	Walker Morledge, Oklahoma City	E. R. Musick, Oklahoma City	Fourth Tuesday
Okmulgee	A. R. Holmes, Henryetta	J. C. Matheney, Okmulgee	Second Monday
Osage	C. R. Weirich, Pawhuska	George K. Hemphill, Pawhuska	Second Monday
Ottawa	W. B. Sanger, Picher	Matt A. Connell, Picher	Third Thursday
Pawnee	E. T. Robinson, Cleveland	R. L. Browning, Pawnee	
Payne	L. A. Mitchell, Stillwater	C. W. Moore, Stillwater	Third Thursday
Pittsburg	John F. Park, McAlester	William H. Kaeiser, McAlester	Third Friday
Pontotoc	O. H. Miller, Ada	R. H. Mayes, Ada	First Wednesday
Pottawatomie	A. C. McFarling, Shawnee	Clinton Gallaher, Shawnee	First and Third Saturday
Pushmataha	John S. Lawson, Clayton	B. M. Huckabay, Antlers	
Rogers	C. W. Beson, Claremore	C. L. Caldwell, Chelsea	First Monday
Seminole	Max Van Sandt, Wewoka	Mack I. Shanholtz, Wewoka	Third Wednesday
Stephens	W. K. Walker, Marlow	Wallis S. Ivy, Duncan	
Texas	R. G. Obermiller, Texhoma	Morris Smith, Guymon	
Tillman	R. D. Robinson, Frederick	O. G. Bacon, Frederick	
Tulsa	James C. Peden, Tulsa	E. O. Johnson, Tulsa	Second and Fourth Monday
Washington-Nowata	J. G. Smith, Bartlesville	J. V. Athey, Bartlesville	Second Wednesday
Washita	A. S. Neal, Cordell	James F. McMurry, Sentinel	
Woods	C. A. Traverse, Alva	O. E. Templin, Alva	Last Tuesday Odd Months
Woodward	C. E. Williams, Woodward	C. W. Tedrowe, Woodward	Second Thursday

THE JOURNAL
OF THE
OKLAHOMA STATE MEDICAL ASSOCIATION

VOLUME XXXVI	OKLAHOMA CITY, OKLAHOMA, AUGUST, 1943	NUMBER 8

Epidemic Poliomyelitis

LUKE W. HUNT, M.D.

Post Graduate Committee
Oklahoma State Medical Association

This report is based on a study of 368 patients with epidemic poliomyelitis, the majority of whom were treated at the John Mc-Cormic Institute for Infectious Diseases. The report includes the initial symptoms, the important physical findings, the frequency and extent of the paralysis, some epidemiologic phases of the disease, the clinical pathologic character, the differential diagnosis and a brief discussion of the treatment.

INITIAL SYMPTOMS

From the symptoms observed in these patients, it is apparent that poliomyelitis has two distinct phases, one of a general, systemic nature and another of specialized expression in form of a disorder of the central nervous system. It is further apparent that the systemic phase may be represented by a variety of symptom complexes. From the point of early symptoms, the disease assumed three main characters. One type , often incorrectly called the dromedary type, showed clearly two distinct periods of illness with an intervening period of well-being. In the second type, often called the straggling type, this period of well-being was not present, but there was a sustained indisposition of varying intensity. In the third type, that with sudden onset, all the symptoms from the start pointed to involvement of meningeal and nervous tissue. The first stage of the dromedary type and the continued course of the straggling group were characterized by a febrile condition, with symptoms falling into three main categories: disturbances of the gastrointestinal tract; inflammation of the tonsils and the upper respiratory passage and; malaise without localization of symptoms. Then, pursuant to a remission of all symptoms in the dromedary group or a varying duration of symptoms in the straggling group, one of two things occurred; the patient either promptly got well or showed sudden evidence of meningeal involvement which might be followed by recovery or paralysis.

In the first two groups, acute poliomyelitis, in the early hours of its clinical course, resembled in general any acute infectious disease of childhood. Fever was almost invariably present; in 307 of the 368 cases there was a perceptible rise in the temperature at the onset. In the majority of the cases the temperature varied from 100 to 103 F. and in a few it was higher. The fever was usually of short duration, and the temperature fell rapidly in from 24 to 48 hours. The initial fever lasted in the majority of cases from four to seven days. Occasionally, however, the curves were irregular or prolonged, and this variation often was caused by some complication.

Aside from the fever, the picture in the individual case was colored by the particular set of organs chiefly involved. Disturbances of the gastrointestinal tract were frequent. Nausea and vomiting occurred in 205 of the patients, abdominal pain in 30 and anorexia in 16. Eighteen of the patients had diarrhea, while 32 gave a history of constipation at the onset. There was an almost universial occurrence of constipation in the second phase, i.e., the phase involving the central nervous system.

Symptoms indicating involvement of the upper respiratory tract occurred in 71 of the 368 patients; 44 of these patients had an acute cold, 20 had sore throat, and 11 gave a history of having had chills.

An eruption of the skin, usually in the form of a simple erythema, occurred in 10 of the patients. There was an entire absence of herpetic and purpuric eruptions.

Incontinence of urine occurred in 4 of the patients and retention in 10.

During the systemic phase of the disease there was an almost entire absence of any sign that the central nervous system was involved. However, when invasion of the meninges ocurred, which marked the second phase of the disease, such symptoms appeared; headache in 137 patients, pains in the back or extremities in 103, rigidity of the neck or back muscles in 20 and great tenderness of the muscles and hyperesthesia of the skin in several. Anesthesia of the paralysed member was not recorded. The behavior of the reflexes was irregular, varying from absence to the most extreme exaggeration. In most instances loss of a deep reflex was the forerunner of paralysis. In a few cases it was observed that the knee jerk and the ankle jerk disappeared for a day or two and then returned, and the patient recovered without paralysis. In two cases of polio-encephalitis there was a positive Babinski sign, indicating that the inflammatory process had extended to the pyramidal tract. There was no general tendency toward impairment of the special senses. Convulsions occurred in 8 patients, 5 of whom were under two years of age. Delirium was recorded in three instances and coma in one. The frequency of the various symptoms is recorded in Table 1.

In the initial stage of the disease the patient presented a striking appearance, especially about the eyes. The sclera and cornea had the quality of glazed procelain; the circumorbital tissue not infrequently showed puffiness. In addition, there was often a peculiar expression in the eyes—a look of mingled apprehension and resentfulness. When this appearance was present, often the patient did not wait to be touched before objecting but cried out when any one approached. More often the eyes were partly or wholly closed, and there was a peculiar tired, wilted expression. Not infrequently the chin was pointed upward a little, indicating a small degree of retraction. From this drowsy or almost sleeping condition the patient could be roused by the gentlest touch or manipulation of an extremity. When meningeal involvement was extensive the patient might assume a typical meningitic posture.

Table 1. Frequency of Symptoms in Cases of Poliomyelitis.

	Cases
Fever	307
Vomiting	182
Headache	137
Pains in the back or extremities	103
Malaise	63
Irritability	44
Cold	44
Constipation	32
Abdominal pain	30
Nausea	23
Sore throat	20
Diarrhea	18
Anorexia	16
Stiff Neck	13
Chill	11
Muscular twitchings	11
Restlessness	9
Dizziness	9
Convulsions	8
Delirium	3
Coma	1
None	3

FREQUENCY AND EXTENT OF THE PARALYSIS

The records of the paralyses are not sufficiently detailed to indicate the relative frequency with which various muscles were paralyzed, but they give some indication of the frequency with which the various parts were affected and to some extent of the degree of paralysis. The extent of the paralysis is indicated as partial or total. Since most of the patients of this series were admitted to the hospital from three to nine days after the onset of symptoms, the paralysis had usually reached its greatest extent at the time of admission. Table 2 indicates the frequency with which the various parts were affected and Table 3 the day of onset of the paralysis.

It is apparent that in this series partial paralysis was much more common than total paralysis, the former occurring in 246, or 67.9 per cent, of the 362 cases. The predominance of partial over total paralysis is of importance, especially in the matter of treatment, because in such muscles there remains some initiative, and with it, the power of developing more muscular volume and new associations through the repeated passages of impulses from the brain to the muscles. All degrees of paralysis were observed in these cases, from definite transient paralysis of an arm or leg, lasting for a few days, to complete flaccid paralysis of one or more extremity, which persisted for a time and then either disappeared or remained as a permanent disability. The progressive ascending form of the disease occurred in 13 of the fatal cases and the bulbar form in 18.

Table 2. Extent of Paralysis in Cases of Poliomyelitis.

	Cases in Which Paralysis Occurred	
	Partial	Complete
All extremities	29	22
Both arms	8	2
Left arm	8	2
Right arm	9	2
Left arm and both legs	18	11
Left arm and right leg	2	
Left arm and left leg	5	1
Right arm and both legs	12	4
Right arm and right leg	9	5
Right arm and left leg	3	1
Both legs	45	41
Left leg	26	9
Right leg	33	9
Both arms and respiratory or abdominal parts	6	7
Both legs and respiratory or abdominal parts	6	2
Respiratory	3	
Facial	10	
Pharyngeal	15	

*In 6 of the 368 cases there was no evidence of paralysis.

Table 3. Day Paralysis Appeared After Onset of Symptoms in Cases of Poliomyelitis.

Day	Cases	Day	Cases
1	44	6	10
2	117	7	13
3	100	8	8
4	47	9	1
5	21	10	1
Total			362

Paralysis of the leg muscles was more frequent than paralysis of the arm muscles. It was also observed that the muscles of the upper extremity were more severely affected nearest the trunk and less severely lower down whereas in the leg, the largest proportion of the severe paralysis was in the lower part of the leg and foot. When the muscle of the upper extremity were involved with out paralysis occurring in the other parts of the body, the paralysis was more severe than paralysis in this region when the muscles of the legs were involved; i|e., paralysis of the arm that was strictly regional was more severe than paralysis of the arm which existed in combination with more general paralysis.

Forty-five patients showed extension of their paralysis after admission to the hospital. This occurred as a rule on the first or second day after admission and was usually observed in the fatal cases.

Since the patients in this series were observed for only from three to five weeks, no accurate record of the ultimate results can be given. However, 295 of the 368 patients showed some improvement during their stay in the hospital; 7 showed no paralysis when discharged; 6, paralysis did not develop; 29 showed no improvement, and 33 died.

INCIDENCE OF THE DISEASE WITH RESPECT TO AGE

Of the 368 cases, 212, or 57 per cent, occurred in children four years of age and under. There were 19 cases in infants under one year. The youngest patient was five weeks of age; the oldest, 39. Of the deaths, 11 (a mortality of 5.2 per cent) occurred in patients under four; 10 (9.9 per cent) occurred in patients from 5 to 9, and 10 (21 per cent) in patients from 10 to 19. One death occurred in a child under one year of age, this child being the youngest patient who died of respiratory paralysis. The death rate for the series was 8.9 per cent. The incidence with respect to age groups is shown in Table 4.

Table 4. Incidence of Poliomyelitis and of Deaths from the Disease in Various Age Groups.

Age Group	Cases of Disease	Deaths	Percentage of Deaths
0- 4	212	11	5.2
5- 9	101	10	9.9
10-19	47	10	21.0
20-29	6	1	16.0
30-39	2	1	50.0

The distribution of cases by months is shown in Table 5. Two hundred thirty-four cases, or 63 per cent, occurred during August and September. An analysis of the death rate by months showed that the greatest relative percentage of deaths occurred early in the season, 12 per cent in July and 15.4 per cent in August. Toward the close of the season the death rate decreased sharply, 6.2 per cent in September and 2.8 per cent in October—which seems to indicate that the disease is most severe in the early cases of an epidemic.

As to race and color, the only data available showed 357 cases in white persons and 11 in Negroes. While Negroes seemed to be less affected than white persons, the difference in number stricken per capita of the blacks and whites is not great enough for one to base an absolute statement as to relative immunity on it.

The type of child which seemed most susceptible to the disease was the large, well developed, lump type. The adolescents and adults in whom the disease was more severe were not similar to the younger patients but appeared more delicate.

CLINICAL PATHOLOGY

The changes in the spinal fluid varied with the stage of the disease and with the reaction of the meninges. In the systemic phase the fluid was usually increased in amount, the cell count was from 30 to 100 per cubic millimeter, and the aggregate of cells was made up entirely of polymorphonuclear leukocytes or of both leukocytes and lymphocytes. The globulin was increased in some cases and not in others. In the stage of paralysis, and most of the patients were in this stage, the fluid was still increased in amount, the number of cells varied from 18 to 2,000 or more, and from 80 to 90 per cent of cells were lymphocytes.

Table 5. Distribution of Cases of Poliomyelitis and of Deaths from the Disease by Months.

	Cases	Deaths Number	Percentage
January	1	0	0.0
April	1	1	100.0
June	5	0	0.0
July	50	6	12.0
August	111	16	15.4
September	113	7	6.2
October	71	2	2.8
November	8	0	0.0
December	8	1	12.5
Total	368	33	

In general, the highest cell counts were shown by the patients showing symptoms of severe meningeal irritation; 201 of the 326 patients whose spinal fluid was examined showed cell counts of from 0 to 100, 80 had cell counts of from 100 to 200, 45 had cell counts of 200 and above, and 6 had cell counts of 1,000 and above. In the fatal cases the cell counts of the spinal fluid were invariably high, the average count being 200 and above. The pressure of the spinal fluid was increased in 279 patients and was normal in 47. Globulin was present in 280 cases. In most cases the globulin was distinctly increased. The blood showed a constant change. In the majority of cases the total white cell counts showed a marked and constant elevation to from 12,000 to 18,000. There was a definite increase in polymorphonuclears of from 10 per cent to 15 per cent, and in most instances, a diminution in lymphocytes of from 15 to 20 per cent. The cell counts of the spinal fluids are given in Table 6.

PATHOLOGIC ANATOMY

Autopsies were made in 13 of the 33 fatal cases. The dura and pia-arachnoid were usually injected and often edematous. The surface of the brain appeared wet, soft and deep gray-pink. In cases in which the cerebral symptoms were pronounced the convolutions showed swelling and flattening, with hyperemia of the gray matter and here and there small hemorrhages. The cord exhibited congestion and a moist condition of the dura and pia-arachnoid, and on cross section the gray matter usually bulged and was dark gray-pink. Microscopically, the earliest change was an infiltration of small round cells around the blood vessels of the leptomeninges, most marked in the lumbar and cervical regions. The infiltration extended into the fissures of the cord and followed the blood vessels. In the cord itself the small blood vessels were distended; there were hemorrhages in the gray matter and a marked perivascular infiltration, chiefly of lymphocytes. In the severe cases the lesions were not confined to the anterior gray matter of the cord but extended to the posterior horns and even to the white matter. Besides the interstitial reaction with its cellular infiltration, hemorrhages and edema, there were always definite changes in the ganglion cells. These showed all signs of degeneration from the slightest swelling and loss of Nissl bodies to complete destruction. With the degeneration process well under way polymorphonuclear and other cells replaced the degenerated cells, forming the so-called neuronophages. Other changes observed in these autopsies were hyperplasia of lympatic glands and of the spleen and general cloudy swelling of the organs. Bronchopneumonia was found in 2 cases.

THE DIFFERENTIAL DIAGNOSIS OF POLIOMYELITIS

The diagnosis of poliomyelitis is usually based on the findings of a short, initial febrile stage of the disease, with headache and vomiting, general tenderness, rigidity of the neck and back, sweating, somnolence, a rather characteristic spinal fluid picture, and the frequent development of a paralysis which is customarily flaccid in type and irregular in distribution, most frequently involving the leg muscles, but in some instances, involving the arm and trunk muscles or those supplied by the cranial nerves. Differentiation from other disease depends on the stage or type of the disease. Someone has said that the best way to diagnose the disease is to think of it and do a spinal puncture.

The preparalytic stage of poliomyelitis with evidences of involvement of the central nervous system must be carefully differentiated from a number of other conditions. The meningeal signs may be sufficiently marked to simulate epidemic or tuberculous meningitis. The former is characterized by more severe headache, neck rigidity and the Kernig sign. The spinal fluid is cloudy, shows a greater number of polymorphonuclears, and the meningococcus is found in the spinal fluid. The fever is higher, herpes is common; there are no flaccid paralyses. Tuberculous meningitis is much slower in its onset; there is often a history of tuberculosis and very often a focus somewhere in the body. Convulsions are not uncommon and there are no isolated flaccid paralysis of the limbs. Examination of the spinal fluid should reveal the presence of tubercle bacilli and a decreased sugar content. Epidemic encephalitis occasionally begins with spinal symptoms but the presence of ocular palsies, pupillary changes, radicular pains, abnormal involuntary movements, paresis of the bladder, and the subsequent course should distinguish the two diseases. The spinal fluid findings are essentially identical. The preparalytic stage of poliomyelitis may also be confused with various general systemic infections such as typhoid fever which, in unusual cases, shows a rapid onset of extreme prostration, high fever, delirium, tremor and headache. The hyperesthesia and fever of acute rhematic fever, and the general body aches of influenza, may cause mistakes in diagnosis.

After paralysis has developed, poliomyelitis must be differentiated from the various other diseases in which paralysis occurs. The paralysis due to post-diphtheritic neuritis is apt to appear at a later period in the course of an acute infection than does infantile paralysis and the pre-existence of diphtheria usually has been recognized. It must be remembered, however, that in poliomyelitis there may be a very considerable degree of faucial inflammation in the preparalytic stage. Diphtheritic paralyses are usually more gradual in development than are those of poliomyelitis, but may be equally rapid. In diphtheria the nerve injury almost invariably affects the soft palate and the muscles of accomodation, and a toxic myocarditis is usually present. The spinal fluid is essentially normal.

Other forms of neuritis, such as those due to alcohol, arsenic and lead, are, as a rule, symmetrical. They develop slowly and lack an initial febrile stage. The causative factors are generally easily determined and the incidence is almost invariably in adults. Acute scurvy and rickets with temporary paralysis merely deserve mention.

Hysteria in young women may also produce deceptive manifestations but the reflexes are normal. Finally, injury of nerves of bones and of muscles must all be considered in the differential diagnosis.

TREATMENT

PROPHYLAXIS

There are as yet no specific remedies in general use for the prevention of the disease. Some investigators have recommended the subcutaneous injection of 10 to 20 cc of pooled convalescent serum in children apparently menaced by the disease. However, the incidence of susceptibility is low (probably not more than 2 per cent of children under 13 years of age are susceptible), and convalescent serum is usually very limited in availability.

In time of an epidemic, there are certain general measures which may well be adopted by all members of a community. First, segregation of individuals should be instituted as far as is practicable. Unnecesary gatherings should be omitted and persons should avoid going into congested places. In the second place, personal contacts such as kissing and handshaking should be omitted. Third, pets should not be handled and steps should be taken for protection against insects of all kinds. Fourth, individuals should keep physically fit, with special attention to proper food, elimination, rest, fresh air and sunshine. Sixth, cleanliness of person and of environment should constantly be enforced. Seventh, swimming in epidemic areas where the water may possibly be contaminated with local sewage should not be permitted. Eighth, a ban should be put on all tonsillectomies in children during the epidemic period.

The use of nasal antiseptics is not advised because immune bodies are normally present in the nasal mucosa and these natural, protective mechanisms may be counteracted by antiseptics.

SPECIFIC TREATMENT

Opinions differ greatly as to the efficacy of various methods recommended for the specific treatment of poliomyelitis. Convalescent serum has been used extensively in the treatment of the disease. Its use is based on the following evidence: 1. an attack of poliomyelitis in most instances confers a lasting immunity to the disease; 2. the blood serum of convalscent persons and of monkeys who have had the experimental disease neutralizes the virus; 3. convalescent serum, when tested in experiments, exerts a protective action against the virus.

Convalescent serum was administered to 52 patients in this series. It was not used in a greater number because most of the patients were seen after paralysis had developed and it is generally agreed that if convalescent serum is to be of value it must be given in the preparalytic stage or very soon after paralysis has developed. In most instances marked improvement was observed after its use. In the majority of patients receiving serum, 20 to 30 cc were given intraspinally and 60 cc intravenously. A few received a second administration. It is difficult to evaluate the effects of convalescent serum. If a patient is given the serum before the onset of paralysis and it does not develop, it does not necessarily indicate that the serum prevented the paralysis. The disease may stop spontaneously after the systemic phase of the disease or after involvement of the central nervous system and no paralysis occur.

Pooled convalescent serum, that is, serum obtained from several donors who have had a frank attack of the disease, is more potent. Neutralizing substances have been found as early as the sixth day of the disease and it is reasonable to presume that blood may be safely drawn after all symptoms of the acute stage, notably fever and muscle tenderness, have subsided.

THE HOT PACK TREATMENT

It is generally agreed that the hot pack method is an advance in the treatment of poliomyelitis. It is based on the symptoms observed in the acute phase of the disease; pain and spasm of the affected muscles, mental alienation of the opposing muscles and muscle incoordination. If these symptoms are not relieved, deformities and functional disability may occur. The muscles in spasm may shorten and have a tense, taut appearance so that the entire outline of the muscle belly and tendon is prominent. Fibrillary twitching may be present and hyperirritability is pronounced particularly if an attempt is made

to move the muscle from the shortened position which it assumes because of spasm. Knowledge of muscle action aids greatly in observing which muscles are in spasm.

Mental alienation is the inability of a muscle to perform voluntary movement even though the nerve paths to the muscle are intact. At first, the muscle is unable to contract because it has been pulled from its normal resting length by its opponent which is in spasm, and because an attempt to contract produces pain. If mental alienation is not overcome, paralysis, atrophy and disuse may ocur. Destruction of the anterior horn cells may occur and if this is extensive, the muscles may not be alienated but paralyzed. True paralysis cannot be distinguished from mental alienation until spasm of the opponent has been completely relieved and muscle re-education given a trial.

Incoordination is the substitution of muscle action by a muscle or group of muscles for the muscle which normally performs such a movement. It may be due to pain when an attempt is made to lengthen a muscle which is in a shortened position because of spasm due to the inability of the opposing muscle to perform the desired movement. Examples of muscle incoordination are: substitution of the toe extensors for the tibialis anticus when an attempt is made to perform dorsiflexions of the foot in the presence of spasm of the calf muscles, contraction of the adductors when the gluteus is unable to perform abduction of the thigh.

The hot pack method of treatment is based on the above mentioned concept of the disease. The treatment is begun immediately after the diagnosis has been made. It is directed first to overcoming pain and muscle spasm. This is accomplished by the application of the hot packs. Muscle re-education is then instituted to develop mental awareness of alienated muscles and re-establish muscle coordination. Early relief of spasm makes it possible to begin muscle re-education much earlier than has been customary in previous methods of treatment.

Naturally, the entire course of treatment should be under the direction of the physician and carried out by nurses and physiotherapists who have had special training in the hot pack method.

A Plan for the Use of Blood Plasma in Rural Communities

A. RAY WILEY, M.D.

TULSA, OKLAHOMA

Medical practice is still making history. We are passing through an era that, in the future, may well be called the blood and plasma transfusion era. While blood transfusions are not new,[1] transfusions of all types have received a tremendous impetus during the present decade. The most advantageous types for the individual needs of the patient are, however, not too well understood. I refrain from being critical of my colleagues, but I do see both whole blood and plasma transfusions given indiscriminately, without thought or knowledge of the needs of a particular case or patient. A knowledge of both whole blood and blood plasma dosage for each patient is as important as the knowledge of the use of any other medicament.

Briefly stated, whole blood is given to provide functioning erythrocytes and to increase the coagulability of the recipient's blood. It also increases the blood volume, thus increasing the plasma volume and decreasing the capillary permeability, thereby preventing the escape of the blood protein. By this action, shock is resisted or overcome. However, these later attributes may be obtained by better and safer methods than the use of whole blood transfusions.[2] If the need is primarily for erythrocytes and/or to increase coagulation, I would list, acute hemorrhage, purpura and hemophilia as the only conditions in which the use of fresh, whole blood transfusions are justified.[3] The indiscriminate use of whole blood transfusions in any anemia, primary or secondary, where bleeding is not acute, is open to justifiable criticsm, and in my opinion, is to be deplored.

The function of the erythrocytes is primarily for carrying oxygen to the tissues. Even in acute hemorrhage, we know that there are tremendous reservoirs of erythrocytes in the spleen and the liver which are sufficient to meet most emergencies of the body. It is much better to use plasma quickly in an acute hemorrhage, than to wait for time-consuming, technical tests required to complete a whole blood transfusion.

Pooled plasma has come to the forefront in recent years as the agent par excellence in transfusions. This seems justified because of its safety and convenience. Since no typing or matching is required in giving pooled plasma, it can be given anywhere that any intravenous injection can be given. Even in acute hemorrhage, one or repeated plasma injections may be all that is necessary as it will tide the patient over a danger period until whole blood can be given, if whole blood is finally required.[5]

There is no hard and fast rule deciding between the use of plasma and whole blood. Clinical symptoms are always the surest guide posts. If an acute hemorrhage has occurred, blood pressure reading, pulse rate and quality and appearance of patient are valuable symptoms. The hemoglobin determination is of extreme importance as well as the red blood count. The hematocrit reading and protein determinations have been of little value in hemorrhages, while just the reverse is true in acute burns.[4] I have, rather arbitrarily, used a hemoglobin reading of 30 per cent as the dividing line between the use of plasma or whole blood. If, with other clinical symptoms given above, the reading is 30 per cent or less, whole blood is used and if the reading is above this point, my experience indicates that plasma will suffice. Some clinicians advocate using a higher percentage level[3] but the above rule has been useful with me.

Stored whole blood has been found useful if less than one week old. If used for functioning erythrocytes, the fresher it is, the better. If it is older than one week it is useless for the red cell function. Swelling of the cell and hemolysis begin within forty eight hours and gradually increases at a mounting rate. Various ingredients have been added to blood in attempts to prevent fractioning of the red cells. The indications are promising, particularly with the use of certain dextrose mixtures.[6] In the past, whole blood has been used for obtaining the natural end for acquired immune bodies. All these qualities are possessed by plasma of the whole blood. By using this plasma, the same effect is obtained and, at times, the plasma can be used to better advantage than the whole blood.

With improved techique in processing plasma, its availability should become widespread and the rural physician should have plasma at his disposal at all times. A modern biological laboratory and trained technicians are necessary for the production and this situation, up to the present time, has left the rural physician in an awkward position. Plasma, of course, may be purchased from commercial houses, but most physicians agree that this has been so expensive as to make it practically prohibitive. Plasma purchased from commercial houses is not returnable.

I want to suggest a plan whereby any member of this Association may have plasma available at all times and without undue expense. It is reasonable to assume that every member has some connection or acquaintance with a hospital that maintains a blood-plasma bank. It has been calculated that any hospital with an average daily census of fifty patients or more should have a blood bank. There are seventeen hospitals in Oklahoma in this group and every one has, or should have, some form of blood-plasma bank. The hospitals of the size given, that do not have a blood-plasma bank, should proceed to set one up immediately. The hospitals with banks and those obtaining them should co-operate with the rural physicians and, for a reasonable deposit, loan the physician a supply of plasma together with a sterile, ready-to-use intravenous set. I suggest that he be loaned two containers of 250 c.c. each (2 units). This set should be kept handy at all times, in refrigeration, when not carried to the patient. If the plasma is not used in three to four months, it should be returned to the hospital and exchanged for a fresher-supply of pooled plasma. It is assumed that the needs for plasma in the hospital will be greater than those of the individual physician in the outlying districts and that the hospital will soon use the returned plasma,

as it is considered useable for one year. This plan would avoid waste. In the event that the loaned plasma was used and a new supply requested, then the members of the family or friends of the patient should present themselves to the hospital as the donors to replace the blood. The ratio of one donor for each 125 c.c. of plasma used should be set. The hospital would then make the same charge as though the patient had been in the hospital. This charge varies but is usually $10.00 for any amount of plasma up to 500 c.c., if replaced by donors furnished by the patient. If only professional donors are available who make their own charge, the cost if from $25.00 to $30.00, however, since the war began, professional donors are not often available.

I believe the hospital will cooperate in such a plan and encourage it. Under recent planning by the State Health Department it is possible that smaller hospitals will be aided so that they, in turn, can help in the plan I have outlined. This may be accomplished by having the hospital produce its own plasma or through State help. In either case, the cost should not be prohibitive. This plan is not perfect, but it will answer most of the problems of the present time.

BIBLIOGRAPHY

1. Clinical Excerpts: Quoting from a Hebrew Manuscript, "Naam, prince of the army of Ben-Adad, King of Syria, when attacked with the leprosy applied to his physician, who, to effect a cure, removed the blood from his veins and replaced it with other blood."
2. Hardin, R. C.: Jour. Iowa St. Med. Ass'n. Vol. 31. April, 1941. Elman, Robert: Jour. A.M.A. Vol. 120, No. 15.
3. Wiener, A. S.: Medical Clin. No. Amer. Vol. 24, No. 3. pp 705. May, 1940.
4. Scudder, John: Shock. J. B. Lippincott Co. 1940.
5. Marsh, Frank B.: Military Surg. Vol. 90, No. 1. pp 76, January, 1942.
6. Kolmer, John A.: Am. Jour. Med. Science. Vol. 200. pp 311. September, 1940.

Lower Abdominal Pain in the Female*

LT. COMDR. CLYDE M. LONGSTRETH,
MC-V(S) USNR

NORMAN, OKLAHOMA

One of the most common complaints encountered in private and clinic practice in Gynecology is lower abdominal pain, bilateral, right or left, which may be associated with many other vague or specific complaints. You are all familiar with these, such as backache, vaginal discharge with or without itching, joint pains, headaches, anorexia, nausea, fatigue, nervousness, and frequently eye

*Read at the Annual Meeting of the Oklahoma State Medical Association, May 12 at Oklahoma City.

signs of blurring or poor vision. Secondary to these complaints is very frequently added the so-called "Vagatonia", syndrome of dizziness, palpitation, and shortness of breath or sighing respirations.

Judging from ten years private practice and clinic work in New York City, it can be said there is a sharp rise in complaints associated with lower abdominal pain immediately after the birth of the first child. Although these complaints must be looked for in the unmarried and virgin type, yet the preponderance of the cases occur subsequent to the birth of the first child. This group of symptoms following childbirth does not reflect upon the type of delivery or the ability of the accoucheur. It was also noted that while heavy housework as experienced by those women in the lower income brackets does aggravate the condition, yet the well-to-do and wealthy patient also presents the same problem. This train of symptoms, if not corrected by proper treatment, will and does become progressively worse with each succeeding pregnancy.

Let us review some of the causes of lower abdominal pain which may be due to normal ovulation, dysmenorrhea, spontaneous threatened abortion, urinary infections or ureteral strictures. These symptoms may be due to certain acute conditions such as specific infections (pelvic inflammatory disease). Also stressed in the literature are many non-specific pelvic infections such as the monilia group, or trichomonas associated with streptococci. Besides these, though not to be taken up in this paper, are the medical problems of gastro-intestinal etiology, so frequent in modern life. Often the patient may complain only of gastro-intestinal symptoms which are aggravated by fatigue and nervousness, but when these symptoms are thoroughly analyzed their origin may be found to be strictly pelvic.

Adnexitis acute, subacute and chronic will be considered. However, specific disease in the female patient must be definitely proven. Also there are cyclic physiological changes occurring monthly in the ovaries of the female patient. Cases have been noted many times in which the ovary is enlarged to the size of 5x6 cm. only to return to normal size after a few weeks observation. The possibility of endometriosis and pathological tumors must be borne in mind, while postural conditions may be ruled out by adequate orthopedic consulation.

The uterus per se is very seldom the cause of lower abdominal pain or backache. The preponderance of cases have shown that retrodisplacement of the uterus alone causes symptoms in not more than five per cent of the cases. Probably 30 per cent of uteri are congenitally displaced. Pain from the uterus itself probably occurs only in the infrequent cases of pan-metritis, uterine tumors such as endometritis and fibroids. The pain usually occurs during the menstrual periods.

Lastly, the most important etiological factor involved in backache and lower abdominal pain in the female is the cervix itself. The pathology involved in these cases is found to be variable from a mild cervical erosion, cervicitis, mild, severe or cystic, and endocervicitis, to old lacerated cervices unilateral or bilaterial, together with many secondary infections involved, bacterial, fungi, or protozoan. The type and severity of the cervical lesion will not so much determine the degree of backache as dictate the type of treatment to relieve the symptoms. A "cervical" backache may be low, mid or high, between the scapulae and even higher. This pain in the region of the scapula often simulates a gall bladder pain.

The lymph drainage from the infected cervix, whether it be mildly, moderately or severely infected, empties into the utero sacral ligaments and the broad ligaments on its way to the hypogastric iliac and periaortic nodes. After a patient has carried an infected cervix for some time, whether months or years, there is always noted, on examination, definite tenderness of the pelvic ligaments. The pain caused by pressure upon these ligaments can be demonstrated to the patient on bimanual examination by pressure with the examining finger up and against the utero sacral ligaments as well as the broad ligaments, the patient is then able to identify it as her particular type of backache and/or lower abdominal pain. In many cases it has been noted that her only complaint may be pain in the right lower abdominal quadrant, often simulating an acute appendix with definite tenderness and history of nausea.

Apparent adnexal tenderness may be occasioned by a loop of bowel which has extended down into the pelvis and been inadvertently pinched by the examining hands. After a short time, this bowel will probably float upward into the abdominal cavity and thus cease to cause this particular pain or discomfort. The explanation for this pain is probably on a basis of gas distension. Also,

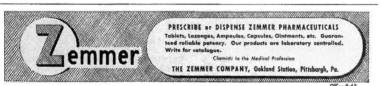

the normal sensitivity of the bowel to the examining finger must not be allowed to confuse the examiner. The examining fingers are pressed up against the ligaments rather than down against the rectum.

Although this condition of the cervix is noted most frequently in the childbearing age of 18 to 40 years, it may occur at very early age as well as be carried over into the later years of the patient's life. A small cervical erosion is not uncommonly found in girls of the early 'teen age and frequently gives lower abdominal pain localized in the right or left lower abdominal quadrant due to drainage from the cervix into the pelvic ligaments. The incidence of cervical erosion in girls under twenty years has been shown to be 10 to 20 per cent, that is, before any pregnancies have occurred. In the young matron, the moderately infected cervix very frequently causes menstrual disturbances, especially menorrhagia, and may be an important factor in sterility, relative or absolute. In the older patient, the cervical condition, having extended over a number of years as a cystic cervicitis, may often manifest itself in joint pains or aggravation of a joint condition already present.

The treatment of lower abdominal pain in the female can be properly carried out only after a complete and thorough examination is made and a definite diagnosis is established. In general, it can be stated that the best treatment and the best results will be obtained by conservative therapy. In the majority of specific pelvic inflammatory cases, it has been shown that with only bed rest the condition will be cured, and the tubes found to be patent after six months, as proven by insufflation. There should be no surgery to the tubes in acute inflammatory disease. We now use the sulfa drugs in the acute stages and short wave therapy in the chronic process of the disease. The great majority of good sized tubo-ovarian masses can be reduced to normal size by short wave therapy properly administered. The Elliott treatment has been found inferior to the short wave in these cases.

Before pelvic surgery is done, it is safer to apply to the vagina and therefore to the cervix, a powder mixture of two-thirds sulfanilimide and one-third sulfathiazole two or three times before the operation. This application will tend to eliminate the dangers from non-specific mixed infection. Douches may or may not be used as their value is questioned.

As to the treatment of apparent ovarian cysts, it cannot be too strongly urged that the operator usually wait and observe his patient for a period of time covering at least one and preferably several menstrual cycles. An enlarged ovary may be found later to be perfectly normal in size. This is due to the frequency of physiological rather than pathological ovarian enlargement. It is normal for the ovulating ovary to increase in size due to follicular or corpus luteum changes. It is also normal for the ovary, like the testicle, to be tender when squeezed.

If it becomes necessary to perform surgery for pelvic pathology it is urged that resection of the abnormal tissue alone be carried out and that the operator save the normal tissue. For following bilateral oophorectomy, as shown by blood studies, the onset of the climacteric starts within a few days, the symptoms starting within a few weeks. The surgical menopause gives us the most marked and incapacitating symptoms of menopause. It must be remembered that only a very small piece of ovarian tissue left in situ may give this woman normal hormone levels, perhaps a child, and prevent long years of semi-invalidism.

Likewise, unnecessary removal of the fallopian tubes not only deprives the patient of the chance for pregnancy but may cause severe embarrassment to the blood supply of the ovaries. Conservative treatment of the tubes should be exercised because tubal plastic operations reported in the literature have given less than seven per cent successful results, measured in terms of subsequent pregnancies.

The treatment of the most common cause of lower abdominal pain and backache in the female, namly lesions of the cervix, may be divided into three groups. First the treatment of erosion in the nulliparous cervix should be applied conservatively by use of the actual cautery. Some form of local anaesthesia may be used for this work. The cauterization need be done only lightly but thoroughly. One thorough cauterization often will suffice. It should not be done more often than once in one or two months and in general not more than one to three times. The treatment should be done a few days after the menstrual period is completed so that as much healing as possible will have taken place before the onset of the next period. Cauterization within a week of the expected period may induce increased or prolonged bleeding. The patient should be warned that 7 to 10 days after cauterization, vaginal bleeding may occur, from exposure of small blood vessels when the necrotic cauterized area sloughs away. After healing has taken place, probably in six to twelve weeks, the cervix must be checked for any possible stenosis. This can easily be done in the office.

Silver nitrate in various strengths has been used very considerably in the past for cervical lesions but I mention it here only to condemn it. In my personal experiences it has proven worthless. But more important, as mentioned by a staff member of the Memorial Hospital, New York City, at a conference, the silver nitrate is not strong enough in even 50 per cent strength to cauterize thoroughly the lesion and yet is strong enough to act as a chronic irritant to the cervical lesion and the cervix itself.

Second, the treatment preferred for cervicitis with associated moderate endocervicitis is conization with application of the cautery to any bleeding points. Before this operation is performed the patient should be protected from any pain by some premedication and a local paracervical infiltration anaesthesia of procain one or two per cent. This cervical repair is not carried out until at *least* three months following delivery and preferably six months post-partum. The operation using the endotherm biopy loop will remove only the inflamed tissue involved. This loop has been found to give the best results from the long wave diathermy machine. In cases of severe endocervicitis, a conization can be carried right down to the internal os. However this procedure requires caution because, in this area, bleeding may occur and is more apt to lead to stenosis later.

Third, in the severely lacerated cervix with associated inflammatory changes of the cervical lips, conization may be impractical for repair and the condition will probably require a unilateral or bilateral trachelorrhaphy in combination with the cautery or possibly some use of the conization principle.

With exception of the trachelorrhaphy all the above surgical procedures on the cervix can be safely carried out in the doctor's office with no pain to the patient. After a short rest the patient may return home and the next day may continue with light housework. She will, of necessity, be as quiet as possible during the first and second menstrual periods following the operation. These cases must all be watched and careful follow-up treatment be administered until the lesion is completely healed, usually two to three months. According to the literature, the average case required two and a half to six months to heal.

After the cervix is healed, careful check must be made to ascertain and cure any cervical stenosis or potential cervical stenosis. Stenosis of the cervix can cause severe lower abdominal pain and frequently cause considerable difficulty in gynecological diagnosis. The treatment, of course, is simple, namely, dilation.

After the cervical lesion has been cured, there is usually some residual tenderness remaining in the pelvic ligaments which also causes lower abdominal pain. This residual tenderness cannot be taken out by the operating knife but it can be cured by judicious use of the short wave therapy.

In conclusion it is again emphasized that the most common complaint met with in gynecologic practice is lower abdominal pain and that the etiologic factor involved in most cases is pelvic in origin and can be cured by minor surgical procedure and conservative therapy safely carried out in the gynecologist's office. Too often, we see patients who have been subjected to one or more major surgical procedures, and are still complaining of their original symptoms.

Recently, at the direction of Captain L. B. Marshall (MC) U.S.N., Commanding Officer of the U.S. Naval Hospital at Norman Oklahoma, Doctor E. S. Burge and myself have begun collecting pertinent cases for study from the "Out Patient Department". These cases, coming from all parts of the United States, give an excellent cross section study of results obtained from various surgical approaches to this problem of lower abdominal pain. After a considerable number have been collected and tabulated, they will be reported in the future.

DISCUSSION
M. J. SERWER, M.D.
OKLAHOMA CITY, OKLAHOMA

Dr. Longstreth has discussed many of the conditions causing low abdominal pain. This can lead to but one conclusion, namely, that pelvic pain is a very elusive symptom. A likely explanation is that the genital organs have few sensory fibers and an abundant sympathetic innervation. The only undue sensitive areas are the pelvic peritonium and the internal cervical os.

We have all seen cervical erosion, cervical cancer, ovarian and uterine tumors, uterine retrodisplacements, ectopic pregnancies, etc., all without any pain whatsoever. Should pain be present, then it can be safely assumed that the internal cervical os or the pelvic peritoneum are involved, either by infection, inflammation, pressure, adhesions and the like. This may explain the apparent discrepancy between the severity of the pain and the degree of pathology.

Therapy, then, should be directed toward an alleviation of the existing pathology. We have all seen uterine suspensions without relief, due to the disregard of the coexisting parametritis or pelvic peritoneal inflammation.

The diagnosis of genital neurosis is one that is used usually to cover up a diagnostic error. Low abdominal pain rarely persists in the absence of a pathologic lesion. As our diagnostic ability improves, the diagnosis of the neurosis becomes less frequent. Much that is diagnosed as neurosis is, in reality, a hormonal disturbance as a result of disturbed ovarian circulation.

I would like to stress the importance of the general practitioner with these patients. Each physician tends to view lower abdominal pain in the light of his own specialty, sometimes to the detriment of the patient. It is surprising how much backache may be cured merely by the wearing of proper shoes. Likewise, much backache occurring after pregnancy could more properly be treated by an orthopedist. Much joint disturbance could be avoided if we were to pay more attention to the patient's comfort when in stirrups on the delivery table.

Recent Advances in Psychosomatic Medicine

CHARLES E. LEONARD, M.D.

OKLAHOMA CITY, OKLAHOMA

This paper presents some of the recent advances in research on the emotional and somatic relationships in various symptom complexes.

It was well established some 40 years ago by Freud and his students that there was an intimate causal relationship of conscious-alien impulses to neurotic symptoms, dreams and other phenomena of normal behaviour. This led to the conclusion that such phenomena coincided with an intra psychic struggle between certain unconscious wishes and the integrated personality, which did not permit their direct and undisguised expression in the conscious life of the individual. From this fact psychoanalysis has extended its investigation into the realm of somatic complaints in individuals who are unstable emotionally and where the somatic complaints were either not relieved or only partially relieved by medicinal treatment. Time does not permit me to go into all of the recent advances made in this line, and since the psychogenic factors that go to form even one case are sufficient to require a lengthy paper, I must limit this paper to a very superficial sketch of a few selected cases and in closing will try to mention some of the conditions upon which much research is being pursued.

I will present the analysis of a case of functional vomiting, as the underlying psychogenic factors are very similar in cases of anorexia nervosa, and peptic ulcers and other gastric conditions. This patient was a white girl 28, single and very well educated. She had suffered from bulimia followed by vomiting for many years. She was the younger of two children, the brother being four years, her senior, and always the object of her jealously as well as admiration. The marital situation of the parents was very unhappy. The father had been married previously and had a son by his first wife. This marriage ended in divorce and the father never told the patient's mother about his first wife and son until she was pregnant with the first child. The wife reacted with tremendous hostility, rejecting the father and showering all her love on her son. The patient was an unwanted child and at birth was placed on the bottle and never given the breast although the brother had been breast fed for some time. The mother was very religious and brought the patient up to live a perfect life and to show none of her hostilities or jealousies. The patient lived in mortal terror of being rejected by her mother, and the mother, realizing this attitude, used it to further her own end and to make the patient obedient. The father, not wanting this child, told her that women were no good and would have nothing to do with her although he was very nice to the older brother. The patient was rather shy but at the same time very self-sufficient, and rebelled at receiving help from anyone. She recalled that all during her life she would have spells of ravenous appetite which could not be satisfied. These were nearly always followed by vomiting as a reaction to her greed. In her every day life she was always doing little favors for people in hopes that they would like her and do bigger favors for her. However, if she did receive more than she gave, she reacted by vomiting. The patient had the idea firmly fixed in her mind that if the mother loved her child she always allowed it to receive gratification at the breast. Her hatred of her brother became more manifest, and she began to recall memories of having to give up the best food to him and being punished by both mother and father for any acts of jealousy on her part.

As this and other unconscious material became mobilized, the patient was brought to see that, in her mind, the receiving of food was likened to being loved and in these periods when she felt rejected she aggressively took what she felt was rightfully hers and her bulimia increased. This she always reacted to by extreme feelings of guilt and attempted to restore what she had incorporated. As the patient began to understand this, by means of her dreams, phantasies and associations, it became clear to her that it was a childish mechanism, and ·that, while it might have been of value to her as an infant, as an adult it was entirely valueless. Following the recognition of this, her life adjustment became very good and symptoms stopped.

The second case is one of rather severe migraine, and it is presented to show some of the many self-punishing mechanisms that have to be dealt with and also to show that similar dynamics are found in cases ranging from mild chronic headache to severe depression with suicidal trends. This patient was a white girl 30 years old, highly educated and doing professional nursing. She had been treated by allergists and numerous medical men with little or no results in the relief of the headache. The headaches had started during adolescence and when she came to analysis they were occurring about two to three times a month and lasting one to two days. This patient also showed some depressive tendencies with alternated with the headache. That is, if she became severely depressed with suicidal thoughts, the headache did not appear. Her mother had committed suicide when the patient was 14 years old. Her memory of this is one of sadness, with an underlying feeling that she did not like to admit to herself, of happiness that she could take care of her father and two younger brothers. All the neighbors commented on what a fine little mother she made, and she could recall phantasies of giving up her entire life for her brothers and caring for them forever.

Some of the disturbing factors that would come out at this time and would always precipitate a headache and severe depression, were earlier memories of being forced to take care of the younger brothers as they came along and how she wanted the mother's care herself and did not want to share it. Several childish unconscious acts were to pinch the brother's finger in the door or allow him to fall out of the buggy. For these she was unmercifully punished and shamed until the time came that she would punish herself for even having hostile thoughts toward the brothers. This unconscious hostility was so completely opposite to her conscious overt acts that she could not bring herself to face these childish hostilities, but she would react with severe headache or marked depres-

sion and at times it was difficult to prevent her from committing suicide. This continued until one day she left several babies in the nursery and did not put them to the breast, for she rationalized that it was more important to bathe the mothers than feed the babies. Her supervisor reprimanded her for this and asking her if she wanted to kill the babies. The patient immediately developed a severe headache that lasted three days, during which time there were dreams of killing children and then herself. Following this, she gained insight into her hostile wishes and her reaction of self punishment. It has been well over a year now since her analysis was completed. As yet there have been no headaches, no depression, and she is adjusting well to her life situation.

The third case is that of a 50 year old man who had worked up to the position of assistant manager of a large company through hard work and the friendly help of the manager. About five years previous to the development of his heart symptoms he had a rather severe anxiety attack which was relieved when he was transferred to another town for a few years. His present attack started when he returned to work under his friend and benefactor again. On admission he showed marked anxiety, weakness and pulse rate of 120. The history was that of paroxysmal tachycardia starting about six months previously. The attacks started during breakfast every day but Sunday, and by the time he reached the office he was so weak he would have to rest for an hour or so during which time the manager would usually leave the office to make his rounds of the different stations, then the patient would be able to carry on his routine work. During the short time this patient was seen, he complained bitterly about his lack of education and that he would be unable to advance any further in his line of work, as the next step was the manager's position. He also went into great detail about how much he owed the manager for the steady increase and favors he had received at his hands. During this time he recalled a dream he had had on several different occasions during the past five years. The dream was that he had killed his uncle to inherit his money. Always following this dream was the feeling that he was going to be fired. In discussing the dream the patient remarked that the uncle's money would help him a lot and he would just as soon see the uncle dead as he had always hated him anyway. But he could never understand why he always had the feeling that he was going to be discharged from his position. He also made the remark that the uncle resembled the manager in appearance but that the resemblance stopped there. It was pointd out that perhaps the dream really ment that it was the manager that he wished to kill in order to secure the higher position. This the patient strongly denied and became panicky. However, the suggestion was followed up by rather mild interpretation until the patient was brought to face his hostility and see that his paroxysmal tachycardia was really a physiological increase in heart rate to supply the body in preparation for combat, and the reaction to this was, of course, anxiety and the weakness, a defense against aggression. This patient made a nice adjustment to his working situation and has had no return of the heart or anxiety symptoms.

The last case I wish to present is that of a 15 year old white girl, who had developed a rather severe globus hystericus 18 months before coming for treatment. She had developed severe choking spells with an inability to swallow which would last from one to five days. There had been a marked loss of weight. She had to be taken out of school and had become a semi-invalid. Her symptoms developed when her father started to pay a lot of attention to her girl friend and called her his adopted daughter. This friend was just the patient's age and came from a very rejecting home. She became very attached to the patient's father, and tried in every way possible to secure the love and attention she desired from this father-substitute. The patient, having been very strictly reared, was taught that her things were to be shared with this unfortunate girl, and so the patient developed a strong conscious love and mother-like attitude toward this girl. During the interviews the patient admitted that at times she was rather resentful of this girl demanding so much attention from the father. Following this admission the choking spells became intensified. The mother aided in the treatment by recalling that when the patient was eighteen months old she saw the baby sister nursing the breast, struck her mother on the knee, tried to pull the sister away and cried, "My breast". Following this she developed a strong father attachment which the mother considered abnormal and could not understand. The parallel between these two situations soon became evident to the patient, and with the aid of some dreams she soon accepted insight into her hatred of this girl friend. It then only remained to show her the mechanism of hostile identification and self-punishing drive that her strict up-bringing had precipitated in order to cause the symptoms to disappear. It has been six months since the completion of this case, and to date there has been no recurrence of symptoms.

These four cases have been very superficially presented, and are of interest only in that they give a little insight into the dynamics of symptom formations.

The analytic literature has lately shown a marked increase in the number of articles on the emotional state in somatic symptoms. Some of the most recent is French's and Alexander's monograph on the "Psychogenic Factors in Bronchial Asthma", which shows that in some cases the central emotional problems concerns separation from the mother. The asthma symptom is related to the suppressed crying for the mother, and it is shown that the sexual conflict is very strong.

Bollmeier, in his unpublished paper on the "Differential Diagnosis of Emotional Glycosuria from Diabetes Mellitus", states that the conflict seems to be tied up with unconscious hostility and that the fluctuations of the sugar output are more influenced by emotional factors than by carbohydrate intake, and that emotional glycosuria is a reversible condition.

Wilson in his paper on "A Study of Structral and Instinctual Conflicts in Cases of Hay Fever", states that the emotional component in hay fever is tied up with the early sexual curiosity in relation to the sense of smell which is deeply repressed into the unconscious.

Benedek and Rubeustein have a monograph in the process of publication at the present time that brings out the relation of phychodynamic processes to the ovarian activity and menstrual cycle.

In Wilson's paper on "Typical Personality Trends and Conflicts in Cases of Spastic Colitis", he states that the unconscious conflict is associated with the desire to retain and keep.

Levey states in his paper on "Oral Trends and Oral Conflicts in a Case of Duodenal Ulcer", that the pain is a masochistic solution of the guilt conflict produced by the desire to receive and retain for himself as long as he can justify his dependence by suffering.

Levine shows in his paper in a case of chronic diarrhea and vomiting that the unconscious dynamics are due to the desire to give or eliminate.

Leon Saul's work on Urticaria, while relatively new and not yet thoroughly investigated, seems to show that the emotional conflict is set up in a rather inhibited individual with an intense longing for love, but who is unable to satisfy these desires by a normal sexual relationship. It was also found that in these individuals there were strong unconscious exibitionistic tenencies.

The last article I wish to mention is the work on "Essential Hypertension" by Alexander, in which he found that in the emotional conflict was tied up with strong unconscious hostile impluses that the individual was unable to express openly.

SUMMARY

1. These clinical case histories have been superficially reviewed. The first two were treated by the classical phychoanalytic procedure for a period of one year. The third case was treated by short psychotherapy involving eight interviews which covered a period of three weeks, and the treatment of the fourth covered a period of four weeks involving ten interviews. These cases were presented to show the emotional component involved in these various somatic symptom complexes.

2. A few of the very recent papers on psychosmatic symptoms have been very briefly covered.

BIBLIOGRAPHY

1. Alexander, Franz: Psychology—A Study of a Case of Essential Hypertension Psychosmatic Medicine. pp. 1-139. 1939.
2. Alexander, Franz; Wilson, George W., Levey, Harry B; Levine, Maurice; The Influence of Psychologic Factors upon Gastro-Intestinal Disturbances—A Symposium. Psychoanalytic Quarterly, Vol. 3, 501-588. 1934.
3. Alexander, Franz & Thomas; Psychogenic Factors in Brochial Asthma. National Research Council. 1941.
4. Alexander, Franz; Bollmeier, L. M., Meyer, Albrecht; The Differential Diagnosis of Emotional Glycosuria from Diabetes Mellitus. Unpublished.
5. Benedek, T. & Rubsustein: Relation of Psychodynamic Processes to Ovarian Activity and Menstrual Phase. Psychosomatic Medicine Monography. 1942.
6. Leonard, Charles E.: The Analysis of a Case of Functional Vomiting and Bulimia. Accepted for publication in Psychoanalytic Review. Unpublished.
7. Saul, Leon J. & Bernstein, Clarence Jr: The Emotional Settings of Some Attacks of Urticaria. Psychosomatic Medicine, Vol. 3, No. 4, pp. 349. 1941.

Epidemic Keratoconjunctivitis

A Summary of the Recent Literature

VICTOR C. MYERS, M.D.

INDUSTRIAL HYGIENE PHYSICIAN

OKLAHOMA STATE HEALTH DEPARTMENT

The disease first appeared in epidemic proportions in this country on the west coast in September, 1941. It is probably endemic in the far east and occurs sporadically throughout the world. Since its first major appearance in west coast shipyards, epidemics have occurred in industrial communities in Connecticut, New York, Michigan and other states. As yet, no definite cases have been reported in the Oklahoma area. We have large aggregations of workers in the state, and an epidemic of this nature could interfere materially with war production. Therefore, it seems advisable to make as many physicians as possible aware of the existence and nature of the disease in an effort to prevent its widespread occurrence.

The etiology is believed to be filterable virus. Sanders and Alexander isolated such a virus from patients with Keratoconjunctivitis. This proved to be pathogenic for mice and rabbits. Its pathogenicity was neutralized by serum from convalescent patients, and mouse virus could be used to produce human infection with specific antibody formation. Conjunctival scrapings from infected patients have shown increased monocytes. Smears and cultures are negative or show contamination.

The incubation period varies from 5 to 10 days and is usually about eight days. Means of transmission are by direct contact and contaminated hands, instruments, towels, etc.

Initial symptoms are frequently indefinite and variable. The disease is easily confused with other acute infections of the eye, especially panophthalmitis, gonorrheal ophthalmitis, streptococcic conjunctivitis, diphtheritic infection, staphlococcus infection, and allergy. Edema of the eyelids and palpebral conjunctiva, and the feeling of a foreign body in the eye are the usual initial symptoms. A foreign body or abrasion may be present, but these are believed to be coincidental. The bulbar conjunctiva becomes edematous early. Lacrimation and photophobia are present to a degree, but real pain and blepharospasm do not appear until the cornea is affected. There is little or no formation of pus. Pre-auricular and sub-maxillary adenitis with tenderness is usually present. Headache, malaise, and fever may occur. In most of the cases there has been unilateral involvement at the onset with infection of the other eye in from five to eight days. The disease is self-limited, and in most cases the conjunctivitis disappears spontaneously in from 14 to 18 days.

Keratitis occurs in from 50 per cent to 90 per cent of the cases and within six to twelve days after the conjunctivitis appears. Discrete gray infiltrates appear in and immediately under the epithelial layer of the cornea. In a large percentage of cases these involve the pupillary area of the cornea. Seldom does erosion of the corneal epithelium occur. The extent of visual impairment is dependent on the number and location of corneal infiltrates. These may disappear in a few days or may last for several months. Permanent visual impairment may result.

At the present time no specific treatment has been found. It is recommended that the eyes be kept clean during the acute stages with irrigations of boric acid, isotonic solution of sodium chloride, or 1:5,000 mermuric oxycyanide. Instillations of 1 per cent atropine and 1 per cent holocaine are recommended for relief of pain and photophobia. Some beneficial results have been reported from the use of 5 per cent sulfathiazole ointment and 5 per cent solution of sodium sulfathiazole sesquihydrate. The most encouraging results have been obtained from the use of convalescent human serum. Further investigations are now under way on the value of this form of treatment.

The most effective preventive measure is complete isolation of the infected individual. The dangers of transmission of the disease at home, as well as in the plant, must be explained to the patient. Extreme cleanliness should be observed. In this respect, personal protective equipment (goggles, respirators, etc.) should be assigned to each worker for his exclusive use. These should be thoroughly sterilized before transferring such equipment to another worker. Physicians and nurses must wash their hands thoroughly with soap and water after each patient. Eye droppers, instruments, and solutions must be sterilized to prevent spread of the infection. The disease has been transmitted through medical personnel. Infection may be spread not only from known cases, but also from those undiagnosed cases suspected of having foreign bodies in the eye.

Outbreaks of the disease, real or suspected, should be reported immediately to the Division of Industrial Hygiene, Oklahoma State Health Department, where further information may be obtained.

BIBLIOGRAPHY

1. Hogan, M. J., and Crawford, J. W.: War Medicine, Vol 2, pp. 984. 1943.
2. Sanders, Murray, and Alexander, R. D.: Journal Exper. Medicine, 71-77. 1943.
3. Joint Report issued by U.S. Public Health Service and Committee on Industrial Ophthalmology, American Medical Association. Jour. A.M.A., Vol. 121, No. 14, pp. 1153. 1943.
4. Walter, F. J.: Jour. A.M.A., Vol. 120, No. 14, pp. 1157. 1942.
5. Braley, A. S., and Sanders, M.: Treatment of Epidemic Keratoconjunctivitis, Jour. A.M.A., Vol. 121, No. 13, pp. 999. 1943.

ARE WE IN GOOD HEALTH?

"When the four limbs are well developed and the skin is clear and the flesh is full, that is the health of the body. When the parents and children are affectionate, the brothers are good towards one another and the husband and wife live in harmony, that is the health of the family. When the higher officials obey the law and the lower officials are honest, the officers have regulated and well-defined functions and the king and ministers help one another on the right course, that is the health of the nation. When the Emperor rides in the carriage of Virtue, with Music as his driver, when the different rulers meet one another with courtesy, the officials regulate one another with law, the scholars urge one another by the standard of honesty, and the people are united in peace, that is the health of the world. This is called the Grand Harmony."—"Between Tears and Laughter" by Lin Yutang.

· THE PRESIDENT'S PAGE ·

"There are times that try men's souls. The summer soldier and the sunshine patroit will, in this crisis, shrink from the service of his country; but he that stands it now, deserves the love and thanks of man and woman. Tyranny, like hell, is not easily conquered . . ."

The Wagner-Murray-Dingell Bill has been introduced in the Senate. It is the American Beveridge Plan—"from the cradle to the grave." Its passage would doom the practice of medicine as we have known it. It would place almost unlimited control of the profession in the hands of one man—the Surgeon General of the Public Health Service. It must not pass! Not because of any selfish interest on our part, but for the good of the health of all the people. An enslaved physician cannot adequately serve the people.

Each of you has a solemn duty as an American Citizen. Write to your Senator today, and ask for a copy of Senate Bill No. 1161. Write now! This is trouble in the land, but "if there be trouble, let it be in my day, that my child may have peace . . . ". Familiarize yourself with the medical provisions of this bill and discuss them with your friends. Congress is in recess and your Senators and Congressmen are at home, perhaps for the last time until the war is concluded. They are home to feel the pulse of the people they represent. Are we anemic—have we a pulse left?

The medical men of Oklahoma will not fail in their obligations as guardians of the health of the people, or as citizens. Let us not wait until the County Societies meet in the fall—let each of us, individually, do his duty now! Eternal Vigilance is the price of Liberty.

James Stevenson

President.

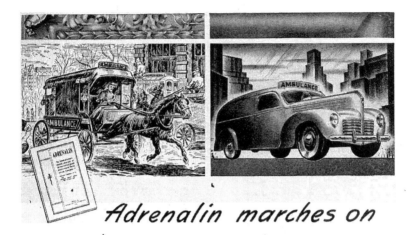

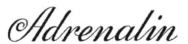

Adrenalin marches on

"The therapeutic applications of adrenalin are already numerous and new uses for it are constantly being found out by different experimenters. Generally speaking, adrenalin, when locally applied, is the most powerful astringent and hemostatic known . . . and it is the strongest stimulant of the heart . . . it will unquestionably attain to a prominent place in the materia medica."

A Parke-Davis publication issued in 1902.

Today—four decades after isolation and crystallization of ADRENALIN* (epinephrine hydrochloride)—a great volume of literature attests to the high place it has attained in materia medica. Physicians know its amazing record as a circulatory stimulant, vasoconstrictor and hemostatic. ADRENALIN is the 20th Century's first great medical discovery. No trade-marked product has found wider acceptance; none enjoys a wider field of usefulness.

*TRADE-MARK REG U. S PAT. OFF.

The active principle of the medullary portion of the suprarenal glands was isolated in crystalline form and its chemical structure determined in 1901 by Parke, Davis & Company

PARKE, DAVIS & COMPANY
DETROIT · MICHIGAN

The JOURNAL Of The
OKLAHOMA STATE MEDICAL ASSOCIATION

EDITORIAL BOARD
L. J. MOORMAN, Oklahoma City, Editor-in-Chief
E. EUGENE RICE, Shawnee
NED R. SMITH, Tulsa
MR. R. H. GRAHAM, Oklahoma City, Business Manager

CONTRIBUTIONS: Articles accepted by this Journal for publication including those read at the annual meetings of the State Association are the sole property of this Journal.

The Editorial Department is not responsible for the opinions expressed in the original articles of contributors.

Manuscripts may be withdrawn by authors for publication elsewhere only upon the approval of the Editorial Board.

MANUSCRIPTS: Manuscripts should be typewritten, double-spaced, on white paper 8½ x 11 inches. The original copy, not the carbon copy, should be submitted.

Footnotes, bibliographies and legends for cuts should be typed on separate sheets in double space. Bibliography listing should follow this order: Name of author, title of article, name of periodical with volume, page and date of publication.

Manuscripts are accepted subject to the usual editorial revisions and with the understanding that they have not been published elsewhere.

NEWS: Local news of interest to the medical profession, changes of address, births, deaths and weddings will be gratefully received.

ADVERTISING: Advertising of articles, drugs or compounds unapproved by the Council on Pharmacy of the A.M.A. will not be accepted. Advertising rates will be supplied on application.

It is suggested that members of the State Association patronize our advertisers in preference to others.

SUBSCRIPTIONS: Failure to receive The Journal should call for immediate notification.

REPRINTS: Reprints of original articles will be supplied at actual cost provided request for them is attached to manuscripts or made in sufficient time before publication. Checks for reprints should be made payable to Industrial Printing Company, Oklahoma City.

Address all communications to THE JOURNAL OF THE OKLAHOMA STATE MEDICAL ASSOCIATION,
210 Plaza Court, Oklahoma City. (3)

OFFICIAL PUBLICATION OF THE OKLAHOMA STATE MEDICAL ASSOCIATION
Copyrighted August, 1943

"THE MILKY WAY"

According to Samuel Johnson's Dictionary, milk is "the liquor with which animals feed their young from the breast". We know that the milk of animal sustenance was making flesh and bone long before the milk of human kindness discovered the therapeutic value of this liquor. Hippocrates recognized the medicinal value of milk and prescribed it on various occasions. In common with other Greek authorities he recommended it in the treatment of phthisis. Galen and Aretaeus, the last of the great Greek physicians, were staunch supporters of the therapeutic use of milk.

Dioscorides, Celsus, Serapion and Paulus Aegineta employed it in various conditions. The latter said, "Whey is possessed of detergent properties, and hence it loosens the belly if separated by boiling", also, "when milk is boiled either by hot pebbles or any other way, it is an excellent remedy for dysenteries and other acrid defluxions of the bowels" and the "milk of a woman is of the best regulated temperament; after which the goat's, and then that of the ass and sheep; and last of all the milk of cows."

The use of boiled milk for "defluxions of the belly" was described by Rufus, after whom Oribasius and Avicenna copied their allegiance to the same; "The method of preparing milk for use by putting heated stones into it, is mentioned by Dioscorides, Pliny and others. Serapion recommends heated iron. It is interesting to note that Galen was aware that milk coagulates in the stomach before it is digested" and that it "is described as the most satisfactory food by all medical writers, and some believe that patients suffering from pulmonary ulcer (phthisis) before it has become large or calloused, can be cured by its use alone.

"Physicians of old advised human milk for patients wasted with phthisis, and recommended it while standing, directly from the breast. This idea appears good to me since human milk is so natural to the human stomach, and, thus taken, has no opportunity to be cooled by the surrounding air. When this proves repellent to the patient, the next best is asses' milk, since it does not curdle and (on account of its thinness) easily penetrates to the lungs, in fact, to every part of the body.

"In any case when milk is advisable, it should be taken immediately after milking with the animal standing alongside. Thus drunk warm it rarely curdles in the stomach and this may be absolutely prevented by adding salt or honey. The proper amount of salt is that to the taste, of honey as much as will sit sweet on the somach."

Galen, who sent his cases of "pulmonary ulcer" down to his beloved Stabiae on the Mediterranean for treatment, gives an interesting account of his observations on the production of therapeutic milk:

"Appropriate now is to speak of milk and not of the milk at Stabiae alone, but everywhere, not only in Italy but other countries. Stabiae, however, has special advantages. It is in an isolated commanding position, the air is dry, and the pasture is wholesome for cattle. Such pasture-land may be artifically created elsewhere, but, even with the cultivation of proper herbs and shrubs on suitable hillsides capable of making the milk healthy and befittingly astringent, it is not possible to change the air.

"It is situated on a hill of moderate height in the lowest position between Sorrentum and Naples looking toward and three miles from the Mediterranean. Sloping gently to the west and protected also from the north, it escapes the disagreeable, rainy and cold winds,—Eurus, Subsolanus and Boreas. Near at hand is another higher hill, called from time immemorial Vesuvius, though now Vesvius, and universally known on account of its eruptions. This not only protects it to the north, but the volcanic action conduces to the drying of the air, and the settling ashes make the air drier still. About are no marshes or stagnant water.

"No doubt there are other dry hills similar to the one on which Stabiae is situated elsewhere on earth in close proximity to the sea, not high enough to be subjected to violent winds and not so low as to be submitted to the rising vapors of the fields. Make sure, however, that your selected elevation face not the north and thus be averted from the sun. If it is a temperate clime like Stabiae so much the better. Let the herbs on the hill be agrostis (bent grass or red top), lotus (clover), Polygonon (of the nature of beggar-weed or cow-grass), melissophylum (bastard balm) and the shrubs lentiscus (?), arbutus, rubus (raspeberry), hedera (common ivy), cytisus (broom) and such like.

"The cattle at Stabiae are cows, and their milk is as thick as the milk of asses is with goat's milk in between. Thinking the milk of other animals might be more beneficial in certain cases, I put feeding on the hill at Stabiae cows, asses and goats. Cow's milk contains most fat, goat's milk less, and ass's least of all."

Though chemical analysis will show that Galen's conclusions were not wholly accurate, we must give him credit for his searching investigations. The record shows that Galen tried to differentiate the milk of "the human being, the bitch, wolf, hyena, bear, sow, ewe, camel and mare."

Note the modern tone of the following paragraph:

"Milk is most wholesome when pure and devoid of acidity, extraneous taste and odor. It should be bland and sweet to the taste. The producing animal should be of a flourishing age, well-fed, moderately exercised, and the off-spring weaned. The milk of sickly or poorly kept animals is harmful. Care must be taken then of their digestion and (he humorously asserts) we will willingly accept the risk of popular ridicule in prescribing a diet for asses."

Aretaeus, who in all probability was Galen's contemporary and whose classic description of pulmonary tuberculosis has hardly been surpassed, gives milk a laudible reputation and calls it a "sweet medicine". The following is from the Adams translation of his works, "For milk is pleasant to take, is easy to drink, gives solid nourishment, and is more familiar than any other food to one from a child. In color it is pleasant to see; as a medicine it seems to lubricate the windpipe, to clean, as if with a feather, the bronchi, and to bring off phlegm, improve the breathing, and facilitate the discharges downwards. To ulcers it is sweet medicine, and milder than anything else. If one, then, will only drink plenty of this, he will not stand in need of anything else. For it is a good thing that, in disease, milk should prove both food and medicine. And indeed, the races of men called Galactophagi use no food from grain. But yet it is a very good thing to use porridge, pastry, washed groats of spelt (alica), and the other edibles prepared with milk."

With the exception of the knowledge gained through the science of bacteriology, we have learned very little about milk since the 2nd Century A.D. It is true that scientific infant feeding with percentage formula awaited the advent of Thomas Morgan Ratch who founded the first milk laboratory (Walker-Gordon) in Boston (1891). This was followed by similar laboratories in London. From this beginning, the movement for clean milk has spread throughout the world.

Wattes said, "That very substance which last week was grazing in the field, waving in the milk pail, or growing in the garden, is now become part of the man."

"ON THE MOVE"

This is the slogan of The Medical Administration Service, Inc. appearing in bold letters on the front page of this organization's prepared discussion of the Medical Planning Research Study on the Beveridge Report. "The Medical Planning Research is an organization of 400 anonymous British physicians, most of them under 45 years of age". On the inside of the front page we find this quotation from the Medical Planning Research Interim General Report; "Medical opinion is on the move and no desire to suspend judgment can alter this fact". In our opinion when all the implications are considered, this is tautomount to saying "to hell with health". In other words, whether the patient lives or dies, the right blanks must be properly filled out.

We wonder if these young doctors realize that medicine moved out of the nebulous realm of magic in the Fifth Century, B. C., and that in spite of all obstructive handicaps, it survived the Dark Ages and has been on the move ever since. What these young men really mean is that lay opinion is just now being moved by designing paliticious and un-informed bureaucrats riding on the adminis-trative omnibus which overides a society temporarily blinded by the confusion and un-rest occasioned by the war. The Medical Administrative Service, Inc. should carefully reread the following confession found in the Medical Planning Research Interim General Report; "The scientific study of administra-tion is in its infancy. Scientific methods are more easily applied to material objects than to sociological ones. As a result, technical achievements have outstripped administra-tive organizatioin in local, national, and in-ternational spheres. In spite of this, tech-nicians who have been forced to work in large organizations have remained inferior in status to the administrators. Science be-gins by observation and the classification of experience. Our proposals for health admin-istration will be preceded by an analysis of past experiences in both administrative and technical organization. All new administra-tive proposals should be regarded as scientific experiments, and ours are no exception. Each phase of their óperation should be watched carefully and modified or altered as proves necessary.

"No-one who has had any experience of large administrative machines denies that direction is necessary inside a broad policy. The disputed question is rather who should give the direction . . .

"In internal structure, any large organiza-tion is subject to a series of mutually opposed forces, on the nice balance of which its effic-iency depends. These are:

"1. The technician v. the administrator.
"2. Parallelism v. hierarchy.
"3. The individual v. the committee.
"4. The centre v. the periphery.
"5. Uniformity v. diversity."

Medicine in the United States is neither in its infancy nor in its dotage. It knows what it is about and where it is going and refuses to be hampered by the vexing problems of outside administration.

The members of the medical profession ac-customed to scientific reasoning know there is no such thing as a nice balance between the above opposing forces. A compromise in the application of medical science to human needs represents a loss and establishes a haz-ard which the conscientious doctor is not will-ing to accept.

Medicine in the United States has demon-strated exceptional administrative ability in its own sphere. It has initiated the most ex-acting educational requirements in the his-tory of the world. It has organized and im-plimented the method of meeting these re-quirements in medical schools and hospitals to the point of ultimate minutia. It has standardized hospitals for the benefit of the sick and it has originated and helped to main-tain a great public health administration. It has brought about the highest health level and the lowest death rate existing in the history of all comparable nations. Within its own ranks it orginated and administered the most stupendous voluntary contribution to the war effort the country has yet witnessed. Must it, with all these accomplishments, be turned over to administrative agencies admit-tedly in their infancy? In the face of emer-gency, the doctor must be free. When the wounded are brought back or when the civil-ian is critically ill, who will dare tell the doc-tor what to do. He bears the responsibility and he must be free to exercise his special skills under the guidance of his own judg-ment. The doctor has won his spurs in the difficult realm of humanitarian medical ser-vice.

Voltaire, the insubordinate friend of medi-cine, after spending his life in an attempt to establish freedom of the soul through the power of the pen, finally wrote Frederick the Great, "It is true, then, sire, that in the end men will become enlightened, and that those paid to blind them will not always be able to put out their eyes."

ADMINISTRATIVE HYPEROPIA

The reports coming from intelligent lay-men who find it necessary or expedient to live in Washington, indicate that civilian med-ical service is hard to secure and often un-satisfactory when well-meaning civilian doc-tors find it difficult to be civil because they are severely overworked by the great influx of government employees and others who come and go because of the exigencies of war.

In Oklahoma, where, with few exceptions, medical care continues to be fairly adequate and the people relatively happy with the ser-vice available, we wonder why Washington should request us to consider making a place for refugee doctors. Let charity begin at home. Give Washington a few of the expend-able doctors. For the duration we must keep faith with the heavy quota of doctors we have loaned to our country. Their patrons await their return. Washington's floating population is made up of people who hope to return to their family doctors but need temporary and emergency care.

May we respectfully suggest that the hub be cooled by applying grease at the axle before disturbing orders are radiated along the spokes to peripheral areas, not adequately explored. May we also suggest that the hyperopic officials be supplied with corrective lenses and sent to a school of recognition.

WAGNERITES TAKE NOTICE

The Medical Advisory Committee for Oklahoma's Aid to Dependent Children, working on a purely voluntary basis, recently reported on 260 cases. After proper investigation the Committee made specific recommendations in 156 cases. Of these, 69 refused to follow the Committee recommendations, 71 of the total number were committed to hospitals for medical or surgical care and 38, or approximately 50 per cent, refused the treatment recommended. Twenty-four were chosen as suitable for vocational rehabilitation. Of these, 5 refused and 7 were found to be mentally incapable of pursuing the necessary training.

If this happens in an agency with the voluntary services of the best doctors working for the love of humanity, what will happen under the bureaucratic set-up with the inevitable cold, impersonal medical service which often amounts to a "take it or leave it" attitude, so long as the right forms are filled out. In addition to the above difficulties, the advocates of compulsory health administration should take account the fact that there may be many conscientious objectors to any plan that takes 6 per cent of the employees' pay and 6 per cent from the employer to provide something which they would not purchase at any price or accept as a gift because it is contrary to their religious teachings.

What of the Christian Scientist, the disciple of the new thought and the faith healer? Are not these people being robbed when they are required to pay for pooled medical care, none of which they will have unless public health takes a hand and requires medical supervision for the control of contagion?

It is unfortunate that we have so many who have no faith in medicine but accept all benefits of public health and sanitation. But with nothing better than bureaucratic medicine, we may expect their number to increase.

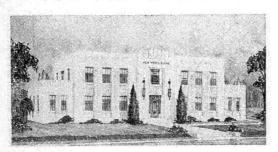

ASSOCIATION ACTIVITIES

SUPPLEMENTARY ROSTER

(*Indicates serving in armed forces.*)

The following is the list of 1943 memberships that have been received in the Executive Office of the Association since the publication of the Roster in the July issue of the Journal:

CADDO

HAWN, W. T. ....*Binger*

LYONS, MASON R. ....*Anadarko*

GARFIELD

CHAMBERS, E. EVANS ....*Enid*

LOGAN

LARKIN, H. W. ....*Guthrie*

MUSKOGEE

*McINNIS, J. T. ....*Muskogee*

OKMULGEE

McCALEB, PHILIP ....*Morris*

TULSA

RAMEY, CLYDE ....*Tulsa*

WOODS

TRAVERSE, C. A. ....*Alva*

APOLOGY

The Editorial Board of the Journal of the Oklahoma State Medical Association extends sincere apology to Dr. C. C. Young of Shawnee for the error made in the Roster appearing in the July issue. Dr. Young was listed as deceased but we are glad to report that he is in very good health.

CRIPPLED CHILDREN'S COMMITTEE AIDS IN POLIO FRIGHT

The Crippled Children's Committee of the Association, in cooperation with the University Medical School, its teaching hospitals and other interested agencies released on July 28 a bulletin to all members of the Association outlining the program in effect at the University Crippled Children's Hospital for the combating of the polio now manifested in Oklahoma.

The following reprint of the bulletin is for the purpose of reemphasizing the principle features of the present onset and to acquaint the profession with the hot pack treatment being given at the Hospital together with preventive measures should be taken by both the public and local communities.

PREVENTIVE

The first essential feature in the control of poliomyelitis is immediate reporting of cases to the County Superintendent of Health by telephone or telegraph. This will enable the health department to study the trend of spread and progress of the disease, and in areas with full-time county health departments. to collect detailed information regarding cases, which will be of definite aid in the accumulation of information leading to complete knowledge of control methods.

Isolation of diagnosed and suspected cases is necessary since our present knowledge of the spread of poliomyelitis is limited to the fact that the causative virus may be recovered from the nose, throat and bowel discharges of cases. This would indicate that the control of this disease is dependent upon measures which are utilized in the control of respiratory diseases and of typhoid fever. *Unfortunately, no vaccine, serum, nasal spray or gargle has as yet been developed which aids prevention in the least.* We are dependent, therefore, on careful sanitary measures. Sanitary disposal of human excreta is of utmost importance. Excreta from cases should even be treated as that from typhoid. Fly

breeding should be reduced to a minimum. Careful safeguarding of food supplies and food handling is essential, and pasteurization of milk should be encouraged.

In all counties having a full-time health department, the health officer is available for consultation on preventive measures. The Oklahoma State Health Department and the Oklahoma Crippled Children's Commission are training as many nurses in the hot pack treatment as can be spared and as far as possible will be available for home instruction *but not for bedside nursing.* These nurses will also be available for instruction in this method *but not for private treatment purposes.* Where there are full-time health departments, contact the medical director for further information. In unorganized counties, nurses from the Oklahoma Crippled Children's Commission will be available in a like manner, and you should contact the county health superintendent for further information.

Arrangements are being completed at once for care of patients in other areas of the State in addition to Oklahoma City.

EARLY DIAGNOSIS

It is important to make a diagnosis without waiting for the development of paralysis. While no age is immune. it is well to remember that over one-half of the cases occur between the ages of one and six years with a tendency for the age incidence to be higher in rural communities.

The early symptoms are not usually striking but the onset is often abrupt with the child being alternately drowsy and irritable but mentally clear. Most patients who are old enough to complain of headache and there may be some vomiting with abdominal pain. Either diarrhea or constipation may be present and neither is characteristic. Pain in the back of the neck and in the mid-dorsal and lumbar regions are important symptoms.

The child appears flushed and the prostration is apt to be greater than one would expect from the moderate fever of 101 to 103. The pulse is generally accelerated out of proportion to the fever. The throat is often infected. An important sign is a tremor of the hands. The most diagnostic signs appear in the stiffness of the neck and back resistance to anterior flexion. Normally a child, in a sitting position, can bend forward and touch his head to the bed between his knees. One with poliomyelitis will maintain the erect position and bend forward from the hips rather than flex his head and trunk; if flexion is forceful attempted, he will complain of pain.

In the presence of the above symptoms and findings, a lumbar puncture should be done. Usually the pressure is moderately increased and, while the fluid appears clear, close examination by transmitted light may show it to be ground glass in appearance. The cell count is usually increased to from 25 to 500 with lympocytes predominating. Globulin is usual and the total protein nearly always increased while sugar is present in normal amounts.

TREATMENT

From the standpoint of this communication, we are dealing chiefly with the treatment of anterior poliomyelitis in the acute stage, since it is felt that late sequela can be best handled at central clinics .

Of course, the problem of treatment is care of the sick child—the child requiring whatever measures may be indicated to combat his symptoms. Many of these children become rapidly dehydrated, need fluids and other medication.

In the past, the standard treatment for the affected parts have been immobilization which is well understood by the medical profession.

Based upon the theory that in the early stage the major portion of the patient's discomfort and a portion of his later disability is due to muscle spasm rather than flaccid paralysis, a newer method is being used and studied in medical centers.

Under the newer method, it is felt that the hot pack treatment has a very distinct advantage particularly in the early stage. Early physical therapy in the nature of muscle stimulation, muscle re-education, etc., is of extreme value, but is not essential in the acute stage. By the acute stage, we mean three to four weeks from the onset.

Throughout this period, the involved portions of the body are painful to movement, tender to touch and the joints show marked restriction of motion due not to the joint but to spasm of the muscles. A careful, but non-traumatic, examination can be made strictly within limits of pain, and will demonstrate the muscles that are in spasm or that are not functioning. The involved areas should be the recipients of the hot pack treatment.

The parts most frequently involved are (roughly in the order of frequency) the back, the neck, the ham strings, the calves, pectorals, abdominals, and to a lesser extent, the other muscle groups. In case of doubt, it is advisable to pack the area in question until all muscle spasm has disappeared.

If there are signs of bulbar involvement, the case, of course, is much more critical and will require much more heroic measures; such as, 15 minute packs to the chest, oxygen inhalation, respirator, etc.

The technic of this new procedure will not be discussed; however, nurses are being trained in the technic, and we hope will become available in most sections of the State.

Some precautions, however, should be noted. The child should be handled very carefully and any movement avoided which causes his discomfort.

The packs should be hot but should be wrung absolutely dry—the lest excessive moisture in the blanket will cause skin burns. The child, of course, should be kept in bed and given physiological rest. Passive motion of the joints, exercising great care to stop before any discomfort is elicted, is permissible and even advisable. This procedure must, however, be done under your direct supervision.

OKLAHOMA CITY TIMES CARRYING HEALTH FEATURE

Available to All Other State Papers

Beginning July 19 the Oklahoma City Times instituted a new feature known as "Is There a Doctor in the House".

This series of health articles which is being written by Elizabeth Wilkins, a feature writer of the Times, are in cooperation with a special committee of the Association and the Department of Health.

The articles are designed to give helpful information to the lay public and to help alleviate unnecessary calls upon the physicians' time. They are written in understandable lay language and are featured by old superstitions concerning cures for certain diseases.

The Times has written to your local paper advising that it may reprint the articles without cost and it is suggested that the local County Medical Societies request the editors of the local papers to consider the offer of the Times.

All articles appearing in the Times with reference to medical conditions have been checked by the Special Committee of the Association before publication.

SOUTHERN MEDICAL ASSOCIATION TO MEET IN CINCINNATI, OHIO

The Executive Committee of the Southern Medical Association has accepted the invitation of the Campbell-Kenton County Medical Society of Kentucky to hold

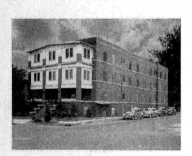
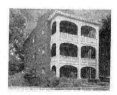

the Annual Meeting November 16, 17 and 18 in Cincinnati with the Hamilton, Ohio County Medical Society as co-host. The Netherland Plaza Hotel will be general headquarters.

The following reprint from the Announcement Bulletin outlines the 1943 program. Oklahoma physicians are urged to make railroad and hotel reservations early.

Program Plans

"Several program plans were considered by the Executive Committee. Exigencies of the times seemed to make it desirable to concentrate and condense all work. The opening day, Tuesday, will be devoted to general clinical sessions, and will be a Kentucky and Ohio Day. The program will be made up of physicians from both the Kentucky and Ohio sides of the river.

"On Wednesday and Thursday two general sessions will meet concurrently. In one, papers will be presented from the Association's sections representing the surgical specialties, and in the other, papers from the sections representing the medical specialties. There will be no formal section meetings this year. All sections will have the same officers for another year. Each of the twenty-one sections of the Association will furnish its proportional share of the papers for the general sessions, and papers will be listed on the program from the sections from which they come. There will be no discussion of the papers, but there will be a question and answer period following each paper. The chairman of the various sections will preside over their part of the program.

"The Executive Committee suggests that all programs be divided about equally between physicians in the armed forces and physicians in civilian practice.

"All activities—meetings, scientific exhibits, hobby exhibits, technical exhibits, and registration—are to be held in the three principal downtown hotels, within a block of each other, so that no local transportation will be needed for convention guests.

"On Tuesday evening there will be a general public session with address of welcome, response, address of the President, and two other addresses. There will be no formal entertainment on Tuesday evining, no President's reception and grand ball as in previous years. In keeping with the spirit of the times the Cincinnati meeting will be devoted strictly to medical and surgical problems with no official or formal entertainment.

Hotels

"Cincinnati has a number of good hotels and it is anticipated that all who may wish to attend the meeting in November can be comfortably housed. Among the good hotels are: Netherland Plaza, Gibson, Sinton, Fountain Square, Metropole, Palace, Alms, Broadway, Kemper Lane, Mariemont Inn, and Parkview. The Netherland Plaza will be General Hotel Headquarters. The Gibson and the Sinton will be headquarters for association meeting conjointly with the Woman's Auxiliary—designations to be announced later."

AMERICAN BOARD OF OBSTETRICS AND GYNECOLOGY ALTERS REQUIREMENTS

The annual meeting of the Board was held at Pittsburgh, Pennsylvania from May 20 to May 25. A number of changes in Board regulations and requirements were put into effect. Several of these changes are designed to broaden the requirements for candidates in Service. Examples are, the allowance of a stipulated amount of credit toward special training requirements for men in Service and assigned to general surgical positions, special training allowances on a preceptorship basis for men assigned to obstetrical or gynecological duties in military hospitals and working under the supervision of Diplomates or recognized obstetrician-gynecologists, as well as credit toward the "time in practice" requirement of the Board to be allowed for time in military service.

The Board will no longer require a general rotating internship, but will now accept a one year interne service, although the rotating internship is preferable.

Such services must be in institutions approved by the Council on Medical Education and Hospitals of the A.M.A. The privilege of reopening applications by candidates who have been declared ineligible has been extended to two years from date of filing the application, instead of one year.

The Board has ruled temporarily to excuse men in military service from the submission of case records at the stipulated examination times, thereby permitting them to proceed without further delay with the Board examinations. This does not obligate the Board, however, to waive the case record requirement for such candidates. Plans have been made to provide similarly for Service men upon their eventual discharge from the Armed Forces.

Applications for the 1944 examinations of the Board are being received at the office of the Secretary, Dr. Paul Titus, 1015 Highland Building, Pittsburgh, Pennsylvania. Booklets of information regarding Board requirements and examinations, together with application forms will be sent upon request.

All applications for the year 1944 must be in the Secretary's Office not later than November 15, 1943, ninety days in advance of the Part 1 examination date. Candidates are required to take both the Part 1 and Part 2 examinations. The Part 1 examination consists of the written paper and the submission of twenty-five case history abstracts, and will be conducted on Saturday, February 12, 1944. This examination will be arranged so that the candidate may take it at or near his place of residence. Upon the successful completion of the Part 1 examination, candidates are eligible for the Part 2 examination consisting of a pathology and an oral examination. This is given at the annual meeting of the Board once each year, the time and place of which will be announced later.

The Office of the Surgeon General has issued instructions that men in the service, eligible for Board examinations be encouraged to apply and that they request orders to "detached duty" for the purpose of taking the examinations whenever possible.

DR. CARROLL POUNDERS APPOINTED TO COUNCIL OF SOUTHERN MEDICAL ASSOCIATION

Announcement has been received of the appointment by Dr. W. T. Cotton, Hot Springs, Arkansas, President of the Southern Medical Association, of Dr. Carroll M. Pounders, Oklahoma City, to the Council of the Southern Medical Association as the Oklahoma representative.

Dr. Pounders succeeds Dr. George Osborn of Tulsa who was appointed to fill the unexpired term of the late Dr. Robert Anderson of Shawnee. The By-Laws of the Association provide that a physician may not succeed himself even though he is filling out an unexpired term.

Dr. Pounders is to be complimented upon his appointment.

DEPARTMENT OF AGRICULTURE STUDYING POST-WAR HEALTH PROBLEMS

The Post-War Planning Committee of the South Central Region, (Texas, Louisiana, Oklahoma and Arkansas), of the Department of Agriculture has appointed a Sub-Committee on Health which is designed to study the health needs of the farmer in the post-war era.

At a meetnig of the Sub-Committee held in Dallas, Texas on June 22, medical, dental and agricultural representatives from the four states were called together to discuss health problems.

Representing Oklahoma were C. R. Rountree, M.D., President-Elect, H. A. Shoemaker, M.D., Acting Dean of the Medical School and Mr. R. H. Graham, Executive Secretary of the Association.

At the meeting, representatives of the Department of Agriculture pointed out that the average yearly farm income, ranging from the western to the eastern boundary of the region, varied from $1,200.00 to $250.00 per family of five. The income fluctuation obviously reflects the type of medical care purchasable by the family.

During the past two years the Department of Agriculture has developed, in seven counties located in six states, experimental plans of medical care wherein each farm family pays a total of $54.00 a year for complete medical, dental and hospital care. The family may choose the physician or dentist and the patient-physician relationship is maintained without the intervention of a third party.

An interesting feature of these experimental plans is the method by which payments to the plan are made by the families. The family is assessed six per cent of its annual income and should this assessment not amount to $54.00, the balance is paid by the Department of Agriculture as a subsidy.

The success of the experimental plans was reported to have met with a variance of success but, in the main, to have been satisfactory where there was complete understanding and cooperation between the participating agencies and the individuals. Fees for professional services were in all instances set by the local county medical society.

Coming in for a part of the discussion was the problem concerning hospital and diagnostic facilities in rural communities. In this field there was a wide variance of statistics and statements which generally tended to point out that these facilities were in ratio to population and economic condition that made their existence warrantable.

No definite conclusions or recommendations were made by the Sub-Committee, it being agreed that further study was necessary.

PREPAID MEDICAL-SURGICAL COMMITTEE MEETS

Dr. John Burton, Oklahoma City, Chairman of the Prepaid Medical and Surgical Committee, has announced that preliminary work concerning a prepaid program were considered by his committee at a meeting held in Oklahoma City on July 15.

The Committee, composed of Dr. Burton; Dr. V. C. Tisdal, Elk City; Dr. W. Floyd Keller, Oklahoma City; Dr. A. S. Risser, Blackwell; Dr. H. C. Weber, Bartlesville; Dr. Finis W. Ewing, Muskogee; Dr. A. W. Pigford, Tulsa and Dr. Ben W. Ward, Tulsa, will now submit the preliminary plan to the Association's attorney for legal interpretation.

The plan, to be operated in cooperation with the Blue Cross Hospital Plan, will incorporate features of other successfully sponsored plans by medical associations in making available to low-income groups a facility for budgeting for their illnesses.

As has repeatedly been pointed out, the success of such undertakings depends upon the full cooperation of the medical profession.

The Journal will carry the Committee's report as soon as it is available.

DR. CLINTON GALLAHER NAMED CHAIRMAN OF ADVISORY COMMITTEE PUBLIC WELFARE DEPARTMENT

Dr. Clinton Gallaher of Shawnee was elected Chairman of the Medical Advisory Committee to the Aid to Dependent Children's Fund at a meeting of the Committee held in Oklahoma City on July 11. Dr. Gallaher has been a member of the Committee since its inception and succeeds Dr. C. R. Rountree, Oklahoma City.

The Committee which has made an outstanding record according to Mr. Jess Harper, Director of the Public Welfare Commission, has reviewed 2,661 cases submitted for examination with reference to the physical or mental eligibility of the applicant for asistance from the Aid to Dependent Children's Fund.

Other members of the Committee are Dr. R. M. Shepard, Tulsa, Dr. Walker Morledge, Oklahoma City,

Dr. Hugh M. Gallbraith, Oklahoma City and Dr. C. R. Rountree, Oklahoma City. Dr. Alfred A. Sugg, who recently resigned, has as yet not been replaced.

All Committee members serve without compensation.

• OBITUARIES •

CALVIN EDWARD BRADLEY, M.D.
1885-1943

Dr. C. E. Bradley, Tulsa, died at his home on July 6 after an illness of several weeks.

After receiving his medical education at Barnes Medical College in St. Louis, Dr. Bradley entered practice in Oklahoma in 1911. During the World War No. I he entered the service and was with the American and the British abroad. For gallantry under fire, he was decorated by the British Army.

After the war, Dr. Bradley returned to Tulsa and resumed his work, becoming a prominent pediatrician in state medical circles. He was active in the interests of organized medicine and medical legislation and, as a result, was appointed on the State Board of Medical Examiners and was serving on the Board at the time of his death.

The passing of Dr. Bradley takes from the profession a tireless worker in the interests of organized medicine and a leading figure in the field of pediatrics.

H. B. WILSON, M.D.
1858-1943

Dr. H. B. Wilson of Wynnewood, born January 25, 1858 in North Carolina, died at his home May 1, 1943.

After graduating from Vanderbilt University in 1893, Dr. Wilson did postgraduate work at the University of Chicago and at Tulane, specializing in surgery. In 1903 he established the first hospital in southern Oklahoma at Wynnewood. Dr. Wilson was the first counselor of the Seventh District and organized every County Medical Society in this District. He was a prominent layman in the Methodist Church and active in the Masonic Lodge. He was an honorary member of the State and American Medical Associations.

Dr. Wilson was buried under Masonic auspices on May 2, 1943.

Classified Advertisements

A Welcome to American Doctors

Australians in every part of the Commonwealth have been encouraged and strengthened in their resolution to bring defeat upon the enemy by the news that members of the American armed forces are arriving in this country in considerable numbers. Americans have been schooled in the same tradition as ourselves, they speak the same language, have the same love of freedom and the same purpose for the future. Every American unit has its medical personnel, and American doctors share with Australian doctors the same ideals in science and the practice of medicine. In the name of the medical profession of Australia we welcome to our shores the medical officers of America's fighting forces. Among the medical officers of the Royal Australian Navy, of the Australian Army Medical Corps, and of the Royal Australian Air Force, and among civilian medical practitioners the Americans will find comrades and collaborators.—The Medical Journal of Australia.

A WORD FROM THE WISE

"Any reorganization of the medical profession that threatens the personal bond between doctor and patient is to be viewed with suspicion, even if the object appears at first sight to be more thorough and careful practice. With the exception of the relationship that one may have with a member of one's family, or with the priest, there is no human bond that is closer than that between physician and patient (or patient's family), and attempts to substitute the methods of machine or organization, be they ever so efficient, are bound to fail.

"Even the most forward-looking medical man must admit that for a long time to come, the main function of the medical profession will be to heal, relieve and comfort those who are sick or in distress, and plans which are devised to readjust the relationship between doctors and laymen must be based primarily on this consideration. New needs and opportunities are to be recognized and met as well as possible, but the chief thing is to be certain that in the name of the newer "Service" with its capital "S," nothing of the old-fashioned, modest but effective service of doctor to patient is lost."—Doctor and Patient by Francis W. Peabody, M.D.

The medical profession deserves the grateful recognition and regard of all other callings in modern life. It has always insisted that the practice of medicine is a profession and not a trade. Trade is occupation for livelihood; profession is occupation for the service of the world. Trade is occupation for joy of the result; profession is occupation for joy in the process. Trade is occupation where anybody may enter; profession is occupation where only those who are prepared may enter. Trade is occupation taken up temporarily, until something better offers; profession is occupation with which one is identified for life. Trade makes one the rival of every other trader; profession makes one the co-operator with all his colleagues. Trade knows only the ethics of success; profession is bound by lasting ties of sacred honor.—President Faunce, of Brown University, in an address to the Rhode Island Medical Society, 1905.

THE GREAT PHYSICIAN

Hans Zinsser said of Francis W. Peabody "Yet as one thinks of him in retrospect, appraising him as a physician, one becomes more and more convinced that his great significance for American medicine sprang from those very qualities which endeared him in his personal relations, applied to and interwoven with his professional life. Intellectual and emotional sanity and integrity, from which wisdom, kindness and courtesy are derived, were the natural endowments which brought him distinction as a human being and which gave him an importance for American medicine possessed by very few of his contemporaries.

"In the history of medicine there are many names associated with the discovery of facts, with learned treatises and with technical achievements of one kind or another; there are relatively few of whom we think especially as physicians in the sense in which this word is used in regard to Suydenham, for instance. It is a rare blending of learning and humanity, incisiveness of intellect and sensitiveness of the spirit, which occasionally come together to an individual who chooses the calling of Medicine; and then we have the great physician."—Doctor and Patient by Francis W. Peabody, M.D.

My concern is not whether God is on our side; my great concern is to be on God's side.—Lincoln.

We can do anything we want to do if we stick to it long enough.—Helen Keller

TANKS A MILLION

Tanks a million is our Uncle Sammy's cry,
And tanks a million shall be our reply,
    There's more to go in them than just iron and steel:
    Loyalty, honor, American zeal.
We'll scrap fears and hatreds, pack sands of desire,
Political differences melt in the fire,
    The Wronged and Oppressed carry such an appeal
    To our standards and rights, our hearts they anneal.
Our Open Hearth fires warm the world with their flame.
Molding armor and men with stout heart and frame,
    Patterned by heroes of pioneer devotion
    From mountain and valley and ocean to ocean.
When they arrive at the line of inspection,
They are headed unswerving in one firm direction
    O'er barbed wires of treachery, barriers of dictators,
    Reducing mock idols to eloquent craters.
We'll heave to our task, and slack not a minute,
Keep them rolling along, put all we've got in it.
    We'll work night and day, buy bonds by the billion.
    To our own Uncle Sam! Here's tanks a million!
(Taken from The Journal of the Indiana State Medical Association, August, 1942, Page 441.)

A Call to Colors

The doctor who remains at home and cares for the sick people there will suffer the real strain of this war. It is necessary to see that the armed forces are furnished with the necessary complement of doctors, whether or not the other responsibilities of the government in such particulars are met fully. That is so because the armed forces will be, presumably and at any time, in a position where they cannot supplement their supply of doctors. They must be able to take care of something like the anticipated peak load at any time.

There has been some criticism of the demand of the Army for six doctors per 1,000 soldiers. That is not a fair criticism, and for the reason just stated. At that, quite possibly the armed forces will not at any time be supplied with medical service one hundred percent. We must remember, in this connection, that it is the Army and Navy which will be primarily concerned in winning the war, and if the war is not won, the lot of the people and their need for medical service will be deplorable, indeed, and that is not to say that the role to be played by the people at home is not important. Indeed, the contrary is true. The people must, through extra endeavor and sacrifice, support the Army in the field, something the Army cannot do for itself.—Texas State J. Med., June '42.

"SUNLIGHT" VITAMIN FOR NAVY

The officers of the new battleship, U. S. S. New Jersey, intend to see to it that the health of its personnel will never suffer through lack of sunlight.

In addition to guns and all the other instruments of destruction, orders have been placed for installation of constructive health-giving ultraviolet ray apparatus that will "shoot" the vitamin D of sunshine into the men. The information comes from the Hanovia Chemical and Manufacturing Co., with the permission of the Navy Department, Washington, D. C. For the first time, ultraviolet sunbaths will be made available to the entire personnel of one of our battleships.

Three group solarium-type ultraviolet lamps and two smaller solarium units are being placed aboard the New Jersey. They are being set up below decks especially to serve men who would be otherwise denied much of the natural benefits of sunshine; in addition the lamps will be used in the sick bays.

United States and British submarine crews have for some time been provided with ultraviolet irradiation, as have the workers in many blacked-out British factories where it has been found helpful in reducing absenteeism, according to Frederick W. Robinson, Hanovia's director of research. Similar lamps are specified for the newest aircraft carriers.

More Doctors Needed For the Armed Forces*

At a conference of the Directing Board of the Procurement and Assignment Service for Physicians, Dentists and Veterinarians, held on July 31 with the War Participation Committee of the American Medical Association and in the presence of Mr. Paul V. McNutt, chairman of the War Manpower Commission, and representatives of the Army and Navy medical departments and the Public Health Service, it became apparent that the medical profession must produce toward the winning of the war an additional six thousand physicians for the armed forces before Jan. 1, 1944. Pursuant to a realization of this objective a directive has gone to the generals in command of the various service commands authorizing them to induct into the service physicians between the ages of 38 and 45 who have been declared available by the Directing Board of the Procurement and Assignment Service for Physicians, Dentists and Veterinarians and who are otherwise subject to Selective Service.

The needs of the armed forces are real. The members of the War Participation Committee raised with the representatives of the various governmental agencies all the questions that have from time to time challenged the need; the challenge seems to have been met effectively. Indeed, the intimation was made clear that the needs of the armed forces will be met by specific regulations of the Selective Service Administration or the enactment of necessary legislation if required. All physicians up to 45 years of age who have been indicated as available have therefore placed on them now the responsibility for an immediate decision as to their enlistment with the armed forces. The need is so positive that questions of essentiality of men in positions of teaching and research and in industrial medicine are likely to be rigidly reviewed in the near fu-

6,000 MORE PHYSICIANS NEEDED NOW!

ture with a view to extracting from civilian life every one that can be spared.

As the war continues and intensifies, new needs for the services of the medical profession become apparent. An army in motion and one engaged in the kind of aggressive combat that now concerns our armed forces needs physicians in even greater numbers than have heretofore been demanded. Many thousands of interned aliens and prisoners are now the burden of the United States and must be given medical care.

If there is any physician who still hesitates under these circumstances, he should realize the added advantage to him of accepting now the commission that is proffered. Should it become necessary in the near future, as seems quite likely, to enlist new activity by the Selective Service Administration and the Officers' Procurement Service to bring in the six thousand physicians that are so certainly required, those recruited by that technic will inevitably begin their service with the minimum commission that is offered, namely that of first lieutenant. Until that technic is installed, the men of special competence and of years beyond those of the recent graduate have the assurance of careful consideration and a commission more nearly in accord with age and experience.

The call here made has the approval of the Directing Board of the Procurement and Assignment Service and of the War Participation Committee of the American Medical Association. The medical profession may well be proud of the fact that it has been the only group given, by directive of the President, the responsibility of maintaining service in civilian life and at the same time supplying the needs of the armed forces. Let us not fail in meeting fully the trust that has been placed upon us.

*Reprinted from The Journal of the American Medical Association, Saturday, August 7, 1943

★ *FIGHTIN' TALK* ★

The following is an excerpt from a letter received from *Captain L. S. Morgan*, Ponca City, now stationed at the Santa Ana Army Air Base at Santa Ana, California:

"When I entered the Army Air Corps on September 29, with my bright and shining uniform and headed for the Army Air Base at Santa Ana, California, I was overflowing with the spirit of adventure, and the usual amount of patriotism. I immediately was enrolled in the Officer's School, for indoctrination. The course lasted four weeks, and finished off with a five day bivouac in the San Bernardino mountains near Lake Arrowhead, which specialized in five and six mile packs, under full pack up broken mountain trails. It was a question of survival of the fittest and fortunately, I survived. Many others took the ambulance route back to camp, much to their humiliation. At the completion of the Officer's School, I was presented with another sheepskin, to add to my collection.

"There are two things uppermost in the minds of all Medical Officers, as I have found it. These two questions are, 'Will I be sent overseas?' and 'When will I receive a promotion?' The answer to the first question is in the lap of the Gods. The answer to the second is just about as uncertain, although the answer can best be illustrated through an example. Two Medical Officers were discussing promotions. One asked the other, 'Which has the most rapid promotions, the Army or the Army Air Corps?' The second officer said, 'In the Army they will tell you promotions are more rapid in the Air Corps and in the Army Air Corps, they will tell you promotions are most rapid in the Army,' so I conclude they are not rapid in either branch of the service, which stands correct."

Moorman P. Prosser, Norman, was recently made a Major at Camp Gruber, Muskogee, and is Chief of Neuropsychiatry at the Station Hospital there.

Captain Chas. G. Stuard, Tulsa, is stationed at Jefferson Barracks, St. Louis. He recently passed the American Board of Ophthalmology.

Major Hervey A. Foerster, Oklahoma City, stationed at Camp Maxey, Brownwood, says that he believes he is the highest ranking major in the Army, having served two and one-half years on June 27, as a major.

Lieutenant Marvin Elkins, Muskogee, is Ward Surgeon at the Station Hospital in Camp Maxey.

Major Francis Dill, Oklahoma City, United States Public Health Service, has been recently transferred to Camp Maxey from Abilene, Texas and is the head of the Paris-LaMar County Health Unit at Paris, Texas.

Colonel R. N. Holcombe, Muskogee, is now stationed at Camp Ellis, Illinois, at Headquarters of the Medical Group of the Army Service Forces Unit Training Center.

After several months on the desert, *Captain Floyd T. Bartheld* has been assigned to the 2nd Battalion, 64th Regiment at Camp Bowie, Texas.

The following is taken from a letter received from *Major E. Rankin Denny*, Tulsa. Major Denny is stationed in Camp McCoy, Wisconsin at the Office of the Medical Sub-Section, Hospital Branch.

"Day before yesterday I had a birthday. It ended my first year as Chief of the Medical Service at Station Hospital, Camp McCoy, and what an experience! I can say that I have seen more mumps than 90 per cent of the men in civil life see in an entire lifetime. Now that doesn't sound very interesting but as most of the physicians know, there is a tremendous amount of research work going on now on mumps, particularly in immunology, and I prognosticate that the time is not too far distant when mumps will be a preventive disease. The most interesting phase of the study of this group of cases has been the complications which have arisen, namely encephalitis. It is called meningo-encephalitis by some although there is relatively little evidence that the meninges are involved. Some of the cases of mumps encephalitis occur in individuals who have had mumps in years gone by and the encephalitis is the only manifestation of the disease. Were it not for the fact that these cases were occurring in the presence of an epidemic, I doubt that one would be able to make a correct diagnosis unless we had access to the very best laboratories that are equipped to carry on complement fixation tests of the blood.

"Our camp is fortunately situated in an area where there are a number of fine streams and one small river. Lt. Col. William T. Pugh, a very fine surgeon from Virginia who is the Chief of the Surgical Service here at the Station Hospital is a most expert fisherman and he is at present teaching me the art. I find it most entertaining and an excellent substitute for golf. In fact, I go fishing about three nights a week. The other night I caught a 14-inch trout. (I'm bragging now because I know damn well it was an accident).

"I can truthfully say that this army experience has been an interesting and enlightening one. I have tried to make it more or less a post-graduate course, and although my administrative duties take up more than 50 per cent of my time, I average seeing eight to ten cases a day. The latter, of course, are the unusual and interesting cases and which usually present some problem for diagnosis or disposition."

Lt. Colonel Dan E. Sewell, Oklahoma City, formerly stationed at the Pecos Army Air Base at Pecos, Texas, has been transferred to the Station Hospital at the Kingman Army Air Field, Kingman, Arizona, where his duties are those of Base Surgeon and Senior Flight Surgeon. He reports as follows:

"On arrival here I was pleasantly surprised to find already stationed here Lieutenants Lum Russell and Pat Murphy, both of whom are former University of Oklahoma graduates, Russell being on my surgical service and Murphy being Flight Surgeon.

"A Sunday or two ago I took off and drove over to Needles, California, about seventy miles away and renewed my acquaintance with all the physicians who are now stationed at Needles under the command of Colonel Rex Boland. As is generally known, the weather in Needles is not cool but the boys seem to be taking it in their stride, as well as a few of their wives and children whom I also had the privilege of meeting at that time. It seems that at Needles the next best thing to getting a leave of absence is taking the weekend off and going to Las Vegas, Nevada for a little relaxation."

Captain Edwin M. Harms, Blackwell, enjoyed hearing about his various friends through our news letter and reports from the Army Air Base at Casper, Wyoming:

"My active duty date was August 25, 1942, at which time I was sent to Salt Lake City to the Eighteenth Replacement Wing and there was appointed as the Wing Surgeon for said Wing, and served in this capacity until November 9, when I was relieved of duty there and assigned as Chief of the Eye, Ear, Nose and Throat Service, Station Hospital, Army Air Base, Casper Wyoming. I served in this capacity until May 26, 1943, at which time our Base Surgeon was assigned to Flight School, and in addition to other duties, I was assigned

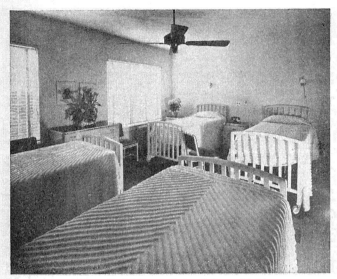

Base Surgeon. Needles to say, I have not had to look for additional work or entertainment. The work has proven most interesting and of a very varied nature."

Captain Floyd Newman, Shattuck, reports that he is still on detached service and is anxious for a boat ride just any time.

Captain Harry Green, Tulsa, is now in charge of dermatology at the Station Hospital, Camp Sibert, Alabama. He has met a "swell bunch of fellows" among the Medical officers there and states that it is more than fair compensation for the lonesome hours when he misses the friends at home and home itself.

Lt. Colonel George Kimball, Tulsa, from somewhere in a nice cool climate, reports that he is working pretty hard but took time out to read our news letter, which he enjoyed.

Captain Jackson Birge, Oklahoma City, is now stationed at Fort Benning Georgia. At present he is Plans and Training Officer and Dispensary Officer. We hear that Captain Birge is really putting out for his Uncle Sam with a lot of hard work. He has been training a lot of medical and surgical technicians to serve as ward men and it is said he is at the top of the list at administration.

Lieutenant R. G. Ray, Tulsa, took the time to drop us a much appreciated note from 'somewhere'.

Lt. Colonel James G. Hughes, who conducted a two-year Postgraduate Course in Pediatrics in the State, reports that he has command of the 225th Station Hospital at Fort Benning, Georgia. Lt. Colonel Hughes says "I'd like more than anything to hear from some of those docs all around the State, but I suppose they're too tied up with their increased work during war time to write much."

Lt. W. B. Newell, Jr., Enid, has proudly informed us that he has a new baby girl, Cynthia Ann Newell, born in Las Vegas, New Mexico on February 25.

Captain George T. Allen, formerly of Oklahoma City, is now stationed at Biggs Field, El Paso, Texas.

Lt. (sg) Frank Woods, Oklahoma City, President of the Oklahoma University Medical School Class of 1935, is located at the Naval Recruiting Office at Jacksonville, Florida.

25 YEARS AGO

JOURNAL, August, 1918

NEW ARMY NEEDS FROM OUR PROFESSION

Four months ago the Surgeon General's office indicated there would be needed immediately 8,000 physicians to equalize the needs of the 800,000 registrants to be called in 1918. This estimate was shortly thereafter reduced to 5,000. Almost immediately the country was electrified by the statement that we "now have more than half a million men in France." Soon the mark reached a million. Every great railway line running across the country bore evidence that there was a constant stream of trained men going to the seaboard for embarkation and coincidentally with the superactivity the Provost Marshal General began his insistent calls for thousands of new men to take the places of those who were leaving the cantonments; these calls came in such rapid succession as to amaze people who had not noticed the work particularly before. In many places Class 1 was exhausted by them.

This preliminary statement is made to show the impossibility of anyone trying to guage the demands of the Medical Department for medical men. We thought we needed the 8,000, but as a matter of fact that 800,000 that we were to have called out leisurely in 1918 has

probably long been sucked into the rapidly expanding and hungry maw of our training camps and when we have case up our figures at the end of the year we will likely find that 3,000,000 for all Army branches will be nearer the number than the first estimate.

To meet this demand we must place more medical men in the field than we ever thought would be needed. Already the number runs far above twenty thousand (estimate) and the American Medical Association, which has completed an exhaustive, grass-roots survey of the situation, believes that we will be called to furnish approximately 40,000 men before we are through with the war if the ratio of men to the number of soldiers in service is maintained as heretofore.

They are now formulating the suggestion to all county organizations to secure at least 20 per cent of their registered practitioners for the service.

A survey has already been made of our State's resources in this respect or is being made, and we should soon know approximately how many men have gone from each county, how many are left and of those how many probably can be spared.

It is suggested that no locality should, unless clearly oversupplied, send more than 50 per cent of its practitioners, for it must not be overlooked that the civilian population at home, after we have an army of five million in France, will approximate more than one hundred million people and they must necessarily have medical attention or the suffering will be incalculable. We have some localities heretofore oversupplied with physicians, but as a rule the rural districts have had localities where there were not enough. Obviously such districts as the latter should be very carefully approached and the committees having charge of the consideration of ways and means should make their suggestions square with the facts and needs of each community. It has been said that some one with supposed authority has promised to send physicians to localities needing them. It must be said right here now that it is a practical impossibility and was a promise made with little knowledge or study of the situation. The rural community now deprived of its physicians will remain in that estate until the war ends, for the attractive lure of the cities will take those who can move, so it follows that the first and severe demands should be made on the cities where hospitals and centralized population makes it easier for physicians to centralize and systematize their work in such manner that they may, in the aggregate, do twice or thrice the work they formerly did. We have remaining in Oklahoma many men who by a little stretch of management could arrange their affairs to make the sacrifice entailed on entering the service of their country. These men should now prepare to answer the call soon to be made on them. We should not forget that the most important thing confronting the free peoples of the world today is winning the war and the efforts toward building up private practices and furthering selfish and personal ends must be relegated until the most important work is finished. Unless we win the war physicians may well look forward to conditions of impoverishment, taxation rates undreamed of and possibly such impossible interference with the intimate and personal affairs of the American family life as to make our lives unbearable.

The only thing we have to suggest in this matter is that each physician must be the sole judge of whether he should go or not, but the man who can go and trumps up this and that trivial excuse for not going is soon likely to become a mark for derision from his fellow man.

Personal News—JOURNAL, August, 1918

Dr. Lea A. Riely, Oklahoma City, has been made a Captain in the Medical Reserve.

Dr. H. T. Ballantine, 1st Lieutenant, M. R. C., Muskogee, was ordered to report for duty August 5.

Dr. A. C. Hirshfield, Oklahoma City, has been commissioned in the Medical Reserve Corps. He has already seen service, having been attached to surgical units in both the Russian Navy and Army earlier in the war.

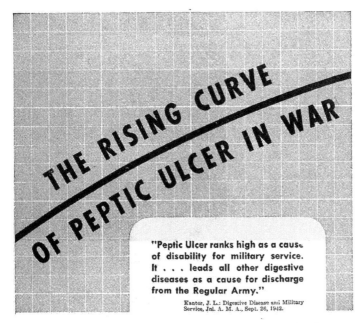

THE RISING CURVE OF PEPTIC ULCER IN WAR

"Peptic Ulcer ranks high as a cause of disability for military service. It . . . leads all other digestive diseases as a cause for discharge from the Regular Army."

Kantor, J. L.: Digestive Disease and Military Service, Jnl. A. M. A., Sept. 26, 1942.

THE increased incidence of peptic ulcer among the armed forces, defense workers and civilians today confronts medicine as a major problem.

Of the various types of therapy used to control this problem none has proved itself more valuable than CREAMALIN, brand of aluminum hydroxide gel.

CREAMALIN, the first aluminum hydroxide gel to be made available to physicians, was also the first to be Council-accepted. CREAMALIN contains approximately 5.5% aluminum hydroxide.

Therapeutic Effects of CREAMALIN

CREAMALIN
Brand of Aluminum Hydroxide Gel

REG. U. S. PAT. OFF.

- Pronounced antacid action of 12 times its volume of N/10 HCl in less than 30 minutes (Toepfer's reagent)
- Prolonged action in contrast to fleeting effect of alkalies
- Non-alkaline; non-absorbable; non-toxic
- No acid rebound; no danger of alkalosis

- Prompt and continuous pain relief in uncomplicated cases
- Rapid healing when used with regular ulcer regimen
- Mildly astringent; may reduce digestive action, thus favor clot formation
- Demulcent; gelatinous consistency affords protective coating to ulcer

Modern non-alkaline therapy for peptic ulcer and gastric hyperacidity

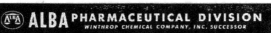

ALBA PHARMACEUTICAL DIVISION
WINTHROP CHEMICAL COMPANY, INC. SUCCESSOR

NEW YORK, N. Y.
WINDSOR, ONT.

WOMAN'S AUXILIARY NEWS

The following excerpt is from an article "Progress of the Woman's Auxiliary to the American Medical Association 1942-43" which appeared in the Bulletin of the Woman's Auxiliary to the American Medical Association.

"Temporary expedients are sometimes necessary to meet emergencies, but let us not forget that such expedients should be temporary; let us not be beguiled into believing that a temporary change in direction should take the place of a permanent service which has proven its worth. Every citizen of this Republic should recognize this principle for the problems of the professions are essentially the problems of America. We all belong to one Commonwealth, which has prospered and grown strong by united effort.

"The Woman's Auxiliary, remembering its purpose, has striven to make its contribution to the war effort within the Auxiliary, rather than outside of it. Not one among you but has given time to one, perhaps several, of such organizations developed to meet a specific need. In many instances such organizations may have seemed to pale the importance of any peace-time endeavor, and this is right, to a certain extent, but so surely as day follows night, peace must come again and we shall be called for an accounting. The trend of thought in post-war planning envisions health as an important factor in our changing social evolution.

"The voice of organization must not be silenced or even dimmed if it is to be heard in the aftermath of war—that day when the men in our armed forces come back to the kind of America for which they have been fighting.

"There must surely appear issues to be decided and no doubt the status of medicine fixed for a long time to come. If we remember this fact in our united strength, we shall have performed a noble service in at least one of the Four Freedoms our men are fighting for. Each of these freedoms must find application at home as well as abroad to be worth the gaining. One of our greatest obligations today is to realize that our responsibilities are not light in 1943. We must have the stamina to apply our high principles to our everyday life, in order to use our forsight to prepare for a future society. So far no way has presented itself which seems so certain of results as keeping the identity of the Auxiliary in all our war effort, and your President earnestly recommends that this means be employed with even greater intensity.

"During the first half of the year, when travelling conditions were not nearly so impracticable as they have since become, engagements in almost every section of the country were fulfilled. There were many and frequent occasions for pride in the way adverse conditions were being met and overcome, It has not been without inconvenience and sacrifice that many of our smaller Auxiliaries have continued to remain organized.

"What more valiant service could we, as Auxiliary members, render than to continue to direct our efforts toward the advancement of health education? The year is well on its way, but, nevertheless, there is still much time ahead to profit by the reports and objectives set forth in this issue of the Bulletin. The foregoing articles, taken together, form therefore a report of progress of the Auxiliary as a nationwide organization concerned with a multiplicity of problems of state and national importance. A more comprehensive report will be given at our annual session.

"This year countless hours of voluntary service to the Red Cross have been given by our members in Nutrition, First-Aid, Civilian Defense, Nurses' Aide and Motor Corps. The Doctors' Aide Corps, which orginated in Atlanta, Georgia, in August, 1942, with the endorsement of their Advisory Council, is having wide-spread interest throughout the States.

"No radical changes of policy or program were planned or attempted, as it was the opinion of our Advisory Council that effective progress could be attained to conservative tradition, making such temporary changes as wartime needs demand.

"Copies of revisions of the By-Laws were not printed, as this Committee asked for alloted time in which to make further changes it deemed necessary. These when printed, along with the Handbook, will be in the Central Office for distribution.

"The year has been filled with unpredictable changes, due to the war emergency, but your President has found this busy year interesting indeed. While the accomplishment of plans and objectives has necessarily been turned temporarily to war work in its many branches, our various departments of health education have not been neglected, as the reports of our Hygeia, Program, Public Relations and Legislation will show. In this field of endeavor our members give their services to their country in the line for which they have been trained and fitted.

"The establishment of a Central Office in Chicago last May, with an efficiently trained secretary, who edits our quarterly Bulletin, secures subscriptions, sends renewal notices and attends to the many routine duties of Auxiliary work, has justified the long range planning by our Board of Directors. This has given your President more time in which to make wider contacts through the demands of other organizations.

"The purpose of the Bulletin (which is self-sustaining even in this war emergency) is purely an informative pamphlet, without thought of expansion into broader fields of journalism. It is to be hoped our entire membership will recognize the value of the Bulletin and subscribe to it annually. This is essential for our progress to a unified, informed membership.

"In carrying out the policies of the national organization, there has been the fullest cooperation on the part of the President-elect, Mrs. Eben J. Carey. Particularly does your President extend appreciation to each officer, to the separate chairman and to the Central Office secretary, who have served so faithfully during uncommon difficulties. A special message of gratitude is sent to the State Presidents, who have had to meet the exigencies of the times with fortitude, and to the Advisory Council whose assistance has been untiring, timely and invaluable.

"What double measure then is the appreciation of your President, since this message must take the place of a warmer, more personal expression of thanks. Only through this printed message will she be able to tell you how gratifying has been the knowledge that you have each measured up to the ideals of the Auxiliary. Together we have given serious and concerted thought to filling our places in the medical world in a way to preserve our usefulness to both our husbands and to our country. The keeping of roll-call up to a high peak and the performance of all public work within the Auxiliary roster are, and shall remain, our aims."

Health may be restored and life prolonged if the public is educated to seek early diagnosis and treatment of abnormalities of the urinary tract—Maurice Meltzer, M.D., New York, declares in a recent issue of Hygeia, The Health Magazine.

Every man owes some of his time to the upbuilding of the profession to which he belongs.—Theodore Roosevelt.

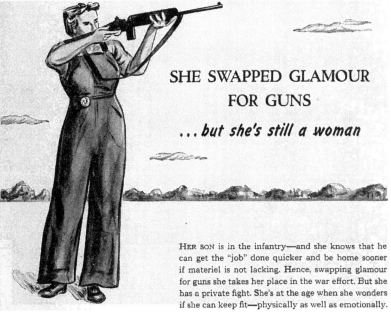

Blue Cross Reports

The threat of Federal legislation to include hospital and medical care on a compulsory basis, has again made its appearance. This time in the form of a bill submitted by Senator Wagner of Illinois, to both Houses of Congress on June 3, 1943 .

This bill, except for minor details, is the same as that submitted previously by Elliott of Massachusetts and Green of Rhode Island. In all cases, the proposed bill was written by the Social Security Board, sponsored by its chairman, Mr. Altmeyer.

In his radio talk on July 28, Mr. Roosevelt made reference to this subject, however, with slightly different application. It is probably reasonable to assume that the general application was inferred.

On previous occasions the Blue Cross Plan has made several mailings to the employers and civic leaders in Oklahoma regarding this subject. At this time we are mailing 2,000 copies of an article which appeared in "Business Week" on July 10. This article urges the cooperation of the employers with the Blue Cross Plans in order that what is being proposed by Federal legislation might be accomplished by individual enterprise on a voluntary basis. In three or four weeks we are also going to mail 2,000 copies of an article which appeared in "Hospitals", written by Dr. C. Rufus Rorem, Commissioner for the Blue Cross Plans in Chicago. This article is very specific in its analysis of this bill and we hope that it will be well read.

On part occasions in sending out literature on this subject, there has been little response, perhaps because most employers are today very busy with many problems caused by the present emergency. However, it seems that the interest in Washington on this subject is being accelerated. If we are to maintain a free health system in our country, there must be a general understanding among hospitals, doctors and business men, and there must be a coordinated effort on the part of all of us, or we shall find ourselves with a 12 per cent payroll tax right in our lap and it will be too late to do anything about it.

Says Many More Accurate Surveys of Vitamin Deficiency Needed

A survey of approximately 400 consecutive patients admitted to the clinic wards of Stanford University Hospital with reference to inadequate diet and signs of vitamin deficiency showed that approximately one-fourth had been taking an inadequate diet but the occurrence of clinical signs of vitamin deficiency was very low, Marcus A. Krupp, M.D., San Francisco, reports in The Journal of the American Medical Association for August 29. Of those with inadequate diets, only 11.4 percent showed definite signs of vitamin deficiency. Only two instances of clinical vitamin deficiency were detected among 297 patients with adequate diets and in the entire group the incidence of definite vitamin deficiency disease was 3.1 percent. Dr. Krupp says that the survey shows that even with a serious disease, such as cancer, deficiency disease does not readily supervene provided the diet remains adequate.

"Recent surveys of vitamin deficiency disease," he explains, "have on the whole shown a disturbingly high incidence. Most of these reports have been made by careful, well trained investigators, and the results seem dependable. However, it is important to take into account the locality in which the survey is made, the particular population group and the criteria for diagnosis. Some of the statements made in the lay press, on the other hand, must be interpreted with caution, such as those claiming that 50 percent of the employees in a certain factory in southern California had clearcut evidence of one or more sorts of vitamin deficiency. It is on this account that many more accurate surveys should be made in various parts of the country. . . ."

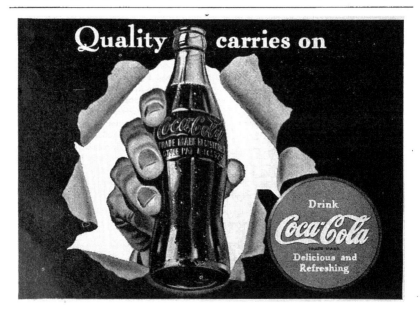

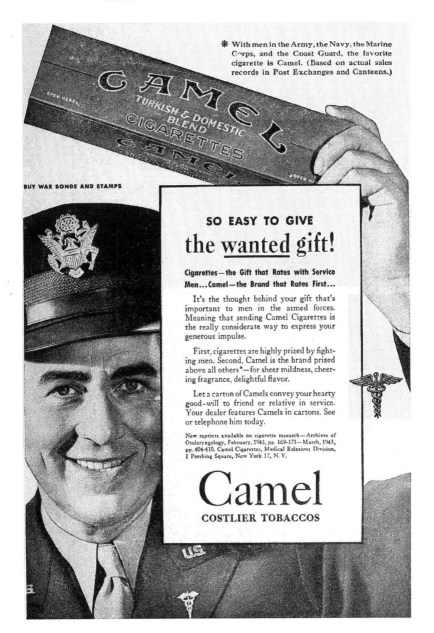

* With men in the Army, the Navy, the Marine Corps, and the Coast Guard, the favorite cigarette is Camel. (Based on actual sales records in Post Exchanges and Canteens.)

BUY WAR BONDS AND STAMPS

SO EASY TO GIVE
the wanted gift!

Cigarettes—the Gift that Rates with Service Men...Camel—the Brand that Rates First...

It's the thought behind your gift that's important to men in the armed forces. Meaning that sending Camel Cigarettes is the really considerate way to express your generous impulse.

First, cigarettes are highly prized by fighting men. Second, Camel is the brand prized above all others*—for sheer mildness, cheering fragrance, delightful flavor.

Let a carton of Camels convey your hearty good-will to friend or relative in service. Your dealer features Camels in cartons. See or telephone him today.

New reprints available on cigarette research—Archives of Otolaryngology, February, 1943, pp. 169-173—March, 1943, pp. 404-410. Camel Cigarettes, Medical Relations Division, 1 Pershing Square, New York 17, N. Y.

Camel
COSTLIER TOBACCOS

360

University of Oklahoma School of Medicine

Dr. Donald B. McMullen, Associate Professor of Hygiene and Public Health and Associate Professor of Bacteriology, has been selected by the Committee on the Teaching of Tropical Medicine of the Association of American Medical Colleges to go to Central America for the month of September to observe methods of tropical disease control. Dr. McMullen will spend about three weeks at a United Fruit Company Hospital and at least a week with the local field unit of the Office of the Coordinator of the Inter-American Affairs. He will make the trip by Pan-American Airways.

Dr. Tom Lowry, Dean, attended the conference of Public Health Divisions in Dallas on Wednesday, July 14, in regard to the poliomyelitis situation in the Southwest.

Dr. H. R. Bennett of Warm Springs, Georgia a representative of the National Foundation for Infantile Paralysis, Inc., is visiting the School and Hospitals in connection with the poliomyelitis situation in this state.

Two wards of the Oklahoma Hospital for Crippled Children have been set aside for the use of poliomyelitis cases. Dr. Charles M. Bielstein, formerly Resident in Pediatrics, University Hospitals, has been appointed Medical Advisor of the Oklahoma Commission for Crippled Children and he is working with Dr. Carroll M. Pounders and Dr. D. H. O'Donoghue who are in direct charge of the poliomyelitis cases in the hospital.

The Naval Specialized Training Unit was activated in the School of Medicine July 1, 1943. Captain J. F. Donelson is the Commanding Officer of the Naval Unit composed of 56 medical students.

A large house at 1407 North Phillips Street has been purchased for the purpose of housing the nurses of the University and Crippled Children's Hospitals. It is to be used as an annex to the present nurses' home and will be occupied when repairs are completed.

Miss Elizabeth Fair has resigned her position as Educational Director of the School of Nursing.

Dr. Samuel A. Corson has resigned his position as Assistant Professor of Physiology.

Miss Dorothy Armstrong has resigned her position as Assistant Librarian effective August 5, Miss Armstrong will take up work along similar lines in California.

HIS OLD FATHER SATISFIED

"Twenty years ago (*Note: now fifty years ago*) a discouraged young doctor in one of our large cities was visited once by his old father who came up from a rural district to look after his boy.

"Well, son" he said, "how are you getting along?"

"I'm not getting along at all," was the disheartened answer. "I'm not doing a thing."

"The old man's countenance fell, but he spoke of courage and patience and perseverance. Later in the day he went with his son to the "Free Dispensary," where the young doctor had an unsalaried position, and where he spent an hour or more every day.

"The father sat by, a silent but intensely interested spectator, while twenty-five poor unfortunates received help. The doctor forgot his visitor while he bent his skilled energies to this task, but hardly had the door closed on the last patient when the old man burst forth:

"I thought you told me that you were not doing anything. Why, if I helped twenty-five people in a month as much as you have in one morning, I would thank God that my life counted for something."

"There isn't any money in it, though," explained the son, somewhat abashed.

"Money!" the old man shouted, still scornfully. "Money! What is money in comparison with being of use to your fellow-men? Never mind about the money; you go right along at this work every day. I'll go back to the farm and gladly earn money enough to support you as long as I live—yes, and sleep sound every night with the thought that I have helped you to help your fellow-men."—National Magazine.

ANY PHYSICIAN MAY EXHIBIT "WHEN BOBBY GOES TO SCHOOL" TO THE PUBLIC

Under the rules laid down by the American Academy of Pediatrics, their educational-to-the-public film, "When Bobby Goes to School," may be exhibited to the public by any licensed physician in the United States.

All that is required is that he obtain the endorsement by any officer of his county medical society. Endorsement blanks for this purpose may be obtained on application to the distributor, Mead Johnson & Company, Evansville, Indiana.

Such endorsement, however, is not required for showings by licensed physicians to medical groups for the purpose of familiarizing them with the message of the film in advance of public showings in the community.

"When Bobby Goes to School" is a 16-mm. sound film, free from advertising, dealing with the health appraisal of the school child, and may be borrowed without charge or obligation on application to the distributor, Mead Johnson & Company, Evansville, Indiana.

Dangers Of Botulism In Home Canning Are Pointed Out By the Journal

The dangers of botulism, particularly during the coming home canning season when many persons who never before attempted home canning will be preserving garden produce, are pointed out by The Journal of the American Medical Association for April 17. The Journal says:

"Meyer and his associates in California have gathered statistics on 367 outbreaks of botulism in the United States since 1899. Only 83 of the outbreaks have been due to commercially canned foodstuffs; with one possible exception, outbreaks have not occurred in nearly twenty years from this source. The other 284 outbreaks have been caused by foods canned in the home. The total cases of the disease for the forty-three years numbered 1,052 with 687 deaths, a fatality rate of 65 per cent. How many other unrecognized cases have occurred is unknown. During the coming canning season many persons who never before attempted home canning will preserve garden produce. The danger from botulism is ever present unless proper precautions are taken. Faust, discussing methods of home canning, emphasizes the necessity of the pressure cooker with an accurate gage or thermometer for nonacid foods, such as string beans and corn. Any such foods that have been processed in any other manner must be reboiled for at least fifteen minutes before tasting or using. Any home canned food that shows the slightest evidence of spoilage should not even be tasted, for the toxin of the botulinus bacillus is the most powerful poison known. The problem calls for concerted effort by agricultural advisers and public health personnel in warning against faulty methods of home canning and alertness of physicians in recognizing symptoms and administering antitoxin early and in adequate amounts."

Dr. Philip Levine of Newark, N. J., announced to the Congress on Obstetrics and Gynecology the discovery of a new factor in the red blood cells which accounts for hundreds of infant deaths before or soon after birth. It is a mysterious substance which makes babies poison their mothers and, in a reaction, kill themselves. The principal use of the discovery to date is in testing the blood of the mother, who may require a blood transfusion during or after childbirth.—Journal Michigan State Medical Society.

Upjohn Diethylstilbestrol Perles

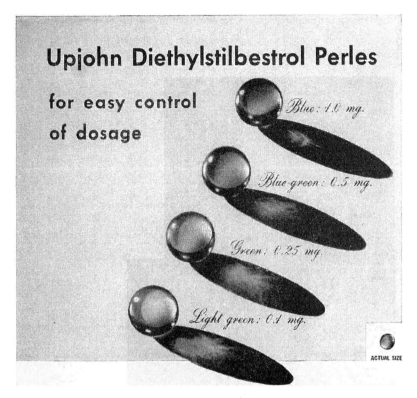

for easy control of dosage

Blue: 1.0 mg.

Blue-green: 0.5 mg.

Green: 0.25 mg.

Light green: 0.1 mg.

ACTUAL SIZE

Rapid relief from vasomotor and mental symptoms of the menopause depends on careful control of dosage. With Upjohn Diethylstilbestrol Perles this dosage control is easy, flexible. For oral use there are now four Perles in different strengths from which to choose. Each Perle is color-coded. It bears a bright, quickly-identified color which helps the physician and the dispensing pharmacist to recognize the potency—light green, 0.1 mg.; green, 0.25 mg.; blue-green, 0.5 mg.; blue, 1.0 mg.

Upjohn Diethylstilbestrol Perles are indicated wherever an estrogenic effect is desired. They have been found of particular value, not only during the menopause, but in senile vaginitis, in gonorrheal vaginitis, and in relieving or preventing painful engorgement of the breasts during suppression of lactation.

"The therapeutic use (of Diethylstilbestrol) has been demonstrated to be effective for all those conditions recognized to respond to the natural estrogens." N. N. R.

Upjohn Diethylstilbestrol Perles are available in each of the four potencies in bottles of 100 and 500

Upjohn
KALAMAZOO, MICHIGAN

ANOTHER WAY TO SAVE LIVES ... BUY WAR BONDS FOR VICTORY

MEDICAL ABSTRACTS

"A TREATMENT OF FRACTURED CLAVICLE BY TRAC-TION." Fred G. Hodgson. Southern Medical Journal. XXXV, 1079. 1942.

This is not a treatment for the ordinary simple fracture of the clavicle, but for those in adults, especially women, where an accurate replacement and maintenance is desired without operation. A number of these patients have to remain in bed on account of shock or of other complications, and others do not object to remaining in bed if they are assured of a good result.

A bed is prepared with a fracture board under the mattress. The head of the bed is raised on shock blocks or a chair. A figure-of-eight bandage is applied to both shoulders with padding in the axilae. On the injured side this bandage is fixed to the head of the bed. As the body slides down in the bed, due to gravity, the fracture is reduced and maintained in place. Usually no anaesthetic is required. Morphia or a sleeping powder is given the first night. The article is illustrated.—E. D. M., M. D.

"THE COCHLEAR RESPONSE AND THE MECHANISM OF THE COCHLEA." Jones H. MacNaughton. (London). Journal of Laryngology and Otology. Vol. 57, pp. 513-526. December, 1942.

When an individual speaks into the ear of an animal the movements of the membrana tympani, produced by sound waves, generate normal impulses in the auditory nerve, accompanied by changes in electrical potential which can be intercepted as they travel towards the brain and, by means of elaborate apparatus, made to operate a loud speaker. The movements of the membrane generate other electrical potentials, which are quite independent of those in the auditory tract and which may also be made to operate a loud speaker. The questions open at present, are, firstly; how are the electric potential in the second category generated? and secondly; do they constitute the stimuli which excite nerve impulses?

The conception now generally accepted appears to be that deformity of the hair cells generates within them a change which constitutes the stimulus exciting the auditory nerve. This conception is now proved by many observations showing that congenital deficiences of hearing are caused chiefly by deficiencies in the organ of Corti, deficiencies in the hair cells. The cells giving the maximum response (frequencies under 1,000 per second) are situated towards the apical end of the cochlea and at a distance from the basilar membrane. The author shows that the hair cell theory of Davis and the so-called membrane theory of Rawdon-Smith are not fundamentally antagonistic, and that differently interpreted, each may play an essential part in explaining the cochlear phenomena.—M.D.H., M..D

"LARYNGOLOGY AND FOLK-LORE." Rolleston, J. D. The Journal of Laryngology and Otology. Vol. 57, pp. 527-532. December, 1942.

Although many centuries elapsed before laryngology reached its full development, there are several references to popular methods of dealing with diseases of the throat. The first in date is found in Celsus: "If a man eat a nestling swallow, for a whole year he will not be in danger from angina." The various local applications mentioned by Pliny may be regarded as examples of folk-lore remedies, such as the use of the dung of lambs before they have begun to graze, the juices of a snail pierced with a needle, the ashes of burnt swallow, mixed with hay, gargles consisting of sheep's milk, etc.

There was a Roman divinity named Angerona. This Goddess was regarded as responsible for an outbreak of epidemic sore throats which might have been diphtheria. In the Middle Ages, St. Blaise was one of the most popular saints. He was frequently invoked in diseases of the throat and his connection with these diseases arose from a legend that he cured a boy who was half dead from having swallowed a fishbone but recovered as the result of the saint's prayer and laying on of hands.

Numerous popular synonyms have been given to a special form of laryngitis occurring in children. The term "croup" was first used in Scotland, and soon adopted by various countries. The old "synanche" or "cynanche" meant any form of sore throat including non-specific laryngitis and diphtheria. Folk-lore suggestions attribute hoarseness to eating nuts, raw fruits, oil and eels.

There are comparatively few prophylactic folk-lore remedies against throat diseases. There is a popular belief that he who eats willow catkins on Palm Sunday will be free from sore throat for the rest of the year. Benediction of the throat is a faithful ceremony performed in memory of St. Blaise in the Roman Catholic Church on February 3. In New Hampshire the belief prevails that a string of gold beads worn on the neck is a preventive of all forms of sore throat.

The folk pharmacopoeia contains various remedies for laryngeal affections, such as animal remedies, plant and mineral remedies, patron saints, and miscellaneous remedies. Liniment of centipedes and painting the throat with the juice of three male crabs have been used. Raw eggs are given as a cure for hoarseness. Horse dung in vinegar has been used as a gargle. A number of plants have been tried for their effectiveness against loss of voice; angelica, bishopwort, blackthorne, cabbage, chervil, garlic, elder, horse radish, lime tree, hyssop, lungwort, mallow, pennyroyal, radish, sage, sorrel, succory and vervain.

A great variety of remedies have been recommended for sore throat such as contact of the hand of a person who has been carried off by an early death, saying the words "crissi, crasi, cancrasi", abstention from meat, rest in a quiet place and ingestion of two spoonfuls of good butter boiled with one spoonful of honey, inhalation of burnt ashes, rubbing the soles of the feet with garlic and lard, tying a black silk cord around the neck, drinking a glass of sea water in the morning, cauterization of the frontal and temporal regions, etc.—M.D.H., M.D.

"X-RAY TREATMENT OF DISEASES OF THE LARNX." Maurice Lenz, New York. The Annuals of Otology, Rhinology and Laryngology. Vol. 52, pages 85-108. March. 1943.

X-ray therapy is an important aid in the treatment of diseases of the larynx. The treatment is based not only upon proficiency in radiotherapeutic technique and adequate x-ray equipment, but as much upon familiarity with the local anatomy, with the natural course of the untreated disease, with the extent of the disease on admission, and the radiosensitivity of the treated normal and pathological tissues.

X-ray treatment is employed chiefly in three groups of laryngeal disease; chronic inflammation, benign tumors and cancer. Inflammatory tissue is more sensitive to x-rays than the adjacent normal tissue, which remains unaffected by the small x-ray doses. The small doses are repeated at weekly intervals or more often until satisfactory regression of the inflammatory infiltrate has been accomplished. Acute laryngitis may react favorably to x-ray treatment, but this is not used for treatment. The disease is self-limited. Irradiation of chronic laryngitis is attempted rarely, and regression of the granulation tissue may be expected. Pachydermia of the larynx should also react favorably. Leukoplakia requires large doses and may recur after it has disappeared, as the x-ray do not attack the cause of the disease. Most often the x-ray treatment had been carried out in tuberculosis,blastomycosis and scleroma. The effect of x-ray on tuberculosis is open to discussion. Blastomycosis improved after irradiation in combination with large doses of iodides. Sclerona has been successfully treated by x-rays.

Benign tumors to not respond to x-ray therapy as readily as inflammatory tissue and some are radioresistant as to make their treatment by x-rays practical. Hemangiomas and various types of papilloma have been treated. Only the cavernous type of hemangioma responds rapidly to x-ray irradiation. The treatment of papilloma depends on its clinical variety. Single papilloma should not be irradiated but remove surgically. In multiple papillomas, treatment by x-rays at times succeeds after the failure of conservative surgery.

Carcinoma of the larynx is usually more radioresistant than either of the first two groups. The x-ray dosage which required to arrest the growth in most cases is close to the maximum tolerated by the normal tissues and produces sloughing of the irradiated epidermis, the laryngeal and pharyngeal mucosa. Unless the dosage has been too intensive, healing follows soon after the slough has separated, leaving little or no clinical evidence of radiation damage of the normal tissues. Because of the danger of injury, x-ray treatment of cancer of the larynx is not repeated except in rare instances. The decision whether a cancer should be irradiated depends on the site, the type and the microscopic anatomy of the tumor. Carcinoma of the band often responds readily to x-ray treatment but not infrequently recurs later. Cancer of the subglottis has the reputation of doing badly with x-ray therapy. X-ray treatment is especially successful in the noinvasive type of cancer of the epiglottis and its folds.

In choosing the best treatment for cancer of the larynx, the advantages and limitations of surgery and x-ray therapy and in a limited way of radium and radon therapy should be considered in each particular case. The best methods of solving the individual problem is by consultation between the laryngologist and the radiologist.—M.D.H., M.D.

"TUBERCULOSIS OF THE GREATER TROCHANTER AND ITS BURSA." Mark S. Donovan and Merrill C. Sosman. The Amer. Jour. of Roentgenology and Radium Therapy. XLVII. 719. 1942.

Bursitis lateral to the greater trochanter is a rare condition, and is frequently caused by tuberculosis involving the greater trochanter. Since this portion of the femur develops as an epiphysis, its cancellous bone is as susceptible to tuberculosis as the femoral head or other epiphyses. An important diagnostic point is the presence of tuberculosis in an active, inactive or healed form in another part of the body.

The authors present the clinical, roentgenographic, operative, and histopathological findings in five cases of tuberculosis of the greater trochanter and the adjacent bursa. All the patients had had symptoms for at least one year before operation. The disease may develop at any age, but the symptoms usually begin during adolescence or early life. The characteristic features are a destructive lesion beginning in the upper part of the trochanter, with formation of a cold abscess and later a sinus. Bursitis is manifested by swelling of the soft tissues over the trochanter and amorphous calcium depositions just lateral to it.

Differentiation from acute infection and from tumors is seldom difficult. In the early stages a light roentgen exposure may be necessary to demonstrate the erosion of the normally thin cortex of the trochanter and the faint calcium deposits in the adjacent bursa. The disease frequently recurs after apparent cure by surgical extirpation.—E.D.M., M.D.

"ANGIOMATOSIS RETINAE (VON HIPPEL'S DISEASE): RESULTS FOLLOWING IRRADIATION OF THREE EYES." American Journal of Ophthalmology, Series 3. Vol. 26. pages 454-463. May, 1943.

The first description of angiomatosis retinae in the literature is by E. Fuchs, who, in 1882, described it under the title of aneurysma arteriovenosum traumaticum. Following this report the disease was described a number of times, under various titles, until 1904, when Hippel established angiomatosis retinae as a clinical entity. In 1927, Lindau demonstrated the close association between angiomatosis retinae and the occurrence of angiomatosis and cystic lesions in the central nervous system, usually cerebellum. He also demonstrated that other viscera are often involved, i.e., kidneys, pancreas, ovaries and the suprarenal glands. Since that time the disease has been known as Hippel-Lindau syndrome. Approximately 160 cases of angiomatosis retinae have been reported in the literature until the present time.

According to Bedell, the earliest photographic sign is fullness of the retinal veins. The first ophthalmoscopic change is a fan-shaped anastomosis between one branch of the central artery and the central vein, which is the beginning of tumor formation. From this rete mirabile a berrylike, redish-colored mass develops that is sharply demarcated from the surrounding area and is supplied by an artery and vein. In a short time it is impossible to differentiate between the artery and vein. The retina surrounding the tumor is slightly elevated. Around the macula and disc, shiny white spots of exudate make their appearance, which later become confluent and show a stellate figure in the macula. Frequently there are collections also along the vessels. A little later a globular detachment of the retinae appears, surrounding the enlarged tumor mass. The condition progresses until there is a massive detachment of the retina, which protrudes into the bitreous. Glistening yellowish-white spots of exudate are present over the entire fundus during this stage. The vessels leading to the tumor become markedly enlarged, the disc becomes atrophic, and the eye amaurotic. Frequently these vascular tumors are multiple either in the beginning or later in the course of the disease. Thus, the circumscribed regions of retinal exudate may produce a picture simular to that of retinis circinata or retinitis albuminurica. Hemorrhages may also occur in the retina and vitreous. Finally, iridocyclitis develops, complicated by secondary glaucoma and eventual opacification of the lens.

Most of the cases of angiomatosis retinae have occurred in growing adults. The average age of the patient is 25 years. Both eyes were involved in 50 per cent of the patients. One-third of the eyes involved had multiple tumors. Lindau reported cerebral involvement in 25 per cent of the cases, these cerebral signs on the average appearing 10 years after the discovery of the ocular lesions. In some cases a familial incidence has been observed; the disease is usually transmitted through the female, although 60 per cent of the cases are reported in males.

The prognosis is poor. At first the visual acuity is good, but later the retina undergoes degeneration. The rate of progression may be very great, and the earlier the disease appears, the more rapidly progressive is the course.

Most of the cases have such a bad prognosis that any therapeutic measures that offer hope of conserving the sight warrants consideration. Formerly, before the disease was understood, intravenous injections of arsphenamine, tuberculin, calcium gluconate and foreign protein therapy were used unsuccessfully. In recent years attempts at therapy have been limited to electrolysis, diathermy and radio-therapy with radium and x-rays.

Electrolysis and puncture diathermy have certain disadvantages in that there is a definite risk of severe hemorrhage, especially if an attempt is made to coagulate the markedly dilated vessels. The resultant destruction of the retinae is extensive. The advantages of radium over x-ray therapy do not seem to be sufficient to warrant the difficulties attendant to its use.

X-ray radiation can be given any competent roentgenologist. It seems safer and less destructive to the retina than do some of the other methods. Three eyes of two patients with angiomatosis retinae were irradiated. In the first patient, who had an early lesion in one eye, there was a marked improvement with retention of 0.8 vision three and one-half years after irradiation. In the second case, both eyes were involved, the right eye being in a well-advanced stage. Both eyes were given 1,800 r. The early lesion showed definite improvement with vision of 1.0 two years after irradiation. During this time, the eye having more advanced lesion became progressively worse, going to anaurosis, complete detachment of the retinae and fliosis.

From the experience of the authors with three eyes and from what is reported in the literature it appears that in early cases x-ray therapy does offer a convenient, safe means of treating these lesions. The advanced lesions have not resopnded to any therapy.—M.D.H., M.D.

"CHILDREN'S FEET. NORMAL AND PRESENTING COMMON ABNORMALITIES." Fremont A. Chandler. Amer. Jour. of Diseases of Children, LXIII, 1136, 1942.

The author states that the medical profession has neglected the field of children's feet, and has left it to some of the cults, shoe manufacturers, and salesmen for development, and in some instances, exploitation. He urges both pediatricians and orthopedic surgeons to be more aware of the problem. He discusses club feet, pronated feet, and cavus feet, and mentions other deformities. He believes that treatment of congenital club foot by manipulation and casts should begin early, preferably the first day of life.

Three functions of the normal foot gradually develop from birth, and reflect regular growth. A prehensile grasping function, similar to the prehensile action of the hand, is present at birth, but, unlike that of the hand, is usually gradually lost. Muscle coordination advances through the rolling and creeping stages to that of standing. Propulsion follows shortly, and a gait is established. The mechanism of walking is described in some detail and is illustrated by drawings and photographs.

A good shoe for a growing foot should afford adequate protection against injury and extremes of temperature; plantar support similar to that afforded by the ground; and an interior which will permit unrestricted variation in size and movement of the foot during all phases of its function.—E.D.M., M.D.

"WEATHER AND OCULAR PATHOPHYSIOLOGY." William P. Peterson, Chicago. Archives of Ophthalmology. Vol. 29, pages 747-759, May, 1943.

It was Duggan who, in recent years, discussed ocular pathology predicated on vascular dysfunction. He stressed the pathologic significance of vascular spasm, which brings in its train a series of local disturbances in water balance, in cellular permeability, in iron balance, with resulting clinical phenomena that may take various forms. The acute episode may be precipitated with chilling or with change in the weather. The author, for the corroboration of Duggan's hypothesis, publishes a series of case histories with a series of corresponding meterograms.

There was, e.g., a recurrent acute iritis in which one acute episode occurred at a sharp barometric crest after low environmental temperatures of the preceding days. Accentuation occurred with the passage of a colder air mass.

Change of weather involves a fundamental change in the air mass in which human beings are living. Polar air is diametrically opposite to tropical air in its character and in its demands on the human body. Polar air is heavy, cold, clear and dry. The body seeks to shut itself off from the unfavorable effect of the cold by a sympathicotonic phase, with increased arteriolar tone, with sugar mobilization, with relative alkalinity, etc. Peripheral tissues become relatively anoxic. The tissue status is reversed when the metabolic products of anoxia begin to enter the circulation; the body is then stimulated. The phase of stimulation may proceed to fatigue, with a reversal of tissue status, and with this reversal the pH is lowered, permeability increased, the blood pressure falls and hydration is augmented.

Obviously any tissue focus that cannot adjust rapidly and adequately to such change begins to reflect local symptoms; swelling may cause pain, there may be hyperemia, an exudate may increase or tissues may undergo rapid autolysis.

Tropical air is warm, moist and lighter in weight, and its effects, unless excessive temperatures are reached, are opposite to those of polar air. The passage of tropical air mass, however, synchronized with the after effect of a polar air mass, may augment the stage of stimulation or of fatigue and result in unusually low blood pressure, in excessive hydration, in low pH, and in pronounced augmentation of digestive phenomea.

In another case of acute iridocylitis, it is seen that the acute inflammation followed a tooth extraction. An anoxic phase will result in swelling about an infected tooth, and, with the passage of a major polar air mass, the anoxemia becomes effective; the patient had his tooth extracted three or four days later when the symptoms became unusually severe. But with such extraction bacteria flood the blood stream, and if any areas of tissue are present where anoxia has existed, foci of dysfunction, with adhesive capilary walls, will be present, and some bacteria may localize and cause an acute inflammatory reaction.

In other cases of episcleritis and scleritis as well as in exudative choroilitis and retrobulbar neuritis it was possible to show that environmental situations normally associated with peripheral vasoconstriction and its resulting anoxia are almost associated with the initiation of the clinical episode or change in the clinical picture. Any extreme in the environmental situation, whether toward cold or toward undue heat, is apt to find reflection in clinical symptoms, for the reason that such changes entail major vasomotor adjustment.

While any one of many environmental factors, e.g., trauma, sensitization, emotion, infection, may act as a precipitating force, the weather episode, on the background of season, is the most common of the energy impacts that are effective, for the biologic effect is apt to be prolonged. The vascular spasm may exist for hours or even days, is subject to summation with repetition of environmental changes and is, in addition, universal in its effectiveness in the population at large, though obviously the individual reaction will be modified by habitus, by shelter, by the condition of the individual, etc.

In a case of retrobulbar neuritis with multiple sclerosis, blindness occurred in one eye with the passage of a major polar air mass, the temperature declining from over 90 F. on June 9 to a low of 47 F. on June 15. Effects of this type should by no means confine the attention of the doctor to the eye or lead to the assumption that one is dealing with a special field of action. The meteorologic episode is universally effective, and the clinical reflection will be found in any organ or tissue. —M.D.H., M.D.

KEY TO ABSTRACTORS

The lowest death rate in the history of the United States was recorded in 1941, according to a recent announcement of the U. S. Census Bureau. Total number of deaths for the entire nation was 1,395,907. Provisional mortality statistics for the year show a death rate of 10.5 per 1,000 population.—Ohio State Medical Journal.

BOOK REVIEWS

"The chief glory of every people arises from its authors."—Dr. Samuel Johnson.

THE INNER EAR. Joseph Fischer, M.D. and Louis E. Wolfson, M.D. Grune & Stratton, Inc. Price $5.75.

This is a thoroughly up-to-date text discussing conditions of the inner ear. The sections on anatomy physiology and applied neurotological physiology are clear, readable and as concise as is consistent with a detailed discussion.

The historical development of the various functional tests, their present most practicable usage and clinical application are so explained that they may be employed and interpreted in the office or clinic.

More than half of the book is devoted to chapters giving clinical discussions of diseased conditions of the labyrinth. Etiology, diagnosis, differential diagnosis, clinical course, medical and surgical treatment as well as a practical review of the significant literature is included in most of these chapters. The discussions of war trauma, the role of the inner ear in aeronautics and the effects of atmospheric pressure changes on the ear include the results of recent studies by military observers.

The problems of deafness, except for otosclerosis, are not included in this work.

This is a valuable book for the library of the otologist and the neurologist.—L. C. McHenry, M.D.

THE NATIONAL FORMULARY: Seventh Edition National Formulary VII. Prepared by the Committee on National Formulary by Authority of the American Pharmaceutical Association. Official from November 1, 1942. Washington, D. C. American Pharmaceutical Association, 1942.

The first edition of The National Formulary of Unofficial Preparations was published in 1888. Since that date a new addition has appeared approximately every ten years. The ambitious Committee of Revision, representing the American Pharmaceutical Association is now proposing to supply a revised edition every five years. Thus the professions of medicine and pharmacy will be supplied with up-to-date information.

In this edition there is a new chapter under the title "Preparations for Use in The Clinical Laboratory." This is of great value to members of the medical profession and laboratory workers because it supplies comprehensive data on ingredients and media. The information contained in this chapter supplemented by that found in the chapter on "Reagents and Preparations for Use in the Clinical Laboratory" supply valuable reference resources. The various reagents are listed in alphabetical order and detailed instructions for the preparation of reagents are provided. The technique of many laboratory procedures is given in detail.

The monumental work of this committee is attested by the fact that 600 pages are devoted to carefully sifted data accurately recorded and thoroughly indexed for the benefit of those searching for information in this field. Approximately 30 pages are devoted to the "History of The National Formulary" and to "Organization and Personnel."—Lewis J. Moorman, M.D.

REHABILITATION OF THE WAR INJURED—A SYMPOSIUM. William B. Doherty and D. Runes. Philosophical Library. New York. 684 pages. Price $10.00.

The editors of this book, which is actually a compilation of various articles written by authorities and published in current standard medical and surgical journals, have recognized the timely value of such work.

The book may well prove a valuable and dependable guide in civil as well as military practice. Rehabilitation of the permanently disabled has always been an important part of treatment but is now increasingly important as the number of war casualties being returned to the hospitals in the United States increases. Since the British medical men have had longer experience in this work during this war, it is only natural that many of these articles are drawn from British sources.

The contents deal in great part with plastic and orthopedic treatment in rehabilitation but also includes physiotherapy, occupational therapy and vocational guidance. Neurologic and psychiatric treatment are included as well as two articles on the legal aspects of rehabilitation. The inclusion of the psychiatric and neurologic chapter is proof of the importance of such rehabilitation which in the past has had all too little emphasis placed upon it.

Perhaps the most interesting as well as timely articles are those from and by the Navy on "Vascular and Neurological Lesions in Survivors of Shipwreck."—L. J. Starry, M.D.

URINE AND URINALYSIS. Louis Gershenfeld, Professor of Bacteriology and Hygiene and Director of the Bacteriological and Clinical Chemistry Laboratories at the Philadelphia College of Pharmacy and Science. Second edition, throughly revised. Lea & Febiger, Philadelphia. 1943. 304 pages, illustrated with 42 engravings. Price $3.25.

This revised book is based on an abundance of new material including recently introduced procedures, with the author's evaluation of the tests.

The book is conveniently divided into three parts; the first part covering general considerations, technique of collecting specimens and a discussion of the abnormal or pathological constituents of the urine. This part will be especially valuable to the clinician, nurse and student.

The second part covers various tests more commonly included in a urinalysis, with the author's evaluation of the tests, their limitations and results that may be obtained from them.

The third part will be particularly benificial to the laboratory technicians performing the more technical or special examinations of the urine. Detailed references are given for those desiring to consult the orginal articles.

This book is concise, authoritative and contains a rich fund of knowledge of practical value.—W. F. Keller, M. D.

PRACTICAL SURVEY OF CHEMISTRY AND METABOLISM OF THE SKIN. Morris Markowitz Associate in Dermatology and Syphilology, Graduate School of Medicine. University of Pennsylvania. The Blakiston Company. Philadelphia. 196 pages. Price $3.50.

For the purpose for which this book is written, to give the dermatologists an accurate conception of the chemistry and metabolism of the skin and its relation to treatment, it is an excellent book. It is well illustrated with charts and data confirming conclusions, especially to show the relationship of the chemistry and metabolism of the skin to dermatological therapeutics.

This survey of fundamental facts is necessary for a better understanding of dermatology. The author has considered the chemistry and metabolism of the skin in detail and has also included a rather extensive study of the chemistry of the blood as it is related to skin disease.

There is also a practical consideration of the hematopoietic changes as related to the problem. It is of interest to compare these studies in relation to the different structures concerned.

From a dietetic standpoint, the author has shown the value of blood chemistry findings with special reference to an increase of glycogen, uric acid, non-protein and urea nitrogens. The value of such therapeutic measures is shown to aid in the disappearance of various eczematous and puritic processes.

A very interesting chapter is devoted to the description of vitamins and avitaminoses as related to skin disease. The various vitamins are considered individually and in combined forms. Their source and something concerning their function is considered along with a study of the relationship with endocrine system and especially with reference to the matabolism of fat, calcium and phosphorus.

The final chapter is devoted to an excellent discussion of avitaminoses. This chapter alone affords a valuable discussion on the typical syndrome, which is called "deficiency disease" and affords information concerning the synergistic interrelationship between the vitamins. This chapter is a logical deduction of the foregoing discussions and is, in fact, a nice conclusion to the book. It is a technical book, interestingly written.—C. P. Bondurant, M.D.

A GUIDE TO PRACTICAL NUTRITION. The Committee on Nutrition and Deficiency Diseases of the Philadelphia County Medical Society with introduction by Morris Fishbein. 1941-1942. John Wyeth and Brother.

This book of less than 100 pages is attractively assembled, although a paper-backed volume. There is a discussion of food requirements in terms of proteins, fats, carbohydrates, and minerals in the first four chapters.

The second section of the book is taken up with a consideration of everyday diets with special diets for pregnancy, childhood and old-age.

A most excellent chapter is concerned with food and nutrition problems as affecting teeth both for the developing period and for protection in later life.

Three chapters are devoted to a discussion of Vitamin deficiencies with particular emphasis on the Vitamin B complex and components, also riboflavin and Vitamin A.

The final chapter is a most concise and practical consideration of nutrition as a problem in war and of public health.

As an appendix there are excellent charts of: 1. Vitamin and mineral requirements, 2. Functional deficiency, symptoms and sources of Vitamins, 3. Carbohydrate content of fruits and vegetables, 4. Table of food composition in weights and measures.

The subjects considered in this book are handled in a concise, readable manner. It should make a convenient and valuable ready reference book for the desk of any practicing physician.—Arthur W. White, M.D.

A SYNOPSIS OF CLINICAL SYPHILIS. James Kirby Howles. C. V. Mosby Co., St. Louis. Illustrated, 671 pages. Price $6.00.

The word synopsis implies a general view. This is difficult to attain in such a broad field as syphilis, however, in this comparatively small volume the author has admirably presented the details essential to the intelligent care of the patient with syphilis. The initial brief discussion of the pathology of syphilis, which is fundamentally the same in each stage except for variations in degree, is clear and concise.

The section on primary syphilis stresses the point, so often forgotten, that chancre may appear on any part of the body except the hair and the nails. In the sections on secondary tertiary syphilis, 39 excellent photographs add much impress upon the reader how variable and imitative the skin eruptions of syphilis can be.

The sections on clinical and laboratory diagnosis emphasize the details of examination so easily overlooked by the busy practitioner and clarify many questions regarding interpretation of various tests.

The section on therapy begins with practical considerations, followed by a discussion of the choice of drugs, including a description of the newer preparation Clorarsen. Immediate and delayed reactions, together with their management, are covered in brief but sufficient detail.

The author's discussion of prognosis and cure is in line with many who have resigned themselves to the horns of the dilemma by denying that either the positive or the negative blood serological test has any bearing on the arrest or activity of a syphilitic infection.

Eleven chapters deal with the description of acquired syphilis of the various systems with special emphasis on syphilis of the central nervous system.

The author closes with a comprehensive discussion of congenital syphilis followed by practical suggestions regarding organization of the syphilis clinic. A list of about six hundred references at the end of the book is especially valuable as a guide to many worthwhile articles in the literature.—A. Brooks Abshier, M.D.

NEW AND NON-OFFICIAL REMEDIES—1943. Issued Under the Direction and Supervision of the Council on Pharmacy and Chemistry of the American Medical Association, Chicago. 771 pages. Price $1.50.

Despite the war and its attendant demand on the energies and time of all doctors, New and Nonofficial Remedies, 1943, published by the Council on Pharmacy and Chemistry of the American Medical Association, is as complete, informative and inclusive as any of its predecessors.

For those who may wish to determine the why of the inclusion or exclusion of certain preparations, the Official Rules of the Council are found following the Preface. In addition, the Bibliographical Index and the Index to Distributors which precedes the General Index, now found at the back of the book, both contribute materially in determining the status of different articles.

Revisions and additions, some of which indicate in a rather striking manner, increasing skepticism of the Council concerning a drug, serve to keep the book up to date with advanced medical knowledge. The most noteworthy additions are those of Nikethamide, first introduced as Coramine; Stilbestrol, the synthetic and more reasonably available estrogen; Trichinella Extract for the diagnosis of trichonosis; and Zephiran Chloride, a new antiseptic agent.

To one who seeks authentic data on any new preparation or to one who wishes clarification of confusing facts from the less dependable sources, New and Nonofficial Remedies, 1943, is the answer. The book well upholds the reputation gained by previous volumes. The grateful thanks of every member of the medical profession should be extended the Council on Pharmacy and Chemistry of the American Medical Association for its work.—L. J. Starry, M.D.

Great men are they who see that spiritual is stronger than any material force; that thoughts rule the world. —Emerson.

Eye injuries in American industry are occurring at a rate of 1,000 every working day and 98 percent of them are wholly unnecessary, according to a study sponsored by the National Society for the Prevention of Blindness (Columbia University Press). It was found that about 1,000 workers lose sight of one eye and 100 or more the sight of both eyes in a year as a result of occupational hazards. Many more have damaged sight. It is pointed out that there is no need for the blinding of workers in American industry. The industrial accident and disease hazards affecting the eyes are now commonly known. Methods of eliminating these hazards or of protecting workers against them have been thoroughly demonstrated. Devices which provide protection against almost every type of eye accident are now available.—Science.

OFFICERS OF COUNTY SOCIETIES, 1943

COUNTY	PRESIDENT	SECRETARY	MEETING TIME
Alfalfa	H. E. Huston, Cherokee	L. T. Lancaster, Cherokee	Last Tues. each Second Month
Atoka-Coal	J. B. Clark, Coalgate	J. S. Fulton, Atoka	
Beckham	H. K. Speed, Sayre	E. S. Kilpatrick, Elk City	Second Tuesday
Blaine	Virginia Olson Curtin, Watonga	W. F. Griffin, Watonga	
Bryan	J. T. Colwick, Durant	W. K. Haynie, Durant	Second Tuesday
Caddo	F. L. Patterson, Carnegie	C. B. Sullivan, Carnegie	
Canadian	P. F. Herod, El Reno	A. L. Johnson, El Reno	Subject to call
Carter	Walter Hardy, Ardmore	H. A. Higgins, Ardmore	
Cherokee	P. H. Medearis, Tahlequah	*James K. Gray, Tahlequah	First Tuesday
Choctaw	C. H. Hale, Boswell	E. A. Johnson, Hugo	
Cleveland	J. A. Rieger, Norman	Curtis Berry, Norman	Thursday nights
Comanche	George S. Barber, Lawton	W. F. Lewis, Lawton	
Cotton	A. H. Holstead, Temple	Mollie F. Seism, Walters	Third Friday
Craig	F. M. Adams, Vinita	J. M. McMillan, Vinita	
Creek	H. R. Haas, Sapulpa	C. G. Oakes, Sapulpa	
Custer	F. R. Vieregg, Clinton	C. J. Alexander, Clinton	Third Thursday
Garfield	Paul B. Champlin, Enid	John R. Walker, Enid	Fourth Thursday
Garvin	T. F. Gross, Lindsay	John R. Callaway, Pauls Valley	Wednesday before Third Thursday
Grady	Walter J. Baze, Chickasha	Roy E. Emanuel, Chickasha	Third Thursday
Grant	I. V. Hardy, Medford	E. E. Lawson, Medford	
Greer	G. P. Cherry, Mangum	J. B. Hollis, Mangum	
Harmon	W. G. Husband, Hollis	L. E. Hollis, Hollis	First Wednesday
Haskell	William Carson, Keota	N. K. Williams, McCurtain	
Hughes	Wm. L. Taylor, Holdenville	Imogene Mayfield, Holdenville	First Friday
Jackson	E. S. Crow, Olustee	E. W. Mabry, Altus	Last Monday
Jefferson	F. M. Edwards, Ringling	L. L. Wade, Ryan	Second Monday
Kay	Philip C. Risser, Blackwell	J. Holland Howe, Ponca City	Third Thursday
Kingfisher	C. M. Hodgson, Kingfisher	H. Violet Sturgeon, Hennessey	
Kiowa	B. H. Watkins, Hobart	J. William Finch, Hobart	
LeFlore	Neeson Rolle, Poteau	Rush L. Wright, Poteau	
Lincoln	H. B. Jenkins, Tryon	Carl H. Bailey, Stroud	First Wednesday
Logan	William C. Miller, Guthrie	J. L. LeHew, Jr., Guthrie	Last Tuesday
Marshall	O. A. Cook, Madill	Philip G. Joseph, Madill	
Mayes	Ralph V. Smith, Pryor	Paul B. Cameron, Pryor	
McClain	B. W. Slover, Blanchard	R. L. Royster, Purcell	
McCurtain	A. W. Clarkson, Valliant	N. L. Barker, Broken Bow	Fourth Tuesday
McIntosh	James L. Wood, Eufaula	William A. Tolleson, Eufaula	First Thursday
Murray	P. V. Annadown, Sulphur	F. E. Sadler, Sulphur	Second Tuesday
Muskogee-Sequoyah-Wagoner	H. A. Scott, Muskogee	D. Evelyn Miller, Muskogee	First Monday
Noble	C. H. Cooke, Perry	J. W. Francis, Perry	
Okfuskee	L. J. Spickard, Okemah	M. L. Whitney, Okemah	Second Monday
Oklahoma	Walker Morledge, Oklahoma City	E. R. Musick, Oklahoma City	Fourth Tuesday
Okmulgee	A. R. Holmes, Henryetta	J. C. Matheney, Okmulgee	Second Monday
Osage	C. R. Weirich, Pawhuska	George K. Hemphill, Pawhuska	Second Monday
Ottawa	W. B. Sanger, Picher	Matt A. Connell, Picher	Third Thursday
Pawnee	E. T. Robinson, Cleveland	R. L. Browning, Pawnee	
Payne	L. A. Mitchell, Stillwater	C. W. Moore, Stillwater	Third Thursday
Pittsburg	John F. Park, McAlester	William H. Kaeiser, McAlester	Third Friday
Pontotoc	O. H. Miller, Ada	R. H. Mayes, Ada	First Wednesday
Pottawatomie	A. C. McFarling, Shawnee	Clinton Gallaher, Shawnee	First and Third Saturday
Pushmataha	John S. Lawson, Clayton	B. M. Huckabay, Antlers	
Rogers	C. W. Beson, Claremore	C. L. Caldwell, Chelsea	First Monday
Seminole	Max Van Sandt, Wewoka	Mack I. Shanholtz, Wewoka	Third Wednesday
Stephens	W. K. Walker, Marlow	Wallis S. Ivy, Duncan	
Texas	R. G. Obermiller, Texhoma	Morris Smith, Guymon	
Tillman	R. D. Robinson, Frederick	O. G. Bacon, Frederick	
Tulsa	James C. Peden, Tulsa	E. O. Johnson, Tulsa	Second and Fourth Monday
Washington Nowata	J. G. Smith, Bartlesville	J. V. Athey, Bartlesville	Second Wednesday
Washita	A. S. Neal, Cordell	James F. McMurry, Sentinel	
Woods	C. A. Traverse, Alva	O. E. Templin, Alva	Last Tuesday Odd Months
Woodward	C. E. Williams, Woodward	C. W. Tedrowe, Woodward	Second Thursday

*(Serving in Armed Forces)

THE JOURNAL
OF THE
OKLAHOMA STATE MEDICAL ASSOCIATION

| VOLUME XXXVI | OKLAHOMA CITY, OKLAHOMA, SEPTEMBER, 1943 | NUMBER 9 |

Naval Medicine*

CAPTAIN LESLIE B. MARSHALL, M.S., U.S.N.
*Commanding Officer United States
Naval Hospital*
NORMAN, OKLAHOMA

The title of this paper has been given as "Naval Medicine". This title, to a certain extent, is a misnomer, for it is manifestly impossible to cover all aspects of naval medicine in the allotted time. However, I propose to tell you something of the Medical Department of the Navy, its organization, functions and duties as they apply to the thousands of personnel now serving in all parts of the world.

Perhaps as good a way as any to begin is to give, at the outset, the mission of the Medical Department of the Navy. That mission is, "To keep as many men at as many guns as many days as possible." This you can readily see, is no small job and requires not only the trained medical officers but also the nurses, the hospital corpsmen, the administrative officers and all of the Civil Service Personnel that go to make up the personnel of our corps.

The Department of the Navy was created by an act of Congress April 30, 1798. Our Navy was but a tiny infant in those days but has grown over the years into the huge organization that it now is. The Bureau system of the Navy Department was established by an act of Congress August 31, 1842. This act provided that the business of the Department should be distributed among five bureaus, including a Bureau of Medicine and Surgery. The present laws provide that all duties of the Bureau shall be performed under the authority of the Secretary of the Navy, and that its orders should be considered as emanating from him and shall have full force and effect as such. The Chief of the Bureau is appointed by the President for a

period of four years by and with the consent of the Senate and, while so serving, holds the title of Surgeon General of the Navy and the rank of Rear Admiral in the Medical Corps.

The Bureau of Medicine and Surgery is organized as follows:

1. Division of Administration.
2. Division of Personnel (Doctors, Nurses, Hospital Corps, Civil Service Personnel.)
3. Division of Dentistry.
4. Division of Physical Qualifications.
5. Division of Preventive Medicine.
6. Division of Aviation Medicine.
7. Division of Material and Finances.
8. Division of Inspections.
9. Division of Planning.
10. Division of Publications.
11. Division of Red Cross and Veterans' Administration.

Each division is a separate unit in the organization, and the head of each unit or division is responsible to the Surgeon General for the proper functioning of his unit. All of these activities must be correlated and all must work closely together to have an efficient Medical Department. This, then, will give you an idea of the framework and the basis of the Naval Medical Corps. From this framework there goes out all of the multitudinous activities of our corps.

Perhaps to try and run the course of Naval Medicine it would be well to trace the career of a Naval Medical Officer from his original entry into the corps until he reaches the goal of every regular Naval Medical Officer —that of having command of his own hospital. If you will give me the privilege, I will trace my own career over some twenty-six

*Read before the Annual Meeting of the Oklahoma State Medical Association, May 11, Oklahoma City.

years of Naval service. My service is fairly typical of the Naval Medical Officer both in war and peace times.

Early in 1917 there appeared in the city of Memphis, Tennessee, a representative of the Medical Department of the Navy. His mission was to interest young doctors in the Navy Medical Corps, point out advantages and disadvantages, conduct the physical examination, check into the professional work of the individual and, if qualified, to recommend that individual for a commission in the Naval Reserve Force. I was one of the fortunate ones that received a commission. Shortly thereafter, orders came for me to report to the Naval Hospital, Philadelphia, Pennsylvania, for an indoctrination course prior to being sent to sea. At the Philadelphia Hospital I joined a small group that had been gathered from other cities and schools. After reporting we were told to get our uniforms and, in a short time, we blossomed forth with our first uniforms—first gold braid—a Lieutenant, Junior Grade, in the Naval Coast Defense Reserve. A short intensive course was given covering Naval Regulations, customs of the service, public health, surgery, medicine, obstetrics, x-ray, tropical medicine, laboratory, sanitation, eye, ear, nose and throat, psychiatry, etc. We had the privilege of knowing and working with such men as DaCosta, McCrae, Holloway, Judson DeLand, Fischer, Stellwagon, Chevalier Jackson, all of these brilliant men who, at that time, were the top men in their profession. I gave anesthetics for Dr. DaCosta and have also stood across the table from him as an assistant. From those men we gained much. The influence of their experience, their ability and their teaching we have carried to this day.

Just about midway of this course we were given the opportunity to qualify for a commission in the Regular Navy Medical Corps. This involved another profession and physical examination, and again I was among the successful ones. At this point I might say that in peace times every Naval Officer must prove his qualifications for promotion by examination at the time promotion comes along. When the course finished, I received orders to report to the Commanding Officer of the U.S.S. Nevada for duty. I became the Junior Medical Officer of the ship and had charge of the ward and laboratory under the Senior Medical Officer. Aboard ship I learned how to find my way around a ship, Naval terms, drills, inspections of personnel and material. I learned that a medical officer is largely responsible for the efficiency of his ship. He looks into everything concerning the ship and its crew from a medical standpoint; cleanliness, food, water, ventilation,

uniforms, vaccinations, as well as taking care of those sick and injured, and he is fully responsible for all supplies and equipment belonging to his department.

Some three months later I suddenly received orders to a new duty, that of placing a ship in commission, and the duty as Medical Officer of that ship when commissioned. The ship proved to be a small yacht that formerly belonged to Horace Dodge, and the Navy was converting her into a sub-marine patrol vessel. This was another aspect of naval medicine, that of obtaining supplies and equipment, getting the sick bay of the ship located and built, examining the crew, records, and other activities. In addition I was made Communication Officer and, as such, I had charge of all secret codes and publications of the ship.

For a year our duty aboard that ship was chasing submarines up and down the coast of France. I was then ordered ashore in France where I had another year. The job there was inspection and fumigation of ships, in addition to caring for all the sick and injured aboard ships without medical officers. Also there was the opportunity to observe and assist in the treatment and care of war casualties and evacuation of casualties by hospital train and ship.

When the work of bringing the soldiers and sailors home was finished, I returned to the States and again to the hospital in Philadelphia, where I had charge of an active medical ward. After a period of time, orders came again to the hospital in Philadelphia, where I had charge of an active medical ward. After a period of time, orders came again, and off to sea as Medical Officer of a repair ship; another aspect of Naval Medicine where I learned industrial medicine, since the ship was a Mother Ship for destroyers and we could do almost any repair work necessary. From the repair ship I was sent to duty aboard a destroyer and finally arrived on the Asiatic station. For two years I was the only Medical Officer of nine destroyers, each with a crew of one hundred men and five to seven officers. There all the problems of small ships, surgery in civilian hospitals, treatment of venereal diseases, health of the various ports visited, seeing cholera, leprosy, leishmanniasis, kala azar, typhus, malaria, dengue, intestinal parasites, schistosomiasis (flukes). There was also the problem of learning how to cope with life in the tropics, tropical foods, clothing and quarters.

From there, I went on a three years' tour of recruiting duty at Minneapolis, Minnesota, a most profitable and instructive period. This included work at the University of Minnesota, visits to Rochester, serving on the staff of the Minneapolis General Hospital in Medicine, as well as carrying on the regular work of examination and enlisting of recruits. There came at that time a deep interest in the Naval Reserve, which also was most instructive. The last two years an interest in Urology developed, and those two years were spent with Dr. Oscar Owre in his large and varied practice where he taught me the basis of all the Urology I know. From Minneapolis I went to San Francisco for a short post-graduate course with Dr. Frank Hinman at the University of California in Urology, and from there to a hospital ship as Chief of the Urological Service. This time we were on the receiving end of the patients and there I learned a method of transportation and reception of patients from ships at sea to the hospital ship. When the tour of duty aboard the hospital ship was finished, I went to the U.S. Naval Hospital, San Diego, California, as Chief of the Urological Department. I remained there for three and one-half years with all the many and varied problems of a large and active urological service, for at that time we were having the veterans of World War No. 1 in large numbers in our naval hospitals. After the three and one-half years in San Diego, I went to sea again, and was ordered back to the Asiatic station as Senior Medical Officer of the U.S.S. Houston, the Flagship of the Asiatic fleet, which was sunk in the South Pacific. At the end of the year, I was sent to the U.S. Naval Hospital, Canacoa, P.I., as Chief of Urology. I then returned home and to the U.S. Naval Hospital, Mare Island, California, as Chief of Urology and Assistant in Surgery. I spent over four years in that hospital, then back to the Orient as Medical Officer of the Marine Embassy Guard, Peking, China. There I learned field tactics, sanitation and camps, as well as carried on the routine work of medicine and surgery. In 1940 I was sent to the Naval Hospital, New York, as Chief of Urology. This was only a short tour of duty. The promotions had come along with the years, and the younger men were coming up, so orders came to a training station as Executive of the Medical Department. From that time on all clinical duties were replaced by administrative work. There came mosquito control, incineration, pest control, detention, inspections, psychiatric problems and construction of new buildings.

In July, 1941, orders came to report to the Chief of the Bureau in Washington, and there orders were issued to proceed to the British Isles to establish a Naval Hospital and to become its Commanding Officer when established. We built two hospitals in North Ireland fully equipped and ready to work.

In the meantime, the war picture changed radically. Pearl Harbor was attacked by the Japanese and our activities were directed to the West instead of the East; therefore, my services were considered necessary elsewhere. So, home it was again to receive orders to proceed to the West Coast as Executive Officer of a hospital that was being converted from a former club, and to assist in the expansion of that hospital. Much valuable experience was gained in construction work along with regular executive work of a hospital that was receiving war casualties. From that hospital sudden telegraphic orders came to proceed to Norman, Oklahoma to establish a Naval Hospital and to become its Commanding Officer when established. We built the hospital, equipped it and placed it in commission in about four and one-half months. The flag was raised on November 15, 1942 and on November 16, there were patients in the hospital. This is now a very active institution covering all hospital care, including an Out-Patient Clinic and hospitalization of dependent personnel.

This short summary of the career of one naval medical officer gives you broadly the many activities included in the term "Naval Medicine." The Medical Officer must always remember that he acts in a dual capacity; he is a Naval Officer as well as a doctor, with all the attendant responsibilities.

SUMMARY

Naval Medicine covers briefly: Indoctrination, interne training, teaching, specialization, sea duty on all types of ships, shore duty in all shore activities, sanitation, public health, recruiting, recruit training, organization, construction of dispensaries and hospitals, temporary hospitals, permanent hospitals, all war casualties ashore and afloat, venereal disease control, administrative duties, and finance and accounting for funds, setting up ship's service stores, welfare for the enlisted personnel, recreation for personnel, submarine duties, aviation medicine, sanitary reports of cities visited, quarantine laws, military, naval and international law, and many others not mentioned in detail.

A good Naval Officer is one who is well grounded in all of these activities; not only one who has acquired skill in one of the various specialities but also one who is capable of carrying on his job and his profession in any duty in which he may be assigned. He is a doctor, a teacher, a leader, a builder, frequently a lawyer, and often in certain areas he takes the place of the priest of any faith.

Trichomonas Vaginalis*

KENNETH J. WILSON, M.D.
OKLAHOMA CITY, OKLAHOMA

The genito-urinary infestation of the protozoan parasite Trichomonas is of increasing significance because of universal prevalence and recognition of its potentialities for producing remote and systemic disease, as well as that of the genitals. Early impressions of the etiology and distribution of this parasite were that it was a transition of the buccal and alimentary types to a morphologically increased stature and virulence, in the more favorable medium of vaginal secretions, that resulted in a troublesome leucorrhea. It was believed to be the product of poor hygenic habits, since its incidence was first observed in the clinic-type patient, rather than of an infectious or communicable nature. More recent observation has disclosed probably dissemination to be through inoculation from contact with infected individuals. The usual mode of communication being through contaminants, particularly toilet seats, and occasionally by direct implantation in coitus, as the male is rarely infected. Furthermore, it is not the product of uncleanliness, although this may be a contributing factor, as it occurs as frequently in the fastidious individual and young females who would seem to have hygenic advantages as in the under-privileged. It is my belief that ignorance of the mode of transmission of this highly communicable malady, contributes to its spread. Likewise, the indifference of our profession, as some have regarded its presence in the genital flora of no importance, is far short of the responsibility charged to us in preserving the health of a populace. The vast number of females seen with the disease presenting symptoms, as well as those who are symptom-free, suggest its epidemic nature.

Apparently school contacts constitute one of the chief sources of infection. Upon inquiry, many mothers recall that a school-age daughter had some unusual vaginal secretion before she noted her own genital irritation. Microscopic examination may verify the presence of trichomonas in the juvenile. Another important observation is that the victims who have been advised that any female may harbor the organism whether she is aware of it or not, are far less likely to return with reinfection.

A study of the epidemic that occurred in Wiesbaden in 1939 disclosed the presence of trichomonads in the blood of domestic animals and fowl as well as the excreta of flies. There was difficulty in finding the parasite in direct blood examination, but its identification was simplified by culture. In this country there has been no verification of these findings, although some of my experiences in clinical observation certainly point toward the likelihood of blood stream invasion with focalization on certain serous structures. I recall a case of acute endocarditis in a very elderly man who had a fulminating trichomonal urethritis and no evidence of other infection. Another case of pleuritis with effusion in a middle aged man with trichomonal urethritis, without respiratory or other infectious processes, showed motile trichomonads in the aspirated pleural secretion. A recent report of a case of pneumonia calls attention to the presence of buccal trichomonas in quantity as the only organism found in the secretion. Of course, these instances do not establish facts, but they lend impetus to curiosity.

While clinicians agree that the habitat of trichomonas vaginalis evidences a predilection for the genital and urinary tracts of females and accounts for many genito-urinary inflammations, there is no satisfactory explanation of how it invades the deeper structures. Many contend that it may invade any tissue. Certainly one sees many pelvic inflammations, that have been classified as perimetritis, which are undoubtedly due to this organism.

From our knowledge of the manner of invasion of the gonococcus and the parellel of clinical evidence in trichomonal cases, it is indicative of similar, if not identical, mode of extension. The known tendency of gonococcic infection to remain a local process, although systemic invasion occasionally occurs through the blood stream, is also imitated by the trichomonas vaginalis.

Trichomonas is too often responsible for urinary tract infection, particularly in the gestational state. Some observers contend that the trichomonas is so commonly demonstrable in the urine of those having vaginal infection they have come to regard every case of vaginal trichomoniasis as involving the

---

*Read before The Doctors Dinner Club of Oklahoma City, Oklahoma, January 19, 1943.

urinary system. Fortunately, in most instances, the distribution is confined largely to the urethra and bladder, so that it is accessible to local therapy. I have been able to identify trichomonads in the urine in most of my cases with this type vaginitis.

For practical reasons most clinicians use the hanging drop method of examination for the organism. I am sure that there is ample familiarity with this technique in the vaginal smear, but I fear a lack of appreciation that in frequent urination there is a constant flushing of the urinary tract that washes away the organism before it reaches anything like maturity, so that one must look for immature forms that may be identified by their motility. Furthermore, great dilution necessitates more diligent search, on account of scarcity of organisms in the specimen. It is mandatory that the urine be obtained by catheterization and that it be examined immediately, before chilling of the parasite, as it loses motility with change of temperature for any appreciable time.

Time will not permit elaboration on symptoms of trichomonas vaginitis, which are already familiar to all. Although one should have in mind the occurrence of genital itching, burning, discharge of a scalding nature and fetid odor, bleeding, sense of weight and soreness in the pelvic structures and occasionally systemic symptoms similar to that of other infectious processes. In urinary tract involvement there may be the usual frequency, burning and tenosmus seen in any infectious lesions of this system.

A flood of literature, reaching the doctors' desks, mostly from commercial sources, may arouse optimism in treatment that is destined to disappointment. Discussion of the subject is directed toward treatment of the symptom leucorrhea, rather than rational consideration of scientific approach. In view of evidence that the infection not only invades the vaginal and urinary tracts, but the endometrium, tubes and accessory genital and urinary glands, therapy must be designed to reach these elusive foci. Therefore, successful management is contingent upon identification of every structure involved. While the organism succumbs to any parasitic or antiseptic agent, there are two general means of attack; local exposure to the remedial agent and chemotherapy. Gynecologists are agreed on desirability of securing and maintaining a normal vaginal pH, to facilitate growth of protective Doderlein bacilli in any vaginal invasion, which is facilitated by introduction of additional acid and glucose to perpetuate an antagonistic flora.

The constant association of a diplo-streptococcus with trichomonas vaginalis has led to a great deal of speculation on its pathogenicity. It was originally suspected of being the real culprit, but late experiments disclose the possibility of inoculation of trichomonas without bacterium, although, none are ready to dispute the likelihood of its being a contributing factor, particularly, in presuming lymphatic extension. However that may be, it is sufficient for therapeutic purposes that we be guided by the distribution of the parasite. In this connection, I should like to call attention to the necessity for differentiation of the gonococcus by the Gram method of staining. It is hardly possible to distinguish these similar cocci, unless one be intracellular, except by the positive staining of the streptococcus in contradistinction to the negative gonococci.

Out of the confusion of suggested procedures and remedial agents one must adopt some form of routine. It should begin with advising the patient of the possible sources of infection and pointing out the means of avoiding recurrence. A careful microscopic study of specimens from the areas, usually involved to determine distribution of the parasite, will enable one to apply therapy where indicated.

In vaginitis daily cleansing with mild acid solutions and the introduction of some preparation containing a parasiticide, acid and glucose, for a period of two weeks will cure most cases. If there is also involvement of the urinary tract it should have simultaneous treatment. When limited to the urethra and bladder, dilation and instillation of silver solutions and others will suffice. If there is higher extension, chemotheraphy is indicated. In the urinary tract it is not known whether the chemotherapeutic agent influences the infection through its effect on the blood or by its presence in the urine, although, it seems certain the beneficial effect on the pelvic infection is blood born. Vaginal and cervical infection does not seem to be influenced by chemotherapeutic drugs.

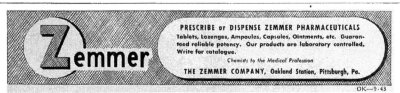

At this juncture I should like to note that neo-prontosil has been the most effective drug used in urinary tract invasion and does not have to be administered in maximum dosage. In pelvic involvement there does not seem to be any appreciable difference between it and the sulfa drugs. Bartholin glands are seldom amenable to treatment unless distended so they can be identified. Cervical involvement, if the glands are invaded, requires eradication of the cervicitis by the thermal destruction. Salpingitis is treated by chemotherapy and pelvic heat.

The known effect of estrogens in increasing cornification of genital epithelium in the treatment of gonococcic infections, particularly in the juvenile and menopausal ages, suggests its indication as an adjunct in the treatment of obstinate trichomal infestation. Most of the cases clear up with about two weeks treatment. Some will require an additional course. A few are almost perpetual, probably because of our inability to locate and reach some foci of infection. All should be advised to use acid douches through the menstrual periods for some four months following the apparent eradication of the organism, as recurrences and reinfection is most likely to appear at this time.

The Transmission of Diseases by Blood Transfusions

A. RAY WILEY, M.D.

TULSA, OKLAHOMA

I have often been asked, "is there any danger of transmitting disease by blood transfusion or plasma transfusion"? The answer, definitely, is, "yes, under certain circumstances." Fortunately, these circumstances are comparatively rare. Any blood-born infection is subject to transmission by transfusion. Of all the diseases possible to transmit, syphilis is the one most feared and may be the one most often occurring.

In 1940 I reviewed the literature on this subject and as far as possible, the case records of 33 cases of syphilis were proven to be due to blood transfusions from syphilitic blood donors. In order to establish transfusion as the source of a patients' syphilis, it must be definitely shown by clinical and laboratory studies, (a) that the recipient did not have syphilis prior to the transfusion, (b) that the recipient does not have nor does later develop a chancre, (c) that the period between the transfusion and the development of secondary symptoms be within reason, and, finally, (d) that the stage of syphilis in the donor was not chronic (late latent) nor influenced by pregnancy of the donor.

In performing transfusions we are apt to feel secure by making a Wassermann test on the donor. I cannot too strongly emphasize the fallacy of this. In reviewing the cases of known transfusion syphilis, many of the donors had negative Wassermann tests at the time of transfusion, only to become strongly positive later. From the time of initial invasion (chancre) until the antibody (reagent) is sufficiently developed to give a positive test, may be from two weeks to two months. It is in this period wherin lies the danger from transfusion. The Wassermann reaction does not depend upon the presence or absence of the spirochetes in the blood stream but upon the presence or absence of antibodies.

Syphilis is transmissable when, and only when, active spirochetes are present in the donors' blood. This occurs only during the acute stage of the disease, even before the donors' Wassermann has time to become positive. The duration of the infectious period in the untreated case is not definitely known. It disappears rapidly in the treated case and certainly is absent in late latent syphilis. The greatest danger is in obtaining blood from a donor who has become infected without his knowledge and the infection so recent that any blood test would be negative at the time of transfusion. Later in the course of the disease, the donors blood may show a positive Wassermann and yet be perfectly safe for transfusion. Note the following: Morgan[1] says, "not a single instance of incontestible 'transfusion syphilis' has been reported in which the disease was transmitted by blood from a donor with latent or chronic syphilis uninfluenced by pregnancy. In repeated instances donors with chronic syphilis have failed to transmit the disease." Eberson and Ergman[2] injected blood from 73 individuals with chronic syphilis into rabbits' testicles and not a single infection resulted; yet, with similar technique, blood from patients with acute syphilis regularly induced syphilis in the rabbits. McNamara[3] deliberately gave 17 transfusions to 10 patients from 6 donors known to have chronic syphilis. No case of syphilis occurred in any of the recipients.

What is a reasonable period for secondary symptoms to appear following transfusion? In a study of the 33 cases mentioned the period varied from 28 days to 120 days, with an average of 70 days. It is reasonable to assume that, if transfusion syphilis has occurred, secondary symptoms must occur between three and a half to four months.

From this point it follows, that an examination of the donor is most important in all transfusions. This brings up the question, and an important legal one, who is responsible for the examination of the donor. Several of my legal advisors, without quoting actual case decisions, are definitely of the opinion that the responsibility rests with the patients' attending physician. Even the furnishing of professional donors by the hospital does not relieve the physician. If the attending physician desires and does have a hospital resident physician or an interne to perform the examination, the attending physician is still responsible for any error by the interne or resident. The technical laboratory or any of the laboratory staff of the hospital has no obligation other than obtaining blood specimens and correctly reporting the true findings for transfusion. This department cannot be charged with the responsibility of questioning nor examining the donor.

The extent of the examination of a donor depends upon the individual judgment of the examiner. I take a very careful history, particularly in reference to any contacts with any contagious diseases. Not only is the donor questioned about syphilis but any and all contacts with acute eruptive diseases, also typhoid, malaria, meningitis, pneumonia, typhus and streptococcic infections. Following the history, a very careful search is made for any evidence of disease. A close search is made in both male and female donors for any evidence of a chancre or beginning chancre. There is no excuse for the all too common practice of simply sending a group of donors to the laboratory without any examination other than a Wassermann test and using any blood that passes the laboratory.

Of the 33 cases already mentioned, seven of the donors had secondary eruptions on them at the time of the transfusion. Such carelessness is deplorable and must be condemned. Do not be misled by the fact that the donor is a relative of the patient. Of the 33 cases, 16 of the donors were relatives of the patients. Syphilis is no respecter of persons.

So far, I have considered transmission of syphilis with whole blood transfusions. What are the possibilities with plasma transfusions? If the plasma of one infected donor is added to a batch of pooled plasma, it would be diluted but all would be contaminated. Does freezing plasma destroy the spirochetes? Freezing does not destroy ordinary bacteria. So far as I know, no research work has been done to determine the viability of the spirochete after a period in frozen plasma. Until this is done we must assume that freezing is no protection against infection. Converting plasma to the dry state should destroy the spirochetes, but here again, new work must be done. It is customary to carefully check the sterility of all plasma before it is reduced to the powder state, but sterility tests for syphilis and malaria cannot be made by ordinary methods.

How can one eliminate all danger of spirochetal or treponemal contamination in blood or plasma? A very good study of this has been made by Kolmer[4]. His conclusions are, "all that is necessary is to dissolve .1 gm (neoarsphenamine) in 10 cc of sterile distilled water and add 1 cc (0.01 gm. of the compound) to each 100 cc of citrated blood, yielding thus a 1:10,000 solution. After mixing and standing at room temperature for fifteen minutes, it is ready for intravenous injection." Kolmer refers to whole blood to be used immediately. If any doubt exists about plasma being contaminated with syphilis spirochetes, that same technique may be carried out just before its use.

SUMMARY

The possibilities of infection from blood transfusions and plasma transfusions have been pointed out. The danger from syphilis and the dangerous and innocent periods of transmission are discussed. The necessity of careful donor examinations is given. The responsibility of these examinations is pointed out. Safety precautions are given.

In conclusion I wish to say that nothing in this paper should deter anyone from performing blood or plasma transfusions whenever clinical conditions justify a transfusion. Rather it is designed to enhance the value of transfusions, to promote safety in transfusions and to stimulate interest.

BIBLIOGRAPHY

1. Morgan, Hugh J.: Amer. Jour. Medical Science, Vol. 189, No. 6. June, 1935.
2. Eberson, F. and Ergman, M. F.: Jour of A.M.A., Vol. 160, No. 76. 1931.
3. McNamara, W. L.: Amer. Jour. Syphilis, Vol. 9, page 470. 1935.
4. Kolmer, John A.: Amer. Jour. Syph., Gon. and Ven. Diseases, Vol. 23, No. 2, pages 150-164 March, 1939.
5. Gilman, Robert L.: Syphilis and Transfusion. Indian Jour of Ven. Diseases, Vol 2, No. 3. September, 1936.
6 Transmission of Syphilis by Blood Transfusion: Current Comment Jour of A.M.A. July 11, 1931.
7 Rein, Chas. R., The Control and Prevention of Transfusion Syphilis. Jour A.M.A., Vol. 110, pages 13-18. January 1, 1938.
8. Mandelbaum, Harry: Transmission of Syphilis by Blood Transfusion. Jour. A.M.A., Vol. 106, pages 1061-1063. March 28, 1936.
9. Cummer, Clyde L.: Transfusion Syphilis. Amer Jour Med Sciences, Vol. CLXXXV, No. 6, pages 787-789. June,1933.
10. Polayes, Silik H and Lederer Max: The Transmission

of Syphilis by Blood Transfusion. Amer. Jour. of Syphilis, Vol. XV, No. 1, page 72. January, 1931.
11. Williamson, G. Richards: Congenital Syphilis from Blood Transfusion to the Mother During Pregnancy. The Amer. Jour. of Syphilis. Vol. XVII, No. 4. October, 1933.
12. Post, Chas D. and Cooney, Gerald C.: Accidental Transmission of Syphilis by Blood Transfusion. Reprint. Jour. A.M.A., Vol. 100, page 258. January 28, 1933.
13. Blood Transfusion from Syphilitic Patient. Jour. A.M.A., Vol. 107, page 303. Reprint. July 25, 1936.
14. Transmission of Syphilis by Injected Blood. Jour. A.M.A., Vol. 100, page 281. January 28, 1933.
15. Jones, Harold W.: The Transmission of Syphilis by Blood Transfusion. Amer. Jour. of Syphilis, Vol. 19, pages 30-38. January, 1935.
16. Straus, R.: Kline Exclusion Test in Prevention of Transfusion Syphilis Reprinted from Archives of Dermatology and Syphilogy, Vol. 36, pages 1039-1043. November, 1937.
17 McCluskie, J. A. W.: The Transmission of Syphilis by Blood Transfusion. The British Medical Jour., Vol. 1, pages 264-266. February 11, 1939
18. Kast, Clara C.: The Treponemicidal Activity of Arsphenamine and Neoarsphenamine in Vitro with Special Reference to Citrated Blood and a Suggested Method for the Prevention of Transfusion Syphilis. Amer. Jour. Syph., Gon. and Ven. Diseases, Vol 23, pages 150-164. March, 1939.
19. Willis, Morton W.: Transfusion Syphilis. New York State Jour. Med., Vol. 37, pages 60-67. January 1, 1937.
20 Klauder, Joseph V.: Accidental Transmission of Syphilis by Boold Transfusion. Amer. Jour, Syph., Gon. and Ven. Diseases, Vol 21, pages 652-666. November, 1937.
21. Averbuck, Samuel H.: Syphilis Transmitted by Transfusion. Jour. Mt. Sinai Hospital, Vol. 5, pages 627-632. January, 1939.
22. Hendrick, Harriet: Diseases Transmitted in Blood Transfusion. The Proceedings of the Inst. of Med. of Chicago, Vol. 10, No. 10, page 185. January 15, 1935.

Etiology of Malignant Neutropenia*

COLONEL WILLIAM H. GORDON, M.C.
BORDEN GENERAL HOSPITAL

CHICKASHA, OKLAHOMA

Malignant neutropenia is a condition characterized by an acute onset of marked malaise, prostration, weakness, and high fever which may or may not be accompanied by ulcertative and gangrenous angina of the buccal mucosa, and occasionally is associated with ulcerations of other mucous membranes of the skin. It often exhibits a partial or total leukopenia accompanied by an absence of polymorphonuclear leukocytes.

At present, the etiology of the disease is debatable. Many writers have considered it to be a chronic Vincent's angina which has suddenly become malignant. Others believe it to be a very severe sepsis, whose causal agent has a definite action upon myeloblastic tissue and the bone marrow. A few believe it to be one of the end results of some chronic illness. Still others consider it to be due to a toxic substance similar to benzol or some other hydrocarbon which depresses or paralyzes activity of the bone marrow and, as a result, causes a marked diminution in the manufacture of granular leukocytes. As a result of this loss of fighting cells, the tissues of the body are invaded by the bacteria which ordinarily exist in its cavities without producing symptoms, following which invasion, gangrene, ulceration, sepsis, etc., occur.

Others have theorized as follows concerning the disease: first, the characteristic ulcerations found in malignant neutropenia are the result of bacterial emboli which have occluded the vessels to the affected area; second, that these lesions are secondary to a septicopyemia. This second theory indicates that this is a specific disease resulting in gangrenous areas caused by a specific toxin against the leukocytes. Thirdly, it is considered to be a primary affection of the bone marrow resulting in a decreased formation of granulocytes, with resulting lowering of resistance of the patient, which terminates in intercurrent infection, necrosis of mucous membranes and skin, and finally death. This is probably the most plausible theory since no emboli are found at autopsy.

The following classification covers all the various etiological factors of neutropenia which have been presented in literature: 1. unknown, 2. chemicals and drugs, 3. bacterial and protozoan (acute and chronic), 4. allergic, 5. embryonic, 6. biological, 7. physical, 8. incidental, 9. endocrine, 10. experimental, 11. splenic neutropenia.

*Read before the Annual Meeting of the Oklahoma State Medical Association, May 11 at Oklahoma City.

CHEMICALS AND DRUGS AS CAUSES OF MALIGNANT NEUTROPENIA

Neutropenia, in recent times has been prominently associated with exposure to benzol, hydrocarbons, and tri-nitro-toluene. Further we find those cases in which it has occurred following the treatment of some conditions with arseno-benzol, bismuth, bismarsen, amidopyrine, barbital, dinitrophenol, one of the sulfonamides, and other drugs. These have all been described in medical literature as definite causes by various authors.

McCord studied benzol poisoning as an industrial disease and found marked similarity between that condition and agranulocytosis. Dameshek has also described benzene poisoning with accompanying agranulocytosis. While under treatment for syphilis, several cases have been reported in patients to whom arseno-benzol and bismarsen had been given. Other cases have been recorded in which bismuth was given alone. An identical picture has been reported in chronic tri-nitro-toluene poisoning. Clyde Brooks reported a case in a young physician which occurred after drinking an excess of alcohol. Many cases have been reported following the carelessness or indiscriminate administration of the sulfonamide series of drugs.

Madison and Squire believe a large percentage of the cases of malignant neutropenia are due to the use of drugs containing amidopyrine and barbital. Watkins has published a few reports of the disease which he considers were caused by the above drugs and their combinations.

However, in our series of 97 cases we find but one which may belong to this group. We have corresponded with many psychopathic hospitals and find that no cases of the condition have been diagnosed in such institutions, although the above drugs had been used in large amounts.

Kracke, in his study of the causes of death from the United States Bureau of Vital Statistics, found that a large percentage of patients who had malignant neutropenia were women, and that a high percentage occurred among physicians, nurses, relatives of people connected with the medical profession, hospital maids, medical students, and laboratory technicians. In the study presented herein, of more than seven hundred cases, including 97 cases seen by the writer and the rest from literature, it has been found that approximately 20 per cent of the patients were from a group closely associated with the medical profession. All these patients and others were closely questioned as to the use of drugs which they may have received as samples, and those prescribed by physicians, and in only a few cases can

the intake of medicines of the benzene series be considered a causative factor of malignant neutropenia and that but indirectly. As a result of this study, in our opinion only a small per cent of these cases of malignant neutropenia cannot be attributed to the careless use of drugs.

BACTERIA AND PROTOZOA AS CAUSES OF MALIGNANT NEUTROPENIA

The following organisms have all been described as accompanying or etiological factors of malignant neutropenia; streptococci of all types staphylococcus albus and aureus, Vincent's aspirillum and fusiform bacillus, pneumococcus, gram negative and gram positive bacilli, bacillus coli, bacillus pyocyaneus, bacillus subtilis, meningococcus, diptheria bacillus, and bacillus Welchii, acute Vincent's angina, severe local and general sepsis, epidemic influenza, pneumonia, malaria and meningitis have been accompanied or followed by this condition.

Cultures from the blood, gums, mouth, and throat of patients suffering from malignant neutropenia have yielded the large and diversified group of micro-organisms mentioned above. However, as is usual in such cases, no single strain of bacteria can be pointed to directly as the specific etiological agent of malignant neutropenia.

Lovett, Klein, Maschke, McKeen, Kahlstrom, Kenny, Hammock, Zeilor, and many others have reported cases from which a pure culture of bacillus pyocyaneus was obtained. We have one case which yields a pure culture of bacillus pyocyaneus and in animal studies with this culture, we have produced leukopenia with agranulocytosis. Hill's case occurred in a woman of 35 years of age after extraction of a molar tooth. Many organisms, including Vincent's spirillum and bacillus were found in the smear from gangrenous gums. Skiles and others have reported the disease after Vincent's angina and also after extraction. Skiles, too, believed that the disease was due to a specific infection in the gangrenous area, which secreted a special toxin against cells of the granulocytic series. . Hirsch and others, however, stressed the point that its origin was not in the tonsil. Several of our cases have had their tonsils removed previous to the onset of granulocytopenia.

Frank and Smiley reported a case during an attack of acute mastoiditis. One case was reported with gas bacillus septicemia. Iberbein writes "Agranulocytosis is tuberculosis of the bone marrow." Others have reported the disease with tuberculosis.

A large number of Detroit cases as well as many of those in literature were sent to contagion hospitals with an entrance diagnosis of diptheria and were later diagnosed as malignant neutropenia by laboratory and clinical tests or by autopsy. Two cases are reported in literature following diptheria. Also, the condition has been reported following pneumonia, malaria, and other infections.

ALLERGY AND NEUTROPENIA

Several investigators have considered allergy as an etiological factor in malignant neutropenia. Several patients among those reported have shown an eosinophilia. However, the evidence in favor of an allergic cause of agranulocytosis is not convincing although asthma has been reported as a possible predisposing cause in the development of a neutropenia. One writer has seen the condition following the use of pentonucleotide while others have expressed a belief that malignant neutropenia may be an allergic reaction following pyramidon therapy. Among our cases was one which did not recover from the third attack of the disease. At post mortem, the intestinal tract showed giant urticarial patches on the mucous lining of the large and small bowel.

THE PRODUCTION OF MALIGNANT NEUTROPENIA BY PHYSICAL AGENTS

The chief physical agent said to have produced neutropenia is the x-ray used in deep therapy. However, in review of literature only one case was reported following Roentgen-ray therapy. Extractions of teeth, and fractures of bones, especially the skull and leg bone, and other injuries of the osseous tissue not infrequently preceded the development of agranulocytopenia.

HEREDITY AS A FACTOR IN MALIGNANT NEUTROPENIA

Some authors, studying the question of neutropenia, have ascribed its cause to a congenital deficiency of the bone marrow or to a maturation arrest of the leukocytes.

Thompson reported seven cases which exhibited the picture of an acute infectious disease with high fever, low pulse, enlarged lymph glands, and a low white count with neutropenia. The majority of these cases recovered but the cause was not determined. Laude, too, has written concerning this group. Fitz-Hugh and Krumbhaar believe it to be a maturation arrest. We believe that in a large per cent of the cases there is a congenital deficiency in the bone marrow. This is supported strongly by those instances in which one member of a family developed malignant neutropenia, while another developed myeloid leukemia, and also by the occurrence of two cases of neutropenia in one family. Hart has also reported the condition in two sisters, as has Zinninger.

MALIGNANT NEUTROPENIA INCIDENTAL TO OTHER CONDITIONS

Malignant neutropenia has developed in individuals while they were under treatment or observation for cholecystitis, cardiac disease, amoebic and ulcerative colitis, furunculosis, syphilis, tuberculosis, and carcinoma. George Blumer in 1930, showed that an agranulocytic blood picture may occur in disease of local and general sepsis other than agranulocytic angina. William Murphy, Leuchtenberger, N. Christoff, and others have confirmed this report. Removal of badly infected teeth is prominent as an incidental condition associated with malignant neutropenia. Edith Peritz' case, together with many others in literature, also three of our cases occurred while being studied at the clinic or hospital for bile duct disease at the time of their initial attack. Mack and Klages write concerning the anemias of cancerous bone marrow. One physician recently had a chronic severe diabetic who developed rectal ulcerations accompanied by severe neutropenia which terminated in death. Autopsy revealed intestinal ulcerations.

ENDOCRINE FACTORS IN MALIGNANT NEUTROPENIA

As with allergy, the evidence in favor of an endocrine dyscrasia underlying the neutropenic state is still scant and unconvincing. Beyond a cursory report describing the menses and pregnancy as contributory etiologic factors the literature supporting this theory is very meager.

SPLENIC NEUTROPENIA

The first series of cases on this interesting condition was reported by Doan and Wiseman in 1942. As stated earlier, this type of neutropenia is believed to be the result of a hitherto unreported cause of neutropenia; namely a pathologically altered physiological function of the normal spleen. Fundamentally it is closely allied to congenital hemolytic acholuric jaundice and thrombocytopenic purpura for the following reasons: in hemolytic jaundice there is an increased destruction of the erythroytes in the spleen; in thrombocytopenic purpura there is an increased destruction of the thrombocytes in the spleen; and in splenic neutropenia there is an increased destruction of neutrophils in the spleen. Further historical aspects of the condition are not available at this time. From the few cases reported it appears that the condition may be subdivided into three classes; acute, sub-acute and chronic. It is devoid of seasonal preference. From the few cases recorded, it evidently parallels malignant neutropenia in the ratio of two females affected to every male. The age incidence likewise appears to be similar, mainly in the fourth and fifth decades.

The symptoms of this condition vary with the severity. In the chronic case the patient complains of little else but tiredness and general malaise. In the acute case there is usually a concommitant hemolytic anemia and thrombocytopenia of varying degrees. Usually in the acute type the onset is characterized by a cold, accompanied by hyperpyrexia, rapid pulse, great prostration, and not infrequently, ulcerations of the tonsillar fossae and buccal mucous membrane. Later on the ulceration may be quite severe, even occurring in the skin. Jaundice with negative direct Van den Bergh is common. When anemia is present it is of the macrocytic hemolytic type with reticulosis. When bleeding is present it varies from a mild purpura to severe epistaxis, black and tarry stools, extensive petechiae and ecchymosis in the skin. The spleen is constantly enlarged but not tender.

The blood picture closely resembles that of malignant neutropenia in that there is present marked diminution in the neutrophils of the peripheral blood and resultant leukopenia. Monocytes and lymphocytes are equally well represented. But unlike malignant neutropenia, thrombocytopenic purpura with low platelet count, and hemolytic anemia are the rule.

Scrapings of the splenic pulp showed a marked increase in the splenic clasmatocytes within which cells were ingested neutrophilic leukocytes, as well as some erythrocytes and an occasional normoblast. No other abnormalities were detected in the spleen.

Sternal marrow revealed a marked hyperplasia of myeloid cells without any appreciable shift to the left. The granular leukocytes seen were the mature polymorphonuclears and the C myelocytes. There was no toxic destructiion of these marrow cells and no maturation arrest.

In malignant neutropenia, therefore, the destructive process affects certain of the myeloid elements of the marrow, causing the inhibition of neutrophil production; in splenic neutropenia the spleen no longer phagocytoses old worn out blood elements along, but on the contrary destroys normal healthy blood elements as well. In the marrow of malignant neutropenia there is a dearth of neutrophils; in the marrow of splenic neutropenia there is usually a hypesplasia of myeloid elements. In malignant neutropenia, anemia and thrombocytopenia are exceedingly rare; in the splenic neutropenia, hemolytic anemia and thrombocytopenic purpura are the rule. In malignant neutropenia the spleen is usually not enlarged; in splenic neutropenia it is constantly enlarged. Malignant neutropenia is unaffected by splenectomy; splenic neutropenia as well as its concommitant hemolytic anemia and thrombocytopenic purpura, is invariably cured by splenectomy.

If these points are kept in mind, there should be no confusion between these two distinctly different types of neutropenia. Splenic neutropenia could only be confused with leukemia of the subleukemic type. But here, splenic neutropenia never shows the alterations in the quality of the myeloid elements despite the fact that myeloid hyperplasia is present in both, while qualitative changes in myeloid elements is the rule in sub-leukemic leukemia.

SUMMARY OF THEORIES OF THE ETIOLOGY OF MALIGNANT NEUTROPENIA

1. Neutropenia following chronic Vincent's angina.

2. Severe sepsis affecting myeloblastic tissue and bone marrow.

3. End result of chronic illness.

4. Toxic substances depressing or paralyzing bone marrow activity.

5. Secondary invasion by bacteria in tissues with lowered resistance.

6. Chemical poisoning—as by benzol, benzene, etc.

7. Drug poisoning—as barbital, amophridine and sulfonamide drugs.

8. Allergy.

9. Endocrine dyscrasia.

10. Possible congenital absence of a necessary substance in bone marrow which makes the individual susceptible to the development of leukopenia.

However, because of the multiplicity of possible etiological factors as presented in the literature, it is believed that the absolute etiology of the disease is still unknown. If we can judge by similar experiences with other diseases, undoubtedly an entirely different cause than has so far been considered may eventually be discovered.

DISCUSSION
HUGH JETER, M.D.

It has been a pleasure to have read Colonel Gordon's manuscript. He has covered the subject of etiology very thoroughly and I have the feeling that what I may say will add very little to his paper.

Permit me to emphasize the fact, which the experience of many has seemed to prove, namely, that the specific etiological agent has not yet been definitely established. The following is a case which I reported in the Southern Medical Journal in 1939, which illustrates the uncertainty and illusiveness of the etiological factors:

A surgical case of Dr. D. H. O'Donoghue's, in St. Anthony Hospital, who had a "dry osteomyelitis." That is the name I gave it because she had a destructive lesion of the femur, later followed by a similar destructive lesion of the opposite femur, both operated and drained and nothing but necrotic material obtained. It was not only dry, but it was also sterile and the only conclusion I could make was that the destructive bone lesion was the result of a tiny embolus in each instance. This is mentioned because there is some reason to believe that the absorption of necrotizing tissue is a factor in the production of malignant neutropenia.

This lady had five successive recurrences of agranulocytosis of neutropenia, each with sudden drop to below one thousand in the total white count with practically no neutrophils and with corresponding elevation of temperature to as high as 104 to 106, and the associated ulcers of the throat, and she was desperately sick each time.

Ample opportunity to investigate different methods of treatment was afforded by the recurrences. Pentanucleotides, transfusions, parenteral liver and other less commonly used forms of therapy were tried and, strange enough, during the last episode or paroxysm no treatment whatever was given and the patient took the identical course as those which preceded. The drainage became very thin and watery as the white count went down and, we thought perhaps somewhat more abundant and again each time more cloudy and less abundant when the white count improved. This lady is still living and well and her white count during the last two years has been checked and is within normal limits.

Vincent's infection and a few other saprophytic types have been known to be followed by, or associated with, malignant neutropenia.

'It is interesting to note that there has been a wave of decreased incidence of malignant neutropenia. Dr Kracke's study and reports in connection with the incidence have surely been a factor in reducing the, shall we say, careless use of amidophrine. When I say the specific etiological agent has been discovered, I do not wish to discount the value of the discovery of such factors, and believe amidopyrine has been a factor.

In one of our cases we obtained repeatedly a gram negative bacillus by blood culture, which proved later to be nonpathogenic to monkeys. I believe with malignant neutropenia we may expect non-specific blood stream positive cultures as we do with leukemia, because the barriers to infection have been weakened and the resistance of the patient permits invasion of most any type of micro-organism which happens to inhabit the area or areas of ulceration. This probably explains the inconsistant reports concerning various bacteria which have been recorded by different observers as possible etiological agents.

I am grateful to Colonel Gordon for this fine paper.

PHYSICIANS AS ARTISTS

"From time immemorial, medicine and art have been closely associated. The same skill that makes the surgeon's fingers deft with scalpel and ligature is at work in the beautiful examples of sculpture and carving shown in this book. The eye that so quickly and accurately evaluates the graduations in color and texture between normal and pathologic tissue coordinates the hand that wields the painter's brush. The man who chooses medicine as his life's work is largely motivated by a love for his fellow man, else he would select a vocation offering greater monetary reward. From the beginning, he is trained to exercise his powers of observations, and in time develops imagination, sympathy, understanding, philosophy and reverence, all of which are the very essence of art. Moreover, he deals with that most exquisite forms of divine art and beauty, the human body.

"An artist-physician has said; "The tendency of most persons is to regard the artist with awe as a superman endowed with talents not vouchsafed to the ordinary mortal. Most doctors have a latent artistic sense which may be purchased for a small sum and any local artist practice. When opportunity affords, slip away to the park or country, sit down on a camp-stool and practice sketching from nature. At first the results may not be satisfying, but in course of time you will be gratified to notice a marked improvement. An ample sketching kit may be purchased for a smal lsum and any local artist will be glad to give you instruction.'

"At the least, every physician is able to develop a sensitiveness to and an appreciation for fine art. He can also cultivate a hobby, which, if not one of the fine arts, is in the class of 'work by the side of work.' Dr. Charles A. Dana, who has always stressed the value of cultural medicine, has advised; "Be a collector, for example, of stamps or automobiles, or old books, or neckties or pins; or find diversion in some collateral branch of science; the lore of birds, of fishing and shooting. Make a garden or cultivate shrubs and flowers. These kinds of activities will make your life happier and your professional character more attractive and effective!"—Quoted from "Parergon," published by Mead Johnson & Company, Evansville, Ind. Free copy available to physicians on request.

Verumontanitis
The Application of the Sex Hormones

ROBERT H. AKIN M.D.

OKLAHOMA CITY, OKLAHOMA

It is difficult to anticipate during one's anatomical studies, that the shriveled structure in the floor of the prostatic urethra, the verumontanum, would ever assume much clinical importance. An apprenticeship in cystourethroscopy clears away part of the haze surrounding this "true mountain" of the pioneer anatomists. A further contact with verumontanitis brings forth a great effort to ascertain the etiological factors and formulate a satisfactory and rational plan of treatment.

Although it is usual to find the sexually active adult males are predominantly involved, verumontanitis and hypertrophic veru are sometimes seen in infants and young children. The symptoms may be obstructive to urination or obstructive to the genital glands, or they may be due to irritation only. Young boys who have frequency or urgency of urination, who pull at their genital organs, or who have enuresis, frequently are found to have enlarged or inflamed verus. Adults often have premature ejaculations, crawling or pricking sensations in the penis and perineum, and painful spermatic cords. The pains may radiate to the femoral regions, or may simulate sacroiliac or sciatic pains from resultant seminal vesicle or prostatic congestion. The symptoms may persist for months or years, or recur at frequent intervals.

Acute Neisserian posterior urethritis certainly involves the veru but such a verumontanitis usually subsides quickly unless overtreated or complicated by non-specific organism. In a series of about 400 cases having chronic or recurrent non-specific urethritis, Moor and Brown were able to culturally isolate and type pneumococci in approximately one-third of the cases. These were the most chronic and persistent of the series. The colon bacillus, the streptococcus fecalis, the staphylococcus aureus and albus, and the pyocyaneus were other organisms cultured. Distant primary foci of infection in teeth, tonsils, sinuses, furuncles, hemorrhoids, gall bladder and lungs must have some importance as pneumococci cultured from apical dental abscesses and the urine were found to be the same type. Syphilis and tuberculosis are possible causes. A survey of the upper urinary tract frequently reveals stones, or hydronephroses with infection.

It is probable that alcoholic drinks or carbonated drinks produce no more than a transitory irritation unless some of the above infections are present. Congenitally small meatus, or stricture of the urethra produce overdistention of the posterior urethra and are contributory factors.

At first glance it would seem trivial to consider such an obscure and small subject. A decade of listening to the story of the traveling salesman who sat on a centipede from one town to the other, and had had his verumontanum coagulated or fulgurated by urologists in each large city to give some relative relief, convinces one of its importance. Cystic degeneration of the verumontanum would seem to indicate the need for fulguration and granulation of the veru, or justify silver nitrate cauterization. These are not ideal, however, because of the atrophy and scarring which may result. The use of sulfa compounds for these non-specific cases usually affords relief but unless urethral obstructions and upper urinary tract factors are cleared up, recurrence is certain. Formed cysts and marked granulation do not readily clear up solely as a result of the sulfa drug therapy. It is for this reason that I mention estrogens and androgens as therapeutic agents. Since 1937, I have not found it necessary to cauterize or coagulate the veru for cysts or granulations, reserving fulguration for benign papillomata only. Both estrogens and androgens increase the height and thickness of the prostatic urethral mucous membrane. In sufficient doses they may even change this mucosa to transitional type, as demonstrated by experiments on monkeys by Zukerman and others. These changes in the mucosa of the posterior urethra are transitory and usually subside in forty days after the discontinuance of the hormone, at least in the case of estrogens in monkeys. Androgens increase the secretory activity of the prostate and seminal vesicles while the estrogens decrease the secretory activity. In verumontanitis with congested seminal vesicles and prostate, secretory activity is undesirable until the patient and his infection has reached a permissible functional state. Estrogens have, therefore, proven more effective and valuable in the actual treatment of inflamed or enlarged veru than the more actively congesting androgens, and appear to have produced no harmful effects. Over-dosage with estrogens may produce bladder atony so that two to five thousand unit doses once or twice a week have been used for four to eight doses. This has usually been sufficient. We do not give ten thousand units and have not used stilbestrol for this treatment as we have not found it necessary.

In summary, it is necessary to determine and eradicate the etiological infection, correct urethral obstructive or upper urinary tract pathology, and restore the normal posterior urethral mucosa. It is unwise to forget that light tonic massages and hot sitz baths have their place in the treatment, and mild deep instillations of protein silver, or mild merthiolate are also helpful. Estrogens are apparently of considerable value.

A Review of the Management of Late Syphilis

C. P. BONDURANT, M.D.
Professor of Dermatology and Syphilology University of Oklahoma School of Medicine
OKLAHOMA CITY, OKLAHOMA

When the average individual thinks of syphilis he thinks of it as a contagious disease, and this is rightly so. The lay public, as well as physician, is seemingly unaware of the death-dealing qualities of late syphilis. I approach the subject of the management of late syphilis with a profound sense of guilt, feeling that if, as physicians, we fastened our eyes upon the chancre and early course of syphilis, and not upon the fixed pupil, the Charcot joint, or the aneurysmal bulge, and turned our writing and thinking to the chancres and their early sequellae, a few decades might witness the extinction of this infection. To focus the gaze of medicine upon the infectious stage of syphilis, the chancre the secondaries and their recurrences, and to secure their sterilization at the shortest interval is then the first great commandment of current syphilology.

To make a distinction between early and late syphilis, it is necessary to call attention to the fundamental pathology which formulates these stages. As the early stage, which is characterized by a uniformity of distribution of organisms and lesions, begins to fade, the successive recurrent outbreaks become less and less and the periods of quiescence become longer and longer, until the disease presents no tangible evidence of its existence then it is said to have become latent. In other words, no clinical evidence of the disease is present and during this period the full course of the disease is below the clinical horizon. This period of latency may vary from a few months to a lifetime but it is by no means a period of inactivity. It is to be considered a state of balance which is the product of a relative immunity maintained by slow, chronic, inflammatory changes. By this immunity process which begins early in the course of the disease, a large majority of the spirochetes which saturate the body are eliminated. The few that remain are lo-

calized in certain tissues and the damage which they are to produce later depends to a great extent upon the site of this localization.

During early latency, recurrent lesions may occur on the surface and require sterilization by treatment, but these are not destructive lesions and are rarely harmful to the patient. Following this part of the latency period the lesions are largely internal, do not contain many organisms, and the relation between these organisms and the tissue is changed. These have acquired the ability to produce destructive lesions and are harmful only to the patient himself. They are characterized by a wide varity of pathological activity, occurring in unpredictable locations with no reference to time, involving almost any structure of the body and impairing its function to any degree from an imperceptible alteration to its complete destruction. The immunological background of the patient, a little understood process, to a great extent is responsible for the degree of this damage. We cannot help but believe that this immunity is to some degree made or altered by the early treatment of the individual. Here it might not be amiss to warn of the complicating factors of recurring late syphilis that might follow the so-called quick treatment of early syphilis now highly recommended and accepted to meet the public fever for speed seen in all war times. The history of syphilis therapy is not without record experience in this respect.

The diagnosis of the late stages of syphilis is often far from simple, and calls for the cooperative endeavor in these diagnostic problems as in no other field of medicine. Syphilis, unlike any other disease, may involve simultaneously many systems of the body. The resulting symptom complex may tax the most experienced. Laboratory methods have been a valuable addition to the clinical diagnosis of syphilis so masterfully practiced by the older syphilologists, but it is regrettable that too many have placed an exaggerated reliance on laboratory methods, and rely exclusively on the laboratory to the neglect of various signs and symptoms of this disease which stand out as leading clues to this infection. There is a tendency to accept blindly the laboratory findings in diagnostic syphilology. To the lay mind a positive blood test means syphilis, and a negative blood test rules it out, and among some medical men this type of diagnosis prevails. We must not forget that in late syphilis in many instances there is positive disease with a negative Wasserman. This percentage has been variously estimated at from 10 to 30 per per cent. There is no substitute in this form of diagnosis for a searching history and a careful and complete physicial examination, supplemented by laboratory findings on both blood and spinal fluid. Our greatest and most dangerous error is to accept as final a negative blood Wasserman.

Once the diagnosis of late syphilis is established we are confronted with the question of therapy, and we are forced to realize that a biological cure is an improbability. Faced with this we ask, "What is then the purpose of treatment?" This is many-fold, with the first aim to afford symptomatic relief. As a rule this is well within reason and fairly easy but the question of relapse has to be reckoned with. To correctly plan the type of therapy necessary, the character of the involvement, the history of previous treatment and the general condition of the individual, all weighed carefully with prolonged treatment in mind, will usually be sufficient. The second aim is the restoration and maintanance of normal anatomy and with this, if possible, the return to normal function. The realization of this, of course, is dependent upon the location, type, and extent of the damaged tissue. When these aims are unattainable, the imperative issue is to stop the pathological progress and to preserve as far as possible a stationary relationship between the disease and the host. The laboratory is of value to us in determining these questions but the serological progress is quite a secondary issue and we must not allow our interest to be focused upon laboratory findings and lose sight of the condition of the patient himself. It has been wisely said that the clinical yardstick is the only measure of success in the management of late syphilis. The amount and type of treatment to be administered can only be determined by careful and complete study of the individual case.

The management of the various types of late syphilis almost demands a special field in each group. Outstanding among these types is the treatment of truly latent syphilis and

the importance of this is only realized when we consider the frequency with which it is seen. This is that great group of syphilitics whose infection has lasped into obscurity and is diagnosed only by repeatedly positive serological tests. Most of the cases of syphilis complicated by pregnancy fall in this group, and it has been estimated that one-third of all luetics are truly latent. The prognosis of the latent case which receives proper and prolonged treatment is not discouraging. The purpose of treatment here is to prevent progression, relapse, and infectiousness with final sterilization. It must be recalled that this part of the course of late syphilis is really a slow but gradual inflamatory process which remains below the threshold of clinical perception. The art of practice is many times taxed to secure the complete cooperation of the apparently well individual, but this, however, is usually done when absolute frankness is maintained and simple explanations are made. Usually this type of therapy is begun with heavy metals combined with the intermittent use of the iodides, later to be followed by full courses of the arsenicals if these are tolerated. The relationship of these should be in a ratio of more of the heavy metals with arsenic than is used in early syphilis. The results are about equal whether intermittent or continuous treatment is used. Again the study of the individual case should decide this point. A rule acceptable to most clinicians is a year of continuous treatment followed by a year of intermittent treatment. In the Wasserman fast cases, fever therapy is an excellent addition to the second year's treatment and this is receiving wide acceptance. There is little doubt that fever raises the tolerance of the patient for the spirocheticidal drugs and definitely increases their efficiency. If the general condition of the patient permits, I usually give small doses of arsenicals during the latter part of the fever course, these being given during the elevation of the temperature. The tolerance for these drugs is usually increased by administering them in glucose and saline. I usually follow the course of fever with potassium iodide and arsenic in a short course. It is not uncommon to find the Wassermann reversed in these cases after a prolonged rest.

From a death-dealing standpoint, cardiovascular syphilis undoubtedly has first place. It has been estimated that once syphilitic disease of the heart has been diagnosed, a life expectancy of four years is all that can be promised. Here, as in no other phase of syphilology, the strict individualization of cases is mandatory. The success of our management of this group is dependent upon the acuteness with which the early diagnosis is made. Conservative therapy is the first rule and the syphilologist should assuredly make use of a free consultation with the internist in this phase of syphilitic management.

Another type of late syphilis of increasing importance is syphilis of the central nervous system. The cellular structure of the central nervous system when considered from the standpoint of its ability to recuperate and recover lost function makes it one of the hardest systems of the body to manage when luetic disease is diagnosed. It has not been long since the syphilitic involvement of the central nervous system was regarded as untreatable except by palliative means. With the newer methods of diagnosis and therapy this structure is seen to yield in a very satisfactory manner and it is not boastful to state that it can be handled by any physician reasonably equipped and sufficiently interested. The advancement in spinal fluid examination and study alone has afforded practical diagnosis with an accuracy which was thought beyond reason a few decades ago. A symptomatic neurosyphilis has come to the front as a diagnosis more and more in the last few decades and constitutes that phase of neurosyphilis where the spinal fluid abnormalities are present with the absence of clinical evidence. The accepted practice of routine spinal fluid examinations in all late syphilis cases has served well in the management of this phase of the disease. The importance of this procedure is further demanded by the fact that abnormalities of the spinal fluid precede by years the appearance of clinical damage and the patient is indeed fortunate who has this information available for the doctor charged with his care. On the other hand, the doctor who manages a case of late syphilis without this information should be ashamed.

Once the central nervous system is involved to a degree sufficient to present a clinical phase, definite types may be recognized. Many more or less elaborate divisions of these have been outlined, but a simple and practical one is as follows: the interstitial type which involves the supportive structures of the brain and spinal cord and the parenchymatous which represents the involvement of the true nervous tissue. It must be understood that both of these can be present in the same case. Of the latter group, the two great divisions are the tabetic and paretic forms, each having its own chain of symptoms and serological formula.

The management and observation of these various types of neurosyphilis form one of the most fascinating chapters in all medical therapeutics. The first thought after clinical and laboratory evidence is obtained is the strict individualization of cases. When we ask what is the management of this type of neurosphilis we should ask what is the management of this case of neurosyphilis. The early management of asymptomatic neurosyphilis is little different from the routine treatment of uncomplicated cases. When the damage has advanced to a degree of moderate abnormalities, the plan is intensified, and the titre of the fluid Wassermann is used as the guide. When the improvement is slow either from the clinical or laboratory angle, a course of tryparsamide is added with the usual precautions, and with the more resistant cases, fever therapy is used. I know of no procedure that pays the dividends of fever therapy in early central nervous system cases.

The diffuse meningovascular cases present such a variety of clinical pictures that it makes it difficult to outline more than a generalized type of management. The lesions are primarily inflammatory rather than degenerative, but soon become degenerative and their management is usually successful when carried out in the regular routine manner. Arsenicals are not to be feared as much in this type as they once were.

When the definite paretic and tabetic formulae are encountered it has been the experience that routine treatment does not produce desired results and to use valuable time for its employment is not permissible. This is not neglected but fever therapy is started at once. Due to the speed with which these lesions progress, and their very destructive nature, the element of time assumes a great importance. The type of fever used in these cases is usually from malaria or typhoid vaccine. The hypertherm, or electric heat box, is effective but hazardous, and its popularity is seemingly on the wane. The old procedure of spinal drainage has been found to be of little benefit and has been abandoned as a method of therapy. The prognosis in central nervous system involvement is entirely dependent upon the type and amount of destruction produced and the general condition of the patient. As in all debilitating disease, rest and general care are of utmost importance. I have made extensive use of typhoid vaccine in the routine care of these cases and find it on a par with malaria in producing fever, and from a prognostic standpoint.

When the treatment of the neurosyphilitic is terminated the responsibility of the physician is not ended. He must remember that in all syphilis, relapse is the rule and the patient's only safeguard against recurrence is post-treatment observation, both from the clinical and laboratory standpoint. Much responsibility of a medical and sociological nature is associated with the care of the syphilitic and there is no doubt that the successful therapist is the one who can correctly correlate these many factors, interpreted and adjusted to the needs of the individual case.

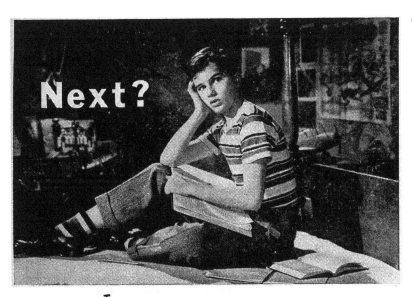

*T*here's no rule about the length of a war, and no telling how great the sacrifices needed to win it. All we know is that it *must be won.*

We hope and pray that the *next* generation will be spared—that our lads of fourteen and fifteen are destined for something else but the horrors of war and the fields of battle.

We hope that we, of this generation, may transmit to the next generation a world in which ruthless savagery and killing have ceased ... a world in which they may live and work in peace.

America must not lose this war—*dare* not lose it! We must win as *quickly* and completely as possible. If we win in time, hundreds of thousands of lives will be saved, and the youths of today will build the greater America of tomorrow.

It takes *money* to provide our fighting men with planes, tanks, guns and ships—tens of billions of dollars. It takes *War Bond* money—from you, and you, and you—regularly—every payday—10% of your income, at least—more, if you can.

Your Government will give you back $4 in 10 years for every $3 you invest now—$25 for each $18.75 Bond you buy. And your investment is backed and guaranteed by all the strength of the world's most powerful nation. The better we arm our *men,* the more lives of our *boys* will be spared, and the sooner will their future be assured.

Knowing this to be true—knowing that War Bonds will help save our country—the lives of our fighting men—yes, even the lives of those who are mere boys now ...

Can you possibly *not* put every dollar you can scrape together into War Bonds?

FACTS ABOUT WAR BONDS

1. War Bonds cost $18.75 for which you receive $25 in 10 years—or $4 for every $3.

2. War Bonds are the world's *safest* investment — guaranteed by the United States Government.

3. War Bonds can be made out in 1 name or 2, as co-owners.

4. War Bonds *cannot* go down in value. If they are lost, the Government will issue new ones.

5. War Bonds can be cashed in, in case of necessity, after 60 days.

6. War Bonds begin to pay interest after 1½ years.

Keep on Buying War Bonds

PUBLISHED IN COOPERATION WITH THE DRUG, COSMETIC AND ALLIED INDUSTRIES BY

LEDERLE LABORATORIES, Inc., NEW YORK, N. Y. — A UNIT OF AMERICAN CYANAMID COMPANY

· THE PRESIDENT'S PAGE ·

CARELESS WORDS

There is a poster on display about the State depicting a dead sailor lying in shallow water. The caption is, "A Careless Word—A Needless Loss".

Robert Hudson, a distinguished attorney, several years ago addressed the Oklahoma Presidents and Secretaries Meeting and spoke very frankly from a long professional experience. He stated that most malpractice suits originate in "another doctor's office". A careless word!

The greatest cement ever poured binds together the bricks and stones that compose great buildings where physicians and dentists office. Here they have to meet in elevators, in coffee shops and drug stores, and they have to speak. They gradually get acquainted and finally learn that the other fellow is not as bad as had been thought— "he's just another man trying to make a living".

And there is a human cement too. The Woman's Auxiliary performs a service in professional relationships of unobtrusive, but enormous value. When Mrs. Jones speaks to Doctor Jones about Doctor Smith's charming wife she met today at the Auxiliary Meeting, it sets Doctor Jones to thinking about Doctor Smith in an altered light. The Old Testament is wrong—it should read "the way of a maid with a man". The writers of old were not acquainted with the captivating guile with which the modern doctor's wife influences the medical profession—for its own good.

Is there a Woman's Auxiliary in your County or in your District—there should be.

James Stevenson

President.

The JOURNAL Of The
OKLAHOMA STATE MEDICAL ASSOCIATION

EDITORIAL BOARD
L. J. MOORMAN, Oklahoma City, Editor-in-Chief

E. EUGENE RICE, Shawnee   NED R. SMITH, Tulsa

MR. R. H. GRAHAM, Oklahoma City, Business Manager

CONTRIBUTIONS: Articles accepted by this Journal for publication including those read at the annual meetings of the State Association are the sole property of this Journal.

The Editorial Department is not responsible for the opinions expressed in the original articles of contributors.

Manuscripts may be withdrawn by authors for publication elsewhere only upon the approval of the Editorial Board.

MANUSCRIPTS: Manuscripts should be typewritten, double-spaced, on white paper 8½ x 11 inches. The original copy, not the carbon copy, should be submitted.

Footnotes, bibliographies and legends for cuts should be typed on separate sheets in double space. Bibliography listing should follow this order: Name of author, title of article, name of periodical with volume, page and date of publication.

Manuscripts are accepted subject to the usual editorial revisions and with the understanding that they have not been published elsewhere.

NEWS: Local news of interest to the medical profession, changes of address, births, deaths and weddings will be gratefully received.

ADVERTISING: Advertising of articles, drugs or compounds unapproved by the Council on Pharmacy of the A.M.A. will not be accepted. Advertising rates will be supplied on application.

It is suggested that members of the State Association patronize our advertisers in preference to others.

SUBSCRIPTIONS: Failure to receive The Journal should call for immediate notification.

REPRINTS: Reprints of original articles will be supplied at actual cost provided request for them is attached to manuscripts or made in sufficient time before publication. Checks for reprints should be made payable to Industrial Printing Company, Oklahoma City.

Address all communications to THE JOURNAL OF THE OKLAHOMA STATE MEDICAL ASSOCIATION, 210 Plaza Court, Oklahoma City. (3)

OFFICIAL PUBLICATION OF THE OKLAHOMA STATE MEDICAL ASSOCIATION
Copyrighted September, 1943

EDITORIALS

SCIENCE HAS ITS LIMITATIONS

The following from Lin Yutang's latest book, "Between Tears and Laughter" is well worth quoting:

"For it must never be forgotten that even in the realm of the physical world, science explains the *how*, but never the *why* and the *wherefore*. It deals with the process, but not the ultimate cause, nor the values of the end results. The process lies within the field of mathematics, the values and primary cause lie without. Science explains how the atoms behave, but does not explain why they so behave. It describes how two molecules of sodium and carbon comes together, but does not explain why they must come together. It describes acids and alkalis, but cannot say anything about the ultimate acidity of acids. It proves that quinine cures malaria, but does not know why quinine kills the malaria germs. It describes to you the laws of gravitation, but does not pretend to tell you what gravitation is, and why it must be. Before the ultimate Door of Mystery, science always stops short and never enters. It sees acorns sprout and grow oaks, but cannot tell why they must do so. It observes and proves the survival of the fittest, but cannot account for the arrival of the fittest. It explains how the giraffe survives by his long neck but cannot explain the chemical and physiological process that produced the first long neck. It tells of the survival value of the spotted leopard, but is at a loss about the arrival of the spots. It explains the survival value of the flower's fragrance, but is bashfully silent as to how lilacs and lemons develop their peculiar fragrance. It tells you that silkworms spin silk from mulberry leaves and bees produce honey from nectar and cows produce milk from common grass, and not much else is really enlightening. For ultimately, bees just produce honey and cows just produce milk and lilacs just create out of the common sod that unmistakable, incomparable perfume. And they all do it simply, finally, and inevitably."

Medical science alone may cure disease but the patient needs that intangible something which only art can supply, which only God can reason why and which only bureaucracy can cause to die. Again we quote from Yutang:

"There is more truth, kindness, heroism, romance, humor, pathos, more depth and richness of life in a country doctor's office than in the Foreign Office of any nation;

and it is of this truth, heroism, romance, and humor and pathos that the stuff of life is made, and by which the stream of human life is carried on."

Though eager to direct it, bureaucrats do not know the meaning of medical science, therefore, they stand ready to plunge headlong through "the ultimate Door of Mystery." Unfortunately, they are planning to drag millions of innocent people in after them.

MEDICAL PRESCIENCE

Let it be a matter of record that doctors who fear socialized medicine in any form are not selfishly reminiscent but as Walter Pater once said, "prescient of the future". Let the politician who would force the issue look upon the record and be prepared for the consequences.

The far-seeing doctors do not claim omniscience but experience has taught them that those who bow to bureaucracy and spend valuable time filling blanks in triplicate do not climb mountains, ford streams and brave storms to save the sick. Let doctors remember that it requires more fortitude to maintain freedom than to accept tyranny.

As a profession, we are at war, fighting for the one and only freedom worth having —the freedom to oppose everything that robs us of individuality in our service to humanity.

We know that medicine is a vital living science with evolutionary ends and that it should not be "rough hewn" by revolutionary trends.

THE PRIMARY ATYPICAL PNEUMONIAS

For the comfort of conscientious clinicians who covet concise bedside knowledge, attention is called to the fact that exhaustive etiologic and epidemiologic studies, including serologic and immunologic experiments have not contributed any definite etiologic or diagnostic data on the primary atypical, or so-called virus pneumonias.

For a current authoritative discussion on this subject, the reader is referred to a report of the investigation of John H. Dingle and his coworkers in a recent issue of War Medicine.[1] The authors present a detailed account of their clinical observations including x-ray findings and a carefully tabulated account of their laboratory investigations. The clinical aspects as reported by these anthors constitute one of the best bedside pictures of this relatively new malady, now available in medical literature. This clinical picture also contains a comprehensive discussion of the x-ray findings which is very

helpful. The discussion of symptomatology is based chiefly upon the study of 69 cases which were carefully observed for this specific purpose. For the complete study, 216 cases were abstracted from hospital records, making a total of 285 cases. A comparison of these two groups failed to show any striking variations in symptomatology, course of the disease, or x-ray findings. The following paragraph under the title "General Description" is so succinctly comprehensive, it is quoted in full: "The characteristics of. atypical pneumonia were those of a mild to moderately severe illness of gradual onset in which constitutional symptoms predominated over symptoms referable to the respiratory tract in the early stages. Physical signs of involvement of the lungs were ordinarily minimal, although evidence of pulmonary infiltration was seen on roentgen examination. The illness persisted for five to fourteen days and was not influenced by chemotherapy. Complications were extremely rare, and the prognosis was excellent."

Recent editorials in The New England Journal of Medicine[2] call attention to the fact that in all probability there are many forms of the virus pneumonias with a varied etiology. In the June 10, 1943 number,[3] there is editorial reference to a "simple clinical laboratory test that may serve to distinguish some of the cases of virus pneumonia." The promise of such a test resides in the findings of cold agglutinins in many cases of this disease during the past months." However, the editorial closes with the admission that it may prove a "means of distinguishing (only) one of the many forms of virus pneumonias."

Also worthy of note, is the fact that Favour[4] has reported three cases of atypical pneumonia which he was able to identify as probably ornithosis (psittacosis) by the compliment fixation test. Favour urges the careful questioning of patients with atypical pneumonia about contact with birds known to harbor the virus. In each of the cases reported, there was a history of contact with such birds.

Additional comfort may be found in the following reflections upon the pneumonias from Henry A. Christian[5]: "Reading between the lines of the reporters of groups of these patients, the author of this volume senses in them the same sensations that he had in 1918 when suddenly confronted with numerous patients with respiratory disease that he never before had seen, the feeling that he was dealing with a disease new to him, and which must compare speedily with descriptions of past observers. To them came the conclusion that a new respiratory disease had appeared. The experience of 1918, compared with that of the present, leaves this author with the feeling that the clinical descriptions of today agree with those he made of many cases in 1918, although the pathological lesions in the few fatal cases and the etiology and period between contact and onset of the present disease differ; all of this suggests to him that clinically this new disease is a variant of the 1918 influenza, capable, were it to assume pandemic proportions, of clinical identity with pandemic influenza."

1. Dingle, J. H., Abernethy, T. J., Badger, G. F., Buddingh, G. J., Feller, A. E., Langmuir, A. D., Ruegsegger, J. M., Wood, W. B. Jr.: War Medicine. Vol. 3, No. 3, p. 226. March, 1943

2. The New England Journal of Medicine. Vol 228, No. 22, p. 729 June 3, 1943.

3. The New England Journal of Medicine. Vol. 228, No. 23, p 770. June 10, 1943.

4. Favour, C. B.: Ornithosis (Psittacosis) Report of Three Cases and Historical, Clinical and Laboratory Comparision with Human Atypical (Virus) Pneumonia. American Journal Medical Sciences. Vol. 205, No. 162. February, 1943.

5. Christian, H. A.: Osler's Principles and Practice of Medicine. Fourteenth Edition. pp 303.

THE OKLAHOMA CITY CLINICAL SOCIETY

The war goes on and Procurement and Assignment calls for more doctors. Civilian medical needs surge about the veterans who are left at home with increasing demands which must be met, not only with courage and fortitude but with skillful dispatch.

The Annual Meeting of the Oklahoma City Clinical Society is going on according to schedule in order that every doctor on the home front may have refresher courses designed not only to polish off the time tried methods, but to add the accumulating accessories in medical science which should help expedite practice with a saving of time and energy . . . and perhaps added preservation of health and extension of life. This opportunity for the acquisition of knowledge and increased efficiency should not be overlooked, especially as it is literally brought to our doorstep.

Since we are so few and must do so much for so many, let us cultivate increased speed and efficiency by earnestly pursuing the "know how".

Speaking of Books

From the writing of Plato we may gather many details about the status of physicians in his time. It is very evident that the profession was far advanced and had been progressively developed for a long period before Hippocrates, whom we erroneously, yet with a certain propriety, call the Father of Medicine. The little by-play between Socrates and Euthydemus suggests an advanced condition of medical literature: "Of course, you who have so many books are going in for being a doctor," says Socrates, and then he adds, "there are so many books on medicine, you know." As Dyer remarks, whatever the quality of these books may have been, their number must have been great to give point to this chaff.—Aequanimitas with Other Addresses. Sir William Osler. 3rd Edition.

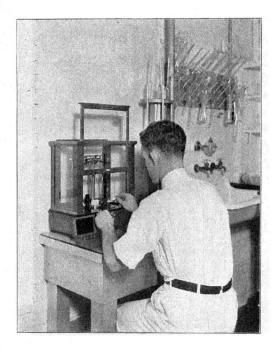

ASSOCIATION ACTIVITIES

13th ANNUAL MEETING
OKLAHOMA CITY CLINICAL SOCIETY
OCTOBER 18-19-20 and 21

The 13th annual and second war time meeting of the Oklahoma City Clinical Society will be held in Oklahoma City, October 18, 19, 20 and 21 at the Biltmore Hotel.

Guest Speakers for the 1943 conference are of the same outstanding stature in the field of medicine as those of previous meetings, according to Dr. J. H. Robinson, President of the Society.

Out-of-city physicians who will appear on the program 'and their specialty fields are as follows:

Dr. A. H. Aaron, Professor of Clinical Medicine, University of Buffalo.

Dr. Vilray Papin Blair, Professor Emeritus of Clinical Surgery, and Professor Emeritus of Oral Surgery, Washington University School of Medicine.

Dr. Louis A. Buie, Professor of Surgery, University of Minnesota, Mayo Foundation.

Dr. Leroy A. Calkins, Professor of Obstetrics and Gynecology, University of Kansas School of Medicine.

Dr. Theodore J. Dimitry, Director, Department of Ophthalmology and Professor of Ophthalmology, Louisiana State University, Professor of Special Anatomy, Loyola University.

Franklin G. Ebaugh, Colonel, Medical Corps, A.U.S. Professor of Psychiatry and Director, Colorado Psychopathic Hospital.

Dr. George B. Eusterman, Professor of Medicine, University of Minnesota, Mayo Foundation.

Dr. Charles Brenton Huggins, Professor of Surgery, University of Chicago.

Dr. Clinton W. Lane, Instructor of Dermatology, Washington University School of Medicine.

Dr. Harry E. Mock, Associate Professor of Surgery, Northwestern University School of Medicine.

Dr. Thomas G. Orr, Professor of Surgery and Head of Department, University of Kansas School of Medicine.

Dr. Louis E. Phaneuf, Professor of Gynecology, Tufts College Medical School.

Dr. Robert D. Schrock, Professor of Orthopedic Surgery, University of Nebraska School of Medicine.

Dr. John A. Toomey, Professor of Clinical Pediatrics and Contagious Diseases, Western Reserve University School of Medicine.

Dr. W. Likely Simpson, Professor of Otolaryngology, and Head of Department, University of Tennessee.

Dr. Charles T. Way, Assistant Clinical Professor of Medicine, Western Reserve University School of Medicine.

Dr. Grayson L. Carroll, Urology, St. Louis University School of Medicine.

Outside activities such as the Annual Smoker are to be held in conjunction with the meeting and the Auxiliary is planning interesting entertainment for the ladies.

Dr. J. W. Amesse, Vice-President, American Medical Association, Denver, Colorado, will be the guest speaker for the Monday night dinner.

The Clinical Society as the Annual State Meeting, provides an excellent opportunity for medical refresher courses and the Clinical Society should have the support of the profession of the entire state.

All physicians who are planning on attending the meeting should make hotel reservations as soon as possible.

ASSOCIATION TO ASSIST O.P.A. ON
FOOD RATIONING PROGRAM

Through the office of Mr. Paul Frost, Associate Food Rationing Officer for the Office of Price Administration has come a request that the Association assist the O.P.A. in the proper administration of the food rationing program as it pertains to the issuing of additional food stamps for special diets.

This particular phase of the food program has from the beginning been misunderstood by both the public and the medical profession and as a result there has been improper use of the regulations.

Dr. James Stevenson, President, has referred the request to the Committee on Public Health with the instructions that Dr. Carroll Pounders, Oklahoma City, Chairman, appoint his own advisory committee.

As soon as the Public Health Committee makes its recommendations they will be sent to the local rationing boards for the guidance of the board members. The recommendations will be published in the Journal.

Physicians should at all times bear in mind that the food rationing program is an intricate part of the war effort and any unnecessary dispensation of food is giving aid and comfort to the enemy—and who wants to help Hitler and Tojo?

Be certain that your patient cannot obtain his necessary special diet in some other manner than through rationed foods.

MILITARY SURGEONS MEETING
October 21, 22 and 23

Rear Admiral Ross T. McIntire, Surgeon General of the United States Navy, and personal physician to President Roosevelt, will serve as honorary chairman for the 51st annual convention of the Association of Military Surgeons of the United States to be held in Philadelphia October 21, 22 and 23.

The announcement was made by Captain Joseph A. Biello, District Medical Officer of the Fourth Naval District, who will act as general chairman for the meeting. The Vice-chairman will be Brigadier General F. Lull, attached to the Medical Corps of the Army, and Commander Edward L. Bortz of the United States Naval Reserve Medical Corps.

The symposium on war medicine will be of vital and direct interest to the health and welfare of the men in the armed forces, to physicians, research specialists and scientists everywhere, as well as to the general public. It is expected that the meeting will bring 2,000 doctors, many of whom have been in active combat, with servicemen in every camp and base throughout the country and on all the fighting fronts.

The announcement of the plans for the convention of military surgeons was made today by Rear Admiral William L. Mann, M. C., of Seattle, Washington, president of the Association of Military Surgeons.

"It is especially appropriate that Philadelphia should furnish the setting for this most important meeting. Philadelphia has long been recognized as the first city of medicine and has made enormous contributions to the advance of medical science. Then, too, it is the birthplace of American freedom, which our military surgeons are now helping our fighting men maintain in this struggle for the survival of democracy throughout the world," Rear Admiral Mann said.

Rear Admiral Richard H. Laning will head the executive committee for the convention, one of the most important ever held by the military services of the United States.

Serving with Rear Admiral Laning on the Executive Committee are: Dr. George Morris Piersol, Dr. Staney P. Reimann, Dr. Gilson Colby Engel, Commander J. R. Tinney, United States Naval Reserve; Major F. D. Creedon, United States Army; and Captain J. R. Kitchell, United States Army retired.

The meeting will be of magnitude and scope never before known in the history of the organization, according to Rear Admiral Mann. Medical officers of the armed forces who have seen actual duties in the various combat zones will report first hand on the United States medical services under combat in climatic conditions new to American arms.

Medicine's methods of meeting the new and complicating factors brought on by mechanized modern warfare will also highlight the sessions. There will be reports and discussions on such new matters as air evacuation, parachute injuries, the physiological aspects of high altitude flying and dive bombing, tropical medicine, blast injuries, amphibious operations, submarine warfare, immersion and temperature extremes, neurosurgical problems and the whole field of rehabilitation.

The military surgeons meeting will be opened with addresses of welcome by Governor Edward Martin, of Pennsylvania, and Major Bernard Samuel of Philadelphia. At the initial evening session, to be known as "Army Night", the President will deliver his greetings to the convention via radio. There will be addresses by the Chinese Ambassador, Wei Tao-Ming, and by Surgeon General Norman T. Kirk, of the United States Navy.

At the following night's session, which will be known as "Navy Night," the principal speaker will be the Hon. Frank Knox, Secretary of the Navy. The presiding officer will be Rear Admiral Ross T. McIntyre, surgeon general of the United States Navy and personal physician to the President.

Nationwide hook-ups will carry reports of the meeting to the public at large and by short-wave broadcast to the people in Allied countries, who will be apprised of the progress of the convention and its meaning to the men in arms and national health in general.

The convention, with its score of exhibits and meetings, will occupy all available floor space in the Bellevue-Stratford during its stay here. The program will list, besides general sessions, a series of forum lectures and teaching panels, as well as a great number of film showings.

PREPAID SURGICAL PLAN TO ATTORNEYS

Dr. John F. Burton, Oklahoma City, Chairman of the Prepaid Medical and Surgical Plans Committee, announced that the preliminary draft of a prepaid surgical plan has gone to the legal firm of Emery, Johnson, Crowe and Tolbert for analysis and legal interpretation.

The plan, which will later be submitted to the County Societies for approval before being offered for enrolment to the lay public in the respective counties, has been prepared from a study of similar plans in operation by other Medical Associations.

The House of Delegates, in instructing the Committee to proceed in the formation of a prepaid plan, while not anticipating the introduction of the Wagner-Murray-Dingell health bill in Congress, nevertheless made possible a combative instrument for the medical profession.

A recent analysis by "Blue Cross" of its first 5,000 hospitalized cases over the entire State, gives an interesting insight to the number of surgical cases that would have been handled through a prepaid plan had one existed at the beginning of "Blue Cross". Of the first 5,000 cases, 2,112 were surgical. The following are their diagnostic divisions:

Infectious diseases	4
Rheumatoid diseases	4
Cancer	3
Tumor and Cyst-benign	129
Fibroid uterus	53

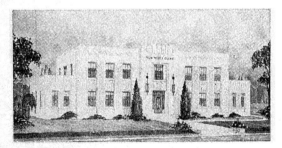

VON WEDEL CLINIC

Other female disorders	114
Goiter	9
Other Glandular disorders	11
Nutritious diseases	1
Ulcer of the stomach of duodenum	10
Other digestive disorders	10
Appendicitis	433
Gall Bladder	18
Hernia	62
Kidneys and ureters	33
Disease of the prostate	9
Disease of the bladder	7
Rectal disorders	128
Diseases of external genitals	5
Disease of the heart	2
Diseases of the blood vessels	4
Respiratory diseases	9
Diseases of the nervous system	1
Diseases of the eye	13
Diseases of the ear	11
Tonsillitis	811
Full term pregnancy	21
Obstetrics	26
Diseases of the bone	16
Burns	2
Injuries due to the accident	67
Poisonings	2
Diseases of the skin	18
Hemorrhages	12
Dental disorders	10
Unknown	9
Miscellaneous	33
Total	2112

Announcement of the completed plan will be made as soon as possible.

WE NEED HELP

The Executive Office is attempting to secure pictures of all the past-presidents and has been unable to obtain pictures of the following:

R. D. Love, M.D., Perry and
R. H. Tullis, M.D., Lawton .

Anyone having information that might be of benifit in finding pictures of these physicians is requested to immediately write the Executive Office.

FOURTH ANNUAL SECRETARIES CONFERENCE
OKLAHOMA CITY, OCTOBER 17, 1943

Dr. A. R. Suggs, Ada, Chairman of the Annual Secretaries Conference, has selected October 17 as the date for the 4th Annual Meeting which will be held in Oklahoma City at the Biltmore Hotel.

The meeting this year will not have a morning session but will have the customary afternoon and evening program with a complimentary dinner.

In addition to the County Secretaries, there will be in attendance the County Chairman of the Procurement and Assignment Service, as a part of the program will be devoted to the profession's participation in the war effort.

Dr. James Stevenson, President of the Association, is also calling a meeting of the Council for the morning of October 17 and anyone desiring to bring any business to the attention of the Council should notify the Executive Officer as soon as possible.

The program of the meeting will include many of the following current topics: Public policy in relation to the Wagner-Murray Health bill (Senate 1161): Report from the Committee on Prepaid Surgical Plan; Maternity and Infancy Program for the families of enlisted men; Farm Security Administration and "Blue Cross Plan"; Procurement and Assignment Service and Post War Planning for returning physicians.

Representatives of the Army and Navy Offices of Officers Procurement will be available to answer questions concerning commissions in the respective medical branches.

The suggestion is made that anyone planning on staying over for the Oklahoma City Clinical Society should make reservations at the hotel as soon as possible.

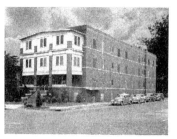
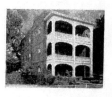

UNIVERSITY HOSPITAL EVACUATION UNIT AT PORT OF EMBARKATION

Word has been received that the Army Hospital Evacuation Unit organized from the staff of the University of Oklahoma School of Medicine has been sent to a port of embarkation and will soon be on duty on a foreign front.

The unit is commanded by Colonel Rex Bolend, Oklahoma City, with the fololwing staff of doctors: F. M. Adams, Jr., D. R. Bedford, Austin H. Bell, S. E. Franklin (Broken Arrow), Allen G. Gibbs, J. A. Graham, Jesse D. Herrmann, George H. Kimball, John F. Kuhn, Jr., Cecil W. Lemon, R. H. Lindsey (Pauls Valley), Paul B. Lingenfelter (Clinton), Bert E. Mulvey, Everett B. Neff, Floyd S. Newman (Shattuck), Robert L. Noell, D. B. Pearson, R. J. Reichert, Harvey M. Rickey, W. W. Rucks, Jr., Chester R. Seba, Evans E. Talley (Enid), James M. Taylor and John P. Wolff. (Note: all are from Oklahoma City unless otherwise indicated).

There is no doubt that this group of Oklahoma physicians will earn for themselves and the State of Oklahoma the same praise for efficiency and resoluteness as has been gained by the 45th Division and the other Oklahoma physicians who are serving in the armed forces.

COUNTY NEWS

The Washington-Nowata County Medical Society has set up the following program for 1943-44. The Society is to be highly complimented on the handling of its future meetings.

Program 1943

September 8
Vacation Talks
Affections of the Myocardium—Dr. Thomas Wells.
Discussion—Dr. F. C. Rewerts.

October 13
Some Common Eye Infections—Dr. O. I. Green.
Discussion—Dr. J. E. Crawford.
Infections of the Hand, Surgical Treatment of—Dr. H. G. Crawford.
Discussion—Dr. H. C. Weber.

November 10
Talk on Harvard Postgraduate Course—Dr. J. P. Vansant.
Poliomyelitis Anterior—Dr. E. M. Chamberlin.
Discussion—Dr. W. H. Shipman.

December 8
Prematurity—Dr. S. A. Lang.
Discussion—Dr. K. D. Davis.
Some Diseases We May Expect After This War—Dr. E. E. Beechwood.
Discussion—Dr. S. G. Weber.
Election of Officers.

Program 1944

January 12
Annual Banquet.

February 9
Some Medical Problems the Result of Aviation—Dr. R. C. Gentry.
Discussion—Dr. S. G. Weber.
Eclampsia—Dr. J. G. Smith.
Discussion—Dr. W. H. Shipman.

March 8
Purpura Hemorrhagica—Dr. L. D. Hudson.
Discussion—Dr. W. H. Shipman
Peptic Ulcer—Dr. B. F. Staver.
Discussion—Dr. G. V. Dorsheimer.

April 12
Otitis Media—Dr. J. E. Crawford.
Discussion—Dr. O. I. Green.
Treatment of Severe Burns—Dr. H. C. Weber.
Discussion—Dr. J. P. Vansant.

May 10
Open Meeting.

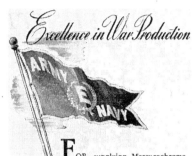
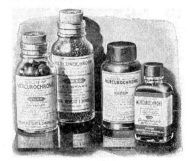

★ *FIGHTIN' TALK* ★

The following promotion has been reported: from Major to Lieutenant Colonel—*Bernard Eugene Bullock*, Clinton.

Lt. Colonel Lee K. Emenhiser, Oklahoma City, and *Major Ed McKay*, formerly of Oklahoma City, collaborated on the following news from their station at Ft. Sam Houston, Texas. Lt. Colonel Emenhiser writes as follows:

"Will write some news from my neck of the woods down here. I am Chief of the Eye, Ear, Nose and Throat Department and several Oklahoma City boys are working with me in their specialties; namely *Major Paul J. Carden* of El Reno and *Major Ed McKay*, previously of Oklahoma City, but who was practicing at Texarkana before coming into the army. *Major J. B. Snow* is the Chief of Pediatrics and is just a few doors down the hall from me. *Major Clyde Kernek*, who was practicing at Holdenville before coming into the army is our Hospital Inspector and his office is just across the hall from me. So, you see, there is a good bunch of ''Okies'' working here under the same roof in one of the greatest, if not the greatest Army Hospital in the country.

"I saw *Lt. Colonel Bob Lowry*, formerly of Poteau and he is now Commanding Officer of the Station Hospital at Brooks Field and working with him is *Captain Frank Joyce* and *Captain Gingles* of Oklahoma. *Lt. Colonel William D. Anderson*, formerly practicing at Claremore dropped by to see me the other day and he is the Commanding Officer of the Station Hospital at Victoria, Texas. *Major Polk Frye*, formerly practicing at Frederick, is now the Commanding Officer of the Station Hospital at San Angelo, Texas. *Captain Bob Roberts*, formerly practicing at Stillwater is stationed here at Ft. Sam Houston, Texas with the First Auxiliary Surgical Group. *Major LeRoy Sadler* came by inspecting us from the Eighth Service Command at Dallas, Texas.

From the Branch School of Aviation Medicine at Nashville, Tennessee, comes the word that *Captain Roy L. Neel* is completing the course for Flight Surgeon of the Army Air Corps. Other Sooners stationed at Nashville are *Lt. Colonel Rayburn*, formerly of Norman and *Captain George Dodson*, graduate of the Oklahoma School of Medicine in 1940. Captain Dodson was sent back from Hawaii to take the course for Flight Surgeon.

Colonel Wallace N. Davidson, Cushing, has just received our first news letter and has written to us from ————. Colonel Davidson says that he is in command of a rather large hospital unit there and it is his opinion that he has some of the best surgical and medical personnel that it is possible to obtain and that they are doing splendid work and a lot of it.

Lt. E. D. Greenberger, McAlester, is busy with maneuvers after a few days vacation which included a little fishing and some swimming "à la natural". Before reporting for maneuvers, Lt. Greenberger was stationed at Camp Atterbury, Indiana.

By V-Mail we hear from *Lt. Logan A. Spann*, formerly of Tulsa. He says that he missed the first State Meeting since 1936, but has plenty to do in a Medical Company in operation in ———— and is doing surgery to his heart's content.

Major Glen W. McDonald, formerly of the State Health Department stationed in Pontotoc County, reports that since last November he has been assigned in Boston at Headquarters, First Service Command as Veneral Disease Officer for that area. He covers the six New England States in his travels but as yet has seen nothing that looks as good as old Oklahoma.

Lt. James D. Martin, Cushing, is now stationed at the Office of the Post Surgeon, Ft. Sam Houston, Texas. Lt. Martin entered the Service on September 23, 1942 and was first attached to a pool of medical officers at Ft. Sam Houston and later was assigned to his present post. He reports that the work there is similar to an office practice as far as the ''sick calls'' are concerned with the addition of a number of outside activities including a civilian dispensary for first aid to industrial accidents and many other allied duties.

Society Note

We are glad to note, by the following report, that the social season has been officially opened in ————. Sorry that there was no enclosure of pictures with which to enhance the report.

"On Friday, August 13, Dr. ''Pat'' Nagle (*Oklahoma City*) (of the Surgical Facility Nagles) entertained *Dr. D. G. Willard* of Norman and Drs. *Bill Klein* and *James H. Melvin* of Oklahoma City.

"Dr. Nagle's lean-to was attractively decorated with luscious Polynesian pin-ups (*Note: ???*) and assorted enemy ampoules. Dr. Nagle was coyly clad in khaki shorts and operating cap. Guests were uniformly dressed in herring-bone twill, the latest creation for evening dugout wear.

"Dr. Nagle also furnished the evening's special entertainment, rendering 'The Guillotine' by B. Welchii.

"A delicious buffet was served, featuring papaya, candied taro and hearts of palm salad. The fragrant aroma of gorgeous bougainvilleas and hospital alcohol enhanced the fond nostalgia for the meandering North Canadian."

The important arrival was heralded on Monday, August 30, 1943, of Miss Sari Dee Frank, new daughter of Captain and Mrs Louis S. Frank. Captain Frank is stationed at Cimarron Field, Oklahoma City. The clever announcement was entitled "United States of America Ration Baby One" and was a most official looking Ration Book—thoroughly enjoyed by the recipients.

The following article appeared in the Oklahoma City Times.

Kisses Greet Healdton Man In Messina

Captain Fred T. Perry, late of Healdton, isn't quite sure whether it was a privilege or a misfortune to be the third United Nations officer to enter Messina.

Describing his entrance into the Sicilian city, Perry, a physician, said he "noticed that every window and every door on the street was opened a little and people were staring at me."

"Finally," he wrote his wife, "one woman gingerly pointed at me and said 'Americano?' I nodded my head and smiled—then all hell broke loose. The people ran out of the houses, grabbed and kissed and hugged me, all of them talking at once."

"Some of them," the letter continued, "said they had been waiting two years for us—why hadn't we come sooner?"

Perry said a favorite radio program of the Yanks in Sicily was a propaganda broadcast by a "sweet-voiced woman from Berlin" whom the soldiers immediately dubbed "Dirty Gerty."

Gerty implores the English-speaking soldiers to "stop this foolish venture," they roar with laughter and make salty comment on her "thin and corny" arguments.

Perry's parents, Mr. and Mrs. J. S. Perry, live at Purcell. Before entering the army with the 45th division, he practiced medicine at Healdton.

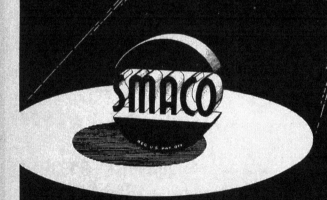

Major John W. Records, Oklahoma City, reports from Carlisle Barracks, Pennsylvania. He is stationed at the Medical Field Service School there.

Lt. Colonel W. D. Anderson, Claremore, has been Post Surgeon for two years at Foster Field, Victoria, Texas. He reports his work as enjoyable as well as interesting.

Major E. R. Vahlberg, Oklahoma City, is now stationed at Randolph Field, Texas, taking the Flight Surgeon's course.

Lt. E. D. Padberg, Ada, is Officer in charge of the Medical Dispensary and Contagious and Quarantine Officer for the Classification Center in San Antonio, Texas. He is looking forward to Flight Surgeon's Training in the near future.

Captain J. Levine, McAlester, has been in North Africa for several months and reports the following by V-Mail after just now receiving our first news letter:

"I have flown on raids over Pantellaria, Sicily and Italy. At times they are commonplace, at others quite dramatic with anti-aircraft setting up a blanket of smoke and fire twenty thousand or more feet in the air—enemy fighters peeling off and coming in with their guns spitting lead and fire—the clatter of your own guns—the shouts over inner-phones—the wail and whine of the rushing wind—the powerful roar of motors—mountainous clouds of dust and smoke thousands of feet in the air from bombed area. A plane suddenly hit, shudders, staggers in flight, bursts into flames and falls downwards, its wild flight forever stilled.

"These and similar moments occurring in split seconds sort of sets ones sympathetic and porosympathetic network in a twitter."

Captain Charles H. Eads, Tulsa, is stationed at March Field, Riverside, California and states that he is the only "Oakie" there. He has completed one year in the service. Captain Eads arrived at March Field last September and spent his first month there doing some basic training and going to school. He was then sent to Carlisle Barracks for another month of school and from there to Edgewood Arsenal, Maryland for . . . . . another month of school! From Edgewood Arsenal, he was returned to March Field where he was given the job as Assistant Executive Officer of the Station Hospital. He continued in that capacity until February at which time he became ill and was sent to Palm Springs for a short time. Upon his return to March Field he was put in charge of one of the Wards and is now serving there.

Record Production of Synthetic Substitute for Treatment of Malaria Disclosed

The price of Atabrine, synthetic substitute for quinine in the treatment of malaria, has been reduced to a new low of $4.50 per 1,000 tablets, Dr. Theodore G. Klumpp, president of Winthrop Chemical Company, announced recently as he disclosed receipt from the U. S. Army of the largest single order on record.

At the same time, he revealed that production of Atabrine in this country was now in excess of 500,000,-000 tablets per year, sufficient for full treatment of 33,000,000 cases of malaria, and was rapidly approaching a rate of 600,000,000 tablets per year, which would be sufficient to treat 40,000,000 cases.

"The new price to the Government," Dr. Klumpp said, "reflects both recent increases in Government orders and improvements in the manufacturing process. The $4.50 price to the Government compares with the former low of $6.00 per 1,000 tablets, with the $66.66 in 1933, when Atabrine was first introduced to the American medical profession.

"At the new low price, it costs about as much to treat a case of malaria with Atabrine as to send an airmail letter. Actually the cost of medication with Atabrine is 6¾ cents per case, as compared with 27 cents for quinine. This is believed to be less than the cost of any other medication for any serious disease."

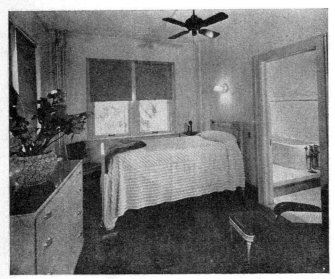

MEDICINE AT WAR

The following article entitled "Wartime Nursing is Different" is an official communication from the War Manpower Commission. It graphically depicts the urgent need for the utmost utilization of nursing manpwer during the war. In its appeal for cooperation from physicians and hospitals it is basically sound and such cooperation must be given if success in this field is achieved.

If you know of a nurse who is inactive in the war effort or if the nurse in your office could be doing more toward the war effort in another field of nursing, ask her to contact the local chairman of the Nursing Council for War Service. Physicians and hospitals must realize that it is their duty to replace registered nurses in their employment with other personnel unless they are absolutely essential to the health of the patients and not merely for the convience of the physician or hospital.

WARTIME NURSING IS DIFFERENT

"It is utterly impossible to provide the necessary volume of wartime nursing service on a peacetime basis. Places where nursing is going on as usual must share with others. Individual nurses who have not made adjustments to wartime needs for their services should understand the necessity for their participation.

"The National Nursing Council has pointed out that the value of any national plan must be judged by its usefulness at the local level, i.e., where nurses live and work—in the country, in the villages, towns, and cities of the nation.

"Wartime nursing is different! That inescapable fact must be generally accepted by nurses, by physicians, and by hospital administrators. Energy and motion now spent in resistance to change must be released for the attack on war-created needs.

"Nurses have wrought many changes, but not enough, in the pattern of nursing service since Pearl Harbor. 'We just do the best we can' is heard more frequently than 'This is our plan.' Generally speaking, educational programs have received more thought than the service programs. Acceleration of the basic course in nursing is an outstanding example. State boards of nurse examiners have initiated others.

"The principles of good nursing have not changed, but nurses are learning to concentrate on the essentials. In the analysis and administration of nursing service radical changes are being made. Tremendously valuable assistance in caring for patients is being secured from the Red Cross nurse's aids and other volunteers as well as from paid auxiliary workers.

"Thus far nursing service has not been rationed; such rationing would be complicated by the differences in individual nurses and the degree of essentiality of needed services. The sharing of services is more difficult than the sharing of goods.

"A critical shortage of nurses exists. Here are the facts:

"Over 36,000 nurses are now with the armed forces and the Red Cross has accepted responsibility for the recruitment of an equal number by June 30, 1944. Our men are receiving skilled medical care of a high order as shown by the high percentage of recovery from injury. Skilled nursing is an important factor in such care. Then, too, the very presence of nurses near the bases of military operations has repeatedly been described as a potent force in maintaining morale.

"There has been an unprecedented increase in the use of civilian hospitals. Hospitals gave fourteen and a quarter million more days of care in 1942 than in the preceding year and the trend still is definitely upward.

This is in keeping with the rapid growth of the Blue Cross (group hospitalization) plans and the Children's Bureau hospitalization program for the care of the families of service men.

"Nursing is essential to the nation's health. The National Nursing Inventories (of nursing resources) of 1941 and 1943, by the U. S. Public Health Service, offer a comparison of data for the two years.

"The total number of nurses graduated in the two years is well in excess of the number withdrawn for military service; this fact is not apparent in the inventory. The returns are apparently incomplete. Active nurses who did not return their questionnaires apparently did not realize the profound importance of the information requested. This information is the basis for present planning and safeguarding the future.

"The relatively small decrease in the number of institutional nurses is much less significant than the increased use of hospitals in creating the serious shortage of nurses. The increased number of nurses in industrial nursing is, of course, not surprising.

"The large number of inactive nurses who reported themselves available is encouraging, but—available for what? Full time? Part time? These nurses and others who are still "hidden" can make a valuable contribution to our nursing resources. Although it requires a little more planning, the service of two part-time nurses can equal that of one full-time one. Wartime nursing puts a tremendous burden on all the administrative nurses.

"Here is the program of the new Nursing Division of the Procurement and Assignment Service. The Red Cross recruitment committees are pledged to recruit 36,000 nurses this year. The new division will (1) determine the availability for military service or essentiality for civilian service of all nurses eligible for military service and submit such determinations to the American Red Cross for use in procurement of nurses for the Armed Forces; (2) promote plans for maximum utilization of full-time nurses and those who are able to serve only part time; (3) develop and maintain a roster of all graduate registered nurses, and (4) develop and encourage sound methods of supplementing the work of nurses with non-professional personnel.

"Through the War Manpower Commission, nursing will not only have the benefit of the experience of medicine in the procurement and assignment of physicians, but means will be found to interpret wartime nursing to physicians and their cooperation secured in effecting desirable wartime adjustments."

Suggested Reading

1. Priorities for Nurses: National Nursing Council for War Service 1790 Broadway, New York, N. Y. May, 1943, revised edition.
2. Distribution of Nursing Service During War: National Nursing Council for War Service, 1790 Broadway, New York, N. Y. May, 1942.
3. Volunteers in Health, Medical Care and Nursing. U. S. Office of Civilian Defense, Washington, D.C.

National Nursing Inventories

	1941	1943
Total returns	289,286	259,174
Active		
Institutional	81,708	77,704
Public Health	17,766	18,900
Industrial	5,512	11,220
Private duty	46,793	44,299
Other	21,276	18,476

Inactive but available for nursing	25,252	38,746 (of these 23,576 are married and under 40 years of age)
Inactive, not available	90,979	49,829
In Nurse Corps of Army and Navy	over 6,371	36,000 (precise data not available)

25 YEARS AGO

It is interesting to compare the handling of the nursing question for the armed forces with 25 years ago. It is apparent that our state has grown very much professionally during this time.

JOURNAL, September, 1918

THE ARMY NURSE QUESTION APPLIED TO OKLAHOMA

The War Department, in calling for nurses over the the United States, has estimated that Oklahoma should furnish more than 400. Oklahoma County, with three rather large hospitals, is called on for 55, while Muskogee County is asked to furnish 35.

We presume this demand is made upon basis of estimated population, at any rate the calculator has overlooked the fact that this is strickly a rural country, that nurses were practically unobtainable before the War in sufficient number to meet the demands and that many of the counties assessed for a certain number of nurses have none whatever to send and have never had them. In such counties as these, mind, if a patient demanded a nurse, the nurse was imported, as a rule very unwillingly on her part, and hurried back to the city, when her task was completed. Attention is called to this condition of affairs now in order that no reflection shall lie upon the state in its failure to come up to the number—it should not be forgotten that in all other things, Liberty Bond sales, Red Cross drives and similar needed activities incident to the War, Oklahoma has done herself proud so far and will likely, as she has heretofore done, carry more than her share of such burdens in the future, thus relieving communities not so fortunately able. But we cannot supply ''Woman Power'' if we have none. We can send all we have in that respect, but will not fill our so-called quota.

The plan to give courses in nursing of a very intensive character, aimed to hurriedly fit the young woman to take the place of a nurse, seems to be the nearest solution of the matter and should be encouraged. It should be encouraged not only to meet the present war needs, but after the war we should have an overplus of nurses as compared with pre-war days in order to give the people adequate nursing service. It is questionable, in view of the shortage of nurses, if there was any good sense in requiring such a long course of training as is required to graduate a nurse. It has long semed to the writer that it was not necessary to place an intelligent young woman in a hospital and have her do the drudgery she is called on to do, go through the same old sing-song of routine daily for three years before she is graduated. It seems that intelligent young women should learn in less time than that to carry out a physician's directions, those most essential to the successful conduct of the average case.

It seems that the medical handling of the local draft boards have been handled very much more efficiently than during World War I and we should be proud of our work at this time.

THE RESPONSIBILITY OF MEDICAL OFFICERS OF DRAFT BOARDS

Not since the War begun has the responsibility of the individual member of Local and Medical Advisory Boards been so accentuated as is now being done by the newly created Medical Section of the Provost Marshal General's Office.

Medical officers of both Local and Medical Advisory Boards are being advised that they must no longer regard their duties as mere matters of form to be carried out when they have the time and inclination to do so, but they must regard them as a most serious obligation toward the Nation. The advices strongly indicate that the authorities are rather tired of the attitude of the certain rare examiner that he is to be pampered with reference to his work. Such men are advised that they must either work or get off the boards and make way for men who will perform the services needed in a proper manner.

The greatest sacrifice imaginable is being made by men who enter the Medical Corps of the Army. With that clearly in mind there should be no delusion in the mind of the man who is permitted to remain happily at home, pursuing his lucrative occupation, as to his duty to the Nation. He should work and work with the very highest efficiency.

Personal and General News. JOURNAL, September, 1918.

Drs. J. E. Hughes and G. S. Baxter, Shawnee, have received Medical Reserve commissions.

Cloudchief and Cowden, neighboring towns in Washita County, are clamoring for physicians. All they had have entered the Army.

Yale citizens are complaining that so many physicians have entered the army from that place that there are not enough left to look after the needs of the sick.

Sapulpa papers indicate that the city authorities of that place have not yet progressed to the point of prohibiting 4th of July foolishness as they report several casualties on that day due to the obsoluete fire cracker and similar relics of the darker ages.

Pottawatomie County physicians recently assembled and drafted resolutions that certain persons in that locality had failed to pay bills due members of the Medical Reserve Corps now in France or in Military Service and that they would hereafter refuse to render any professional service to such delinquents unless they paid the debt due to the absent physician.

• OBITUARIES •

CHARLES T. SCHRADER, M.D.

1879-1943

Dr. Charles T. Schrader died at his home in Bristow, August 27, of a heart attack.

In the early 1900's, Dr. Schrader came to Oklahoma and has been a resident of Creek County for 40 years. He was born in Indiana. Active in the civic affairs of Bristow, Dr. Schrader was three-time mayor. He was a member of the Bristow Methodist Church and a Mason.

Dr. Schrader is survived by his widow and six children: Mrs. Marjorie Rainwater, Drumright; Mrs. Betty Lou Wade, Bristow; Billie Katherine Schrader, Washington, D. C.; Mrs. Georgia Rose Sands, Alexander Va.; Ted Schrader, Bristow; and Charles Schrader Jr., in service with the Air Corps stationed at Fort Worth, Texas.

Woman's Auxiliary

The Woman's Auxiliaries to the various County Medical Societies over the State are just beginning this month to make their plans for the coming year's work. The summer months have been filled with individual members taking active part in the various war activities of their community and they are now making the necessary readjustments in their programs to fit in with the Auxiliaries regular program and war work for 1943-44.

Changes in their personal and county needs has made planning in advance difficult this year and as we go to press we have not received names of officers or committee chairmen from all the organized County Auxiliaries.

Mrs. F. Maxey Cooper of Oklahoma City, as our new State President, will have a message in the October issue which will be of assistance to the County Auxiliaries in completing their programs.

OKLAHOMA COUNTY OFFICERS FOR 1943-1944

President—Mrs. Gregory Stanbro....220 Edgemere Court.
President Elect—Mrs. Walker Morledge..200 N.W. 18th St.
Vice-President—Mrs. Jess Herrmann..1147 N.W. 38th St.
Corres. Secretary—Mrs. Oscar White....609 N. W. 41st St.
Record. Secretary—Mrs. Gerald Rogers..524 N.W. 15th St.
Treasurer—Mrs. Bert Mulvey.........2632 N. W. 27th St.
Ass't. Treasurer—Mrs. John Pine........423 N. E. 16th St.
Parliamentarian—Mrs. Floyd Keller..1213 Larchmont Lane
Press & Publicity—Mrs. Joel Price........912 N. W. 36th St.

Mrs. Gregory Stanbro, President of the Oklahoma County Auxiliary, has called a meeting of the Board for September 9. The Board will make plans for the Woman's Program or the Board for September 9. The Board will make plans for the Woman's Program of the Clinical Society, which will be held in Oklahoma City, October 18. The dates for the Registration Tea and the regular October meeting of the Auxiliary will be decided at the meeting.

TULSA COUNTY OFFICERS FOR 1943-1944

President—Mrs. John C. Perry......2928 S. Columbia Pl.
President Elect—Mrs Carl Hotz............2234 E. 22nd Pl.
Vice President—Mrs. David L. Garrett....1308 E. 27th St.
Record. Secretary—Mrs. M. O. Nelson...1534 S. Norfork
Corres. Secretary—Mrs. L. C. Northrup..1828 E. 22nd St.
Treasurer—Mrs. A. H. Ungerman.......1718 E. 37th St.
Historian—Mrs. J. Fred Bolton.............212 E. 27th St.
Parliamentarian—Mrs. Frank L. Flack..1747 S. Florence.

University of Oklahoma School of Medicine

During the past month Dr. H. A. Shoemaker, Acting Dean, has been twice to Dallas, Texas, for a conference with the Chief of the Army Specialized Training Branch, Eighth Service Command, regarding selection of students for premedical and medical training in the Eighth Service Command. Most of the medical schools and dental schools in the Eighth Service Command were represented and plans were formulated which will facilitate the selection of students to be assigned to this training.

The Naval Specialized Training Unit at the School of Medicine was activated July 1, 1943, with 56 trainees.

Final examinations for the summer semester ended August 23 and a new semester will start September 6, 1943.

A recent issue of the Journal of the American Medical Association reports that Dr. Thirl E. Jarrett, Class of

---

1936, was awarded the Silver Star for gallantry in action.

Dr. George N. Barry, Medical Director, and Mr. Howard R. Dickey, Chief Clerk, University Hospital, will attend the meeting of the American Hospital Association, Buffalo, New York, September 15-17 inclusive.

The Oklahoma Hospital for Crippled Children has 125 cases of poliomyelitis where they are being treated under the direction of the Department of Orthopedics and Pediatrics. The care of these patients has involved considerable additional expense and the various County Chapters of the National Foundation for Infantile Paralysis have come to the aid of the hospital. The Red Cross, the State Health Department, Oklahoma Commission for Crippled Children, and other agencies have co-operated in this work.

Dr. Charles M. Bielstein, formerly resident in Pediatrics and since July 1 has been serving as Special Physician, has been ordered to active duty with the Army on September 5, 1943. Dr. Bielstein has been very active in caring for poliomyelitis cases and will be greatly missed.

Classified Advertisements

FOR SALE: Complete office fixtures for physician's office. For further information address Mrs. J. D. Pate, Duncan, Oklahoma.

Golden Maxims

In the pocket of Hon. Stephen Allan, who was drowned on the "Henry Clay" was found a printed slip, apparently cut from a newspaper, from which the following is copied. It is worthy to be engraved on the heart of everyone.

"Keep good company or none.
"Never be idle; if your hands cannot be usefully employed, attend to the cultivation of your mind.
"Always speak the truth.
"If anyone speak evil of you, let your life be such that none will believe him.
"Drink no kind of intoxicating drinks.
"When you retire to bed, think over what you have done through the day.
"Avoid temptation through fear you may not withstand it.
"Earn money before you spend it.
"Do not put off till to-morrow that which should be done to-day.
"Never speak evil to anyone.
"Keep pure if you would be happy.
"Save when you are young, to spend when you are old."
Read the above maxims at least once a week.

I said, I will take heed to my ways, that I offend not in my tongue. I will keep my mouth as it were with a bridle. Psalm xxxix. 1,2.

Culture and Medicine

One cannot practice medicine alone and practice it early and late, as so many of us have to do, and hope to escape the malign influences of a routine life. The incessant concentration of thought upon one subject, however interesting, tethers a man's mind in a narrow field. The practitioner needs culture as well as learning. The earliest picture we have in literature of a scientific physician, in our sense of the term, is as a cultured Greek gentleman. —Aequanimitas with Other Addresses. Sir William Osler. 3rd Edition.

Blue Cross Reports

The enrolment of Farm Security Administration families in Oklahoma is finally under way.

The ward plan created to serve these people will be offered at this time to District No. 2 which includes the following counties; Alfalfa, Blain, Canadian, Creek, Garfield, Grant, Kay, Kingfisher, Lincoln, Logan, Major, Noble, Okfuskee, Oklahoma, Okmulgee, Osage, Pawnee and Payne.

The enrolment will be conducted on a county basis. Creek County was the first to complete its enrolment. They had 270 farm families as borrowers; 152 of them have been enrolled and their group went into effect September 1. The other 17 counties will enroll as the county supervisors find time to do so. The plan has been presented to all counties but due to local plans and lack of time it may take six months before all counties will get the job done.

As yet we have no information on when the plan will be submitted to the other districts in the state. Experience in District No. 2 will probably determine when the rest of the State will be offered the plan.

From time to time bulletins will be sent to all member hospitals keeping them informed of the progress we make.

Mr. V. E. Bishop, Regional Director in charge of the Oklahoma City office, and Mr. N. D. Helland, State Director, spent three days in Okeene, Oklahoma, as guests of Dr. L. R. Kirby. The purpose of this visit was to offer the Blue Cross Plan to Okeene and the surrounding community on a community basis.

Meetings were held with the Kiwanis Club, the Senior Chamber of Commerce, the Junior Chamber of Commerce, and the farmers. Our movie, "The Common Defense" was shown in the local theaters and the weekly paper cooperated by running an article about the plan.

The residents of Okeene and the surrounding community pay their light bills monthly through the two local banks. The banks agreed to permit local residents to pay their Blue Cross dues on the same basis. The banks will in turn remit to the Blue Cross office for the group each month.

After discussing the program with the local leadership it was decided that the Junior Chamber of Commerce would conduct enrolment as a civic activity. Any gainfully employed person living in Okeene (a town of 1100) or any farmer within the Okeene shopping area is eligible. One-third of the residents are required to make the required group. The enrolment is to be conducted from September 1 to September 20, services to be effective October 1. The results of this enrolment will be available in October.

Dr. Kirby is to be complemented on the fine cooperation he enjoys from his community. Going through his hospital would be an inspiration to anybody. In our humble opinion the cleanliness and efficient manner in which this hospital is run constitutes a fine example of what can be done in a small community. May we also recommend Dr. and Mrs. Kirby as excellent hosts.

The Measure of Progress

Measure as we may the progress of the world—materially, in the advantages of steam, electricity, and other mechanical appliances; sociologically, in the great improvement in the conditions of life; intellectually, in the diffusion of education; morally, in a possibly higher standard of ethics—there is no one measure which can compare with the decrease of physical suffering in man, woman, and child when stricken by disease or accident. This is the one fact of supreme personal import to every one of us. This is the Promethean gift of the century to man.—Aequanimitas and Other Addresses. Sir William Osler. 3rd Edition.

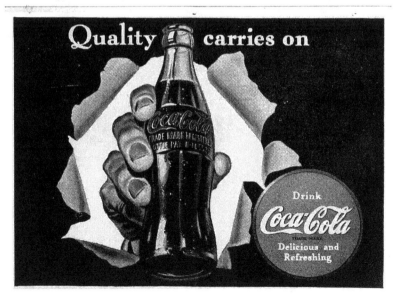

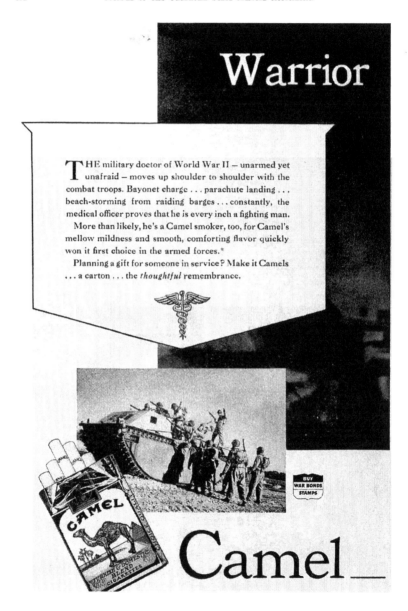

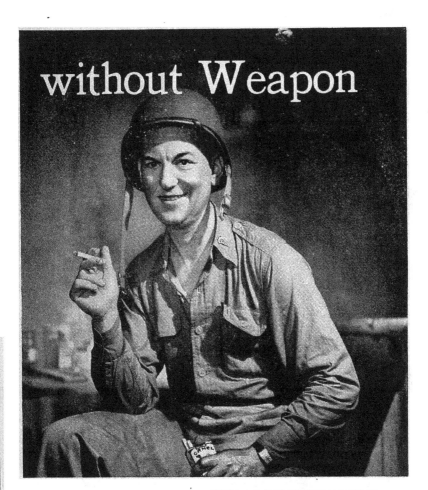

without Weapon

1st in the Service

*With men in the Army, the Navy, the Marine Corps, and the Coast Guard, the favorite cigarette is Camel. (Based on actual sales records.)

New reprints available on cigarette research—Archives of Otolaryngology, February, 1943, pp. 169-173—March, 1943, pp. 404-410. Camel Cigarettes, Medical Relations Division, One Pershing Square, New York 17, N. Y.

_Costlier Tobaccos

BOOK REVIEWS

"The chief glory of every people arises from its authors."—Dr. Samuel Johnson.

THE BOY SEX OFFENDER AND HIS LATER CAREER. Lewis J. Doshay, Psychiatrist, Children's Courts, New York City. Foreword by George G. W. Henry, Associate Professor of Clinical Psychiatry, Cornel University Medical College. Grune and Stratton, New York. 1943.

This is a discussion pertaining to a study and follow-up of 256 juvenile sexual cases that had been treated at the New York City Children's Court clinics between June, 1928 and June, 1934.

The author classifies the cases into two groups; a "primary" group, having no known involvement in any offensive behaviour other than sexual, consisted of 108 cases; a mixed group of 148 juvenile sex offenders who were known to have engaged in various offenses in addition to their sexual abnormalities. The study revealed that the primary group responded one hundred per cent and not a single one of the 108 cases repeated a sexual offense after treatment was given. The treatment consisted of initial psychiatric study, followed by a visit or visits to the court and court clinics where latent forces of shame and guilt were mobilized into activity by the attitudes of the clinic and court toward the offenders. The follow-up studies showed that of this group there were no further sexual offenses and only three petty general offenses occurred later in life.

In the mixed group of 148 cases, after similar therapy, there occurred 10 sexual and 99 general violations, 84 of the latter being felonies, including 34 burglaries, 19 larceny cases and 4 serious assaults, many crimes being accompanied by the use of dangerous weapons.

The text is strongly biased in favor of environmental influences being responsible for juvenile delinquency. The tables and statistical information would impress some toward believing that the treatise is "scientific". However, on page 14, the author quotes from an article published by himself in 1930 with a title, "Evolution Disproves Heredity in Mental Diseases". The quotation would infer that no undesirable trait can be inherited because it could not be carried on in accordance with survival of the fittest, ergo, no undesirable or regressive traits can be inherited. This faulty logic has certainly been disproved, for example, by studies of Slye on the inheritance of cancer in mice. No one could say that cancer is a desirable trait.

It would seem quite possible that the "primary" group of cases were likely incidental victims of the law, indulging possibly much the same as many juveniles do. Juveniles also indulge in the matter of "primary", non-sexual encroachments and a follow- up on these individuals would reveal that many of them have not indulged further after having been caught in the act or having been admonished by proper authorities. These "primary" cases happened to be caught while indulging their offenses and responded to the matter of shame and guilt. It is quite possible that the sexual crime would not have been repeated in any one of them, even though not apprehended, arising out of the sense of guilt and shame that would have been mobilized as a result of individual personal reflection on the matter after the act had been committed.

Those involved in mixed crimes were obviously more psychopathic, and a study of their background shows a more serious environment for them. However, the question may be asked; was the environment not a part of the constitutional make-up of the persons from whom these mixed group cases arose?

This study is only a further demonstration that sociological treatises serve more to provoke questions rather than to offer a solution for any of them.

The book may be summarized by saying that some juvenile deliquent boys make sociological adjustments later and some do not, even through their formative period they indulge in aberrant behavior. We do not have scientific explanation either for the adult successes, or for the adult failures.

However, the book is well written and the cases are interestingly presented. There are also some potentially practical points, provided that the "primary" group were not merely juveniles who would have corrected their abnormal behavior spontaneously without treatment anyway.

The theoretical components of the book are exemplary of the bases of action taken by current sociological theorists who would lead us to believe that they know and have the key to "social security".—Coyne H. Campbell, M.D.

___

COLLECTED PAPERS OF THE MAYO CLINIC AND THE MAYO FOUNDATIONS. Edited by Richard M. Hewitt, A. B. Nevling, John R. Miner, James R. Eckman and M. Katharine Smith. Vol. XXXIV, 1942. Published July, 1943. W. B. Saunders Company.

This well indexed volume of 1000 pages contains much valuable information for the diagnostician and the general practitioner as well as for the general surgeon. In fact, this particular volume devotes more space to medicine than to surgery.

The contents are listed as follows: Recent Advances in Chemotherapy; Alimentary Tract; Genito-Urinary Organs; Ductless Glands; Blood and Circulatory Organs; Skin and Syphilis; Head, Trunk and Extremities; Chest; Brain, Spinal Cord and Nerves; Radiology and Physical Medicine; Anesthesia and Gas Therapy; Miscellaneous.

The general scope of this work can be judged from the above listing of subjects but under these various headings 513 articles are presented. Obviously it is not possible to consider each topic in this brief review but in addition to the routine treatment of many well known subjects with the added knowledge of recent advances, there are valuable papers on the newer aspects of chemotherapy including experimental studies; on vitamin therapy; and of great interest at this time are the papers on the "Dangers of Aerial Transportation". The latter refers particularly to intrathoracic conditions including artificial pneumothorax.

There is a valuable discussion of the "Clinical Applications of Oxygen Therapy". This subject is receiving more and more attention and is assuming a position of increasing importance in therapy. This volume is equally interesting from a surgical viewpoint and any surgeon who takes time to read it will be well rewarded.

Considering the book as a whole, it is refreshing to think a work of such wide interest and particularly so rich in general medical lore, should emanate from a clinic built around a family surgical career.

The reviewer recommends this volume not to specialists but to all doctors who wish to be well informed.—Lewis J. Moorman, M.D.

___

SURGICAL PRACTICES OF THE LAHEY CLINIC. W. B. Saunders Company, New York. 1942. 900 pages.

Here is a book which contains, within its covers, a wealth of surgical information easily available to the seeker because of an excellent index. The material, workmanship of the book, format, type, paper and printing, are worthy of the publishers. The illustrations really illustrate; line drawings, diagrams and tables add to the value of the text. There is a commendable lack of x-ray reproductions which are so often ambiguous.

It is manifestly impossible to adequately review such a book within the limits of the space available, and any review is bound to be colored by the interests and experiences of the reviewer. Certain psychologists tell us that even the character of the morning repast may influence one's reactions. This reviewer was interested to read the Lahey book from the point of view of the younger surgeons or surgeons-in-the-making, and those with perhaps a less wide field of experience. What sort of guide is it for such?

For one thing, this book illustrates the fact that the true surgeon is interested above all in the welfare of the patient, the comfort, and the safety compatible with the largest ultimate benefit of any surgical procedure, even the morale. So this "Surgical Practice" includes all ancillary studies, the patients' history, symptomatology, etiology, surgical pathology, laboratory and x-ray procedures and established principles for pre-operative and post-operative care. Numerous, acceptable case histories illustrate and add interest as well as information to the text, and so increase its clinical value.

To mention specifically the especially excellent articles would seem almost like numbering the chapters—a mere "catalogue of ships". However, the reviewer ventures a few observations.

The section on the Thyroid is a textbook in itself and can be read with profit by every surgeon doing goitre work. In the section on the Pelvis, the paper on "Cancer of the Cervix" deserves praise for its brevity in assigning the treatment of these cases to the roentgenologist; the paper on "Vaginal Hysterectomy" is to be commended for the clearness of detail of both text and illustrations. In the opinion of the reviewer, more of our hysterectomies should be done by the vaginal route.

Both in the section on Anesthesia and throughout the text is given much information on the newer materials and methods of inducing narcosis. The space given to nupercain seems large in proportion, while the use of pentothol sodium is mentioned only in connection with encephalography, transurethral, proctatectomy, "by others", and in combination with fractional spinal anesthesia. Many surgeons in the smaller clinics are finding an increasingly large field of usefulness for pentothol sodium.

For the surgeon-in-the-making, some of the most valuable articles in this comprehensive "Practice" are those dealing with the common, every-day diseases and lesions, hallux valgus, diseases of the bile passages, breast cancer, sciatic pain (not "sciatica"), empyema and hemorrhoids. We find expressed in these papers what may be called the philosophy of the causation of these diseases as well as a clear and concise, yet sufficiently complete statement of the principals of proper treatment which is commendable. If physicians would carefully examine all patients who present themselves with symptoms of hemorrhoids there would be less need for extensive resection of rectum and colon, for colostomies and ablative operations which the authors of this "Practice" have so well developed.

Also, if surgeons generally absorbed the implications recurrent throughout the book on the importance of early diagnosis there would be fewer of the chronic and complicated, and often intractable cases, to be referred to the larger clinics later. But, in view of this book, perhaps even this would entail a loss to surgical science.—A. S. Risser, M.D.

MEMOIR OF WALTER REED: THE YELLOW FEVER EPISODE. Albert E. Truby. Paul B. Hoeber, Inc., New York. 239 pages.

This memoir of Walter Reed, inspired and nurtured by the untiring researches of Dr. Phillip S. Hench and told with captivating facility by the veteran eye witness Brigadier General Albert E. Truby, constitutes one of the most dramatic human interest stories in the history of medicine. Aside from its scientific interest, its stirring spiritual values carry an intriguing appeal for both medical and lay readers.

Though practically every page possesses the readability of romance, the thread of authenticity is never lost. The observant medical reader cannot fail to note the fact that while this unprecedented bit of research, which resulted in the control of yellow fever, was directly under the auspices of the United States Government, it could not have been successfully consummated if it had not been for the convergence of high minded, humanitarian purposes which prompted Surgeon General Steinberg, Governor General Wood and Walter Reed to follow their instinctive medical urge without seeking or awaiting governmental approval. Historically, this is in line with the fact that all great medical discoveries have been individually inspired and independently pursued.

The following letter from Walter Reed to his wife, written at 11:50 P.M., December 31, 1900, from Columbia Barracks, Quemados, Cuba, should inspire an immediate desire to read this most interesting little volume:

"Only ten minutes of the old century remain. Here I have been sitting reading that most wonderful book, "La Roche on Yellow Fever" written in 1853. Forty-seven years later it has been permitted to me and my assistants to lift the impenetrable veil that has surrounded the causation of this most wonderful, dreadful pest of humanity and to put it on a rational and scientific basis. I thank God that this has been accomplished during the latter days of the old century. May its cure be wrought in the early days of the new! The prayer that has been mine for twenty years, that I might be permitted to do something to alleviate human suffering has been granted! . . . Hark, there go twenty-four buglers in concert, all sounding "taps" for the old year."

This book, in handy, attractive format, is easy to hold and easy to read. It constitutes a delightful bedside companion for the busy doctor in want of a stimulus for tomorrows duties.—Lewis J. Moorman, M.D.

AIR BORNE INFECTIONS: SOME OBSERVATIONS UPON ITS DECLINE. Dwight O'Hara, M.D., Professor of Preventive Medicine, Tufts College Medical School. The Commonwealth Fund. E. L. Hildreth and Co., Inc. 1943. 114 pages. Price $1.50.

This little tome is based upon the study of six diseases in the Commonwealth of Massachusetts which killed 300 per 100,000 in 1917 and now account for barely 100 deaths. In war times and crowding of people, the possibility of another pandemic of influenza as in 1918 makes a public health problem. The incidence of respiratory infections is found to be higher in overcrowded or confined areas, in barracks, in prisons or other institutions.

The decrease in mortality often preceded the development and application of preventive methods. "Can preventive methods be coordinated with other factors to achieve even greater improvement."

He emphasizes the fact that it is not so much the polluted air but that the mucous membranes are good air conditioning devices. On this account, artificially conditioned air is just as good a vehicle between throats as their being polluted. Natural immunity and acquired immunity is discussed at length and this is as fundamental as any one thing in medicine. "One thing seems certain, however, that specific antibody formation is stimulated only by exposure natural and artificial. This acquired immunity is obtained in one generation and lost in the next and their epidemics take on a malignant character."

The reactions are given of the nasal mucous membranes to climatic variants such as humidity and barometric pressure together with the vascular adjustments of nasal mucous membrane. The cilia of the respiratory tiact (cilia escalator) are continually cleansing it of offending material.

One does not realize the lessened incidence of Pneumonia Tuberculosis, Diphtheria, Measles, Scarlet Fever and Whooping Cough as shown in the author's graph covering the period of 1900-1940. Diphtheria seems to have gone like the wild pidgeon; measles less so; tuberculosis less than 50 per 100,000; pneumonia a very downward but irregular course. Hence it looks like the student of Geriatrics must be the doctor of the future.
—Lea A. Riley, M.D.

Tyrothricin Found Beneficial in Treating Local Infections

Tyrothricin, a bactericidal substance recently isolated from a soil bacterium, applied to ulcers resulted in sterilization and healing if the local infection was caused by Streptococcus haemolyticus, Staphylococcus aureus or Streptococcus faecalis and encouraging results were obtained when it was applied to mastoid cavities following mastoid operations, Charles H. Rammelkamp, M.D., Boston, reports in the current issue of War Medicine. The latter is published bimonthly by the American Medical Association in cooperation with the Division of Medical Sciences of the National Research Council.

Dr. Rammelkamp's findings are based on the use of the substance in the treatment of 58 localized infections, most of them located on the arms or legs of patients, and its application at the time of operation to 15 mastoid cavities infected with hemolytic streptococci.

"Early in the present studies," Dr. Rammelkamp says, "it was noted that in an infection associated with a mixed flora, that is, both with gram-negative and with gram-positive organisms, it was impossible to rid a lesion of the gram-positive component, even though large amounts of the bactericidal substance were applied...."

He says that the results obtained in the mastoid group justify further trial of the substance in the treatment of mastoiditis following operation.

"The value of tyrothricin in the treatment of other forms of infection has not been established," Dr. Rammelkamp says. "Superficial streptococcic infections of wounds, burns or skin should respond to the local application of the bactericidal substance; staphylococcic infections are likely to be much more resistant...:"

He says that inasmuch as gramicidin, a substance obtained from tyrothricin, has been shown to be less toxic and at the same time more potent against gram-positive organisms, "it appears likely that this substance may prove more useful in treatment of certain localized infections."

Tuberculosis "Cure"?

Successful vaccination of children against tuberculosis, reported recently in newspapers, holds no immediate hope of a "quick cure" of adult victims of the disease. This was the statement released by the Department to newspapers shortly after an announcement of an experiment among Chicago children with Bacillus Calmette-Guerin vaccine.

The Department pointed out that experiments with this tuberculosis vaccine have been carried on since 1906. Efforts of experimenters have been to weaken a virulent strain of tuberculosis organisms produced in cattle to a point where a vaccine made from them will confer immunity in humans. There is always the possibility that the vaccine may become virulent and dangerous to use and European experiments were halted for several years after disaster attended the vaccination of infants in Lubek, Germany, in 1922. Careful work has been carried on at different points in the United States over a period of years, and the results obtained have been disputed by other equally careful workers. Similar reports of success have been made previously.

Until such time as the use of this vaccine is sanctioned by the American Medical Association, said the Department, people should not place many hopes on its effectiveness as a tuberculosis cure or preventive.

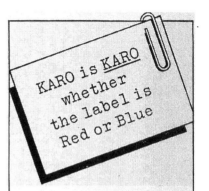
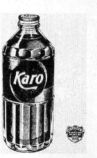

MEDICAL ABSTRACTS

"LESIONS OF THE SUPRASPINATUS TENDON. DE-GENERATION, RUPTURE AND CALIFICATION." C. L. Wilson. Archives of Surgery. XLVI, 307. March. 1943.

The author emphasizes that degeneration, rupture of, and calcification within the supraspinatus tendon may cause disability for as long as two years.

He discusses the gross anatomy of the supraspinatus tendon, the other short rotator muscles of the shoulder, the tendon of the long head of the biceps muscle, and the subacromial bursa.

The function of the supraspinatus tendon is primarily that of abduction of the arm. When the deltoid muscle is paralyzed, the arm can be abducted. Even after rupture of the supraspinatus tendon, injection to remove pain makes abduction possible though much weakened. This tendon acts as an abductor of the arm up to the horizontal position, and from there as a stabilizer of the shoulder joint.

In microscopic study, muscle cells are seen to end abruptly in tendon cells. The supraspinatus tendon is inserted into the greater tuberosity of the humerus through a layer of fibrocartilage, called "the palisades" by Codman. The "critical portion",—the rupture point of the supraspinatus tendon, is the half-inch proximal to the palisades.

Rupture occurs as a transverse tear in the fibers of the tendon. Incomplete rupture may occur on the joint side, where it is called a rim rent, on the bursal side involving the floor of the subacromial bursa, or within the substance of the tendon. A stub of the tendon, found attached to the greater tuberosity of the humerus after rupture, gradually wears away, and the tuberosity suffers erosion. The subacromial bursa is thick. There is exposure of the tendon of the long head of the biceps muscle.

Histological degeneration changes in the supraspinatus can be shown by staining. Degeneration leads to weakening of the tendon and eventual rupture under slight strain. It was demonstrated that a pull of 1000 pounds ruptured a normal supraspinatus tendon three millimeters thick and two centimeters wide.

Incidence of rupture is higher in males than in females, and though it is bilateral, it is generally on the right side. Fracture of the greater tuberosity, instead of rupture, usually occurs in persons under fifty years of age. Degenerative changes and vascularization, accompaniments of old age, may be the cause of the high incidence of rupture in persons over fifty. Trauma and wear may be precipitating factors. Whether occupation causes ischaemia or attrition still remains to be proven.

The clinical signs of rupture are pain at the insertion of the supraspinatus muscle, and inability to abduct the arm. Roentgenographic evidence is best obtained by chemical injection into the shoulder joint one centimeter anterolateral to the coraco-acromial joint, in the direction of the center of the head of the humerus. Rupture is indicated by either a finger-like projection flowing out of the joint cavity, or a free communication between the joint and the sub-acromial bursa.

Operation is the best treatment. A vertical incision one and one-half inches long is made over the anterior aspect of the head of the humerus with its upper end near the acromioclavicular joint and its lower end at the top of the bicipital groove. Repair is not difficult and the recovery period is two weeks.

Calcium deposits in the supraspinatus tendon are painful and irritate the surrounding muscles, tendons and the subacromial bursa. Rupture into the bursa often results in cessation of pain and symptoms. The incidence of calcium is higher in males than in females, and highest in occupations requiring constant use of the arm in abduction. Trauma may be a contributing factor, but is not the cause of calcification. Onset may be insidious or acute. Roentgenograms do not always show deposits. The best treatment is immediate excision of the deposit. In chronic cases diathermy results in absorption of the calcium.

Subacromial bursitis never arises as a primary condition, but is the result of rupture of the supraspinatus tendon or other lesions in the surrounding tissues. It may be treated by hyperabduction of manipulation.—E.D.M., M.D.

"RELATION OF HEMATOLOGY TO OTOLARYNGOLOGY." Goodlatte B. Gilmore, New York. Archives of Otolaryngology, Vol. 37, pages 691-698. May, 1943.

The author makes an attempt to show the relationship between hematology and otolaryngology by the enumeration of specific examples. Emphasis is laid on the fact that a disorder in one field may manifest itself by lesions of the other field. Blood dyscrasias, such as the leukemias, purpura, polycythemia, granulocytopenia and hemophilia, have at times otolaryngologic signs that may mislead the observer into overlooking the cause by paying too much attention to the effect. The changes in the blood in sepsis, Vincent's angina, the Plummer-Vinson syndrome and infectious mononucleosis and the pathologic changes of congenital multiple teleangiectasia are discussed.

Epistaxis persistent or repeated can be the initial sign of leukemia. There may be also hemorrhage in the external meatus, tympanic membrane, middle ear and labyrinth. Leukemic patients may complain of vertigo, tinnitus or deafness owing to the leukocytic infiltration or hemorrhage involving the acustic nerve. Lesions may be also found in the oral cavity. Bleeding gums resembling those of Vincent's infection and lesions imitating scurvy and stomatitis are common. Necrotic or membranous areas may also occur.

In infectious mononucleosis or glandular fever of Pfeiffer angina is a more or less constant symptom, and cervical adenopathy is always out of proportion to the extent of the lesion in the throat. In sepsis there may be a number of pathological conditions which are of interest to the otorhinolaryngologist. Polycythemia may occur in patients which chronic tracheal stenosis, in victims of chronic carbon monoxide poisioning and in persons suffering from repeated small hemorrhages. Epistaxis and bleeding from the gums are characteristic signs. Due to thrombosis of a vessel of the inner ear, Meniere's syndrome may also occur.

Hemorrhagic diathesis is often accompanied by epistaxis. Hemophilia is often first diagnosed by the rhinologist. In congenital multiple teleangiectasia recurrent epistaxis in members of a family through as many as four generations has been reported. There exist many red and purple nevi in the oral cavity and on the mucous membrane of the nose. In granulocytopenia caused by the administration of certain coal tar derivatives, aminopyrine, barbiturates, dinitrophenol, membranous or ulcerative infections in the mouth or pharynx regularly occur. The atypical peritonsillat abscess should be viewed with suspicion, that is, an abscess from which incision does not liberate pus as expected. Following the widespread use of sulfanilamide or its derivatives, leukopenia had frequently been reported and occasionally fatal cases of granulocytopenia. The Plummer-Vinson syndrome with its anemia, glossitis and dysphagia, borders the fields of otolaryngology and bronchoesophagology.

Tests for the coagulation time and bleeding time prior to tonsillectomy were at one time considered as a vital precaution. The value of these tests in lowering the incidence of postoperative bleeding is not doubted. A few well chosen questions about the family and personal history have far greater value. The blood sedimentation test has not been made much use of in otorhinolaryngology. The sedimentation rate is increased in direct ratio to the amount of tissue destroyed. It is a reaction too general to place much emphasis on it in the otolaryngological field.—M.D.H., M.D.

"DECOMPRESSION OF PROTRUDED INTERVERTEBRAL DISKS, WITH A NOTE ON SPINAL EXPLORATION." Arthur Ecker. Jour. A.M.A., CXXL 401, Feb. 6, 1943.

Exploration of the cauda equina in the region of the fifth lumbar vertebra for intractable low-back pain gives prompt and persistent relief in properly selected patients. Exploration should be adequate, and should usually include the anterior aspect of the spinal canal above and below the fifth lumbar vertebra in the midline and far laterally near the intervertebral foramen on each side. The author suggests the interlaminar approach to the spinal canal after bilateral stripping of the sacrospinalis from the spinous processes and laminae, and decompression of small intraspinal protrusions of intervertebral discs without removal of any of the disc structure. The importance of not opening the dura is stressed.

The author considers a disc protruded only if it bulges more when the lumbar spine is extended as a result of the anaesthetist's lifting of the patient's shoulders. It is not the protrusion of the disc which causes sciatic pain, but the compression of the nerve root between the disc and the posterior wall of the intervertebral foramen.

Questionable, slight, and moderate protrusions of the intervertebral discs should be left alone, and the overlying nerve root should be adequately decompressed. This procedure has yielded results as satisfactory as removal of the protruded portions of each discs, and it may minimize the incidence of the recurrence of symptoms.—E.D.M., M.D.

"CHEMOTHERAPY WITH SULFANILAMIDE: CLINICAL RESULTS." Otto Gsell, St. Gallen, Switzerland. Helvetica Acta, Vol. 10, pages 177-202. April, 1943.

It is now three years that clinical research on the effect of sulfanilamide preparations has begun in Switzerland. During this time it became evident that only three or four preparations can be considered as having the optimal clinical effect. These are as follows:
1. Sulfapyridine (M&B 673, Dagenan, Eubasinum) discovered by Evans and Phillips and introduced in 1938 by Whitby.
2. Sulfathiazole (Cibazol , M&B 760, Thiazamide) discovered by Hartmann, also by Foszbinder in 1939.
3. Sulfapyridine (sulfadiazine and Pyriminal) discovered by Finestone in 1940.
In addition as equally preparations have to be mentioned the following sulfathiazole derivatives:
1. Methylsulfathiazole (Ultraseptyl).
2. Sulfaethylthiodiazole (Globucid).
For the treatment of specific infections other preparations are also recommended, though their effect cannot be evaluated with as much certainty as the effect of the above named preparations against pnuemococcic, meningococcic and gonococcic infections. These preparations with specific effect are:
1. Sulfaguanidine and succinylsulfathiazole against intestinal infection.

2. Sulfones, e.g. tibatin (galactosid of 4.4 diaminodiphemylsulfone against streptococcic infections.
3. Marfanil against anaerobe infection.
The earliest sulfonamide preparation such as prontosil, rodilone, septacine are no more considered as first choice for the treatment of pneumococcic and meningococcic infections.

The three best sulfonamide preparations, in fact all sulfonamide derivatives, must be evaluated on the basis of their effect upon pneumococci, meningococci and gonococci. Against these micro-organisms the effect of the three preparations is specific and almost equivalent. Their effect in streptococcic and staphylococcic infections depends not only upon the chemosensibility of the pathogenic cocci but also upon various other factors such as site of the infection, the individual resistance of the body, and individual characteristics of the attacking germs. Hence, the results of sulfonamide therapy in streptococcic and staphylococcic infections show a great variation. The success often depends on the bascularization of the focus of infection.

Erysipelas responds to sulfonamide therapy quickly, and even the earlier types of sulfonamide preparations give good results if used in high doses. Infections of the skin are also easily influenced if they are superficial, such as impetigo, folliculitis, and ulcerations. But as soon as the infective focus becomes encapsulated by a thick wall of inflammatory products and necrotic tissue, as in furuncles and abscesses, or if the blood supply of an infective focus is diminished as in wounds, a good result cannot be expected with certainty.

Streptococcic and staphylococcic infections of the throat and of the cavities of the ear and nasal sinuses are often favorably influenced by sulfonamide preparations, yet the evaluation of sulfonamide therapy in the otorhinolaryngology is not easy, and the opinion of clinicans are still not uniform. One is rarely certain whether the quick recovery was due to sulfonamide drugs or it would have come spontaneously without chemotherapeutic remedies.

How difficult it is, for instance, to find the truth in the sulfonamide therapy of lacunar angina! The author treated 44 cases of acute lacunar tonsillitis with large doses of sulfonamide for two days; in 36 patients the fever ceased and there was complete recovery within from 24 to 48 hours, and in two patients within 72 hours. For the six cases which did not answer to sulfonamide it is assumed that the tonsillitis might have been caused not by cocci but by spirilla or certain types of virus, and such micro-organisms do not respond to sulfonamides. It also happened according to the author's observations that acute lacunar angina with high fever developed in a patient who has been under sulfonamide therapy against a gonococcic infection.

He mentions also recurrent tonsillitis as a new after effect of sulfonamide therapy. This phenomenon is of about the same nature as recurrent pneumonia attacks seen after successful treatment of lobar pneumonia. Recurrent tonsillitis develops after an interval of from 4 to 7 days; it is not a new infection but a local affair due to either an incomplete destruction of bacteria or an incomplete development of antibodies.

In streptococcic and staphylococcic infections of internal organs, as in meningitis, osteomyelitis, sinusitis, no more effect can be expected from sulfonamide preparations if necrotic tissue is present. In such cases a treatment in two phases is the best; high doses of sulfonamides moderate the infection and often prevent general sepsis; the second phase of therapy is the surgical removal of infection localized by chemotherapy. In case of osteomyelitis this therapeutic plan was frequently successful. In meningitis the two-phase therapy reduced the mortality of the disease from 100 per cent to about 30 per cent.

The effect of sulfonamide in focal infection is still waiting for proper evaluation. In influenza infections sulfonamide preparations proved valuable, especially in influenzal meningitis of small children, and at the Pediatric Clinic of Zurich the mortality of the disease was reduced from 92 per cent to 43 per cent.

In only three virus diseases was there any evidence of success of sulfonamide therapy; in trachoma, lymphogranuloma inguinale and smallpox. It happens that these are the virus diseases most often complicated by secondary coccal infections. It is therefore hard to decide whether sulfonamides have any effect on the virus itself. This is true also for common cold and its complications. If sulfonamide is used in common cold at all, it should be administered only against a secondary coccal infection. As a non-specific remedy or as an antipyretic substance, sulfonamide is definitely contraindicated; it is an abuse to prescribe sulfonamides for catarrh or for febrile diseases indiscriminately.—M.D.H., M.D.

CLINICAL AND BACTERIOLOGICAL RESEARCH ON THE TONSILLAR ORIGIN OF FOCAL INFECTIONS: ASSAY OF A DIAGNOSTIC METHOD FOR CUTANEOUS STREPTOCOCCIC ALLERGY AND ITS RESULTS. Roger Max Tuscher. Bern, Switzerland. Revue medicale de la Suisse Romande, Vol. 72. pages 903-960. December, 1942.

There are many observations on the existence of focal infection in the tonsils. If the clinical anamesis and the object findings are properly studied in a particular case, it is possible by these simple means alone to diagnose at least 80 per cent of tonsillar focal infections. On the other hand, there is little to go by in the rest of the cases, especially if the patient is in a status of general allergy. In such cases especially, only the bacteriologic examination accompanied by skin tests for allergy will lead to correct diagnosis.

Throughout the years various diagnostic tests have been elaborated and recommended for recognizing tonsillar focal infection, such as the method of Schmidt-Viggo, lymphopenia after massage of healthy looking tonsils, leukocytosis with lymphopenia after massage of focally infected tonsils; the shift to the left of neutrophil leukocytes in the blood picture (Gording, Reidar, Hakon, Bjorn-Hansen), the tonsilar test of Worms and LeMee; yet, none of them is sufficient to establish with certainty the diagnosis of tonsillar focal infection. On the other hand, an intradermal test with the patient's own bacteria taken from the tonsillar crypts will help greatly in arriving at a correct diagnosis.

The sample taken from the bacterial flora of the tonsillar crypts is inoculated in bouillion of Rosenow. Antigen is prepared and one tenth of a cc is injected intradermally into the anterior face of the forearm. The skin reaction is observed after 24 hours and 36 hours. Preparation of the antigen or vaccine is made according to a slightly modified standard technic.—M.D.H., M.D.

"BLOOD FLOW IN EXTREMITIES AFFECTED BY ANTERIOR POLIOMYELITIS." P. I. Abramson, K. Flachs. J .Freiberg and I. A. Mirsky. Archives of Internal Medicine. Vol. LXXI, page 391. March. 1943.

This work tends to disprove the theory that after poliomyelitis the blood flow of an affected extremity is diminished, and it casts doubt on the rationale of therapeutic methods attempting to improve a supposedly weaker circulation. Twenty-seven patients, who had recovered from active poliomyelitis for varying lengths of time, were the subjects. The peripheral circulation of the affected limb as opposed to the unaffected limb was studied by determining: (1) blood flow by the venous-occlusion plethysmographic method, (2) the response to arterial occlusion, and (3) cutaneous temperature. The blood flow per unit of tissue was not significantly altered on the affected side, being about as often increased as it was diminished. Critical analysis of the other findings also showed no significant differences.

The experiments were performed in the winter time, the patients being brought indoors for the purpose. It was found, particularly in the case of skin temperatures, that before the subject was thoroughly warmed the circulation on the affected side was smaller. Therefore,

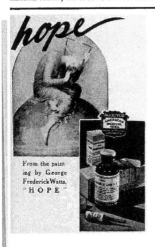

theie was some evidence to conroborate the clinical impression of cooler skin surface and cutaneous varoconstriction in the paralyzed extremity. The authors would do well to pursue their work by the study of dynamic changes in the circulatoin caused by heat, cold, and emotion, and by further study of the control of the autonomic nervous system.

Rigidly controlled experimental woik requires the most caieful considered before being taken over by the clinic as useful fact. Interpretation is everything. In this case the authors have demonstiated beyond much doubt that under ordinary conditions there is not significaut alteiation in the circulation of paralyzed extremities in poliomyelitis. Clinically, it seems that methods designed to improve circulation in this disease, or otherwise to bring back useful function, should not be abandoned.—E.D.M., M.D.

"INTERNAL FIXATION IN INJURIES OF THE ANKLE." Harold G. Lee & Thomas B. Horan. Surg., Gyn. & Obst.. Vol. LXXVI. page 593. May. 1943.

The authors have discussed the necessity for accurate ieduction in fiactuies about the ankle, and have pointed out the frequency with which open reduction is necessary in order to accomplish an anatomical restoration. They have taken up separately; fracture of the lower end of the fibula ,tiimalleolar fracture, fracture of the anterior tibial surface, fiacture of the internal malleolus, Pott's fractuie, separation of the tibia and fibula, and recurrent dislocation of the personal tendons. In each of these various conditions the authors have pointed out the impoitant disalignments to be corrected and the necessity for internal fixation. In nearly every instance, they have accomplished this fixation by the use of a stiategically placed bone sciew. They feel that it is impoitant that operative indications be recognized promptly, and that manipulative treatment be avoided. A classification of those injuries which require operative treatment is presented, and methods that have given excellent results are described.—E.D.M., M.D.

"THE RELATION OF TRAUMA DIABETES." Elliott P. Joslin. Boston. Mass. Annals of Surgery. April. 1943.

Diabetes ranks eighth as a cause of death in the United States, and approximately one individual in 165 of the total population has the disease. No age, sex, iace or social status is immune. Its incidence is increasing and presumably will continue to grow until the average age at death of the population exceeds the decade 44-55 years, in which it is most apt to begin. This makes the date of onset of the disease in relation to the time of the trauma a crucial factor.

There are about 800,000 diabetics now living in the United States.

To prove that trauma is the cause of diabetes in any individual case, evidence must be at hand to show (a) that the disease did not exist befoie the trauma; (b) that the trauma was severe, injuring the pancreas; (c) that the symptoms and signs of the disease developed within a reasonable period following the trauma, the etiologic importance of the trauma waning with the prolongation of the interval; and (d) that the symptoms and signs of diabetes were not transitory but permanent.

Within a very few months after the use of Insulin in human beings, instances of infection at the site of injection if Insulin ceased to occur. Among 1,838 admissions to the George F. Baker Clinic during 1941 there were but eight who entered for abscesses following injection of Insulin. When one consideis that only this small number of incidents occurred among many million injections in patients both inside and outside the hospital, it is evident that both the manufacturers and the patients use care. Needles broken in the skin during injection have never led to serious trouble in the author's experience, and such occurrences are even more rare than abscesses.

More serious are those in which an Insulin reaction has been mistaken for diabetic coma and, in consequence, a dose of Insulin has been given which resulted in death. Fortunately, such instances are few; in fact, but nine are known among 15,000 or moie patients who have had Insulin administered. Four of these received additional Insulin while in shock, one undoubtedly, took a lethal dose of Insulin with design, and the circumstances regarding the iemainder were somewhat obscure. None of the cases were cbseived in Boston, but five were in consultation.—H.J., M.D.

"DIABETES MELLITUS." Elliott P. Joslin. Boston. Mass. New England Journal of Medicine. May 20. 1943.

The year 1941 witnessed the first break in the upward curve of mortality from diabetes mellitus in the iegistration areas of the continental United States during the last seven years. The mortality rates from 1935 to 1941 are as follows:

1935	22.2 per ceut per 100,000
1936	23.7 per cent per 100,000
1937	23.7 per cent per 100,000
1938	23.8 per cent per 100,000
1939	25.5 per cent per 100,000
1940	26.6 per cent per 100,000
1941	25.4 per cent per 100,000

The explanation undoubtedly lies first of all in the prolongation in the lives of diabetic patients, and secondly in the causes of death of these patients becoming more and more those of the population in general and not specifically related to diabetes. A death from diabetic coma is now a rarity. The possibility exists that statistics of diabetic mortality will not represent in the future so good a guide to the incidence of diabetes will be increasingly recorded as a secondary cause of death or, perhaps, be totally omitted from the death certificate. For the true mortality among diabetic patients and for the incidence of the disease in the country, it is probable that privately gathered statistics will be increasingly valuable. Perhaps afer the war the American Diabetes Association with its growing membership of physicians will attack the problem. That the number of living diabetic patients in the country is rapidly advancing there can be no question.

Diabetic Coma:

On March 30, 1943, in the Baker Clinic, there had been 83 consecutive cases of diabetic coma since August 21, 1940, with the carbundioxide content of the blood 20 volumes percent or less, without a fatality.

Adrenal Gland in Carbohydrate Metabolism:

Evidence pointing to the importance of the adrenal gland in carbohydrate metabolism has advanced considerably in the last few years. A review of recent articles is given.

Piegnancy:

The problem of pregnancy complicating diabetes is controversial in four primary respects. First, as regards fetal survival . . . does it deviate significantly irom the normal? Secondly, as to the characteristics of the infants of diabetic mothers, is there an infant recognizable as one so produced? Thirdly, as to the clinical couise of the mother, it is normal or abnormal, and does it affect the fetus? Fourthly, what is the need for special care of the infants and the mother?—H.J., M.D.

KEY TO ABSTRACTORS

E. D. M. ....Earl D. McBride, MD.
M. D. H. ....Marvin D. Henley, M.D.
H. J. ....Hugh Jeter, M.D.

Real Knowledge

"The knowledge which a man can use is the only real knowledge, the only knowledge which has life and growth in it and converts itself into practical power. The rest hangs like dust about the brain or dries like rain drops off the stones."—Froude.

Removal and control of Dropsy

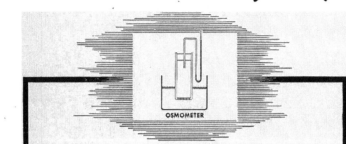

OSMOMETER

*P*assage of fluid from the blood into the tissues occurs in cardiac decompensation, nephrosis, and many cases of chronic nephritis. Disturbance of osmotic pressure relations prevents return of the "leaked" fluid to the systemic circulation, and dropsy results.

In these circumstances Salyrgan-Theophylline solution is customarily employed parenterally. This highly potent mercurial promotes the excretion of excess tissue fluid. In most cases urinary output is increased within a few hours and the edema disappears within a matter of days.

Salyrgan-Theophylline solution is preferably administered intravenously, but may also be given intramuscularly. It is generally well tolerated and injections can be repeated at appropriate intervals without loss of potency.

Supplied in ampuls of 1 cc., boxes of 5, 25 and 100; ampuls of 2 cc., boxes of 10, 25 and 100.

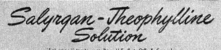

Salyrgan - Theophylline Solution

"Salyrgan," trademark Reg. U.S. Pat. Off. & Canada
Brand of MERSALYL with THEOPHYLLINE INJECTION

 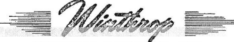

CHEMICAL COMPANY, INC.
Pharmaceuticals of merit for the physician
NEW YORK, N. Y.   WINDSOR, ONT.

OFFICERS OF COUNTY SOCIETIES, 1943

★

COUNTY	PRESIDENT	SECRETARY	MEETING TIME
Alfalfa	H. E. Huston, Cherokee	L. T. Lancaster, Cherokee	Last Tues. each Second Month
Atoka-Coal	J. B. Clark, Coalgate	J. S. Fulton, Atoka	
Beckham	H. K. Speed, Sayre	E. S. Kilpatrick, Elk City	Second Tuesday
Blaine	Virginia Olson Curtin, Watonga	W. F. Griffin, Watonga	
Bryan	J. T. Colwick, Durant	W. K. Haynie, Durant	Second Tuesday
Caddo	F. L. Patterson, Carnegie	C. B. Sullivan, Carnegie	
Canadian	P. F. Herod, El Reno	A. L. Johnson, El Reno	Subject to call
Carter	Walter Hardy, Ardmore	H. A. Higgins, Ardmore	
Cherokee	P. H. Medearis, Tahlequah	*James K. Gray, Tahlequah	First Tuesday
Choctaw	C. H. Hale, Boswell	E. A. Johnson, Hugo	
Cleveland	J. A. Rieger, Norman	Curtis Berry, Norman	Thursday nights
Comanche	George S. Barber, Lawton	W. F. Lewis, Lawton	
Cotton	A. B. Holstead, Temple	Mollie F. Seism, Walters	Third Friday
Craig	F. M. Adams, Vinita	J. M. McMillan, Vinita	
Creek	H. R. Haas, Sapulpa	C. G. Oakes, Sapulpa	
Custer	F. R. Vieregg, Clinton	C. J. Alexander, Clinton	Third Thursday
Garfield	Paul B. Champlin, Enid	John R. Walker, Enid	Fourth Thursday
Garvin	T. F. Gross, Lindsay	John R. Callaway, Pauls Valley	Wednesday before Third Thursday
Grady	Walter J. Baze, Chickasha	Roy E. Emanuel, Chickasha	Third Thursday
Grant	I. V. Hardy, Medford	E. E. Lawson, Medford	
Greer	G. P. Cherry, Mangum	J. B. Hollis, Mangum	
Harmon	W. G. Husband, Hollis	L. E. Hollis, Hollis	First Wednesday
Haskell	William Carson, Keota	N. K. Williams, McCurtain	
Hughes	Wm. L. Taylor, Holdenville	Imogene Mayfield, Holdenville	First Friday
Jackson	E. S. Crow, Olustee	E. W. Mabry, Altus	Last Monday
Jefferson	F. M. Edwards, Ringling	L. L. Wade, Ryan	Second Monday
Kay	Philip C. Risser, Blackwell	J. Holland Howe, Ponca City	Third Thursday
Kingfisher	C. M. Hodgson, Kingfisher	H. Violet Sturgeon, Hennessey	
Kiowa	B. H. Watkins, Hobart	J. William Finch, Hobart	
LeFlore	Neeson Rolle, Poteau	Rush L. Wright, Poteau	
Lincoln	H. B. Jenkins, Tryon	Carl H. Bailey, Stroud	First Wednesday
Logan	William C. Miller, Guthrie	J. L. LeHew, Jr., Guthrie	Last Tuesday
Marshall	O. A. Cook, Madill	Philip G. Joseph, Madill	
Mayes	Ralph V. Smith, Pryor	Paul B. Cameron, Pryor	
McClain	B. W. Slover, Blanchard	R. L. Royster, Purcell	
McCurtain	A. W. Clarkson, Valliant	N. L. Barker, Broken Bow	Fourth Tuesday
McIntosh	James L. Wood, Eufaula	William A. Tolleson, Eufaula	First Thursday
Murray	P. V. Annadown, Sulphur	F. E. Sadler, Sulphur	Second Tuesday
Muskogee-Sequoyah-Wagoner	H. A. Scott, Muskogee	D. Evelyn Miller, Muskogee	First Monday
Noble	C. H. Cooke, Perry	J. W. Francis, Perry	
Okfuskee	L. J. Spickard, Okemah	M. L. Whitney, Okemah	Second Monday
Oklahoma	Walker Morledge, Oklahoma City	E. R. Musick, Oklahoma City	Fourth Tuesday
Okmulgee	A. R. Holmes, Henryetta	J. C. Matheney, Okmulgee	Second Monday
Osage	C. R. Weirich, Pawhuska	George K. Hemphill, Pawhuska	Second Monday
Ottawa	W. B. Sanger, Picher	Matt A. Connell, Picher	Third Thursday
Pawnee	E. T. Robinson, Cleveland	R. L. Browning, Pawnee	
Payne	L. A. Mitchell, Stillwater	C. W. Moore, Stillwater	Third Thursday
Pittsburg	John F. Park, McAlester	William H. Kaeiser, McAlester	Third Friday
Pontotoc	O. H. Miller, Ada	R. H. Mayes, Ada	First Wednesday
Pottawatomie	A. C. McFarling, Shawnee	Clinton Gallaher, Shawnee	First and Third Saturday
Pushmataha	John S. Lawson, Clayton	B. M. Hackabay, Antlers	
Rogers	C. W. Beson, Claremore	C. L. Caldwell, Chelsea	First Monday
Seminole	Max Van Sandt, Wewoka	Mack I. Shanholtz, Wewoka	Third Wednesday
Stephens	W. K. Walker, Marlow	Wallis S. Ivy, Duncan	
Texas	R. G. Obermiller, Texhoma	Morris Smith, Guymon	
Tillman	R. D. Robinson, Frederick	O. G. Bacon, Frederick	
Tulsa	James C. Peden, Tulsa	E. O. Johnson, Tulsa	Second and Fourth Monday
Washington-Nowata	J. G. Smith, Bartlesville	J. V. Athey, Bartlesville	Second Wednesday
Washita	A. S. Neal, Cordell	James F. McMurry, Sentinel	
Woods	C. A. Traverse, Alva	O. E. Templin, Alva	Last Tuesday Odd Months
Woodward	C. E. Williams, Woodward	C. W. Tedrowe, Woodward	Second Thursday

*(Serving in Armed Forces)

THE JOURNAL

OF THE

OKLAHOMA STATE MEDICAL ASSOCIATION

| VOLUME XXXVI | OKLAHOMA CITY, OKLAHOMA, OCTOBER, 1943 | NUMBER 10 |

Radium Therapy in the Treatment of Cancer of the Skin

LOUIS M. PIATT, M.D.

COLUMBUS, OHIO

Radium therapy, as one method of combating cancer, has, without doubt, been recognized and its value in treatment established. Radium therapy developed more slowly than roentgen therapy because it was expensive and difficult to obtain. Now, with few exceptions, the majority of authors in the United States, England, and on the Continent, agree that irradiation , the object of which is to administer a lethal dose to each neoplasm and to destroy every malignant cell, has proven of such value that it has displaced most of the other methods in the treatment of cancer of the skin. The selection of x-rays in preference to radium is made apparently only by those who have no facilities for radium therapy or whose evaluation of the more exacting dose determination by the mathematical method based upon the unit of intensity and expressed in r units, is limited. There is no doubt that a number of cases have been successfully treated by x-ray, but this achievement is by no means as constant as that of radium therapy.

Although the cosmetic effect is secondary, nevertheless it is worthy of consideration. The selection of the method of treatment which destroys the malignant cells and at the same time gives a satisfactory cosmetic result, should be the method of choice. Better permanent results, as well as excellent palliative effect with negligible risk of injury, gives radium this distinct advantage.

FUNDAMENTALS

It is not the purpose of this paper to discuss the varieties, etiology, or pathology of malignant disease of the skin, except to mention the most common histological types as: 1. Basal Cell Carcinoma or Rodent Ulcer, 2. Squamous Cell Carcinoma or Epithelioma, 3. Malignant Melanoma, and to ascertain that the squamous cell type is the more resistant and the melanoma the most malignant of these neoplasma.

The mathematical method of determining dosage has as its basis a unit of intensity rather than a unit of dose. The unit of intensity is defined as the unit of radiation at a distance of 1.0 cm. from 1.0 mg. point source of radium element filtered by 0.5 mm. of platinum. By this means Sievert, Paterson, Parker and others derived the dosage from various arrangements of radium applicators. Of the many types of applicators the most commonly used are needles or tubes arranged in plaques, triangles, squares and rectangles with radium in varying amounts; 5 or 10 mg. in needles and 10 to 50 mgs. in tubes. (See Fig. 1.) One milligram point source of radium filtered by 0.5 mm. of platinum, at a distance of 1.0 cm. gives 8.3 r per hour, (r/hr).

Biologically it requires 120 hours at 8.3 r/hr. to produce a threshold erythema dose or 1000 r. A threshold erythema dose is defined as a biological reaction indirectly measuring the amount of radiation received. This is to a certain extent variable depending on:

1. The size and shape of the radium source.

2. The distance of radium from the skin.

3. The filter.

4. Rate of administration.

5. Size of the area irradiated.

6. Anatomical site of the field.

7. Pathological condition of the tissue.

The application of radiation to a lesion is mainly governed by the fundamental law that the intensity of radiation is inversely proportional to the square of the distance between the source of radiation and the area irradiated. This, however, is only true of point scource. Radium, as used in needles or tubes, is a distributed series of sources for which the distribution factor in percentage must first be calculated. The greatest intensity can be assumed therefore to be below the center of the line source of radium. (See Fig. 2.) The same holds true for variously shaped applicators such as triangles, squares, rectangles, octagons, etc. When radium is filtered by 1.0 mm. of platinum, the intensity is diminished by approximately 10 per cent.

damage to healthy surrounding tissue. Various methods are employed in the treatment of skin cancer, namely:

1. Interstitial or Needling, 2. Surface Radiation, 3. Combination of both.

INTERSTITIAL METHOD

The object of the treatment is to deliver 5000 to 6000 r to the tumor and tumor bed. Needles of comparative small quantities of radium are used over a prolonged radiation time. These are spaced at from 1.0 cm. to not more than 1.5 cm. distance to produce the best results. It has been our custom in most cases to use 2 mg. needles of varying lengths of 15.0 mm.-23.0 mm.-35.0 mm. The quantity required depends upon the surface extent of the lesion. A margin of healthy tissue around the lesion must be included in

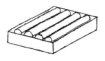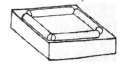

Figure 1.

Homogeneity of radiation should be the aim of filtration. To obtain 100 per cent gamma rays, at least 0.5 mm. of platinum is necessary according to Quimby as given in the table of "Relative Amounts of Radiation Transmitted by Various Metal Filters." In our experience and that of F. H. McKee of New York, most cases of telangiectasis and scarring were caused in insufficient filtration and therefore the effect of emitted beta rays.

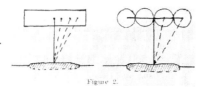

Figure 2.

METHOD AND TECHNIQUE

The distribution of radiation in tissue depends on the method employed, the aim being to obtain equal distribution. For satisfactory clinical results it is necessary to administer a sufficient dose to produce disintegration of the tumor with the least possible

the area treated. In small lesions the periphery only is needled. In more extensive lesions central needles are used to insure even intensity of radiation, contrary to the former belief that the implantation of needles within the tumor tends to produce metastasis. This, too, is in accord with the opinion of Ewing, McKee, Francis Carter, Wood, Quick and others. The usual surgical asepsis with or without anesthesia is taken.

In small cystic lesions we use 1 to 3 small 5 mg. needles spaced at 0.5 distance and implanted at the base for two to one and one-half hours respectively. One week later we apply 2000 r by the surface method and repeat the application in one week for a total of 6000 r. We find that if less is given the possibility of recurrence remains. In some instances, 7000 r units are necessary. A rather marked erythema, sometimes with slight necrosis, may occur. Unless a satisfactory reaction takes place, the result will not be as beneficial. Resultant healing usually takes place in three to four weeks after the application. When an occasional latent healing takes place, no alarm need be manifested.

SURFACE METHOD.

Radium is placed not in contact with the

lesion but at varying distances from it interposed by a secondary filter of wood, cork, rubber, etc., to get the necessary radium skin distance. The radium skin distances in turn depends upon the depth of the lesion treated and the depth dose desired. We find that when we calculate the radium skin distances so that the half value layer, (H.V.L.), is approximately at the level of the base of the lesion, our results are much more satisfactory. The H.V.L. is defined as the depth in centimeters in any material at which the incident beam is reduced to 50 per cent of its surface value.

In surface radiation our most favorable results are obtained when we apply 2000 r units to the lesion at weekly intervals and within two weeks for a total of 6000 r. Occassionally 7000 r units are required to produce a satisfactory reaction. Less than 6000 r has often produced insufficient reaction with the result that complete irradiation of the neoplasm does not occur. Invariably it was necessary in these cases to apply more radiation. In applying surface radiation, it is important to see that the radium not only covers the lesion but that it extends well over its margins and includes some surrounding healthy tissue. We have made it a rule to daily use some bland ointment such as lanolin, cold cream, or vaseline on the lesion to keep the scab soft and to make it easy to remove before applying radium. This permits of more radium absorption as the cornifield layers are known to be radio-resistant.

SUMMARY

1. Radium therapy is one satisfactory method of treating skin cancer.

2. Results obtained by this method are equally as satisfactory, if not better than with any other one method.

3. A more accurate calculation of intensity of radium irradiation in r units is possible with the mathematical method.

4. Cosmetic results are as a rule excellent.

5. A clear perception of the physical properties of radium, biological reaction, computation by the mathematical method and a clear conception of the fundamentals of radium is a basic necessity for lasting results.

BIBLIOGRAPHY

1. Cade, Stanford: Malignant Disease and Its Treatment by Radium. John Write & Sons, Ltd., Bristol. 1940.

2. MacKee, George M.: X-Rays and Radium in the Treatment of Disease of the Skin. Lea & Febiger, Philadelphia. Third Edition. 1938.

3. Quimby, Edith H.: Syllabus of Lectures—The Physical Basis of Radiation Therapy. Edwards Brothers, Ann Harbor, Mich. 1939.

4. Poppe, Erick: Carcinoma Cutis. Amer. Jour. Cancer, Vol. 36, page 179. 1939.

5. Quick, Douglas: President of Radium Therapy. Amer. Jour. Roentg. Vol. 47, pages 607-612. April, 1943.

The Role of Medical Short Wave Therapy in Otolaryngology*

E. H. COACHMAN, M.D.

MUSKOGEE, OKLAHOMA

The light spectrum, of which short wave is but a small segment, is as old as time, yet not until within our life span has it's properties been understood sufficiently well to make it useful in the treatment of diseases.

The spectrum is made up of both invisible and visible rays which measure from a fraction of a millimeter to over 100 meters in length. For convenience the spectrum has been divided into eight segments.[1] The first two we know very little or nothing about, except they are very short waves.

The third segment is represented by the radium rays, with which Pierre and Marie Curie are identified; the fourth, the x-ray

*Read before the Annual Meeting held in Oklahoma City, May 11-12, 1943.

which Roentgen discovered; the fifth, the ultra violet segment which Finsen used in treating Lupus, and later found by others to help control the calcium-phosphate ratio in the cure of rickets; the sixth, by the visible light rays; the seventh, by radiant heat, as secured from the fire or furnace, which has the infra-red rays; while last, but not least, comes the radio wave, which contains both the short and long wave used in diathermy.

It was D'Arsonval[2] who showed in 1891 that high frequency currents when passed through the body, produced an increased metabolism with increased oxygen absorption, and CO_2 exhaled along with increased secretion of urea and heat loss. This he attributed to the effect of the current upon the vasometer nervous system, causing the blood vessels to become dilated, with at first, a fall in pressure, followed by a subsequent rise. He further proved that the single cell itself was affected when he passed the current through unicellular yeast and bacteria, as well as vegetable cells, producing their destruction as well as atttenuation of toxins.

Contrary to D'Arsonval's views there are those who feel high frequency current effects are best explained solely by thermal elevation of the tissues, and to support this, many users have taken thermometer readings in the nose, antra, and general body temperatures, which have varied from actual lowering of temperature, both locally and generally, to elevations ranging several degrees. On the average, though, both the local and general temperatures have risen one-half to one and one-half degrees, which in the routine infection is sufficient to explain the relief secured. There are some whose dramatic results cannot be so easily accounted for, clinically, and to this smaller group we feel D'Arsonval's unicellular findings are applicable.

It was not until 1926 when Schilephake[3] reported his results with regional short wave therapy that the method gained widespread acceptance. Then the commercial demand for better radio tubes gained enough momentum to manufacture stronger short wave diathermy machines, which gave improved results. In contrast to regional therapy, as a joint, arm or leg, the method in America up to this time had been chiefly confined to whole body treatment for purposes of fever therapy.

The majority of us now in practice finished our medical training before short wave therapy became a part of the curriculum, and have been loath to accept it's claims, but today, it, like the sulfonamides, has become a definite part of our medical therapy, and furnishes us with a potent means of rendering an easier, more comfortable, and speedier recovery to the patient.

Short wave diathermy[4] is designated as waves having a length 10 to 30 meters, and depending upon the strength of the present machines, deliver a frequency from 10 to 100 million cycles per second on a wattage of 100 to 450, from an indirect current of 110 to 120 volt of 50 to 60 cycles, although these are units made for direct current. Most short wave machines now carry a wave length around 10 to 12 meters, to lessen radio broadcasting interference, and for practical purposes this is sufficient for our medical needs, since no special property is attached to the different lengths of the short waves.

You will note that the frequency is spoken of in millions rather than hundreds or thousands, which along with the penetrating power of the short wave, is the key to this form of therapy. With frequencies of a few thousand, painful muscle contractions are produced, in fact up to a million cycles these stimuli may be painful. By the time they reach 10 to 100 million cycles the rate of stimulus has far outreached the muscle's capacity, which renders the tissues inert, and makes the application painless. This you can see is comparable to success in large doses where smaller ones are ineffectual.

The office routine with short wave therapy is to precede (or follow) it with whatever medical procedures are suitable to the case, as ephedrine nasal tampons in acute sinusitis, or sprays, vaccines and systemic medications of your choice. Have the patient recline on a wooden top couch or table, on which rests a thin mattress or rubber padding. Metal top tables produce burns as well as lessen the current passing through the head and neck. For the same reason all metals, such as hairpins, ear and neck jewelry are removed, and the patient given a pillow for confortable reclining.

The short wave pads, which measure 10 x 13 inches, are covered with four or six folds of a rough dried bath towel, so that they are held some one and one-half to two inches from the skin of the patient's face. The electric cords, connecting the pads to the machine, are then seperated widely by fastening them with wooden clothes pins to the mattress, which prevents current loss between cords.

The machine now is turned on it's lowest reading to allow the tubes to warm, for 20 to 30 seconds, before the power is turned into them. This gradual warming up process greatly increases the life span of the tubes. Once the current is increased the milliameter on the machine is watched until it registers it's highest point, following which the meter hand will drop back if more current is applied. This dropping back means over-loading of the machine for this particular application. The meter hand should be kept just short of it's highest reading or point of resonance, as it is usually called.

The patients are then asked to keep still for 10 minutes, which they usually do by falling asleep in a few minutes, following the production of warmth throughout the head and neck area, which will start almost immediately the point of resonance is reached.

A time clock shuts off the current and then the pads and towels are applied to front and back of the central chest and back for purposes of including the chain of lymph glands which are always affected in these cases. This takes another five minutes, following which the tight sensation in the head, neck and chest are relieved, the nose aeriated, and the turbinates shrunken, which means increased comfort to any acute upper respiratory infection.

The following day the patient usually shows considerably less redness and engorgement of the turbinates, epipharynx, and throat, has slept much better, and has improved appetite. The course is made much easier, more comfortable, shorter, and evidently safer.

Over a period of eight years, this routine has been followed in both acute and sub-acute sinusitis, tubo-tympanitis, otitis media, mastoiditis, spipharyngitis, tonsillitis, adenoiditis, pharyngitis, laryngitis, tracheitis, bronchitis, and so called colds with satisfying response in the great majority of cases. During this time I have increased my confidence and reliance upon the acceleration and comfort derived from short wave therapy. Incidentally, I've personally experienced it's relief and have no qualms about recommending it.

Children who are frightened and cry, should be watched as their tears may wet the towel and cause a sting from the current. If this happens, the treatment should be discontinued. If the patient reaches over and touches a radiator or metal pipe, a burn may follow, but by far, the greatest number have no trouble. Where the pads are kept well separated from the face, by the towels, nothing need be feared, the only sensation is a pleasant warmth.

To be sure there are cases in which short wave diathermy does not relieve pain, in fact it increases pain! This led to using it as a diagnostic means as well as a therapeutic one, for like many things it can be put to more than one use. In the frequency encountered, these conditions have been classified as follows:

1. Allergy in season, such as ragweed hay fever from mid-August to frost, nasal congestion, mucoid discharge and discomfort is increased, but the same case can be treated successfully in mid-Winter, when a cold or sinusitis is present, the same as any other case. Oftentimes a patient with a greyish mucous membrane suggesting an inactive allergy, with nose dry, can be given ephedrine nasal tampons and diathermy for a few minutes, when they will then show the mucilaginous watery nasal discharge which gives increased eosinophile count on smear examination.

2. Empyema of a sinus; especially in frontal or macillary sinuses, the patient will have increased pain with short wave therapy, but puncture, transillumination, or x-ray will invariably show the affected sinus. This simply means the heat of the diathermy caused the pus and material within the closed sinus to expand, creating pressure, which could only be relieved by opening.

3. Diphtheria carriers; your guess here is as good as mine but increased toxin absorption from the increased circulation should be considered.

4. Ozena; perhaps the same is true as with diphtheria carriers.

5. C. N. S. Lues; again I do not know why the pain is increased.

6. Endocrine dyscrasia; this seems especially true of women with ovarian trouble and has led to relief by injection of mixed ovarian hormones in a few cases. Some hypothyroids of both sexes will react poorly to diathermy.

7. Histamine headaches; nothing but desensitization to histamine seems to help these.

Generally in chronic conditions short wave therapy is of no aid, and in reviewing the conditions above in which pain is increased, it is seen that all except acute empyema of a sinus, is usually classed as a chronic condition. Relief may be expected mostly in acute and sub-acute cases and it is here it's need is greatest.

DISCUSSION
L. C. KUYRKENDALL, M.D.
MCALESTER, OKLAHOMA

I appreciate very much having heard this valuable paper. It is clear that the doctor knows much of the theory as well as the practical application of short wave therapy in otolaryngological conditions.

It is true a high frequency current of interruption sufficiently high does not produce contractions in contractile tissue when passed through this tissue.

As I understood the treatment by short wave, the object is to get heat to an affected part, and since the cells are well supplied with lymph, it is necessary to pass the current through this in order to reach the cells which are involved in the pathological process. These short waves passing through this fluid produces heat because of the resistance of the fluid, in turn producing a sense of well being and comfort, ability to breathe through the nose very much better and the pain either entirely relieved or at least materially reduced. It does not cure the condition but renders the tissues more amenable to local and constitutional treatment.

The analgesic and sedative effect on sensory nerves results in nervous sedation, probably due to the soothing effect of the heat on the irritated and sensitive nerve endings.

There is a note of caution sounded by Dr. Coachman which is important, viz., that those using short wave therapy exercise

every precaution against burns. These, I am sure, can be avoided if proper insulation and contacts are made before the current is turned on. The treatment should never be left to an assistant.

While short wave therapy is and has been of material help to the otolaryngologist, it is by no means a cure-all and should not be so regarded , but when judiciously used, it is of benefit in the relief of many of the acute conditions which we see and treat.

BIBLIOGRAPHY

1. Krusen: Light Therapy. Paul Hacker & Co., Inc., New York.

2. Bierman, William: Medical Application of the Short Wave Current. Williams and Williams. Baltimore.

3. Morgan, J. D.: Electrothermic Methods in Neoplastic Disease. F. A. Davis Company. Philadelphia.

4. Kovac, R.: Electrotherapy and Light Therapy. Lea & Febiger. Philadelphia.

Comparative Symptoms in Peptic Ulcer and Cholecystitis in 200 Cases*

ANDRE B. CARNEY, M.D.

TULSA, OKLAHOMA

It is my privilege, and I consider it an honor, to bring to your attention a resume of the comparative findings, both symptomatically and clinically, in disease of the gall-bladder and gastric ulcer as noted from a review of 200 consecutive cases from the records of one of our local hospitals. It shall not be my purpose in this discussion to distinguish between gastric or duodenal lesions per se, nor to bring out the different characteristic findings associated with cholecystic disease alone, but to endeavor to refresh your memory with a few of the salient facts with which you, as clinicians, are familiar insofar as the two above mentioned diseases are concerned. To attempt to discuss, in such a short time, two diseases upon which volumes have been written, reminds me of a recent radio program in which it was mentioned that in the case of the American joke, much is left to the imagination of the audience.

I need not delve into the history of these two diseases but suffice it to say that during the last fifty years, volumes have accumulated on each. As you already know, most

of this experimental as well as practical work with which we are familiar has originated in the large medical and surgical centers of the country, especially the teaching centers where clinical material is easily available and where there has been sufficient assistance among the undergraduate and interne staffs to put into print the findings of the different well - known investigators. Through a systematic study of these writings we are early taught to associate certain findings with certain diseases. If this would only hold true in practical experience the practice of medicine and surgery would be greatly simplified. However, such is not the case. We find, as we advance practically, that many of the clinical findings and symptoms as represented by the patient do not run true to our former teachings, and that many of these findings are overlapping and confusing, thereby complicating our deductions, even to say the least. I believe that the most common group of overlapping findings are those which I shall attempt to enumerate at this time. These findings were taken from a series of consecutive records from the files, and since they are not the expression of any one clinician, I am inclined to think

*Read before the Annual Meeting held in Oklahoma City, May 11-12, 1943.

that they give us a fair cross section of what the average physician must encounter in arriving at a working diagnosis in either or both of these diseases.

In diseases of the gallbladder, exclusive of acute biliary colic, we encounter as the first major finding—gastric distress. In breaking this symptom down we find the patient has been complaining of a vague pain in the upper abdomen, not localized nor acute. There is a feeling of fullness coming on almost immediately after eating which is invariably associated with belching of gas. Neither nausea nor vomiting are common factors, though they do occur occasionally. There is a particular aversion to such foods as cabbage, onions or excessively rich or greasy foods. This distress seems to be, in the majority of cases, centered in a wide area in the mid-epigastrium. The second most common disturbance noted is a late feeling of fullness in the upper right abdomen about two inches to the right of the mid-line. This disturbance ordinarily makes itself most noticeable about three hours after eating and is aggravated by excessive walking or long automobile rides. Associated with this is in most cases a rather deep tenderness immediately over the gallbladder area and one which the patient readily describes, in fact even goes so far as to assist in the examination and show how the tenderness is elicited. It has variously been described by some patients as feeling like a ruober ball, over distended and swinging loose in the upper abdomen. The third most common symptom is pain in the right back at a point just above the normal kidney area. Less than five per cent of one hundred gallbladder cases complained of pain in the right shoulder and only one complained of pain in the left shoulder. Seventy per cent complained of constipation ranging from mild to obstinate. Having noted these major disturbances in diseases of the gallbladder, I shall now enumerate the most common findings as noted in this review in proven cases of gastric ulcer.

We find, first, that these patients also present themselves complaining of gastric distress. While the distress varies in many respects it also presents the problem of minutely differentiating the actual feelings of the patient. This distress, as in gallbladder disease is, as a rule, noted almost immediately after eating. Like gallbladder disease it is also associated with much gaseous eructation. Unlike gallbladder disease, however, it is associated with more of a feeling of real pain. As time goes on we come to the second phase of this distress, as previously mentioned under cholecystic disease, that is, the latent after-eating feeling that all is not well. When the stomach begins to empty there is a feeling of deep uncertainty, which is also aggravated by much riding or walking. This uncertain feeling is in most cases, as the records show, also slightly to the right of the mid-line in the epigastric area. The third most common comparative symptom is that of pain radiating to the back. This symptom was common in approximately 50 per cent of these cases and the radiation occurs, insofar as we can tell clinically, in the same area, that is, near the upper pole of the right kidney.

Now if we take these major symptoms, most common to both diseases, it is readily understood why not only the diagnostician but even the roentgenologist becomes confused in the absence of positive findings. It is a well-known fact that many lesions such as small gastric ulcers or, for that matter, fairly large gastric lesions, on the posterior wall escape detection under x-ray study. Frequently these lesions may be brought out by a lateral x-ray study which we think is advisable in all cases of suggested gastric lesion unless otherwise demonstrable. Neither is the interpretation of the cholecystogram done with carefree abandon. It is not common for an exploratory operation to reveal the presence of many cholesterin stones even in the face of an apparently normal functioning gallbladder.

While I have dealt briefly with the major findings noted in both gastric ulcer and cholecystic disease, I do not want to leave the impression that we should conclude the examination at this point. After eliciting these major findings we should then conclude the examination through the process of elimination, such as noting the exact location of pain or distress, the exact time as to occurrence, the exact time as to disappearance of pain, the general condition of the patient, whether anaemic, obese, emaciated, the facial expression, etc . These, with our x-ray findings, gastric analysis and other laboratory work, should in a great measure help us to differentiate the conditions. Time, as you know, will not allow a full discussion of either disease. I have purposely omitted the similarity of symptoms occurring in some cases of acute gallbladder colic to those occurring in some cases of perforating gastric ulcer though I am sure that most of you, especially those doing surgery, have experienced this embarrassment.

In conclusion, I shall attempt to briefly outline the salient points as brought forth in this review of the above cases. These cases represent the findings of 52 physicians. No reference is made to medical treatment, surgical procedure or post-hospital care. It is interesting, however, to note the similarity of certain findings in these cases.

CHOLECYSTIC DISEASE	GASTRIC ULCER
1. Epigastric distress after eating.	1. Epigastric distress after eating.
2. Eructation of gas.	2. Eructation of gas.
3. Delayed sense of insecurity in upper right abdomen.	3. Delayed vague pain in upper abdomen — almo·· in mid-line.
4. Occasional pain in back.	4. Rather constant pain in back.
5. Occasional pain in right shoulder.	5. No referred pain to shoulder region.
6. Nausea, occasionally.	6. Nausea, fairly constantly.
7. Vomiting, rarely.	7. Vomiting, rather frequently.
8. Aversion to certain foods:	8. Aversion to certain foods:
a. Greasy or fatty foods.	a. Greasy or fatty foods.
b. Cabbage, onions, radishes, etc.	b. Cabbage, onions, radishes, etc.
9. Intestinal	9. Intestinal
a. Constipation as a rule.	a. Constipation not the rule.
10. General condition of patient:	10. General condition of patient:
a. Well nourished	a. Usually not well nourished
b. Appears healthy.	b. Usually appears chronically ill.
11. Laboratory.	11. Laboratory.
a. Gastric analysis normal to moderate hyperchlorhydria	a. Gastric analysis usually hyperchlorhydria
b. No blood.	b. Blood may or may not be found.
c. Blood findings variable.	c. Occasional anaemia otherwise not of value.
d. Stool—negative findings.	d. Stool—may indicate presence of blood.
12. X-ray.	12. X-ray.
a. Function of gallbladder	a. Gastric defect.
b. Presence or absence of stones.	b. Pyloric obstruction.

DISCUSSION

A. S. RISSER, M.D.

BLACKWELL, OKLAHOMA

Dr. Carney deserves great commendation for the preparation of this paper. Improvement would be greatly enhanced if all medical men would record, group and analyze their cases as Dr. Carney has done in this excellent study.

Time was not sufficient for him to separate the peptic ulcer cases into gastric and duodenal with their frequent variation in symptoms nor to divide the various forms of cholecystic disease according to their pathology and symptomatology.

He has, however, succeeded in emphasizing a fact which surgeons generally appreciate, more or less, that diseases of the gallbladder and diseases of stomach and duodenum, do give what he calls overlapping symptoms. So in many cases only intensive study, aided by x-ray and laboratory, and continued observation will yield a cor-

rect differential diagnosis. Also, while Dr. Carney does not so specify in his paper, he does not separate the milder, more chronic cases from those of the acute abdominal catastrophes such as perforation of peptic ulcer or gall bladder, or some of the complications of cholecystic disease such as cholelithiosis with colic and biliary obstruction, hepatitis, cholangitis or pancreatitis. Suffice it to state here that these do occur, and that they alter the symptomatology accordingly.

Another fact which Dr. Carney implied but did not state definitely is that the symptoms of these diseases, once they are recorded in the consciousness of the patient, are already the results, the culmination of a chronic process. There is a progressive pathology, and the symptoms are the signs of advanced disease. Only by the use of this knowledge will we appreciate the fact that the dyspepsia, gas, belching and indigestion, to use the patients' words, the discomfort after certain foods which may not yet be interpreted by the patient as actual pain—these to the observant physician are sure signs of trouble.

The so-called "instinctive" avoidance of certain foods is not instinctive but is the result of experience, and comes from repeated disturbances of the digestive economy by these foods, manifested by physical discomfort, even before the discomfort becomes actual pain. That stage depends much on the psyche and the mental habitus of the patient. Hence, when pain does occur, in epigastrium, back shoulder—and often we are not consulted by the patient before this stage —we should be on our way to finding the exact cause of these symptoms with a view to halting a destructive process.

Specifically, it seems to me that a larger proportion of the gall bladder cases in my experience complain of pain in the region of the point of the scapula than the right shoulder, and a smaller percentage of peptic ulcer cases have had pain in the back than Dr. Carney's record shows, but I must plead guilty in not having kept exact statistics. In peptic ulcer cases a fair proportion give a rather typical ulcer history, a pain, food, ease, pain sequence, frequently also a seasonal variation of symptoms; the patients average younger than in cholecystitis, and hyperchlorhydria is common. The stools frequently show occult blood, and in gall bladder disease the urine frequently contains bile.

In closing, may I emphasize again some of the points stated or implied in Dr. Carney's paper. A careful history is as important as is a careful physical examination. In my opinion even the roentgenologist will be aided by having a history of the case being studied.

The dictum, "fair, fat and forty" is not now sufficient for a diagnosis of cholecystitis. All the facts pertinent to the case, such as history, physicial, laboratory and x-ray findings, even the mental reactions of the pa-

tients, are to be determined, analyzed, evaluated, correlated, to the end that we may determine the nature of the disease in question and the more promptly institute efficient treatment.

Sanitation in War Time*

MR. H. J. DARCEY
Chief Engineer of Oklahoma State Health Department
OKLAHOMA CITY, OKLAHOMA

Sanitation in war time might be a misleading subject, as it infers that sanitation is a field of work evolved from war time conditions. To the contrary, a sanitation program in war time embraces all the phases of work which are included in a well rounded peace time public health program. It is true, emphasis has been focused on sanitation work in areas where there has been a concentration of population, due to the de opment of Army camps or war industries. Many cities and towns, and even rural areas, have suddenly awakened to find an influx of people greatly overtaxing all the facilities available in the community. Water supplies have had to be built, or expanded, sewer systems and treatment plants constructed, milk supplies increased, eating and drinking establishments provided, and malaria control and rodent control programs initiated.

The Federal Government, realizing the burden placed upon the local governing units to provide the needed facilities, enacted legislation known as the Lanham Act, and appropriated funds to make grants, in whole or in part, to cover the cost of constructing water and sewer improvements, and many other types of projects. The provisions of this Act were carried out under the Federal Works Agency, in cooperation with the other Federal and State agencies directly interested in the program.

WATER SUPPLY

Water supplies are taken as a matter of fact and no thought is ever given to the production and treatment of water by the average individual until the water service fails. Then, a cry usually arises to know the cause of the trouble. In war times, it is more important than ever to see that the supply does not fail and the quality is not impaired.

With the beginning of war, all water

works officials in the State were instructed to exclude visitors from the plants, to erect barriers around all vulnerable parts of the system, to increase chlorine treatment, determine loyalty of all workers, and provide for emergencies by locating auxiliary supplies, equipment, and personnel to be used when needed. In addition, the State has been divided into five Districts, each served by an Engineer of the State Health Department who is subject to call in an emergency. The advantage of this system is that the District Engineer will have information available on the location of equipment, chemicals, and personnel available within the District which can be used, and will arrange to have it made available without delay.

Emphasis must be given to the necessity for keeping trained water works personnel in their present positions, and for regular and frequent examinations of water supply, both bacteriologically and chemically. Suggestion has also been made to increase the chemical treatment, as a factor of safety and to overcome chance contamination of the water after it leaves the treatment plant. This is a good practice for peace time as well, for there are many unknown cross-connections in existence which might permit contaminated water to enter the water system.

Provision must also be made to provide water during the time a water system might be out of service. This can be done through the use of approved private water supplies or from central water points to which treated water will be transported. In all cases, the emergency supply must be under the constant supervision of a trained worker, either a regular employee of the water company or a trained auxiliary worker. The first action to be taken in any emergency is to warn the public not to use any water from an unapproved supply, then to make known the location of all approved supplies in the community.

*Read before the Annual Meeting held in Oklahoma City, May 11-12, 1943.

MILK CONTROL

Providing an adequate, safe milk supply, particularly for use at the military camps and in communities which have had a large increase in population, creates one of the most serious and confusing problems for the public health worker, the confusion resulting from the number of agencies concerned with the production and use of milk.

The milk supply for any community is built up over the years, and for economic reasons is based on a planned program to provide only sufficient milk for the needs of the community. A sharply increased demand cannot be provided overnight, for dairy farms must be expanded or constructed, plant capacities increased, and additional cows brought into the milk shed, or milk must be shipped from another approved source. Lacking the supply, which in many cases was further curtailed by the sale of milk cows for slaughter because of the high price of beef, shortage of farm labor, and the ready sale of milk and cream for the manufacture of butter and cheese at a price nearly equivalent to the fluid milk market price, devious plans were suggested to supplement the dwindling supply. The programs followed to accomplish this goal varied from one community to another. Some have prohibited the sale of anything but Grade A milk, even though such a requirement resulted in the rationing of milk; others have permitted the sale of different grades of milk under the proper grade label, thus allowing all available milk to be used. In still other places, temporary permits were used. Under this plan, the milk from a farm dairy would be accepted for pasteurization and sale as Grade A pasteurized milk, if it was produced under the emergency standards specified by the United States Public Health Service.

The important points to consider in this entire program are the need for correctly labeling the milk according to grade, so the consumer will know the quality of milk being purchased, and to stimulate interest and action in developing an additional supply of graded milk. Milk is one of our valuable food items, and the production of milk should be increased, to provide a substitute for some of our rationed foods. Extreme caution must be excercised to avoid the use on any unsafe milk, and greater care should be exercised in supervising the production and processing of it. If there is any question or uncertainty about the quality of the milk you are using, remember, it can be pasteurized and made safe at home.

FOOD SANITATION

Food sanitation in war time should and is receiving the serious and constant attention of the persons charged with the responsibility of supervising the operation of the food handling establishments, for they realize the dangers and consequences of a food-borne epidemic. Many of you have, no doubt, noticed within recent months, newspaper accounts of outbreaks of food poisoning. Such reports will occur rather frequently, if there is any attempt to minimize or relax the enforcement program.

Numerous factors enter the picture to complicate the food handling problem. First, it has been difficult for the restaurant owner to retain competent trained help, owing to the opportunity of making higher wages in other types of work. The continual turnover of workers has brought untrained help into the restaurants, help without any knowledge of sanitation. Second, the rationing of food has encouraged many people to eat away from home, placing an additional burden on an already over-loaded, and in many cases, under-staffed restaurant business. And third, in an attempt to conserve food, there is the temptation to use food which in ordinary times would be destroyed. All together, they make serious trouble for the restaurant owner. Yet, the consumer must be protected, and rapid strides toward that goal have been made through the adoption of the Standard Eating Establishment Ordinance sponsored by the State Health Department. This ordinance provides for the grading of the restaurants, based on compliance with certain items of sanitation.

SEWERS AND SEWAGE DISPOSAL

Since the beginning of the war, rapidly changing conditions have had their effect on the construction of sewers and sewage treatment plants. In the earlier stages, it was possible to build sewers and sewage treatment plants to serve the increased population in what are known as "War Areas". As the material situation became critical, a limitation was placed on the construction of sewage treatment plants, to those cases where the sewage had a direct effect on a city water supply. This resulted in very few plants being constructed for the municipalities.

The shortage of plumbing fixtures and supplies has made it necessary to limit their use to housing projects sponsored or financed by the Government. This means that existing properties must continue to use the same facilities available prior to the war. With crowded housing conditions, it is important to properly maintain the individual excreta disposal units, to avoid the spead of filth-borne diseases.

Mention should also be made of the need for adequate garbage collection and disposal systems. Uncontrolled handling of garbage has already created a demand for rat control programs in several communities. Failure to heed this warning may easily be the cause of much loss of life, as well as a tremendous economic loss.

MALARIA CONTROL

For years malaria has been a problem in certain parts of the state, a problem which because of the low mortality rate did not receive very much attention from the people. The military authorities recognize the disabling effects of malaria. For that reason, malaria control programs have been established in the vicinity of all army camps or places where military personnel are stationed, whenever field surveys disclose the presence of the Anopheline mosquito. Two such programs are in operation at this time in eastern Oklahoma. In addition, other areas are under regular inspection to obtain information on the need for control program.

SUMMARY

Little of the information I have given is new to the public health worker, but taken as a whole, it is what can and must be done to protect the health of our people, conserve our vital manpower, and ease the strain on the members of the medical profession who are doing an excellent job, under trying circumstances.

What have you done to improve sanitary conditions in the community in which you live?

Modern Aids in the Treatment of Appendicitis

FORREST M. LINGENFELTER, M.D.
OKLAHOMA CITY, OKLAHOMA

JOHN W. CAVANAUGH, M.D.
TOPEKA, KANSAS

LT. HARVEY RICHEY, M.D.
MEDICAL CORPS, ARMY OF THE UNITED STATES

We had, as a basis of study, 1800 cases of appendicitis cared for by the Surgical Staff of the University Hospital during the last 8 years. An attempt has been made to review these accumulated statistics and find out what effect the institution of certain modern aids in treatment has upon the course of appendicitis.

During the first year, 1934 or 1935, the gross mortality, as will be shown by the slides, was 7 per cent. We contrast this with a mortality rate of 1.7 per cent during the year 1942. This is a striking contrast and we are confident that the improved results are due to many different factors. However, if we are called upon to chose the one most important, we would turn to chemotherapy, with suction drainage falling to second place.

Remarkable, as has been the apparent surgical improvements in the treatment of appendicitis, in fairness, one must consider the type of case seen over this period of years. We have heard it discussed many times and we believe it to be true that during 1934 and 1935, because of the financial condition of the people who attended the clinic, cases were brought in at a much later date and on the whole, were in worse shape than those in recent years.

The real value of this study, is in consideration of the factors which we ourselves may influence. Among these are the more accurate diagnosis, more exact preoperative preparation, the exercise of sound surgical judgment as to the time of operation, and careful postoperative care.

Accuracy in diagnosis does not convey the true meaning of the attitude toward appendicitis which I believe should be maintained. The diagnosis of these doubtful abdomens is probably one of the most difficult tasks which we are called upon to perform. One should operate these cases when there remains a doubt in his mind as to the possibility of the existence of an acute appendix. Certain facts in diagnosis stand out in one's experience over the years. Pain in the abdomen is the only symptom that occurs in 100 per cent of the cases of appendicitis. If the pain is persistent the patient should be operated. Localized tenderness is an excellent indication, however, one must not forget, that, with a gangrenous appendix the anesthesia produced by the gangrene may cause the patient to show little evidence of tenderness. In those suspected cases, one should reflect upon the severity of the gastro-intestinal symptoms, and if they are predominant, one should be strongly influenced toward operation. It is heartening to note, from these records, that in only two instances in the last two years was the diagnosis overlooked and the cause of death labeled appendicitis by the pathologist. In one of these cases there was evidence of considerable inflammatory reaction about the pancreas, and although pus was found around the appendix, a review of the chart leaves considerable doubt as to whether the death was not in connection with suppurative pancreatitis.

With reference to preoperative preparation, much consideration in past years has been given the fluid balance and the maintenance of electrolytes. These measures are well understood and nothing is to be gained by an extensive discussion of them.

Collier[1] has established certain requirements for water balance. The factors to be taken into account are 1. The insensible loss of water, 2. The water required by the kidney to excrete body waste, 3. Water lost in stool, 4. Water lost in sweating.

The insensible loss is covered by 1000 cc in inactive individuals. The water necessary to excrete the average of waste in the body (35 grams) amounts to about 500 cc with the normal kidney. The insufficient kidney requires more, for an adequate margin of safety, 1000 cc should be considered the minimum urinary secretion in the surgical patient. Due allowance must be made for fever, increased metabolism, etc. Thus the average surgical case requires 3000 to 3500 cc of water for the 24 hour period.

Yr.	Acute Cases	Deaths
'34-35	219	14
'35-36	179	13
'36-37	196	18
'37-38	217	12
'38-39	184	8
'39-40	196	5
'40-41	254	5
'41-42	156	3

With regard to electrolyte balance. it is startling to note that man has no sensation of chloride deficiency, no salt hunger to warn him. The ox develops salt hunger as the sodium chloride of the body is depleted and will make a supreme effort to get the needed salt.

It is recognized by Collier that neither the hematocrit nor the plasma chloride levels,

serve as an adequate measure of extracellular fluid volume, especially in pathological states, such as shock, in which electrolyte imbalance occurs. The relative chloride loss is influenced by the character of the fluid loss. For example, in vomiting, with alchlorhydia the relative chloride loss is minimal; with hyperchlorhydia, it is marked. It is fortunate that simple water deficiency and simple electrolyte deficiency, although seen as separate entities, are very commonly combined. A fairly satisfactory clinical approach to the correction of both of these conditions may be attained by the adequate use of saline. The average case not sweating and not incident to fever requires 3000 to 3500 cc of water daily. A fairly satisfactory rule is to give enough water to hold the urinary output around 1000 cc daily. It is the concenus of opinion that cases receiving sulfonamides should have a urinary output of at, or above, 1200 cc.

Mortality Rate University Hospital

Yr.	Abscess Cases	Deaths	Mort.
'34-35	36	5	13.4
'35-36	10	0	0
'36-37	13	0	0
'37-38	19	3	16.0
'38-39	13	2	15.0
'39-40	9	1	11.0
'40-41	9	1	11.0
'41-42	10	0	0

With regard to surgical procedure, it seems to me that the term, emergency appendicitis should be restricted. These are surely not emergencies because we feel that the patient is in actual danger of death. If the term is to be applied to them at all, it must be realized that the emergency is in preventing the patient from having peritonitis by the removal of an acute appendix, and not, in the institution of operative procedures to immediately save life. A few hours of rest, the administration of fluids, and in some instances even transfusions may enable these patients in borderline critical conditions, to stand operation well.

The greatest excercise of surgical judgment is not required in the early acute case of appendicitis. That the treatment of these is operative is conceded by everyone. Attempts have been made for the last 20 years to establish criteria for procedure in the late case and many of us have felt that we were satisfied to treat these cases conservatively, with interference only in minor groups, notably children and the aged. We are now wondering if chemotherapy may not materially affect the management of the late case? How important it is to immediately remove the source of contamination in the late case?

Such a procedure can undoubtedly be accomplished with more safety than in previous years. After careful consideration we believe, in the late case, it would be safer to limit the spread of infection by chemotherapy without surgical interference. Limitation of the spread of infection can better be affected by chemotherapy than by surgical means. We must remember that we can use chemotherapy without surgery. Two of our cases were operated, one at 140 and one at 190 hours.

We like to think of A. J. Ochsner's plan for the management of late appendicitis as a plan for the preparation of patients for operation and in this original work he so labeled it. Recently there has been a tendency because of chemotherapy, to throw out this monumental advance and proceed to operate every case of appendicitis, without regard to the existing pathological condition.

Mortality Rate University Hospital

Yr.	Chronic Cases	Deaths
'34-35	13	0
'35-36	13	0
'36-37	11	0
'37-38	16	1
'38-39	8	1
'39-40	6	0
'40-41	10	0
'41-42	3	0

Lungren, Garside, and Boyce[2] have recently, again, brought forth Ochsner's statistics and they show that, with a few facilities at his command he was able to reduce his mortality to a striking degree. Ochsner reported on 1000 cases, between July 1, 1901 and April 1, 1904, with a mortality rate of 2.2 per cent.

Guerry, in a series of 2,959 consecutive cases at about the same time, and by conservative treatment of his late cases, reported a mortality rate of 5.4 per cent. These results obtained almost 40 years ago by treating late cases conservatively seem almost incredible. We hope that we are not too much inclined to look backward, but if these records were based upon sound statistics, we have reason to pause and contemplate them, they would indicate that from the present review of our cases, with all the modern aids, we have gained little. With the things now at our command, we should be able to improve on these results.

Lehman[3] has written at length concerning the widening possibilities, through recent developments, in chemotherapy. He has expressed some views which might alter our conception of the inherent pathology when estimating the status of these patients. He considers the difference between contamination of the peritoneum and peritonitis. The peritoneum, contaminated, may escape the effects of infection, if proper measures are taken, and if the contamination is removed within a reasonable time. Contamination, with reference to rupture ulcer, is readily recognized. We have been slow to get the same conception, in appendicitis. The appearance of the peritoneum, in contamination, may represent defensive reactions which may comprise injection, dulling, febrin deposits, and free fluids. Mere inspection, or even a positive culture, will not definitely determine whether or not an infection will follow.

If we dilute our cases of peritonitis with those suffering from contamination only, our figures will be distorted and we will come to regard peritonitis with an unwarranted sense of security. To quote Lehman; "It is not the unmistakable fact of perforation, which should govern the classification, it is a consideration of the more serious complication, peritonitis."

Penberthy's paper[4], April 1942, reported; "Acute unruptured appendicitis, mortality .4 per cent.' '

"Acute ruptured appendicitis with local peritonitis, mortality 5.5 per cent."

The latter group Lehman believes is not peritonitis, but largely made up of cases of peritonial contamination only.

Lehman and Parker[5], in a series of cases of all ages, reported 40.6 per cent mortality in their group of true peritonitis.

Penberthy's mortality in children with true peritonitis was 64.9 per cent. True peritonitis is a very fatal disease, the control of which is unsatisfactory with or without chemotherapy.

Radvin, Rhodes, Lockwood[6] reported in 1940, on a series of 809 cases. In the first 552 cases, their mortality was 1.5 per cent and in the last 257 cases, their mortality was brought down to .4 per cent.

These excellent results have been largely due to the use of sulfanilamide. K. Toshiro,[7] et. al., discussing sulfanilamide, states that it is bacteriostatic in dilutions up to 1-10,000 and higher. No tissue damage was demonstrated in parenteral injections of 1 per cent.

The local use of sulfathiazole has not been advocated as freely as has the use of sulfanilamide. It has been stated, sufathiazole is more apt to cake, and thus produce foreign bodies.

Sutton[8] states that sodium sulfathiazole produces dense peritoneal adhesions in the dog. He further reported a case of acute perforation, with peritonitis, in which the intraperitoneal use of sulfathiazole was followed by adhesions, intestinal obstruction and required a secondary operation for acute obstruction.

Work by Fox and Jensen[9] would indicate that sulfanilamide is so solvent in the urine that little attention need be paid to alkali therapy in its use. However, with reference to sulfathiazole and sulfadiazine, alkali therapy can readliy produce a urinary ph of between 7.0 and 8.0, which greatly facilitates the solution of these drugs. With regard to sulfapyridine the solubility is not materially affected until the ph of the urine is raised beyond its normal physiological range, (90 to 100), hence the failure of alkali therapy in connection with sulfapyridine.

Mortality Rate University Hospital

Yr.	Cases	Deaths	Mort.
'34-35	268	19	7.0%
'35-36	202	13	6.4
'36-37	220	18	6.3.
'37-38	253	16	6.3
'38-39	205	10	4.8
'39-40	211	5	2.3
'40-41	273	6	2.1
'41-42	169	3	1.7

O. B. Pratt,[10] White Memorial Hospital laboratory, has worked out blood concentration curves with the local implantation of known quantities of sulfanilamide. He has shown that for 1 gram used intraperitoneally, approximately 1 mg. per 100 cc concentration, is achieved in the blood stream. This concentration was reached in about three hours. The concentration gradually declines, to end in a period of about 30 hours.

In connection with these cases it must be remembered that we started with the use of sulfanilamide, went through the period of sulfapyridine and in the last few cases sulfadiazine was employed.

In reviewing the charts, some variation in technique was observed. However, the general plan seemed to be that sulfanilamide

powder was used, about two-thirds being placed in the abdominal cavity and one-third in the wound. The average dose was 120 grains in the adult and in smaller individuals one and one-half grains per pound of body weight were used.

Cases in Age Groups
1940-'41-'42

Age	Cases
0-10	34
10-20	237
20-50	301
50-60	20
60 and over	1
Total	560

We noted a distinct tendency to follow with sulfapyridine after operation. This seemed to suggest a lack of confidence in sulfanilamide alone in the treatment of appendicitis. Most often the sulfapyridine was given by mouth. The intravenous use of sulfapyridine was soon discontinued because of severe reactions. In about 73 instances sulfapyridine was given intravenously usually 120 grs. in 500 cc of normal saline.

We had one death from chemotherapy. This occurred with the use of sulfapyridine. The patient developed an anuria in about 36 hours and died despite ureteral catherization. Examination of the chort showed that adequate intake was maintained. Recently one of the authors has been giving sodium sulfathiazole subcutaneously and sulfadiazine by mouth. The patients appear to get along as well with less toxic effects. I am informed that Dick, of St. Louis, gave a patient with endocarditis 15 grams of sulfadiazine. He stated that the blood concentration went to 2000 mg per 100 cc of blood and was maintained at 1800 by the concentration of fluids. He stated that the patient lived. I give this report to show that sulfadiazine is probably the least toxic of the group.

Chemotherapy takes advantage of the variable toxicity of a given drug for a specific infectious agent, and the cells of the host. The local application of sulfonamide crystals is contrary to the fundamental concept of chemotherapy in two respects. There is established locally a concentration of the drug known to be toxic systemically. Second, it is proposed to broaden the action of the drugs to include an effect upon relatively insensitive bacteria, by increasing the concentration of the chemical agent. Hence the proposal to use sulfonamides as a prophylactic agent against polymicrobial infections marks another departure from conventional thinking.

With the widespread establishment of blood banks throughout the country, it is logical that someone would turn to immune serum therapy in the treatment of peritonitis.

J. O. Brawer[11] et. al., has reported his results, both in clinical use, and experimentally in dogs. He stresses the point that patients with generalized peritonitis are at shock levels because of fluid and protein loss, due to the enormous amounts of fluids collecting in the abdominal cavity. We have all seen these abundant collections in the abdomen.

Hospitalization

All Cases Average 10.8
Ruptured Appendix with Peritonitis 20.3
Abscesses without drainage 21.3
Abscesses with drainage 26.5

He turns to lympholized serum for replacement and states that his results were better than any other type of therapy. He states that lympholized convalescent peritonitis serum was kept in ampules for periods of 15 months. His average dose of serum was approximately 250 cc every eight hours. He states that he has frequently seen patients with general peritonitis, restore peristalsis in 24 hours and rapidly go on to recovery. Perhaps with the establishment of more blood banks throughout the country, stores of convalescent peritonitis serum may be had, and another aid to these very sick patients may become available.

We wish to apologize for the fact that we have been unable to discuss all the measures made available in the management of appendicitis during the last 8 years. Gastric suction deserves more prominent mention. Incisions have been shown a gradual tendency toward McBurney and away from right rectus. Auchincloss[12] has recently violently condemned right rectus incisions and has shown that the McBurney type can be extended inward and downward by the retraction of the rectus medially for more adequate exposure.

The treatment of abcesses has shown little improvement. The mortality, as shown by slides, varies from 10 per cent to 19 per cent. Owing to the diminished blood supply to the walled off abscess, concentration of chemotherapy at the sight of the inflammatory process cannot be attained and theoretically at least nothing can be expected from chemotherapy. If the abscess is large or if fever is becoming more elevated, surgical drainage should be instituted.

In conclusion we wish to emphasize the fact that surgical judgment is still the best aid in the management of appendicitis.

Cause of Death
1940-'41-'42

Generalized peritonitis 5
Pulmonary embolism 2
Pulmonary atelectasis 1
Multiple liver abscesses 1
Septicomia 1
Late postoper-hemorrhage 1
Collulitis of abdominal wall 1
Auria (Sulfapyridine) 1
Anaesthesia (Spinal) 1

DISCUSSION
C. E. NORTHCUTT, M. D.
PONCA CITY, OKLAHOMA

I have enjoyed the presentation of this subject and note the reduction in mortality rates with interest. This is illustrative of many reports from other medical centers, showing remarkable reduction in the mortality rate, due largely to the more modern aids available at this time in the treatment of appendicitis.

All of the mentioned factors are important and it is difficult to state which has been the most important in the reduction of the present mortality rates. No doubt chemotherapy has played a most important part, as well as the continuous use of the suction. However, I feel that the medical profession as well as the laity has realized the importance of early diagosis and operative interference. We know that the mortality rate can be greatly reduced by early diagnosis and surgical removal of the appendix. The layman has become so familiar with the symptoms of appendicitis that he presents himself much earlier for surgery.

I feel that we too frequently consider all appendectomies as emergencies and do not give full consideration to the pre-operative preparation to make the patient a more safe surgical risk by analyzing the clinical symptoms to determine what type of appendix we are dealing with, and the restoration of the normal fluid and chloride balance, proper sedation, large doses of sulfa drugs pre-operatively and choosing the proper sulfa drug to be placed in the abdominal cavity in the routine appendectomy, as well as the proper dose considering the nature and extent of infection.

I have not limited myself to the use of any one drug for all cases, as my experience has proven the strep strain responds more favorably to sulfanilamide. The pus forming organisms such as colon bacilli and staphylococci respond more favorably to sulfathiazole or sulfadiazine. By applying from 5 to 10 grams over a larger area in the peritoneal cavity, there is a tendency to avoid clumping and interference with the normal tissues. Post-operatively, the selected drug is given per orum as soon as the patient is able to tolerate it, and if considered advisable is given parenterally, more especially where suction is used. It should be continued as long as there is any possibility of further infection.

So far, in my experience, I have had no occasion to fear overdosage, or any deleterious effects. It is most important to replace the fluid and chloride loss, especially in suction cases, keeping the urinary output from 1000 cc to 1500 cc. Give frequent and fairly large doses of opiates to promote intestinal rest. The combination of proper diagnosis, pre-operative preparation, well planned and well executed appendectomies with suction and chemotherapy, will not only reduce the mortality in ruptured cases, but will also reduce the total mortality to around 1 per cent or less.

BIBLIOGRAPHY

1. Collier: Review of Studies in Water and Electrolyte Balance in Surgical Patients. Surgery, page 192. August, 1942.
2. Lundgren, A. T., Garside, Earl and Boyce, William A.: Conservative Treatment of Appendiceal Peritonitis. Surgery, page 812. June, 1939.
3. Lehman: Editorial. Surgery. August, 1942.
4. Penberthy's Paper: American Surgical Association, Cleveland. April 8, 1942.
5. Lehman and Parker: Annals of Surgery, Vol. 108, page 833 and 856. 1938.
6. Radvin-Rhodes-Lockwood: Annals of Surgery, pages 3-53. 1940.
7. Toshiro, K., et. al.: Surgery, page 690. May, 1942.
8. Sutton, Henry V.: Journal of A.M.A. June 13, 1942.
9. Fox and Jensen: Journal of A.M.A., page 1147. April 3, 1943.
10. Pratt, O. B.: Report Memorial Hospital Laboratory.
11 Brawer, J. O., et. al.: Journal of A.M.A., Vol. 118, No. 15, page 1284.
12. Auchincloss, Hugh: Drainage and Wound Closure Technique in Appendicitis Operations. Annals of Surgery, page 435. September, 1942.

Consultants

Poll the successful consulting physicians of this country to-day, and you will find they have been evolved either from general practice or from laboratory and clinical work; many of the most prominent having risen from the ranks of general practitioners. I once heard an eminent consultant rise in wrath because some one had made a remark reflecting upon this class. He declared that no single part of his professional experience had been of such value. But I wish to speak of the training of men who start with the object of becoming pure physicians. From the vantage ground of more than forty years of hard work, Sir Andrew Clark told me that he had striven ten years for bread, ten years for bread and butter, and twenty years for cakes and ale; and this is really a very good partition of the life of the student of internal medicine, of some at least, since all do not reach the last stage.—Aequanimitas with Other Addresses. Sir William Osler. 3rd Edition. tion.

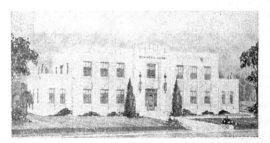

Special Article

HOW FIRM THE FOUNDATION,
HOW FRAIL THE SUPERSTRUCTURE

LEWIS J. MOORMAN M.D.
OKLAHOMA CITY, OKLAHOMA

George Washington (1732-1799), elected without opposition as first President and in possession of every reason for self assurance and popular confidence, wrote Alexander Hamilton, "If I should be prevailed upon to accept it, (the Presidency), the acceptance would be attended with more diffidence and reluctance than ever I experienced before in my life." . . . In his inaugural address he declared that "the preservation of the sacred fire of liberty and the destiny of the republican model of government are justly considered as DEEPLY, perhaps as FINALLY, staked on the experiment intrusted to the hands of the American people." When urged to accept a third term, he firmly declined. In his Farewell Address he said, "the batteries of internal and external enemies will be directed covertly and insidiously against the fortress of that very liberty which you so highly prize." Even so, he trusted the people of the United States and did not consider himself indispensable.

Marshall's summation of Washington's character makes us proud of our past and fearful of our future. "In him, that innate and unassuming modesty which adulation would have offended, which the voluntary plaudits of millions could not betray into indiscretion, was happily blended with a high and correct sense of personal dignity, and with a just consciousness of that respect which is due to station."

Thomas Jefferson's (1743-1826), position on individual liberty is admirably expressed in the Declaration of Independence which, according to Edward Everett, "is equal to anything ever born on parchment or expressed in the visible signs of thought." "The heart of Jefferson in writing it," adds Bancroft, "and of Congress in adopting it, beat for all humanity." Likewise his own epitaph stands as an eloquent testimony to the fact that he had a fallow spot in his heart for all humanity. "Here was buried Thomas Jefferson, author of the Declaration of Independence, of the Statute of Virginia for Religious Freedom, and Father of the University of Virginia." "Slavery he considered a moral political evil, and declared in reference to it that he 'trembled for his country when he remembered that God is just'."

The honor system at the University of Virginia serves as an outstanding survival of Jefferson's democratic principles with emphasis on individual initiative and responsibility. This youthful demonstration of personal honor and integrity should put to shame our inert, submissive citizenry. In the light of our present trend toward governmental paternalism it is interesting to note that one of the maxims of Jefferson's father was "never ask another to do for you what you can do for yourself."

Patrick Henry (1736-1799), a daring exponent of liberty or death, opposed the famous Stamp Act with eloqent emphasis, "Caesar had his Brutus, Charles the First his Cromwell and George the Third may profit by their example." He became Viriginia's War Governor and his fear of Administrative curtailment of personal liberty was so great that he even opposed the adoption of the Federal Constitution because he thought it contained "an awful squinting toward monarchy."

It is noteworthy that Patrick Henry, after repeated failures in business and an unsuccessful attempt at farming, figured as a potent factor in our freedom from oppression and the development of our country. If he had been handicapped by W.P.A., paid for plowing under farm products, offered farm subsidies or forced to accept social security with an old age pension in the offing, he would never have had the courage to study law, or the power to electrify his countrymen with the determination to fight for liberty and to establish the national foundation of which we are so proud and so negligent.

John Marshall (1755-1835), who in common with James Madison, was largely responsible for Virginia's adoption of the Federal Constitution, wielded a stabilizing power in Congress and in 1801 was appointed Chief Justice of the Supreme Court of the United States. His just and liberal interpretation and construction of the Constitution over a period of 34 years helped to establish our government's firm foundation and his towering intellect, his moral courage, his profound wisdom and his luminous opinions on constitutional law commanded universal respect.

James Madison (1751-1836), this intellectual giant who was a close personal friend of Thomas Jefferson and shared his democratic convictions, was the author of a series of resolutions adopted by the Assembly of Viriginia and known as the Resolutions of 1798, which protested against all attempts to increase the power of the Federal Government by forced construction of general clauses of the Constitution. He was appointed Secretary of State by President Jefferson in March, 1801, and filled that office for eight years in such a manner as to inspire the confidence and approbation of the people." His election as President of the United States in 1809, indicated that the people approved his policy of restricting Federal powers.

Benjamin Franklin (1706-1790), came up from the ranks the hard way. His rise to fame was largely due to fear and want. His struggle with environment led to individualistic convictions and love for the common people. His first trip to England was for the purpose of freeing the people from the oppression of the proprietary governors. On his second trip after failing to reconcile our political and commercial differences with England, he returned to take an active part in the cause of independence. On September 3, 1783, with Adams and Jay, he signed the Treaty of Peace, which according to Washington was "the most liberal treaty ever entered into between independent powers."

Franklin's phenomenal accomplishments in behalf of liberty and science are expressed in the following line from Turgot—"He wrested the thunder bolt from heaven and the sceptre from tyrants."

John Adams (1735-1826), who said "sink or swim, live or die, survive or perish with my country, is my unalterable determination" was imbued with patriotic zeal through the influence of a speech delivered by James Otis as early as 1761. Later, referring to this speech, he said "American Independence was then and there born." Not political ambition, but the passage of the Stamp Act in 1765 precipitated his participation in political affairs. He never was truly a politician but always a powerful proponant of the people and a faithful guardian of their interests. According to Jefferson, he was "the ablest advocate and champion of independence on the floor of the House" and he was the first to propose George Washington as Commander-in-Chief of the Army. In 1796 he was elected President of the United States. In addition to his personal services in this capacity, he bequeathed his son, John Quincy, to the Presidency of the United States and later to a powerful and sound position in Congress where he was known as "the Old Man Eloquent".

Daniel Webster (1782-1852), the Statesman, expressed the spirit which should animate the actions of every true American citizen today, when he said, "I shall exert every faculty I possess in aiding to prevent the Constitution from being nullified, destroyed, or impaired; and, even though I should see it fall, I will still, with a voice feeble, perhaps, but earnest as ever issued from human lips, and with fidelity and zeal which nothing shall extinguish, call on the PEOPLE to come to its rescue." These remarkable patrons of our priceless liberties, who laughed at fear and want and considered it a privilege to fight for personal freedom and national integrity, would have spurned so-called social security including socialized medicine. These great Statesmen believed in the integrity of the medical profession and the individual pursuit of medical practice as the only way to preserve the intimate relationship between the patient and his physician. The records show that when they were ill they had the satisfaction of having the doctor of their choice.

Franklin was a great scientist and maintained a profound interest in medicine. In addition to his varied contributions to medical science, Garrison said, "He was the principle founder and the first President of the Pennsylvania Hospital (1751) of which he wrote a history, by request, printed at his own press in 1754." Through his friendship with European doctors he helped to place a number of young American doctors in European universities for graduate work in medicine thus materially advancing the cause of medical education in this country.

Thomas Jefferson became one of the nation's chief exponents of vaccination against small-pox and did all he could to forward the interests of American medicine because such interests were in line with general welfare. Physicians signed the Declaration of Independence and helped to frame the Constitution. With "reliance on the protection of Divine providence, they pledged their lives, their fortunes and their honor to the cause of independence and they have a right to demand full protection under the provisions of the Constitution.

If there had been a W.P.A. and a social security program including old-age pensions with sufficient personal depravity to make them acceptable, the spirit of "liberty or death" would have died with the dole and there would be no Declaration of Independence.

What Jefferson said about slavery might well be said of our present trends toward socialization, "What an incomprehensible machine is man, who can endure toil, famine, stripes, imprisonment, and death itself, in vindication of his own liberty, and the next moment be deaf to all those motives whose power supported him through his trial, and inflict upon his fellowmen a bondage, one hour of which is fraught with more misery than ages of that which he rose in rebellion to oppose!"

With our present knowledge of evolution and our close proximity to the American Revolution, it seems incredible that we should have permitted the insiduous agencies of devolution to land us on the very brink of a new Dark Age. If we desire to rescue the expiring ghost of our personal liberties from the asphyxiating grasp of bureaucratic control we must defeat the annulling social legislation proposed by the Wagner-Murray-Dingell Bill. If we fail to raise our voices against this sweeping suppression of our treasured rights and privileges "government of the people, by the people, for the people, shall perish from the earth", and we shall be left groping in the shade of our vanishing birthright.

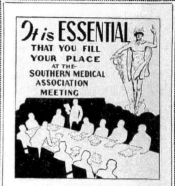

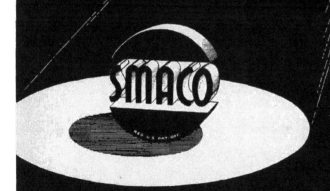

· THE PRESIDENT'S PAGE ·

"There are two dangerous factions in medicine as you know. One is the Old Guard which says that things must stay as they are. And there is the radical section that wants to scrap the entire system and start over. Neither of those factions can do this job.

"If medicine just sits back and resists, resists, resists — the professional reformers are going to ride roughshod over our bodies and nothing can save our precious freedom."

This quotation is from an extraordinarily frank and earnest address given at the ninetieth annual dinner of the Minnesota State Medical Association by Dr. Walter H. Judd, Congressman from Minnesota.*

Acting under instruction from your House of Delegates, the Committee on Prepaid Medical and Surgical Insurance is hard at work—studying other plans which are attempting to solve the problem of these people in the low income group who find serious illness an economic as well as physicial catastrophe. The Oklahoma plan, which will emerge from the Committee soon, will be merely our contribution in medical economic research that is being conducted by many other State and County Societies throughout the United States. It is an experiment—and all the progress that has been made in scientific medicine has been based on experiment. Such an experiment, on a voluntary basis, will be more scientifically conducted than a compulsory plan managed by the Federal Government. It will preserve the right of the patient to a free choice of his physician, and preserve the doctor-patient relationship. Let all of us, conservatives and liberals alike, let these middle-of-the-road men who constitute your Committee join the nationwide effort being made by medical men to solve a problem, rather than have the Federal Government in the picture.

This is post-war planning, looking forward to the day that our present artificial prosperity will collapse, and conditions of the early thirties may return.

We have a responsibility to the many doctors in the service of their country—and a responsibility to the next generation. Let us all be prepared to make a little sacrifice now, that those who follow us will remain as we have been—Free!

*Reprinted on page 443.

James Stevenson

President.

The JOURNAL Of The
OKLAHOMA STATE MEDICAL ASSOCIATION

EDITORIAL BOARD
L. J. MOORMAN, Oklahoma City, Editor-in-Chief

E. EUGENE RICE, Shawnee

NED R. SMITH, Tulsa

MR. R. H. GRAHAM, Oklahoma City, Business Manager

CONTRIBUTIONS: Articles accepted by this Journal for publication including those read at the annual meetings of the State Association are the sole property of this Journal.

The Editorial Department is not responsible for the opinions expressed in the original articles of contributors.

Manuscripts may be withdrawn by authors for publication elsewhere only upon the approval of the Editorial Board.

MANUSCRIPTS: Manuscripts should be typewritten, double-spaced, on white paper 8½ x 11 inches. The original copy, not the carbon copy, should be submitted.

Footnotes, bibliographies and legends for cuts should be typed on separate sheets in double space. Bibliography listing should follow this order: Name of author, title of article, name of periodical with volume, page and date of publication.

Manuscripts are accepted subject to the usual editorial revisions and with the understanding that they have not been published elsewhere.

NEWS: Local news of interest to the medical profession, changes of address, births, deaths and weddings will be gratefully received.

ADVERTISING: Advertising of articles, drugs or compounds unapproved by the Council on Pharmacy of the A.M.A. will not be accepted. Advertising rates will be supplied on application.

It is suggested that members of the State Association patronize our advertisers in preference to others.

SUBSCRIPTIONS: Failure to receive The Journal should call for immediate notification.

REPRINTS: Reprints of original articles will be supplied at actual cost provided request for them is attached to manuscripts or made in sufficient time before publication. Checks for reprints should be made payable to Industrial Printing Company, Oklahoma City.

Address all communications to THE JOURNAL OF THE OKLAHOMA STATE MEDICAL ASSOCIATION, 210 Plaza Court, Oklahoma City. (3)

OFFICIAL PUBLICATION OF THE OKLAHOMA STATE MEDICAL ASSOCIATION
Copyrighted October, 1943

EDITORIALS

THE VOICE OF THE PEOPLE

Medicine in the United States, sharing in the freedom vouchsafed by the courage of Patrick Henry, the principles of Thomas Jefferson, the sword of George Washington and the wisdom of Benjamin Franklin, has made phenominal progress, meeting all the demands, arising through improved transportation, rapid industrialization and urbanization in such a way as successfully meet the successive hazards and at the same time providing the highest health level, the lowest mortality rate and the most rapid rise in longevity experienced by any country in the world.

Having followed the swift changes arising in a mechanized world with adequate response, medicine can cover the post-war period with its wonted initiative and efficiency if not handicapped by governmental control. We are at war with Germany for the purpose of preserving our own way of life, yet our Commander-in-Chief has championed the principles laid down in the Wagner Bill which are virtually those foisted upon the unthinking, subservient German people sixty years ago by Bismarck and his malleable Emperor, William I. Must we suffer the shame of having our hard-won freedom replaced by this child of the Reichstag which was sired by the designing Bismarck with the consent of Germany's first Emperor, the power-loving, war-minded, presumptive vice-regent of God?

May the shades of our patron fathers inhabit the halls of Congress and protect our personal liberties. Since shades do not vote, a baptism of letters and telegrams protesting the Wagner Bill may bolster their influence. Politicians know that the voice of the people is the voice of God.

THE CHALLENGE

Those who write for the Journal are urged to give time and thought not only to scientific but to literary composition as well. Our commonwealth is young and our State Medical Journal is relatively immature. We must try to give it character and cast worthy of our advanced professional accomplishments. The world should know that Oklahoma is not lagging in medical progress. The State Journal constitutes the chief medium for the dissemination of this knowledge.

It has been said that in 1820 Sydney Smith

made this challenging remark, "In the four quarters of the globe, who reads an American book; what does the world yet owe an American physician and surgeon?" Stung by this remark, Nathaniel Chapman of Virginia, then teaching medicine in the University of Pennsylvania, joined Matthew Carey to found the "Philadelphia Journal of Medical and Physicial Sciences" which later became the "American Journal of Medical Sciences."

The world is challenging the medical profession of Oklahoma. We must take our place in the record of scientific medicine as well as in its practice .

COUNTING THE COST

Since we live in a world where progress has become ultramaterialistic and since, in the United States, we are facing a move to make medical service economic, mathematical and universal, society should be apprised of the fact that under the proposed plan, the cost will be doubled and the quality divided by two. Adding the latter to the former and saying the cost will be quadrupled is not sufficient. Cutting the quality strangles the spirit of service and multiplies suffering and death in a way so subtle that they defy accurate dollar and cent estimates.

At the risk of posing as a spiritual prophet in an age of materialism, we predict that the bureaucratic freezing of medical service will lead to a sour utopia with a sad defrosting.

ON THE LEVEL

If this leveling process goes on without interruption all the peaks will bow down to meet the dusty plateaus and the beckoning lights of unselfish, individual human endeavor will go out all over the world. When we all are homogeneously housed on a horizontal line with an administrative club for every head that bobs and a bureaucratic buoy for every soul that sinks, we may thank our stars that we have reached the level of indispensable morons, with four freedoms and a vote; not merely something to be plowed under or rolled back.

But if the toboggan for perdition should come whizzing by, grab it! Hanging on a strap, initiative is better than social security static, which would keep you away from the big fire. Even a moron should enjoy seeing the bureaucrats burn.

"We must beware of trying to build a society in which nobody counts for anything except a politician or an official, a society where enterprise gains no reward, and thrift no privileges."—Winston Churchill.

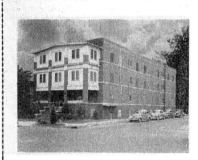
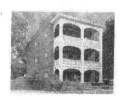

ASSOCIATION ACTIVITIES

OKLAHOMA PHYSICIAN TO APPEAR ON POSTGRADUATE PROGRAM AMERICAN COLLEGE OF PHYSICIANS

The American College of Physicians has announced its Postgraduate Courses for Fellows and Associates of the College to be held in Chicago, New York and Philadelphia.

A course in Endocrinology will be held in Chicago October 11 through October 16; Allergy, New York, October 25 through October 30; Special Medicine, Philadelphia, November 8 through November 19.

Henry H. Turner, M.D., Oklahoma City, is one of the instructors in the Endocrinology Course. Dr. Turner will present papers on ''Pituitary Infantilism'' and ''End Results of Prolonged Treatment of Hypogonadism with Testosterone Propionate''.

ANNUAL LEROY LONG MEMORIAL LECTURE HELD SEPTEMBER 30

Harry Alexander, M.D., Dean of Internal Medicine, Washington University, St. Louis, Missouri and Editor of the National Journal of Allergy ,was the guest speaker at the Fourth Annual LeRoy Long Lectures held at the University of Oklahoma School of Medicine on September 30.

The lecture, which is sponsored by the Alumni and Undergraduates of Phi Beta Pi, is a tribute to the late LeRoy Long, M.D., Oklahoma City, who was Dean of the Medical School from 1915 to 1931.

Dr. Alexander spoke on the subject of ''The Present Status of Chemotherapy in the Treatment of Diseases.''

OPTICAL COMPANY ACQUAINTS EMPLOYEES WITH WAGNER-MURRAY BILL

The following bulletin was distributed to the employees of the Barnett and Ramel Optical Company, Inc., of Kansas City, Missouri. The bulletin explains the dangers of the Wagner-Murray Senate Bill and urges each employee to do his part to forestall its passage.

SPECIAL MESSAGE TO ALL B & R MEMBERS!

If you make $80.00 a month, which deduction would you rather have made from your salary . . . $4.80 per month, or $1.48 per month?

If you make $200.00 a month, which deduction would you prefer to have made . . . $12.00 per month, or $2.43 per month?

Well, it's up to you which amount is to be deducted, so Please Read Carefully!

A bill proposing to broaden the present Social Security Act by IMPOSING AN ADDITIONAL TAX OF 6 per cent on wages of ALL INDIVIDUALS earning up to $3,000 per year is expected to be voted on by Congress when it convenes.

This Wagner-Murray Senate Bill No. 1161, is a new SCHEME to socialize Medical, Hospital, Dental and Nursing care in the United States. In addition to the 6 per cent which ALL EMPLOYEES will be taxed, employers must pay a tax of 6 per cent. This 12 per cent added to the present income tax of 20 per cent makes a total of 32 per cent tax upon payrolls, IN ADDITION to the various other deductions, and will result in an estimated 3 billion dollars a year for *Political Medicine*. Furthermore, this gigantic sum will be under the control of only one man (a ''Surgeon General of the Public Health Service''!). This man will have the power to spend your money in any way he choses!

Should this bill become a LAW, you will have to pay this 6 per cent of your earnings—BESIDES the withholding tax and others YOU'RE ALREADY PAYING! Under this law, if your earnings are $250.00 per month, $15.00 will be deducted from your pay each month ($180.00 per year!). If you earn $200.00 per month, the monthly deduction will be $12.00 ($144.00 per year!). If you earn $150.00 per month, $9.00 will be deducted every month ($108.00 per year!). AND SO ON, DOWN THE LINE!

And What Do You Get For Your Money?

Let's compare the cost to you—and the returns—with the Group Insurance Plan B & R has made available to you.

The Government Bill 1161 will provide medical, dental, hospital and nursing care (when needed) with certain time and cost per day LIMITATIONS AND PROVISIONS: X-ray and laboratory costs are thrown in, and, when needed, a pair of glasses. Supposing you earn $250.00 per month, the COST TO YOU for the above is $15.00 each month, WHETHER ANY OF THESE SERVICES ARE NEEDED OR NOT.

Unless you want to have to pay the much higher Government Tax, you have to do something about it. Once that bill becomes a LAW, you have to pay for socialized medicine . . . WHETHER YOU WANT TO OR NOT!

What Can You Do To Prevent Having To Pay This Tax?

Write your Congressman and tell him how you feel. He's representing YOU in Washington, and he expects the people at home to tell him what they want him to do!

But You'll Have To Hurry!

Congress reconvenes September 15 or earlier. This Senate Bill 1161 will probably be one of the first to be voted on. So let's get busy and write to our Congressmen and tell them how we want them to vote—and that we don't want such an UN-AMERICAN SCHEME put over on us!

Then let's all plan to take advantage NOW of the company plan for hospital and accident insurance. Why take a chance? Why have to bear the full burden, when this simple, inexpensive plan takes care of your illness—and that of your dependents, if you like?

LET'S DO OUR PART TO FORESTALL A TYRANNOUS BILL

Sincerely yours,
s / J. F. Ramel, President.

(For complete information on the Wagner-Murray Bill, and the far-reaching consequences it will have, read the articles in the August 7 Saturday Evening Post; August 1 Forbes Magazine; and the August Reader's Digest. They'll show you what you can expect if this bill becomes a LAW!)

OKLAHOMA CITY DOCTORS ATTEND CONVENTION

The following Oklahoma City doctors and their wives will attend the meeting of the Academy of Ophthalmology and Otolaryngology in Chicago on October 9. Dr. and Mrs. William L. Bonham, Dr. and Mrs. Tullos O. Coston, Dr. and Mrs. L. Chester McHenry, Dr. and Mrs. Harvey O. Randel, Dr. and Mrs. O. Alton Watson and Dr. J. C. McDonald.

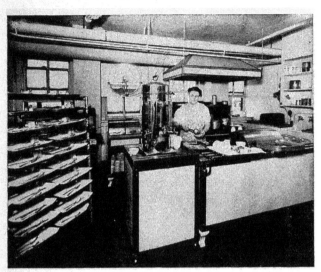

DR. OLYMPIO DA FONSECA, JR. TO LECTURE AT UNIVERSITY SCHOOL OF MEDICINE

At the invitation of the Pan-American Sanitary Bureau, Dr. Olympio da Fonseca, Jr., medical director for Brazil of E. R. Squibb and Sons Intra-American Corporation, has arrived in the United States for an extensive tour. He is appearing before the faculties and students of medical schools throughout this country, discussing Tropical Medicine with special emphasis on malaria, African sleeping sickness, amebic dysentery and ring worm infection.

Dr. da Fonseca is a professor at the National School of Medicine of the University of Brazil and is connected with the Medical Centre of Ceara and the Department of Health of that state. He has attained worldwide renown as a mycologist, both as teacher and as a director in this field at the Institute of Manguinhos. He is the author of the textbook, ''Medical Parasitology''.

Dr. da Fonseca will lecture at the University of Oklahoma School of Medicine in Oklahoma City on November 3.

ADVISORY COMMITTEE TO WOMAN'S AUXILIARY APPOINTED

Dr. James Stevenson, President, has appointed the Advisory Committee to the Woman's Auxiliary. Dr. C. R. Rountree will serve as Chairman and the following as Committee members: Dr. J. A. Rieger, Norman; Dr. A. C. McFarling, Shawnee; Dr. J. C. Peden, Tulsa and Dr. D. Evelyn Miller, Muskogee.

OKLAHOMA CITY PHYSICIANS TO ATTEND PARLEY

The Convention of the South Central Branch of the American Urological Society is being held in Lincoln, Nebraska, October 5 through October 11. The following physicians and their wives plan to attend: Dr. and Mrs. A. M. Brewer; Dr. and Mrs. Elijah S. Sullivan; Dr. and Mrs. Ellis Moore and Dr. Basil A. Hayes.

SAFETY IN BATHTUBS

''We take pride in our millions of bathtubs, yet there is much that can be done to render them safe'' Guy Hinsdale, M.D., Charlottesville, Va., declares in Hygeia, The Health Magazine for October. ''Architects and designers of tubs and fixtures must recognize the dangers and provide foolproof safeguards before bathtub accidents can be eliminated entirely.

''Danger lies in the installation of the tub and electric light fixtures he points out. Architects should be aware of this danger and never allow the electric fixtures or even the switches or buttons to be within reach of the bather. When the bather is in the tub or standing on a wet floor, it is possible for him to receive a fatal shock if he touches a broken or frayed electric wire, most certainly if he tries to use a massage machine. . . .''

CIVILIAN PHYSICIANS INVITED TO ATTEND WARTIME GRADUATE MEDICAL PROGRAMS

The program of Wartime Graduate Medical Meetings for military installations in Oklahoma has recently been announced by Dr. Henry H. Turner, member of the committee for Area 16, which includes Arkansas, Kansas, Missouri and Oklahoma. Other members of the committee are Dr. Frank D. Dickson, Kansas City, and Dr. O. P. J. Falk, St. Louis, Missouri.

This is part of the Wartime Graduate Medical Meetings organized by and under the auspices of The American Medical Association, The American College of Physicians and The American College of Surgeons, and

authorized Surgeons General of the Army, Navy, and Public Health Service for the purpose of providing postgraduate instruction to the professional personnel assigned to the Wartime services who, by reason of their duties in these services, are deprived of the opportunities for such instruction which are usually available to them.

The Commanding Officers of the Station Hospitals have extended a cordial invitation to members of the County Medical Societies in this area to attend these meetings. During the month of October programs were given at Fort Sill, Oklahoma; Will Rogers Field, Oklahoma City, Oklahoma; Borden General Hospital, Chickasha, Oklahoma; Camp Gruber, Oklahoma, and Camp Chaffee, Arkansas.

November and December programs are now being arranged and those for Camp Chaffee, Arkansas, on November 17, and Camp Gruber, Oklahoma, on November 18 are as follows:

2:30 P.M. ''Symptoms Associated with Pathology of the Feet.''
Earl D. McBride, M.D., F.A.C.S., American Board of Orthopedic Surgery, Oklahoma City, Oklahoma.

3:10 P.M. ''Newer Concepts in the Treatment of Venereal Infections.''
Anson Clark, M.D., American Board of Urology, Oklahoma City, Oklahoma.

3:50 P.M. ''The Constitutional Psychopath in the Community and in the Army.''
Charles A. Brake, M.D., American Psychiatric Association, Central State Hospital, Norman, Oklahoma.

4:30 P.M. ''Maxio-facial Surgery.''
Curt Von Wedel, M.D., F.A.C.S., American Board of Plastic Surgery, Oklahoma City, Oklahoma.

5:10 P.M. ''The Management of Hypertensive Cardiovascular Diseases.''
Wann Langston, M.D., F.A.C.P., American Board of Internal Medicine, Oklahoma City, Oklahoma.

Anesthesia

In his Grammar of Assent, in a notable passage on suffering, John Henry Newman asks, ''Who can weigh and measure the aggregate of pain which this one generation has endured, and will endure, from birth to death? Then add to this all the pain which has fallen and will fall upon our race through centuries past and to come.'' But take the other view of it—think of the Nemesis which has overtaken pain during the past fifty years! Anesthetics and antiseptic surgery have almost manacled the demon, and since their introduction the aggregate of pain which has been prevented far outweighs in civilized communities that which has been suffered. Even the curse of travail has been lifted from the soul of women.—Aequanimitis with Other Addresses. Sir William Osler. 3rd Edition .

Doctor and Nurse

There are individuals—doctors and nurses, for example—whose very existence is a constant reminder of our frailties; and considering the notoriously irritating character of such people, I often wonder that the world deals so gently with them. The presence of the parson suggests dim possibilities, not the grim realities conjured up by the means of the persons just mentioned; the lawyer never worries us—in this way, and we can imagine in the future a social condition in which neither divinity nor law shall have a place—when all shall be friends and each one a priest, when the meek shall possess the earth; but we cannot picture a time when Birth and Life and Death shall be separated from the ''grizzly troop'' which we dread so much and which is ever associated in our minds with ''physician and nurse.''—Aequanimitis with Other Addresses. Sir William Osler. 3rd. Edition.

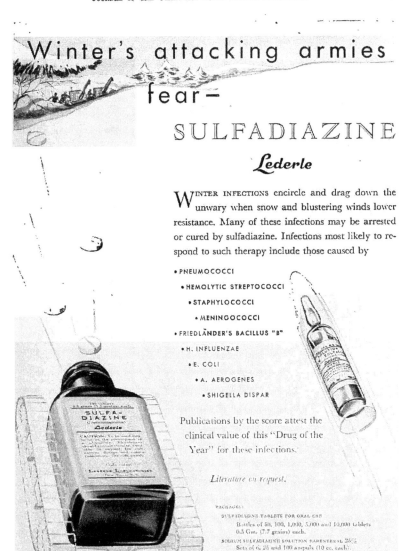

Woman's Auxiliary

The Woman's Auxiliary to the Oklahoma County Medical Association has emerged from a summer of heat, drouth, canning, house cleaning and Red Cross work to begin another war year. As our husbands serve to the limit of their capacities, so we, their wives, stand beside them to sacrifice and to assume even greater responsibility than ever before.

The year ahead brings us a three-fold challenge. First, we must meet immediate war needs. Second, we must carry on as normally as the time will permit. Third, we must plan for peace and a better world of the future.

As to war needs, whether it be in the field of surgical dressings, canteen work, nurse recruiting, or in any one of a dozen fields, each Auxiliary is finding the greatest need of her Country and is filling that need. If no immediate field is open, each Auxiliary stands ready to respond to an emergency. After taking care of the needs of our forces in the field, we turn to the homefront and our own over-worked doctors. We plan to save them time and energy by disseminating health information as approved by the Medical Association. We can be "Doctor's Aides" in many ways. The wives whose husbands are serving in the Armed Forces need us and we need them. The wives who have moved into our community "for the duration" are being welcomed and we hope to keep them as 'informed members'.

Our second challenge is to carry on as normally as possible. Due to the loss of doctors and their families, some Auxiliaries will have a small membership. In some groups the working wives may be unable to leave war jobs to attend meetings. Discouraging as it may be, Auxiliaries are planning to go ahead rather than to disband, which is a step backward. Programs are being streamlined to fit war needs. Meeting times are shifted to evening or luncheon sessions. In some cases fewer meetings are held but work is going ahead. Our common aims and ideals will hold us together.

The greatest challenge of this year and of the years to come is that of molding the future. We, as Auxiliary members, realize that we must study the plans for peace and have a part in formulating those plans. We must look forward to the kind of world we want in the future and, by beginning with a better home community, we must and will ultimately build a good world.

MRS. F. MAXEY COOPER, President

University of Oklahoma School of Medicine

Dr. H. A. Shoemaker, Acting Dean of the School of Medicine, is attending an Orientation Course for civilian representatives of colleges participating in the Navy V12 Program, which will be held at the Naval Reserve Midshipman's School, Columbia University, New York City, from September 16 to September 30. The purpose of this course is to make a wider understanding of the Navy itself, its operation and its mission.

Lt. Victor H. Kelley, U.S.N.R., has been named Assistant to the Commanding Officer for the Naval V-12 Unit at the University of Oklahoma School of Medicine. In civilian life Lt. Kelley served as Director of Appointments at the University of Arizona.

Dr. Allan J. Stanley has been appointed Assistant Professor of Physiology at the School of Medicine. Dr. Stanley was formerly connected with the State University of Louisiana. However, during the past year he has been on leave of absence from the institution

to assist in establishing a curriculum in Biology at St. John's College, Annapolis, Maryland. Dr. Stanley has published extensively on the physiology of endocrines. He has had papers published in the Journal of Morphology, Anatomical Record, Proceedings of the Society for Experimental Biology and Medicine, and Proceedings of the Louisiana Academy of Science.

Registration for the first fall term took place on September 3 and 4. Both the Army and Navy Specialized Training Units are now well established and the school has a real military air with 161 soldiers and 61 sailors in evidence.

Profession or Trade?

The Medical profession deserves the grateful recognition and regard of all other callings in modern life. It has always insisted that the practice of medicine is a profession and not a trade. Trade is occupation for livelihood; profession is occupation for the service of the world. Trade is occupation for joy of the result; profession is occupation for joy in the process. Trade is occupation where anybody may enter; profession is occupation where only those who are prepared may enter. Trade makes one the rival of every other trader; profession makes one the cooperator with all his colleagues.—President Faunce, of Brown University, in an address to the Rhode Island Medical Society, 1905.

Polypharmacy

Now of the difficulties bound up with the public in which we doctors work, I hesitate to speake in a mixed audience. Common sense in matters medical is rare, and is usually in inverse ratio to the degree of education. I suppose as a body, clergymen are better educated than any other, yet they are notorious supporters of all the nostrums and humbuggery with which the daily and religious papers abound, and I find that the farther away they have wondered from the decrees of the Council of Trent, the more apt are they to be steeped in taumaturgic and Galenical superstition. But know also, man has an inborn craving for medicine. Heroic dosing for several generations has given his tissues a thirst for drugs. As I once before remarked, the desire to take medicine is one feature which distinguishes man, the animal, from his fellow creatures. It is really one of the most serious difficulties with which we have to contend. Even in minor ailments. which would yield to dieting or to simple home remedies, the doctor's visit isn't thought to be complete without the prescription. And now that the pharmacists have cloaked even the most nauseous remedies, the temptation is to use medicine on every occasion, and I fear we may return to that state of polypharmacy, the emancipation from which has been the sole gift of Hohnemann and his followers to the race. As the public becomes more enlightened, and as we get more sense, dosing will be recognized as a very minor function in the practice of medicine in comparison with the old measures of Asclepiades.—Aequanimitas with Other Addresses. Sir William Osler. 3rd Edition.

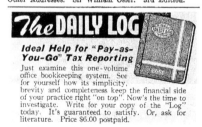

MEDICAL ECONOMICS

A MEDICAL CONGRESSMAN REPORTS TO HIS COLLEAGUES

*Reprinted from Minnesota Medicine, Vol. 26, No. 6, June, 1943.

Dr. Walter H. Judd made his first home appearance since he took his seat as newly elected congressman from the Fifth District, at the Minikahda Club in Minneapolis, Tuesday, May 18, as guest speaker at the ninetieth annual dinner of the Minnesota State Medical Association.

The dining rooms of the club were packed to capacity for the occasion and many more who had sought in vain for tickets to the dinner were admitted to standing room in the rear. They were rewarded by a report which, for its wit and frankness, its earnestness and timeliness will undoubtedly go down as unique in the annals of the association dinners.

The excerpts which follow will indicate to some extent the extraordinary character of the address. It is to be hoped that Dr. Judd's advice will be soberly heeded by his medical colleagues in Minnesota.

Said Congressman Judd:

I am very happy to have this opportunity to make my first home appearance before my colleagues. This will be in the nature of a case report and a clinic. It is addressed to you, first, as doctors and, second, as citizens.

Medicine Praised

First, I want to say now that we do not realize what an outstanding job we have done in this war, as doctors. I didn't realize it, myself, until I saw so many others, down there, in Washington, taking advantage of the war crisis to increase their own preference, standing and power. Not a single profession nor a single trade has organized itself as medicine has, seeing the need ahead even before the Army, Navy or Selective Service saw it, and working out in advance the fundamentals of providing medical service for the maimed in this war. There has been criticism, of course. Politicians took it for granted that doctors were like themselves and some of them even declared that the reason doctors were seeing to it that a sufficient number applied for service was that the older men were getting rid of the young men who endangered their practice that way. They couldn't believe, naturally, that anyone could sacrifice his personal interests for the sake of the sick and wounded of his country. It is discouraging, indeed, how few people there are in Washington who are capable of rising to the ideals which normally actuate the doctor.

Acute Problem

The war, of course, has created an acute problem in medical service. First—the Army demanded 7.5 doctors to every 1,000 men. They have modified that demand to a ration of approximately six per 1,000. But the lack of coordination and wisdom in Army planning for medical service has been disturbing. For instance, our own General Hospital Unit No. 26 sat and rotted for eight months before any use at all was made of its skilled medical personnel. There are many instances even more flagrant. The reason for it lay in bad planning, to begin with, and in unfortunate competition between military departments and the various arms of the service, each one striving for more and more men, regardless of over-all needs, and of the immediate uses to which they are to be put. Such striving is a characteristic of Washington, to be sure, and not confined to the Army. There are sections of the State Department, I am told, which haven't spoken to each other in years, though

they speak about each other frequently and loudly. Medicine, I am glad to say, is head and shoulders above that kind of petty contentiousness.

No Epidemics Yet

Now, the point of this doctor situation is this; We have had the good breaks lately. We have been freer of epidemics in the last six months than at any time for which there are records. In 1942 there was not even the usual seasonal rise in the respiratory infections.

But one day we will get an epidemic. And you know, as well as I do, that we won't be able to stand a big epidemic on the basis of our present distribution of doctors.

The Doctor's Job

It is our job, therefore, to work out the problem of distribution more equitably before, not after, the epidemic comes.

Part of our problem in public health today arises out of our very progress. There is no more enlightenment about the fundamental needs for health and there is a greater demand for hospitals, though in Washington today, not even the President's daughter could get more than four days, in case of childbirth, in any hospital in the city.

There are going to be changes affecting medicine after the war. There is no doubt of it. And I want to see our profession right up in the front lines directing and shaping those changes. Certainly, neither you nor I want the professional philanthropists spinning out the alterations and calling the turn, though that is just exactly what will happen unless we take it over.

Danger In "Old Guard"

There are two dangerous factions in medicine as you know. One is the Old Guard which says that things must stay as they are. And there is the radical section that wants to scrap the entire system and start over. Neither of those factions can do this job.

If medicine just sits back and resists, resists, resists . . . the professional reformers are going to ride roughshod over our bodies and nothing can save our precious freedom.

There are borderline cases where help is needed. We all know and must recognize that. There are areas of maldistribution where action must be taken now. And it is a fact, too that there are not enough doctors for this emergency. It's just a case for rationing, like sugar and meat. I want the medical profession to do its own job of rationing. If we don't it's certain that the "smart" boys will.

Larger Responsibility

We've done a fine job already in this war and before. But out of it comes a greater responsibility. We can accept and carry that responsibility. What we have to fear in so doing, is the "diehards" on the one hand, who will hang back, and the scrappers on the other who want to give everything for nothing. Here is a case in point.

When I went to China, western doctors had been there forty years and still there were no Chinese students studying medicine. Chinese boys were studying law, economics, trades, however, and so I asked a Chinese father one day why he was not educating any of his sons for medicine. "We can't afford it," the father said. "We can't possibly meet the competition of the mission hospitals where everything is given free."

Exploiting the Chinese

You know that many missionaries went to China just to get stars for their own crowns—and at the expense of the poor Chinese. They measured achievement in terms of what they could give away and not in the solid lasting good they could do. They over-looked the fact that, if a medical system in China or anywhere else is not self-supporting, it is not sound. The Rockefeller Foundation made that mistake initially when it established a medical center in Pekin, for instance, which is one of the best in the world. The Chinese knew they couldn't approach what the Foundation had done, so naturally they gave up at the start and did nothing. We were trying to import and force upon them a model which it was impossible for them to reach. We forget that self-respect and independence are engendered only when you pay your own way and those qualities are enormously more valuable than anything you can hand to people. You don't build personality or self-respect by giving things and making people take them.

We Ask for Payment

In our own hospital we came to realize that truth and we began to ask payment for our services. The amounts were small and they were adjusted to what the people could pay, but it made all the difference in the world in the attitude of our people and the effectiveness of our service. We were not popular for it, either, with the old missionaries.

Like the missionaries, the people in our government at Washington do not always understand what constitutes real help. They forget that the objects of their assistance are human beings, with a human being's ambitions and yearnings for prestige.

Washington Headquarters Needed

We doctors have known that always, but we've been too modest to say so. We must remember, though that the "Smart boys" are not modest. They are quite willing to go ahead without advice. And the fact is there has been nobody, up to date, to advise them. I was amazed when I went to Washington, myself, to find that there were no headquarters anywhere in Washington where either the Congress or the departments or agencies could get authoritative advance on medical matters. Small wonder that they made mistakes, and such mistakes are serious. It's the hardest thing in the world to correct a mistake once it is enacted into law by the Congress and even harder once it has been publicity released as a department directive.

What we medical men must do is to establish a headquarters and provide advice on the spot in Washington, not in the sense of lobbying at all, but with the object of giving counsel. You know, most of us in Congress are trying to do right, at least if our own interests aren't too seriously involved. But we need help and the medical profession must provide it.

Congress' Doctors Get Together

There are now seven of us doctors in Congress, by the way.

All of us got together, a while back, in the hope of fostering some sort of over-all scheme to take care of the medical situation. We hoped, at least, to be on the inside so as to survey the situation in the hospitals, in the Army and the Navy and Public Health Service and make an over-all plan. But we didn't get anywhere.

We Need to Study Failures

First let us say we need the *autopsy type of mind* which is willing to look at its own failures and accept them without hunting around for a scapegoat. We need the type of mind which is willing to study its failures and ask itself questions so as to avoid the same failures in the future. If the trouble is in the stomach or liver, it makes no difference to the doctor whether the patient is a republican or a democrat; it is still in the stomach or the liver.

Did We Think it was Harmless?

Second, we need the *biopsy type of mind.* In medicine we don't wait for the malignant growth to kill the patient before we do something about it. We take a sample of the growth as early as possible to see how those cells are growing. We don't say: "Oh, it's only in the toe. Let's wait until it gets to the knee to find

out how it's going to spread." But in government and politics we have been doing just that. We saw what happened in Manchuria in the East and to the Jews in the West. But we waited until the growth spread to Pearl Harbor. We knew it was malignant at the start. Did we think its malignancy would disappear and it would suddenly become harmless and benign when it reached us?

Third, we need the *type of mind which deals with things impersonally.* We doctors may argue about the need for an operation and one of us may lose the argument. But both of us want to see the patient get well. It is discouraging in the extreme that so many men in Washington should care so much less about seeing the patient get well than about their own vanities. They are afraid of this and afraid of that until finally they become afflicted by a kind of dry rot. They are all stooped over from keeping their ears to the ground.

Nobody Can Smear Congress

You know they try to keep a Congressman silent during his first year, knowing well that he will atrophy if they do. Soon he will acquire the universal spirit of looking out for himself first.

Save me from that! I am fortunate in having a profession for the future and no need to think about holding my job. So I am going to have a good time and do what I like. If I am sound, I believe the people will agree with me. If I am in error, it will be over in two years before the dry rot creeps up on me.

There is a great deal of talk about "smearing Congress." The fact is that nobody can smear Congress as Congress smears itself. A young friend on leave from the Army visited the House one day and he was amazed at what he heard there. "Imagine an Army," he said to me, "as disorganized as that."

We have no right to be as disorganized as we are. Of course we are bound to get undeserved blame and undeserved praise. Doctors get it every day, understand it and let it pass. Congress must have the same detachment.

No Sense of Balance

Fourth, we must have *the habit of thinking in terms of alternatives.* As it is, we have no sense of balance in Washington. We take a course of action and it turns out to be a mistake. What do we do? We scrap the whole thing. We do not try to save what is good and substitute other measures for what is manifestly bad. Furthermore, we think only for the present, in the present. We consider how to get rid of the ruins before the building is completed and not at all in terms of building for posterity. And yet the truth is in government as well as in medicine, that nothing we do is worth anything unless we are building for the future. Whether we like it or not—whether we are ready for it or not—we are now on the threshold of a new world. Our future is quite likely to be decided for a generation or more in the next six months.

If we doctors take our share of the general responsibility, if we work as a team now, perhaps we can help find an answer that will last to the question: How are we going to live in this new world?

Jefferson and Medical Education

Jefferson made a lasting contribution to medical education in establishing at the University of Virginia a chair of medicine. Among the five professors imported from England who, with three Americans, constituted the first faculty, was Robley Dunglisson, "a fine looking and agreeable young man." His chair, or "Bench," as one writer called it, embraced no less than seven subjects. Ostensibly he was the only teacher of medicine, but in reality Emmett, the professor of natural history, gave instruction in the cognate subjects of chemistry, botany and comparative anatomy. The chair of medicine as established by Jefferson was purely theoretical in its teachings.—"Medicine in Virginia in the Eighteenth Century." Wyndham B. Blanton, M.D.

★ FIGHTIN' TALK ★

Major and Mrs. Meredith Mercus Appleton announce the birth of a son, Meredith Mercus, Jr., on September 6. Major Appleton, Oklahoma City, is now somewhere in England.

The following bits of news come to us from the South Pacific:

"*Lt. Comdr. D. G. Willard,* Norman, is Commanding Officer of a .Company here and associated with him as his executive officer he has *Lt. Bill Klevn,* a former resident in the orthopedic department at the University Hospital.

"*Lt. Phil Devanney,* Sayre, and *Lt. Logan A. Spann,* Tulsa, are executive officers of another Company and a new addition to the staff is *Lt. (jg) J. H. Brady,* formerly of Fairview, but understand he calls California his home now.

"*Lt. Comdr. Willard, Lt. Spann* and *Lt. Devanney* have all been doing surgery in the Southwest Pacific Area.

"We won't be disappointed when we are relieved by some of our dear brethern for we have been in the service near a year and away from home that long."

We hear from *Major J. Wendell Mercer,* Enid, that he is enjoying a very fine course at the Mayo Clinic. He states that it was good to see Dr. Kelly West and Dr. Wendell Long not long ago.

Lt. Col. William P. Neilson, Enid, writes the following from his station ——————.

"There isn't much for me to write that would be of interest—I do have a great deal of work to do and on the whole am enjoying it. Military medicine is decidedly different from civilian medicine but certainly no less important and there is a mass of information which one must continuously grasp for if he is to do a good job of it."

Lt. Frank M. King, Woodward, is in North Africa and reports that he has been a lot of places and has seen many interesting things. He is now anxiously awaiting the next move.

The following excerpt is from a letter received from *Major Horton E. Hughes,* Shawnee, from 'somewhere' over-seas:

"Keep the home fires burning for Wagner's goat—and drop me a line if you can."

Captain J. K. Lee, Tulsa, is now stationed at Camp Hatheway, Washington. He reports his work as quite interesting.

The following letter was received from *Captain Aubrey E. Stowers,* Sentinel, who seems to be enjoying (as much as possible) the sunny clime of Sicily;

"I received your letter No. 2 and enjoyed it very much. I have been away from Oklahoma for almost three yars now and news, such as was in your letter, is very welcome.

"I am sitting here in an olive grove looking out over the Mediterranean sea, I have gone swimming almost every day since the campaign ended and am getting a tan that I seldom had in the States; however, don't let these words fool you, I don't like it, in the first place I can't understand the language over here. I studied German and Spanish in school, however, I hope that I will have an opportunity to use the German soon. The towns are dirty and the people are dirty, however, I suppose the war effort has been draining these people for several years, they were being taxed to death and the Germans who were here took anything that they wanted. There is absolutely nothing worth while to buy in the stores. The people were definitely ready for a change and glad to see us. The island as a whole could be a very pretty place with a little Americanizing. They grow about everything imaginable, olives, figs, bananas, oranges, lemons, almonds and a great quantity of grapes. They drink wine instead of water and speaking of wines, they produce some of the finest.

"Most of the Northern coast is very rugged, the mountains drop right off into the sea. Palermo, the capitol of Sicily and a city of about 450,000 has quite a number of rather modern buildings but in general is as ancient and as un-modern as the Romans themselves. Fishing over here is quite an industry with the Sicilians. I counted one hundred small sail boats a morning or so ago here from my bunk. They seem to stay out all night. There are very few cars, the people travel mostly by two wheel carts. These carts are really something to see, they are painted with beautiful paintings from the wheels on up. The horses pulling them are decorated with tassels and various other highly colored decorations.

"As to the campaign, you have read already more than I could tell you, but we are ready for another one. This marking time is getting tiresome and it is not getting us back to the States, the one thing that we are all looking forward to.

"There are still a lot of doctors from Oklahoma with us and none of us has seen anything we would trade Oklahoma for. Hope that I will have the opportunity of seeing you in the not too distant future."

Captain Paul H. Hemphill, Pawhuska, now in Sicily, had quite an experience after landing. He and two Colonels found a military hospital that was being operated by two Paratroopers. Captain Hemphill was left at the hospital while the two Colonels went on and the two Paratroopers left to join their units. The following paragraph from his letter describes what followed:

"Alone except for three Italian doctors and 18 corps men who were prisoners of war. I spoke no Italian and they no English and all their supplies and medicines were labeled in Italian. A lot of wounded civilians were brought in—had to amputate a woman's leg—do dressings, intravenous, etc. The pantomine and sigu language to try and get what I needed was really something to see. Was sure glad to see the clearing platoon pull in as one of the officers is an Italian whose folks used to live in Sicily. With him as an interpreter we were able to make good use of the Italian doctors and corps men. Hospital was hardly the name for the place. No lights, or running water, no sterilizers and no screens on the windows or doors and you have never seen flies until you see Sicily—they are everywhere.

"By means of mosquito bars we managed to get the operating room fairly free of them. That is the only time we have used a building since we hit the island."

Major John B. Miles, Anadarko, is now in India and states that it is very interesting country from a medical standpoint. The only other 'Okie' he has seen is *Captain W. L. Shippey,* Poteau, who was a class-mate in the Class of '27.·

CIGARETTE DIFFERENCES

as shown by the rabbit-eye test

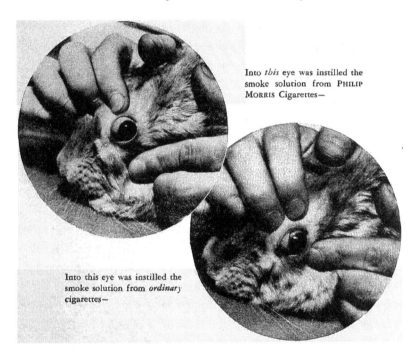

Into *this* eye was instilled the smoke solution from PHILIP MORRIS Cigarettes—

Into this eye was instilled the smoke solution from *ordinary* cigarettes—

NOTE THE DIFFERENCE in Edema. Average produced by *ordinary* cigarettes: 2.7. Average produced by PHILIP MORRIS: 0.8. CLINICAL TESTS showed that when *smokers* with irritation of the nose and throat due to smoking changed to PHILIP MORRIS, every case of irritation cleared completely or definitely improved.

From tests published in Proc. Soc. Exp. Bio. and Med., 1934, 32, 241-245
Laryngoscope, 1935, XLV, No. 2, 149-154

From 'somewhere in the South Pacific' writes *Captain Myron C. England*, Woodward, that he has been very fortunate in his work and has been doing Eye, Ear, Nose and Throat work' all the time. He is getting a lot of varied experience that will be valuable to him upon his return to the states. Captain England says he is sharing his Oklahoma news with *Major F. S. Etter*, Bartlesville.

(*Editor's Note: The office will be glad to supply army addresses of any of the physicians in the service to anyone desiring them*).

The Delilah of the Press

In the life of every successful physician there comes the temptation to toy with the Delilah of the press—daily and otherwise. There are times when she may be courted with satisfaction, but beware! sooner or later. she is sure to play the harlot, and has left many a man shorn of his strength, viz., the confidence of his professional brethren. Not altogether with justice have some notable members of our profession labored under the accusation of pandering too much to the public. When a man reaches the climacteric, and has long passed beyond the professional stage of his reputation, we who are still "in the ring" must exercise a good deal of charity, and discount largely the on dits which indiscreet friends circulate. It cannot be denied that in dealings with the public just a little touch of humbug is immensely effective, but it is necessary. In a large city there were three eminent consultants of world-wide reputation; one was said to be a good physician but no humbug, the second was no physician but a great humbug, the third was a great physician and a great humbug. The first achieved the greatest success, professional and social, possibly not financial.—Aequanimitas and Other Addresses. Sir William Osler. 3rd Edition.

CHANGE OF ADDRESS

NAME ....

....

....

ADDRESS ....

....

....

....

(*Please use this blank if you have a change of address.*)

Chauvinism

With our History, Traditions, Achievements, and Hopes, there is little room for Chauvinism in medicine. The open mind, the free spirit of science, the ready acceptance of the best from any and every source, the attitude of rational receptiveness rather than of antagonism to new ideas, the liberal and friendly relationship between different nations and different sections of the same nation, the brotherly feeling which should characterize members of the oldest, most beneficent and universal guild that the race has evolved in its upward progress—these should neutralize the tendencies upon which I have so lightly touched.—Aequanimitas and Other Addresses. Sir William Osler. 3rd Edition.

• OBITUARIES •

JOHN L. FORTSON, M.D.
1878-1943

Dr. John L. Fortson, Tecumseh, died at his home on September 10 of a heart attack.

In 1910, Dr. Fortson came to Oklahoma from Marshall, Texas and practiced medicine at Kiowa and Clinton, moving to Pottawatomie County in 1913. He served in the medical corps during World War I as a first lieutenant. Dr. Fortson was a member of the First Presbyterian Church, the Masonic Lodge and was active in civic affairs.

Services for Dr. Fortson were held in Tecumseh and burial was in the Tecumseh cemetery. He is survived by his widow, two sons, Lt. John L. Fortson who is stationed at the Naval Training Station at Quonset Point, R. I., and Sgt. Vaughan Fortson, stationed at Westover Field, Mass; one daughter, Elizabeth Fortson of Tecumseh and one brother, Robert Fortson, Marshall, Texas.

SAM H. WILLIAMSON, M.D.
1879-1943

Dr. Sam H. Williamson, Bethany, died September 14 at his home.

A native of Arkansas, Dr. Williamson came to Oklahoma and practiced medicine in Duncan where he operated a hospital for several years. From Duncan, Dr. Williamson moved to Bethany, and practiced medicine there and in Luther and Harrah for eight years.

He is survived by his widow; one daughter, Mrs. Jackie Lenertz, Los Angeles, California; two sons, W. F., Mt. Pleasant, Mich., and L. C., of Wewoka; two brothers and four sisters.

MARION O. BRICE, M.D.
1875-1943

Dr. Marion O. Brice, Okemah, died in Wesley Hospital in Oklahoma City on September 7.

Dr. Brice came to Okemah fifteen years ago to practice medicine. Before that time he was a physician and druggist in Castle.

He is survived by a nephew, Cicero Smith of Tulsa. The Hahn funeral home is in charge of local arrangements and burial will be held in Rock Springs, Ga., Dr. Brice's boyhood home.

Small Town Versus Large City

The environment of a large city is not the essential to the growth of a good clinical physician. Even in small towns a man can, if he has it in him, become well versed in methods of work, and with the assistance of an occasional visit to some medical center he can become an expert diagnostician and reach a position of dignity and worth in the community in which he lives.—Aequanimites with Other Addresses. Sir William Osler. 3rd Edition.

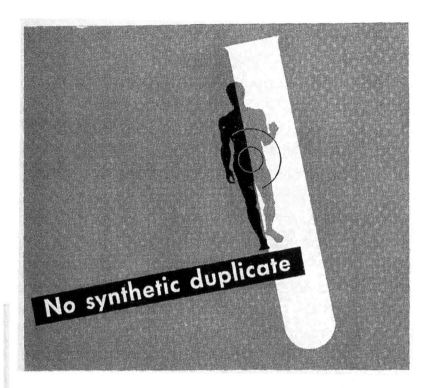

No synthetic duplicate

ADRENAL CORTEX EXTRACT (UPJOHN) is distinctive in its therapeutic action in that it affords the multiple actions of the many active principles of the adrenal cortex. This makes possible more effective, potent therapy for increasing muscle tone and capacity for work, for improving resistance, and for alleviating apathy and depression in adrenal cortical insufficiency.

There is no one synthetic duplicate which can influence carbohydrate metabolism, capillary tone, vascular permeability, plasma volume, body fluids and electrolytes.

ADRENAL CORTEX EXTRACT (UPJOHN) can be given intravenously, as well as by subcutaneous and intramuscular injection. Whenever potent replacement therapy is indicated—

Adrenal Cortex Extract (Upjohn)

Sterile Solution in 10 cc. rubber-capped vials for subcutaneous, intramuscular and intravenous therapy

• 25 YEARS AGO •

JOURNAL, October, 1918

THE PHYSICIAN AND THE NEW SELECTIVE DRAFT REGULATIONS AND LAW

The Journal and its Editor and the Adjutant General's Office had been the recipient of many communications as to the status of Oklahoma physicians under the new draft law or what is commonly called the 18 to 45 draft.

We will attempt here to make some comment on the situation and the probable line of action to be taken as to physicians affected. Of course it is to be positively understood that it is only an opinion, subject to error and modification, and, positively also subject to special regulations which may hereafter be promulgated by the Provost Marshal General after consultation with the Surgeon General's Office.

Legally and technically a physician is entitled to the same treatment as a bricklayer, blacksmith or lawyer at the hands of the Exemption Board. But it should not be forgotten that exemption boards have the power to inquire, and should inquire into the status of each registrant as such—not considering for a moment that he is a physician or whatever he may be, but that he is potentially a soldier—a fighting man physically fitted for trench work or other active army service. While the board should not take into consideration the possibility that the physician registrant could secure a commission in the Medical Corps by application therefore, the board members are simply human and will take into consideration such facts. The boards in some instances may err in this respect and send to active service a physician with many dependents, such as a wife, mother, father or children, but it is extremely likely that should such physician appeal to either the State Adjutant General or to the Provost Marshal General, the case will be remanded with the advice to treat the registrant exactly as other registrants are to be treated—to forget that he is a physician.

This opinion is based solely on the theory that our Constitution and basic law treats all citizens alike. Ours —identical basically with that of the British Empire— makes no distinction when it comes to citizenship. If the Army needs so many electrical workers, bricklayers, stenographers or physicians, the various state adjutant generals are called on to supply their proportionate share or number of each. This demand is based on the United States Constitutional provision which makes amenable for military service every male subject within certain ages. It is our opinion that any physician, having no dependents, qualifying as to the physical fitness and usual average intelligence, and within the draft age, will be and should be drafted, not as a physician, but as a soldier. Many observers in certain localities will add the hope that those in that class may be assigned as privates in the Medical Department to assist the self-sacrificing physician who long ago closed his office, sent his wife and one or more babies to the farm or back to the folks at home, accepted his commission and with it hundreds or thousands of dollars less income and is patriotically serving his country.

Draft boards have the power, and will use it—to inquire if a physician and his wife jointly have enough income to provide for such physician's wife and children when he may be called into the service as a $30.00 a month private. The fact that he drove a several thousand dollar car, technically, cuts no ice in the inquiry. The decision should be based on the joint means of the family estimate what they will have to live on should he and the Government send the dependents the monthly stipend allotted to the private soldier.

It is possible that the regulations may be so amended as to give the Provost Marshal General (Draft Boards and the Adjutant General of the State) the power to decide if a physically fit, single physician with no dependents is not imperatively needed in his location, rather than in the Army; this idea, of course, is purely speculative and is based on the information that already certain localities in Oklahoma are woefully short of physicians due to the universal call to enter the Medical Corps. It does not apply to most Oklahoma cities or average sized towns, but in many instances the rural community is already hard hit. Some have lost all their doctors.

It is our opinion that the State Council of Defense, Medical Section, should resurvey the State, that the committee of each county society should carefully estimate probable needs and be warned in time to not, in their enthusiasm, milk any particular community dry of doctors and leave the women and children to suffer for medical attention hereafter. In those cases where the physician subject to the draft is really more needed at home, where he cannot be adequately replaced—and we must forget that competent physicians are now unobtainable for new locations—such physicians should not only be advised to do so, but should be ordered by his board and the committee to stay where he is and serve his people.

JOURNAL, October, 1918

OKLAHOMA DRAFT BOARD EXAMINERS MAKE A CREDITABLE SHOWING

Medical members of Local and Advisory Boards are to be congratulated on the very good results achieved in sending thousands of men to contonment. Official information just issued discloses that Oklahoma sent; from February 10th to July 13th, 1918, 16,903 men. Of these 16,256 were accepted and 647, or 3.82 per cent, rejected.

Comparatively this is very good. Alabama stood highest in the matter of rejections having 17.46 per cent returned. South Carolina, South Dakota, Vermont and Georgia had more than 10.00 per cent returned, the average of all states being 5.84 per cent.

New Jersey stood first with only 1.93 per cent returned. Oklahoma stands twelfth from the top and while we are proud of that record every effort is being made by the proper officers to reduce the returns from cantonment to the vanishing minimum point.

A comparative statement showing the number rejected by the draft boards of each state might throw some additional light on the subject. Possibly the boards in some states hewed so closely to the line that they sent only what they deemed the physically perfect man.

Not bearing at all on the matter, but as a piece of pleasing information all the states sent to contonment and had accepted during the time 809,138 men. This looks like a very good record for a country lamentable unprepared twelve months ago.

PERSONAL and GENERAL NEWS, JOURNAL, October, 1918

Pawnee, Oklahoma and Grady county medical societies have passed resolutions disapproving in general of any movement of physicians into their counties to take the place of physicians absent in war work.

Grady County Commissioners refused to pay for expenses incident to operation of the Chickasha "Dentention Camp", holding the camp to be beneficial to Chickasha rather that the county—a clever distinction indeed.

NEWS FROM THE COUNTY SOCIETIES

The Woods County Medical Society met in Alva on Tuesday, September 28, with twenty-two present. Dr. P. B. Champlin, Enid and Captain Kimbrough from the Enid Air Flying School were guests. Dr. Champlin spoke on "Disorders of the Back and Treatment", illustrating his most interesting lecture with X-Ray films.

The Wagner-Murray Bill (S-1161) was discussed and there was also a report on the Council Meeting that was held Sunday, September 26, in Oklahoma City.

The next meeting will be held on November 22 and is to be in connection with the Crippled Children's Committee.

There were quite a few out-of-the-county physicians and their wives at the meeting of the Woodward County Medical Society that was held on September 9th at Shattuck. Dr. J. D. Osborn, Frederick and Dr. Oscar Templin, Alva were guests at the meeting. The Wagner-Murry Bill was discussed by Dr. Osborn.

Mr. R. H. Graham, Executive Secretary of the Association, spoke on the Wagner-Murray Bill at the meeting of the Kay County Medical Society held on September 16 at the City Hall, Blackwell, Oklahoma. The next meeting of the society will be held at Tonkawa on October 28.

On September 15 the Seminole County Medical Society met at Wewoka. The Okfuskee, Hughes and Pontotoc County Societies were invited to the meeting and representatives from all three counties were present. Dick Graham discussed the Wagner Bill and did a good job of explaining the Bill and answering the many questions asked by various doctors present.

The next meeting will be held on October 20 at Seminole.

"A Symposium of Poliomyelitis" was the topic for discussion at the Tulsa County Medical Society meeting held on September 13 at the Mayo Hotel in Tulsa. Dr. Luvern Hays, Dr. Theo S. Williams and Dr. Ian MacKenzie were speakers on the subject and a demonstration of the Kenny Method of Treatment of Poliomyelitis was made by local physio-therapists. Discussion followed with additional remarks by Dr. D. L. Garrett, Dr. M. J. Searle and Dr. H. A. Ruprecht.

Shawnee was the meeting place of the Pottawattomie County Medical Society on Saturday, September 18. Dr. J. E. Huges spoke on "Evolution in Medicine."

Ten members were present at the September meeting of the Garvin County Medical Society held in Pauls Valley. The Wagner-Murray Bill was discussed by the membership and sentiment was decidedly unfavorable to the Bill. The next meeting will be held on October 20.

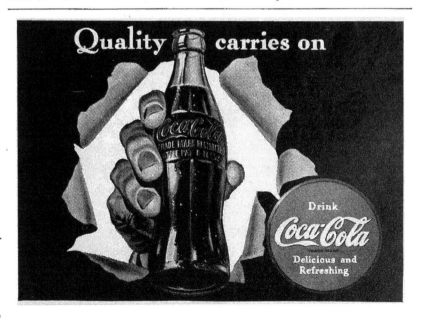

The Grady and Caddo County Medical Societies met on September 16 in Chickasha. The members enjoyed a talk on "Management of Minor Eye Conditions Seen by the General Practitioner" by Captain Sanders K. Stroud of the Borden General Hospital, and a talk on "Neuroses and Psychoses Encountered in General Practice" by Captain Richard C. Cooke, also of the Borden General Hospital.

"Affections of the Myocardium" was the subject chosen by Dr. Thomas Wells, speaker at the meeting of the Washington-Nowata County Medical Society meeting, September 8. The discussion was opened by Dr. F. C. Rewerts.

October 13 is the date of the next meeting. Dr. O. I. Green and Dr. H. G. Crawford will be the speakers.

Cushing was the meeting place of the Payne County Medical Society on September 16. Dr. R. E. Leatherock reviewed summaries of current literature on diagnosis methods of treatment and their evolution in sinus conditions.

The members of the Osage County Medical Society enjoyed a program consisting of an address by Dr. Arnold H. Ungerman of Tulsa, on the "Relationship of the General Practitioner to the Psychiatrist."

The Okmulgee-Okfuskee County Medical Society met on Monday, September 13, at Okmulgee with fifteen members present. Dr. Isom spoke on "Laboratory Diagnosis" and Dr. Peters on "The Public Health Doctor and the Private Practitioner."

A tour through the Government Hospital in Okmulgee is contemplated for the October meeting.

Naval Medical Officers from the Clinton Air Base were guests at the September meeting of the Southwestern Oklahoma County Medical Society at Elk City. Dr. John Lamb, Oklahoma City, discussed "Common Skin Diseases" and Dr. J. F. McMurry of Sentinel, spoke on "Breast Tumors".

News From The State Health Department

KEEPING WORKERS IN GOOD HEALTH

Outline of Scope and Function of Oklahoma's Industrial Hygiene Services With Features of a Plant Program

Modern Medicine and Public Health resources have made it possible to safeguard the health status of the men behind the guns, but modern war makes it no less important to maintain the fitness of the workers and others who are behind the machines that make the guns and carry on the home front. An industrial hygiene program involves the correlation of activities, needs and viewpoints existing between labor, management, nurses, official and non-official agencies, dentists and physicians. The chief function is the promotion and maintenance of the health of workers in industry, which includes manufacturing, sales, and service. The following paragraphs emphasize a few of the immediate possibilities.

The establishment of a medical division in any combined group of 100 or more office and factory workers is indicated. In fact, such attention should be given to even smaller groups. There is little fundamental difference in the kind of medical program for a large establishment, excepting the quantity. All health and medical matters should be coordinated and vigorously

developed to operate under the supervision of a plant physician or medical consultant. It is believed that such a qualified industrial physician should assume more of a health officer function, becoming less and less a private therapist. As the health officer of the plant, the physician will outline for himself many duties of an administrative and professional nature—emergency treatments, medical examinations, rehabilitation, plant inspections, health and safety education, maintenance of confidential medical records, study of all plant health problems, etc.

It is the function of the nurse in industry, to assist the physician in his duties as health supervisor of the plant. Her initiative in the matter of health education is of great value in many fields, as, for example, absenteeism, home visitation, nutrition, sanitation, etc.

Dental services in industry, consisting primarily of education and oral examinations, holds out an opportunity for a kind of prevention that really prevents, and a startling need for preventive measures will usually be found.

The promotion of a nutritional health program should become one of the activities of the medical department. Absenteeism usually results from poor health or personal reasons. General illness is responsible for fifteen times the amount of lost time compared to that resulting from occupational conditions. Work room conditions are frequently the cause of occupational disabilities of workers. Small plants especially seldom have facilities to conduct analysis and determinations or enviromental surveys, due to a lack of proper laboratory and engineering equipment, and trained personnel.

Sanitary facilities, such as toilets, urinals, wash basins and showers are often inadequate and deplorably unkept. The medical department of the plant is ideally situated to emphasize adequate and appropriate methods of taking care of such conditions and units.

The Oklahoma State Health Department, with its well established Division of Industrial Hygiene, is in a position to render valuable assistance to industrial and professional groups, and will render impartial and confidential counsel in matters of plant health problems and the public health.

Osler, "The Young Man's Friend"

He advanced the science of medicine, he enriched literature and the humanities; yet individually he had a greater power. He became the friend of all he met—he knew the workings of the human heart metaphorically as well as physically. He joyed with the joys and wept with the sorrows of humblest of those who were proud to be his pupils. He stooped to lift them up to the place of his royal friendship, and the magic touchstone of his generous personality helped many a desponder in th rugged paths of life. He achieved many honours and many dignities, but the proudest of all was his unwritten title, 'the Young Man's Friend'.—The Life of Sir William Osler. Harvey Cushing. Oxford at The Claredon Press.

The sacrifice of individual initiative and growth to society, the repressing of the culture of the great individuals for the purpose of maintaining the welfare of the great masses, may be compared to a mother who would devour her own children, and the individual who, by his intense egocentric exploits, would weaken the social bonds between himself and the mass is comparable to a heedless child who to warm himself, sets fire to the house of his fathers (Sabatier). The moral dignity, the cultural standard, and even the econimic progress of the mass is justly measurable by what it does to produce the great personality from out of its members and it is a self-evident fact that the dignity and worth of the individual is measurable by what he does for the social body, but whilst the latter is perfectly evident in all truly great men, the opposite relationship, namely, what the mass does for the great individuals, is frequently not detectable.—John C. Hemmeter. "Master Minds in Medicine."

COUNTY HEALTH SUPERINTENDENTS

County	Name	Part-Time Full-Time	Address
**Adair	Church, R. M.	P-T	Stilwell
Alfalfa	Lancaster, L. T.	P-T	Cherokee
*Atoka	Huntley, H. C.	F-T	Atoka
**Beaver	Long, L. L.	P-T	Beaver
**Beckham	Baker, L. V.	P-T	Elk City
*Blaine	Anderson, H. R.	F-T	Watonga
*Bryan	Sizemore, Paul	F-T	Durant
*Caddo	Wright, Preston E.	F-T	Anadarko
Canadian	Johnson, A. L.	P-T	El Reno
*Carter	Canada, J. C.	F-T	Ardmore
**Cherokee	Wood, W. M.	F-T	Tahlequah
**Choctaw	Gregg, O. R.	F-T	Hugo
**Cimarron	Hall, Harry B.	P-T	Boise City
*Cleveland	Nielsen, Gertrude	F-T	Norman
Coal	Hipes, J. J.	P-T	Coalgate
Cotton	Baker, G. W.	P-T	Walters
*Comanche	Parker, Wm. P.	F-T	Lawton
Craig	McPike, Lloyd H.	P-T	Vinita
*Creek	Joseph, P. G.	F-T	Sapulpa
**Custer	Doler, Clahoun	P-T	Clinton
**Delaware	Walker, C. F.	P-T	Grove
Dewey	Seba, W. E.	P-T	Leedy
Ellis	Beam, J. P.	P-T	Arnett
Garfield	Rempel, Paul H.	P-T	Enid
Garvin	Monroe, Hugh H.	P-T	Pauls Valley
Grady	Renegar, J. F.	P-T	Tuttle
Grant	Hardy, I. V.	P-T	Medford
Greer	Lowe, James T.	P-T	Mangum
Harmon	Lynch, R. H.	P-T	Hollis
Harper	Walker, Hardin	P-T	Buffalo
Haskell	Turner, T. B.	P-T	Stigler
Hughes	Floyd, W. E.	P-T	Holdenville
Jackson	Spears, C. G.	P-T	Atlus
Jefferson	Wade, L. L.	P-T	Ryan
**Johnston	Looney, J. T.	P-T	Tishomingo
*Kay	Kinnaman, J. H.	F-T	Ponca City
*Kingfisher	Meredith, A. O.	F-T	Kingfisher
Kiowa	Watkins, B. H.	P-T	Hobart
Latimer	Harris, J. M.	P-T	Wilburton
*LeFlore	Wright, R. L.	F-T	Poteau
Lincoln	Norwood, F. H.	P-T	Prague
*Logan	Hill, C. B.	F-T	Guthrie
**Love	Gray, Wm. J.	P-T	Marietta
McClain	McCurdy, Wm. C.	P-T	Purcell
**McCurtain	Williams, R. D.	P-T	Idabel
McIntosh	Little, D. E.	P-T	Eufaula
Major	Johnson, B. F.	P-T	Fairview
**Marshall	Holland, J. L.	P-T	Madill
**Mayes	Wood, W. M.	F-T	Tahlequah
Murray	Slover, G. W.	P-T	Sulphur
*Muskogee	Brooks, G. L.	F-T	Muskogee
Noble	Francis, J. W.	P-T	Perry
Nowata	Roberts, S. P.	P-T	Nowata
Okfuskee	Spickard, L. J.	P-T	Okemah
*Oklahoma	Hunter, George	F-T	Oklahoma City
*Okmulgee	Peter, M. L.	F-T	Okmulgee
Osage	Aaron, W. H.	P-T	Pawhuska
Ottawa	Hughes, A. R.	P-T	Miami
Pawnee	Haddox, C. H.	P-T	Pawnee
*Payne	Moore, Clifford W.	F-T	Stillwater
*Pittsburg	Powell, Paul T.	F-T	McAlester
*Pontotoc	Mayes, R. H.	F-T	Ada
*Pottawatomie	Haygood, Chas. W.	F-T	Shawnee
Pushmataha	Patterson, E. S.	P-T	Antlers
Roger Mills	Cary, W. S.	P-T	Cheyenne

County	Name	Part-Time Full-Time	Address
Rogers	Meloy, R. E.	P-T	Claremore
*Seminole	Shanholtz, Mack I.	F-T	Wewoka
**Sequoyah	Newlin, W. H.	P-T	Sallisaw
*Stephens	Berry, T. M.	P-T	Duncan
**Texas	Obermiller, R. G.	P-T	Texhoma
Tillman	Childres, J. E.	P-T	Frederick
Tulsa	LeMaster, D. W.	P-T	108 W.6, Tulsa
Wagoner	Riddle, H. K.	P-T	Coweta
Washington	Shipman, W. H.	P-T	Bartlesville
**Washita	Weaver, E. S.	P-T	Cordell
Woods	Templin, O. E.	P-T	Alva
Woodward	Pierson, O. A.	P-T	Woodward

* Full-time county health department
** Full-time district
Note: P-T—Part-Time County Superintendent of Health
 F-T—Full-Time Health Officer

Counties	Director	Address
Bi-County Health Department (Choctaw-McCurtain)	O. R. Gregg, M. D.	Hugo
Tri-County Health Department (Beaver, Cimarron, Texas)	J. L. Nicholson, M. D.	Guymon
Tri-County Health Department (Beckham, Custer, Washita)	R. W. Anderson, M. D.	Clinton
Tri-County Health Department (Johnston, Marshall, Love)		Madill
Five-County Health Department (Adair, Cherokee, Delaware, Mayes, Sequoyah)	Wood, W. M., M. D.	Tahlequah

Jefferson on Vaccination

Jefferson's part in introducing Jennerian vaccination into this country forms another chapter, and an important one, in the history of his contributions to scientific progress. An authority on the history of vaccination wrote in 1881; "Thomas Jefferson was not only a patron and student of vaccination but an active practical disciple of Jenner and the direct introducer of vaccination into Viriginia, Pennsylvania and the whole south . . . Waterhouse and Jefferson were the two men to whom the introduction of vaccination in America was wholly due."

He wrote Dr. Rush on December 20, 1801; "I am happy to see that vaccination is introduced, and likely to be kept up, in Philadelphia; but I shall not think it exhibits all it's utility until experience shall have hit upon some mark or rule by which the popular eye may distinguish genuine from spurious virus. It was with this view that I wished to discover whether time could not be made the standard, and supposed, from the little experience I had, that matter, taken at 8 times 24 hours from the time of insertion, could always be in the proper state. As far as I went I found it so; but I shall be happy to learn what the immense field of experience in Philadelphia will teach us on that subject." Wyndham B. Blanton, M.D., "Medicine in Virginia in the Eighteenth Century." Ford, "Writings of Thomas Jefferson", Vol. 8.

Finest Physical Specimens

American soldiers, sailors, and marines are the finest physical specimens of military men in the world. The average American soldier is 5 feet, 8 inches tall and weighs 152 pounds; during the World War he averaged 142 pounds and during the Civil War only 136 pounds. —Digest of Treatment.

"As luxury, degenerated into weakness and debauchery, begins to range in the bones of man and plagues develop which contaminate the atmosphere, then harrassed man as he hurries from one kingdom of nature to another to seek out alleviating drugs; it is then that he discovers the divine bark of cinchona, then he takes from the bowels of the earth the powerful mercury and squeezes the invaluable juice from the Oriental poppy. The most hidden corners of nature are searched; chemistry breaks up the products into their final elements and credites for it new universes; alchemists enrich natural history; the microscopic vision of Swammerdam taps nature's most sacred processes. But man goes still further. Need and curiosity leap beyond the bounds of superstition. He bravely seizes the knife and reveals that greatest masterpiece of nature, Mankind. This the worst helped him to attain the greatest. So did disease and death force us to attain the gnothi scauton (know thyself). Death and plague educated our Hippocrates and Sydenhams, just as warfare brings forth generals, and it is to the devastating venereal plague that we are indebted for a total reformation of medical taste."—Schiller, "Essays in the History of Medicine."

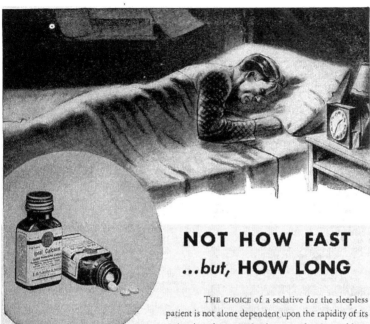

NOT HOW FAST
...*but,* HOW LONG

THE CHOICE of a sedative for the sleepless patient is not alone dependent upon the rapidity of its action, but also upon the duration of action and how the patient feels when he awakens.

Ipral Calcium—a moderately long-acting barbiturate—induces a sound restful sleep closely resembling the normal. One or two tablets, administered orally approximately one hour before sleep is desired, provides a six- to eight-hour sleep from which the patient awakens generally calm and refreshed.

Ipral Calcium is a plain white tablet—and one not easily identified by the patient. It is readily absorbed and rapidly eliminated and undesirable cumulative effects may be avoided by proper regulation of dosage.

HOW SUPPLIED

Ipral Calcium (calcium ethylisopropyl-barbiturate) in 2-grain tablets and in powder form for use as a sedative and hypnotic. ¾-grain tablets for mild sedative effect throughout the day.

Ipral Sodium (sodium ethylisopropylbarbiturate) in 4-grain tablets for pre-anesthetic medication.

Elixir Ipral Sodium in pint bottles.

For literature address the Professional Service Dept., 745 Fifth Avenue, New York 22, N. Y.

MEDICAL ABSTRACTS

"ADVANCES IN THE TREATMENT OF CHRONIC NASAL SINUSITIS." James Harper, Glasgow. The Practitioner, London. Vol. 149, pages 364-372. December, 1942.

During recent years there have been marked and striking advances in the conception and treatment of nasal sinusitis. The sinuses are lined with the same mucous membrane as that which lines the nasal cavities. When the nasal mucous membrane is affected by an acute rhinitis, the sinus mucosa is also affected and goes through the same stages. This helps to explain the severe pressure in the head, which may accompany acute rhinitis. It helps to explain the toxic symptoms which so frequently occur, and why these general symptoms, which may be severe, cause a great many cases of acute rhinitis to be labelled as influenza.

In the case of the sinuses, the openings of which are small and which are in most cases to a large extent closed, owing to the great swelling of the mucosa which occurs in the second stage of the acute inflammatory condition, drainage is poor. Drainage of the cavities is carried out mostly by means of the ciliated cells which line the cavity. If the mucosa is damaged by the infection that it is not possible for it to recover, or if there is a blockage of the ostium by some malformation of the nasal passages, a chronic infection is liable to be set in these cavities.

Observations showed that a large number of patients was not satisfied with the results of nasal surgery. In many of these cases definite nasal abnormities were found. The nasal symptoms were many and varied. Nasal obstruction was often a prominent symptom: frequent attacks of acute rhinitis; a discharge from the nose anteriorly, or the constant hawking of mucous from the throat owing to the discharge dropping down from the post-nasal space.

In many of these cases the operation of submucous resection of the septum was performed. The turbinal bones were trimmed and the patients were given what appeared to be satisfactory nasal passages. There were a good many cases in which the operation failed to relieve the symptoms. In some the maxillary antrum was found to be infected, but in the majority, investigation of the antrum and of the other sinuses gave a negative result. Yet, when nothing was found, finally the antrum was opened in the canine fossa and changes of a definite character were discovered in the antral mucosa. It was rare to find pus in the antral cavity itself, but in some cases little bags of pus were found within the mucous membrane. It was found that all these cavities were infected and the infection was in most cases by a virulent micro-organism. Microscopic examination made it possible to separate the mucosal changes into two main classes.

In the first type of case, the bone in the canine fossa was found to be markedly thin, it had a bluish appearance, and on raising the soft tissues off the bone along with the periosteum, the elevator would penetrate into the antral cavity with only very slight pressure. In this type of case the mucosa was found to be thin. It was of a glistening appearance, and small polypi were found in the inner wall of the canine fossa and on the lower part of the nasal wall. In some cases there were large polypi growing from the mucous membrane generally. The blood vessels were scanty and showed atheromatous changes. Microscopic examination of the mucosa showed marked fibrotic changes in the subepithelial layer and thickening of the periosteum.

In some cases the destruction of the surface epithelium was complete.

In the second type of case, the bone in the canine fossa appeared to be normal, it was, however, hard, with a very rich blood supply. The antral mucous membrane was generally thickened, dark in color, with the consistency of wet blotting paper. The general thickening of the mucous membrane might be as much as one fourth of an inch. The constant feature of the pathological changes was the attack on the sub-epithelial layer, which varied from round-celled infiltration to almost complete fibrosis. In some cases there was degeneration of the surface epithelium with finger-like outgrowths, degeneration of the subepithelial layer, and a deposit of calcium in the mucous membrane itself.

In dealing with the antrum, the Caldwell-Luc operation was performed and the whole of the lining membrane of the antrum removed. The results of this treatment were very satisfactory. The general symptoms, which were many and varied, improved or completely disappeared. Many of these patients suffered from frequent colds associated with bronchitic attacks. In others, asthma was a frequent complaint, and the nasal symptoms though present were not outstanding. There were patients with gastro-intestinal symptoms of varied character. Some of them exhibited symptoms suggesting a duodenal ulcer: others, symptoms suggestive of chronic appendicitis, whereas in others the symptoms did not suggest any definite lesion but rather a general upset of the gastro-intestinal tract.

In a large number of cases the mental condition of the patient was extremely interesting. Patients frequently complained of loss of memory and of great difficulty in concentration. Some were compelled to rest after a comparatively short period of mental exertion. In not a few cases depression was an outstanding symptom. Sometimes going on to melancholia.

Although the results were undoubtedly vastly improved by the treatment of the infected antra, they were by no means satisfactory, and it was concluded that in unsatisfactory cases other sinuses are also affected in addition to the maxillary antrum. The importance of the fundamental fact that the nasal mucosa and that of all the sinuses is continuous was then realized. Thus when sinus infection takes place all the sinuses may be infected. In all cases of antral infection the ethoidal cells are also infected. When the frontal or the sphenoid are infected the ethmoid is also involved.

Treatment should be extended to these sinuses, especially to the ethmoid sinus. One cannot expect much from vaccine therapy in chronic sinus infection. The author recommends regular opening of the antrum through the canine fossa. The middle turbinal is then removed through the nasal passage and any ethmoidal cells round about the opening in to the frontal sinus. This part of the operation must be carried out as thoroughly as possible. The posterior ethmoidal cells which were attacked through the antral opening are investigated then, and any tags of mucous membrane, or any cells which have not been effectively dealt with, are removed with biting forceps. The nasal passages are lightly packed with gauze soaked in an oily medium, and a small piece of packing is inserted into the opening which has been made in the lateral wall of the nose underneath the inferior turbinal. The packing is allowed to remain in situ for 48 hours, when at all possible, this procedure should be carried out in one operation. After-treatment is of the greatest importance.

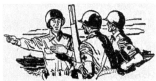
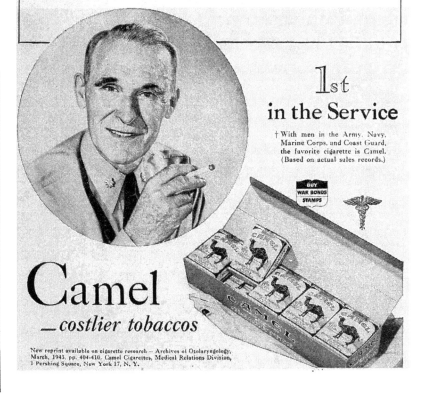

"AMPUTATION ANAESTHESIA BY FREEZING." Edwin A. Nixon. Northwest Medicine. Vol. XLII. No. 131. May, 1943.

There are several advantages arising from this form of anaesthesia: less shock, lower mortality, less postoperative pain, healthier tissues healing, and theoretically lessened bacterial growth in infected cases. A sedative, such as a small dose of morphine or an H. M. C. No. 2, is given thirty minutes before icing. The refrigeration is accomplished by packing the part in ice for from two to two and one-half hours, until the skin temperature has reached two to five degrees centigrade. A pneumatic tourniquet with a gauge is imperative and does no harm to arteriosclerosis, even when left on for from two to four hours.

After amputation, ice bags are placed around the stump for four days. Defrigeration is gradual, and the after pains are lessened. The stitches must remain longer than usual because of the slower healing. This form of anaesthesia is most suitable for patients who are bad risks, including those with diabetic gangrene. It is also suitable for skin-grafting operations.—E.D.M., M.D.

"LEG LENGTHENING OPERATIONS: ITS PRESENT STATUS." Alvia Brockway. California and Western Medicine. Vol. LVIII. No. 11. January, 1943 .

As a result of twelve years' experience with 150 leg-equalization operations, the author believes that each of the five methods has its place. Amputation with prosthesis is valuable in cases of poliomyelitis with severe paralysis and marked shortening, when the patient has sufficiently strong abductor and extensor muscles to control an artificial leg. It is also valuable in a patient with a congenital shortening of four inches or more, and a small deformed club foot.

While epiphyseal stimulation in the short leg has support from some surgeons, the results on the whole have been disappointing. It is best used in the young child with a congenital short leg, when the leg discrepancy is increasing.

Epiphyseal arrest is gaining in favor. The operation is safe and the convalescence is short, but the results are not known until the end of the growth period, and the height at maturity is shortened.

Leg shortening, which should be done in the femur, has fewer complications and a shorter convalescence than leg lengthening, but it decreases stature and involves risk to the good leg.

Leg lengthening, which should be done below the knee, restores the stature which nature intended, and places the operation on the limb of poor function, but it may be accompanied by various complications. Of the author's 150 leg-equalization operations, 109 were for leg lengthening. He believes that leg shortening above the knee and epiphyseal arrest are now more common than leg lengthening.—E.D.M., M.D.

"TOXICITY AND EFFICACY OF PENICILLIN." H. J. Robinson. Jour. Pharmacol. and Exper. Therap., Vol. 77, page 70. January, 1943.

Extensive studies of the acute toxicity and efficacy of penicillin were made in certain bacterial, virus, and protozoan infections. In toxicity studies, penicillin was injected intravenously or subcutaneously into mice in the form of a 10 per cent aqueous solution. Single doses of 0.5, 1.0, 1.5 and 2.0 gm. per Kg. were given intravenously at the rate of 0.1 cc. per minute, the doses being equal, respectively, to 30, 60, 90 and 120 Florey units per Kg. of animal body weight. (The Florey unit is that amount of penicillin which when dissolved in 50 cc. of meat extract broth just inhibits completely the test strain of Staphylococcus aureus.) Penicillin was also given subcutaneously at three-hour intervals day and night for a five-day period. The total daily doses given subcutaneously were 0.8, 1.6, and 3.2 gm. per Kg. which were, respectively, approximately

16, 32 and 64 times the effective therapeutic dose. Tables show the mortality over a ten-day period.

After intravenous injection of 0.5 gm. per Kg., the mice became inactive, depressed, and then became restless and evinced some respiratory distress. All the mice had watery eyes; with the higher dosages, the veins of the cornea and ear appeared to be dilated. Tissues of all mice were yellow. With higher dosage levels, a significant drop in body temperature occurred after intravenous injection. With daily doses of 3.2 gm. per Kg. given subcutaneously in divided doses for five days, all mice appeared sick and 4 out of 10 died. All showed signs of necrosis at the injection site. Mice treated in the same manner with daily doses of 0.8 or 1.6 gm. per Kg. appeared normal with the exception of a slight local reaction at the injection site. The toxic dose of penicillin appears to be about 64 times the effective dose as determined by subcutaneous injection in mice. In the experiments on mice with a more highly purified preparation of penicillin (400 Florey units per mg. as compared with 60 Florey units per mg.), the purer preparatioins were shown to be less toxic than crude ones.

The in vitro effect of penicillin on a large number of pathogenic organisms, including gram-negative, gram-positive, and anaerobic bacteria, was studied by several different methods, and data on the inhibitory effects of penicillin on the individual organisms are presented. There was a striking contrast between the action of penicillin on gram-negative and on gram-positive organisms. Dilutions of 1:1000 were required to inhibit the growth of most gram-negative strains, whereas a dilution of 1:1,000,000 inhibited all gram-positive strains, with the exception of streptococcus viridans and lactis, and one strain of staphylococcus aureus. Among both types of organisms there was considerable difference in resistance to penicillin. Thus, two strains of streptococcus haemolyticus (1685, C-203) were completely inhibited at 1:2,000,000 dilution, whereas S. viridans and S. lactis were only partially inhibited at 1:128,000. Likewise, of the gram-negative group, strains of escherichia coli and bacterium aerogenes were unaffected by penicillin, whereas strains of the salmonella and bacillary dysentery group were inhabited in dilutions of from 1:1,000 to 1:4,000. Penicillin was very effective against the anaerobic bacteria tested (clostridium welchii, tetani, botulinum, and chauvoii).

The effect of penicillin on gram-negative and gram-positive infections in mice was also studied. In daily doses of from 2 to 4 mg. (120 to 240 units) per 20 gm. of mouse, it afforded excellent protection to those infected with gram-positive organisms when treated at three or six hour intervals. Doses of from 0.25 to 0.5 mg. (15 to 30 units) afforded some protection but eventually the mice died. Penicillin was not effective against gram-negative bacterial infections. The data are recorded in tables and compared with the effects of sulfanilimide, sulfathiazole, or sulfadiazine given at three-hour intervals. In general, the protection afforded by penicillin was greater than that of the sulfonamides, particularly if the observation period was extended over ten days. The effect of penicillin appeared to be more permanent, suggesting that it is more bactericidal in vivo. Furthermore, the rapidity with which penicillin is absorbed constitutes an advantage over the sulfonamides. Mice infected with 10,000 L.D. of pneumococci and treated six to seven hours later survive the infection. Under similar conditions, the sulfonamides are not effective. Penicillin was tested in mice infected with mycobacterium tuberculosis, trypanosoma equiperdum, or the influenza virus, PR8, and was found to be ineffective.—H.J., M.D.

KEY TO ABSTRACTORS

E. D. M. ....Earl D. McBride, MD.

M. D. H. ....Marvin D. Henley, M.D.

H. J. ....Hugh Jeter, M.D.

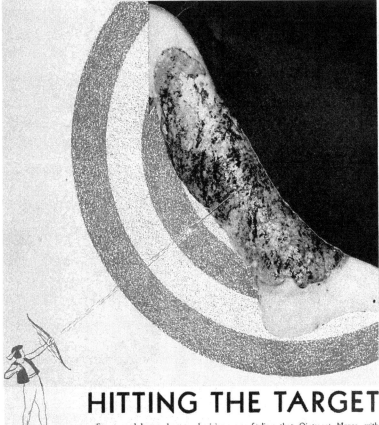

OFFICERS OF COUNTY SOCIETIES, 1943

★

COUNTY	PRESIDENT	SECRETARY	MEETING TIME
Alfalfa	H. E. Huston, Cherokee	L. T. Lancaster, Cherokee	Last Tues. each Second Month
Atoka-Coal	J. B. Clark, Coalgate	J. S. Fulton, Atoka	
Beckham	H. K. Speed, Sayre	E. S. Kilpatrick, Elk City	Second Tuesday
Blaine	Virginia Olson Curtin, Watonga	W. F. Griffin, Watonga	
Bryan	J. T. Colwick, Durant	W. K. Haynie, Durant	Second Tuesday
Caddo	F. L. Patterson, Carnegie	C. B. Sullivan, Carnegie	
Canadian	P. F. Herod, El Reno	A. L. Johnson, El Reno	Subject to call
Carter	Walter Hardy, Ardmore	H. A. Higgins, Ardmore	
Cherokee	P. H. Medearis, Tahlequah	*James K. Gray, Tahlequah	First Tuesday
Choctaw	C. H. Hale, Boswell	E. A. Johnson, Hugo	
Cleveland	J. A. Rieger, Norman	Curtis Berry, Norman	Thursday nights
Comanche	George S. Barber, Lawton	W. F. Lewis, Lawton	
Cotton	A. B. Holstead, Temple	Mollie F. Seism, Walters	Third Friday
Craig	F. M. Adams, Vinita	J. M. McMillan, Vinita	
Creek	H. R. Haas, Sapulpa	C. G. Oakes, Sapulpa	•
Custer	F. R. Vieregg, Clinton	C. J. Alexander, Clinton	Third Thursday
Garfield	Paul B. Champlin, Enid	John R. Walker, Enid	Fourth Thursday
Garvin	T. F. Gross, Lindsay	John R. Callaway, Pauls Valley	Wednesday before Third Thursday
Grady	Walter J. Baze, Chickasha	Roy E. Emanuel, Chickasha	Third Thursday
Grant	I. V. Hardy, Medford	E. E. Lawson, Medford	
Greer	G. P. Cherry, Mangum	J. B. Hollis, Mangum	
Harmon	W. G. Husband, Hollis		First Wednesday
Haskell	William Carson, Keota	N. K. Williams, McCurtain	
Hughes	Wm. L. Taylor, Holdenville	Imogene Mayfield, Holdenville	First Friday
Jackson	E. S. Crow, Olustee	E. W. Mabry, Altus	Last Monday
Jefferson	F. M. Edwards, Ringling	L. L. Wade, Ryan	Second Monday
Kay	Philip C. Risser, Blackwell	J. Holland Howe, Ponca City	Second Thursday
Kingfisher	C. M. Hodgson, Kingfisher	H. Violet Sturgeon, Hennessey	
Kiowa	B. H. Watkins, Hobart	J. William Finch, Hobart	
LeFlore	Neeson Rolle, Poteau	Rush L. Wright, Poteau	
Lincoln	H. B. Jenkins, Tryon	Carl H. Bailey, Stroud	First Wednesday
Logan	William C. Miller, Guthrie	J. L. LeHew, Jr., Guthrie	Last Tuesday
Marshall	O. A. Cook, Madill		
Mayes	Ralph V. Smith, Pryor	Paul B. Cameron, Pryor	
McClain	B. W. Slover, Blanchard	R. L. Royster, Purcell	
McCurtain	A. W. Clarkson, Valliant	N. L. Barker, Broken Bow	Fourth Tuesday
McIntosh	James L. Wood, Eufaula	William A. Tolleson, Eufaula	First Thursday
Murray	P. V. Annadown, Sulphur		Second Tuesday
Muskogee-Sequoyah-Wagoner	H. A. Scott, Muskogee	D. Evelyn Miller, Muskogee	First Monday
Noble	C. H. Cooke, Perry	J. W. Francis, Perry	
Okfuskee	L. J. Spickard, Okemah	M. L. Whitney, Okemah	Second Monday
Oklahoma	Walker Morledge, Oklahoma City	E. R. Musick, Oklahoma City	Fourth Tuesday
Okmulgee	A. R. Holmes, Henryetta	J. C. Matheney, Okmulgee	Second Monday
Osage	C. R. Weirich, Pawhuska	George K. Hemphill, Pawhuska	Second Monday
Ottawa	W. B. Sanger, Picher	Matt A. Connell, Picher	Third Thursday
Pawnee	E. T. Robinson, Cleveland	R. L. Browning, Pawnee	
Payne	L. A. Mitchell, Stillwater	C. W. Moore, Stillwater	Third Thursday
Pittsburg	John F. Park, McAlester	William H. Kaeiser, McAlester	Third Friday
Pontotoc	O. H. Miller, Ada	R. H. Mayes, Ada	First Wednesday
Pottawatomie	A. C. McFarling, Shawnee	Clinton Gallaher, Shawnee	First and Third Saturday
Pushmataha	John S. Lawson, Clayton	B. M. Huckabay, Antlers	
Rogers	C. W. Beson, Claremore	C. L. Caldwell, Chelsea	First Monday
Seminole	Max Van Sandt, Wewoka	Mack I. Shanholtz, Wewoka	Third Wednesday
Stephens	W. K. Walker, Marlow	Wallis S. Ivy, Duncan	
Texas	R. G. Obermiller, Texhoma	Morris Smith, Guymon	
Tillman		O. G. Bacon, Frederick	
Tulsa	James C. Peden, Tulsa	E. O. Johnson, Tulsa	Second and Fourth Monday
Washington-Nowata	J. G. Smith, Bartlesville	J. V. Athey, Bartlesville	Second Wednesday
Washita	A. S. Neal, Cordell	James F. McMurry, Sentinel	
Woods	C. A. Traverse, Alva	O. E. Templin, Alva	Last Tuesday Odd Months
Woodward	C. E. Williams, Woodward	C. W. Tedrowe, Woodward	Second Thursday

*(Serving in Armed Forces)

THE JOURNAL
OF THE
OKLAHOMA STATE MEDICAL ASSOCIATION

| VOLUME XXXVI | OKLAHOMA CITY, OKLAHOMA, NOVEMBER, 1943 | NUMBER 11 |

Some Clinical Observations on Coronary Sclerosis*

WANN LANGSTON, M.D.

OKLAHOMA CITY, OKLAHOMA

Coronary sclerosis is a pathological state of the coronary arteries occurring in and beyond middle life, chronic and progressive, and leading ultimately to impairment of the coronary circulation and myocardial nutrition. This results in a variety of clinical syndromes. These vary with the rapidity and the completeness of the interference with the circulation and the presence or absence of collateral anastamoses. While coronary arteriosclerosis is the predominant cause of inadequacy of the coronary circulation, identical syndromes sometimes occur from coronary obstruction due to other pathology. The diagnosis of coronary sclerosis depends upon the recognition of the syndromes of coronary inadequacy and the elimination of other causes of these syndromes.

In the beginning I want to digress long enough to point out that coronary sclerosis is not diagnosed by inspection of the electrocardiogram. Let me emphasize that advanced arteriosclerosis of the coronaries may exist without symptoms and without alteration in the appearance of the electrocardiogram, with symptoms and without electrocardiographic changes, without symptoms and with electrocardiographic changes and with symptoms and with alterations in the electrocardiogram. Also, may I point out that there is no characteristic appearance of the electrocardiogram in coronary sclerosis and furthermore, that there are many pathological processess that cause changes in the electrocardiogram identical with those commonly seen in cases of coronary sclerosis. It

*Read before the Annual Meeting held in Oklahoma City, May 11-12, 1943.

is, therefore, impossible to make the diagnosis of coronary sclerosis from the electrocardiogram alone. Grave injustices have been committed through such looseness in electrocardiographic reporting.

In the time allotted, it is possible to discuss but a few of the syndromes associated with coronary artery disease. I shall, therefore, pass over the subject of congestive failure except to mention briefly, acute left ventricular failure, paroxysmal dyspnea or cardiac asthma. While this syndrome may occur in connection with aortic valvular lesions and in hypertension, it is predominantly associated with coronary artery sclerosis. It is a dramatic episode, coming on suddenly without apparent provocation, frequently at night. It starts with oppression in the chest which rapidly increases to a sensation of intense suffocation with extreme dyspnea. The patient is frightened, pale, cyanotic and clammy. The accessory muscles of respiration are called into play and the labor which the patient undergoes is most distressing. He feels that he cannot possibly survive. Expiration may be prolonged and noisy and resemble that of bronchial asthma from which it must be differentiated. The victim assumes the upright position with legs hanging down. This position lessens the return of blood to the heart and gives some measure of relief. The attack may be brief and recovery spontaneous, or prolonged and require active measure for relief. This syndrome may be the only manifestation of coronary occlusion and may occur following an occlusion, or without an occlusion.

ANGINA PECTORIS

Angina pectoris is one of the common syndromes of coronary sclerosis and, in typical form, is readily recognized. The sequence, effort, pain, rest and relief is so characteristic as to be almost unmistakable. Too much emphasis has been placed on the localization of pain over the precordium and radiation into the arms and not enough on the character of the discomfort and the method of provocation. Perhaps in a majority of cases, this discomfort is localized behind the middle of the sternum, but just as characteristic is the pain in the spigastrium, in the neck, the shoulder, at the elbow or the wrist, with or without discomfort in the chest. The discomfort may be of almost any character and degree, mild or severe, aching, burning, crowding, crushing, tearing, cutting or prickling. It is provoked by exertion, emotion, eating, cold, hypertensive crisis, epinephrine, insulin. It is relieved by removal of the provocation and the administration of vaso-dilator drugs. The pulse is not affected, the blood pressure is either not affected or slightly elevated, the temperature, leucocyte count and sedimentation rate are not altered. The episodes are of brief duration, lasting from a few seconds to a few minutes, occurring at short or long intervals and are usually NOT accompanied by fear of impending death. The victim often learns by experience to predict the onset and thereby lays the foundation of management, avoidance of provocation. In the intervals between attacks the electrocardiogram is either negative, or the abnormality is that of myocardial damage. There is no characteristic electrocardiogram of the anginal patient. On the other hand, if one is fortunate enough to secure a tracing during an attack, which is very seldom the case, definite alterations in form frequently occur. This fact is sometimes utilized in the diagnosis of obscure cases. Most cases of angina pectoris culminate in coronary occlusion. Increasing frequency and severity of attacks portend early occlusion, and one can sometimes predict the onset of this catastrophe.

The vagaries of angina pectoris frequently are interesting and puzzling. Symptoms appear under circumstances that represent very slight effort while the patient can perform strenuous exercise of another type, or at another time, with impunity. A most interesting case is that of a seventy year old physician who had never had cardiac or gastric symptoms until one morning, after his usual breakfast, he started to walk a block to see a patient. After about half a block he was seized with a severe distress in the spigastrium and had to sit down for a few moments, after which he was able to continue, and he had no more trouble that day. However, the following morning and succeeding mornings he had the same experience. At all other times this man was able to walk without discomfort even after a hearty meal, and was able to drive long distances and to work in his yard and garden. He simply could not walk after breakfast. After being advised to take a tablet of nitroglycerine before starting the walk he experienced no more difficulty. A year after onset he is still active and the disturbance has ceased.

An accurate history, taken by the clinician himself, is the most valuable procedure in the diagnosis of angina pectoris. The family history is exceedingly important. We get a positive family history of vascular disease in about 80 per cent of our angina cases. There may be no abnormal objective findings. More often than not there is no considerable enlargement of the heart to be demonstrated even by fluoroscopy and usually there are no abnormal sounds. In a great many instances the resting electrocardiogram is essentially normal. If abnormal, there is no characteristic finding and all one may say is that there is evidence of myocardial damage. One is never justified in diagnosing angina pectoris from the electrocardiogram alone. Any number of abnormalities may show in tracings from patients with angina pectoris but they are the reflections of damage to the myocardium and not of the anginal syndrome. The electrocardiogram can be of value in the diagnosis of obscure but suspicious syndromes. The test is carried out in the following manner: a resting tracing is made, the patient is then required to exercise until he develops slight pain or discomfort and an immediate tracing is made; he then rests for five to ten minutes and a third tracing is made. In many angina cases, very striking displacements of the RS-T segments downward, or flattening or inversion of T waves are found.

CASE 1. A 68 year old man was seized suddenly with excrutiating pain in the chest while opening his garage door on February 1, 1942. This was accompanied by mild shock and followed by slight fever for a few days. The electrocardiogram on the first day was inconclusive, but later indicated a posterier infarction. After a stormy course, he made a fairly satisfactory recovery, but when he began to get around he developed angina of effort. Later he began to have severe episodes without apparent provocation. It was observed that these episodes were accompanied by marked elevation of blood pressure, and we regarded these as hypertensive crises. These attacks were relieved by nitroglycerine, by inhalation of oxygen and by whiskey, but were not influenced in the least by continuous administration of large doses of aminophyllin. Attacks occurred with increasingly frequency until he was having four to eight a day. On February 4, 1943, in my office, immediately after I had made a resting electrocardiogram, he was seized with an attack and I was fortunate enough to get an electrocardiogram during the attack and another immediately after relief by nitroglycerine. Figure 1 shows very well what happens to the electrocardiogram during an anginal episode, and also shows the return to previous appearance after vaso-dilatation. This man died suddenly without pain several days after this tracing was made.

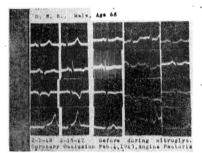

Fig. 1

CASE 2. A 51 year old male had had chest pain for several years according to the formula: exertion, pain, rest, relief. In January of this year he had a severe episode of chest pain associated with distressing dyspnea. He was put to bed for six weeks and then got up and around without difficulty. On March 9 he had another severe bout of pain and during the day several minor episodes produced by walking and relieved by nitroglycerine. On March 10 he came to my office for examination. He had a normal blood pressure and pulse rate, the heart only slightly enlarged, no abnormal sounds and no evidence of congestive failure. The electrocardiogram is extremely interesting. See Fig. 2: left, resting; middle, immediately after slight exercise; right, after five minutes' rest. This undoubtedly represents severe ischemia of the myocardium, and one has no difficulty in prognosticating catastrophe. Three days later he had a severe attack and died suddenly while talking to his physician.

While these cases illustrate the reactions in some cases of angina pectoris I could cite others just as striking in which no such electrocardiogram changes occurred.

CORONARY OCCLUSION

Coronary occlusion is the most dramatic and most tragic of the syndromes associated with coronary sclerosis. It is usually on the

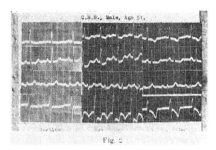

Fig. 2

basis of a thrombus on an atheromatous area, but may be due occasionally to a sub-intimal hemorrhage in a coronary artery, or from the blocking of the ostium of one of the coronaries by syphilitic involvement of the aorta; and rarely from an embolus, usually from valve vegetations of bacterial endocarditis. The end result of occlusion is usually infarction with necrosis. Sometimes necrosis occurs without demonstrable occlusion. If collateral circulation is adequate, occlusion may occur without infarction. The process of thrombosis is gradual but occlusion is sudden. Upon these conditions depends the type of episode encountered.

The typical attack is readily recognized. The sudden onset, usually without provocation, of excrutiating pain in any portion of chest or upper abdomen, anginal in character but persistent, with waxing and waning, with or without radiation to the arms, shoulder, neck or back, with or without rapid drop in blood pressure, with or without shock, followed in a few hours by fever and leucocytosis, in a day or two by increased sedimentation rate of the blood, and sometimes with early, oftener with later, characteristic alterations in the electrocardiogram, make the diagnosis comparatively simple. There is a considerable group of cases however in which the diagnosis is not so clear, and it is of some of these particularly that I wish to speak for a few minutes.

CASE 3. R. C. M., male, age 53, consulted me on October 2, 1942, because, on two days previous, he had severe substernal discomfort coming on after a hearty meal. During the past two weeks he had had several minor episodes of discomfort which he attributed to indigestion. He carried an insurance policy which provided for an annual examination, and a few days before he consulted us he had this examination including an electrocardiogram, and had been pronounced sound in health. His past history was not relevant but his family history was, in that a number of paternal relatives including his father had died of heart disease. The physicial examination likewise was negative. The electrocardiogram was negative in the limb leads, but the T wave was inverted in 4F. This together with the history lead us to suspect and predict a gradually progressive occlusion. He was given relative rest, aminophyllin, and sedatives, nitroglycerine and alcohol with some apparent alleviation of symptoms for a week or two. We repeated the electrocardiograms frequently, and watched the progressive alteration, particularly in leads 1 and 4F. On October 25, about six weeks after first symptoms, and three weeks after we had first seen him, he had a typical coronary syndrome with prolonged pain and shock, followed by fever, leucocytosis, increased sedimentation rate and a characteristic electrocardiogram. He had a mild course and an uneventful convalescence, was allowed up at the end of six weeks, was fairly active at the end of three months, and now after six months is carrying on his regular occupation as an executive in a large firm, and is symptom free. See Fig. 3.

This case is interesting because of the gradual onset and progession to complete occlusion, the relatively mild course and prompt recovery. We believe that in such a case there is development of collateral circulation that serves to limit the size of the infarct, prevents severe shock, and makes more prompt recovery possible.

The next case is similar in some respects but has other interesting aspects.

CASE 4. M. G. S., male, age 45, experienced his first discomfort in the chest while on a Boy Scout hike last summer. On his first visit to us on January 9, 1943, he complained of pain in the chest, shoulders and arms on walking short distances, and over some period of time. It required less and less provocation to produce distress. He developed pain much more quickly after eating, or walking against a cold wind, and finally, just exposure to cold wind without any exertion whatever produced attacks. Physical examination was negative, blood pressure and pulse rate normal, heart was not enlarged and there were no abnormal sounds. The past history was unrevealing, but the family history was significant in that father, mother and a brother had died of heart disease. The electrocardiogram on January 9 was negative. By March 9 when we next saw him, in spite of the conventional treatment for angina pectoris, the attacks had become more frequent, even sometimes waking him from sleep. The electrocardiogram on this date showed slight inversion of T in lead 3. There is also very slight elevation of the S-T segment, neither significant in the isolated electrocardiogram, but very significant when compared with the one made two months before. We were sufficiently impressed that he was hospitalized for observation. Complete bed rest was not enforced. He continued to have episodes for about a week when they ceased altogether. This aroused our suspicions in spite of the fact that he had had no fever, no drop in blood pressure, no change in pulse rate. Electrocardiogram on April 8 showed some progression. On April 18 the electrocardiogram was characteristic, there was leucocytosis, rapid sedimentation rate but no fever. Blood pressure did not, at any time, show any significant drop and there was never any shock. This man has had no discomfort whatsoever since about April 8, has had an uneventful course and appears to be well on the way to recovery.

Coronary sclerosis is an arteriosclerotic process of the coronary arteries, a part of a more or less generalized arteriosclerosis. The

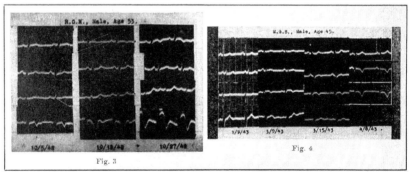

Fig. 3

Fig. 4

cause of arteriosclerosis is as yet undetermined. Certain factors apparently play a part. Heredity cannot be ignored. Strain is probably a factor. Lipoid metabolism seems to be disturbed, and may be a causative factor. The condition is insidious and progressive. Extensive damage may be done before symptoms appear. Coronary sclerosis may masquerade under the guise of indigestion, neurasthenia, fatigue syndromes, etc. Its symptoms may be simulated by many organic and functional disturbances, as intercostal neuritis, spinal arthritis, gastro-intestinal and other digestive disturbances, etc. Its syndromes vary with the type of pathological disturbance. If the smaller arterioles are mainly involved with repeated small occlusions, myocardial fibrosis occurs and congestive failure and paroxysmal dyspnea are likely to occur. When there is disparity between blood demand and blood supply due to narrowing of the larger vessel, angina pectoris in some of its forms occurs. If there is complete occlusion of a larger branch with necrosis of the myocardium we recognize the state of myocardial infarction. Apparently if the occlusive process is gradual in developement collateral circulation has an opportunity to develop and milder episodes with better prognosis occur.

MANAGEMENT

It is not my purpose to discuss the management of the various syndromes of coronary sclerosis in detail. For the most part it is well known. I shall call attention only to a few procedures that have given me some satisfaction. As to the pathological process, I know of no therapeudic procedure that will affect it or its progress in the least. I have had no convincing experience with xanthines, iodides or vaso-dilators.

Cardiac Asthma: Opium, particularly morphine, is specific for the attack. Aminophylline, intravenously, gives prompt relief in many cases and venesection sometimes works dramatically. Nitroglycerine frequently will relieve the paroxysm, especially when associated with hypertension. One of the most satisfactory procedures in cardiology is the use of mercurial diuretics intravenously as a prophylactic in cardiac asthma. One cubic centimeter of Salyrgon-Theophylline will frequently insure relief for from one to three or four weeks, and the patients come back for more. In spite of the untoward effects reported, I have failed to see any such and have no hesitancy in commending it to your use in this situation. It goes without saying that these patients will be kept digitalized.

Angina Pectoris: . The most important therapeutic principle is avoidance of provocation. Patients learn by experience what activity to avoid. If it becomes necessary to perform some act that he expects to produce an attack, a tablet of nitroglycerine will frequently enable him to carry on without distress. Amyl nitrite seems to me to have no important place in the therapy of this condition. It will do nothing that nitroglycerine will not do as well with less disagreeable side effects. The other nitrites have been of no help in my hands. Alcohol is of definite value in the management of these cases. I have been greatly disappointed in the xanthines in the prevention of discomfort or improvement of reserve. Testosterone has been used and there are some favorable reports. I have used it in a few cases with some satisfaction. Its value cannot yet be evaluated. Peculiarly some cases of angina pectoris appear to recover spontaneously in so far as the paroxysms of provoked pain is concerned. Rest is fundamental, excesses must be avoided, smoking should be eliminated, diet must be moderate, rest periods after eating are important, hurry and worry should be eliminated.

Coronary Occlusion: Coronary occlusion is usually a painful and shocking episode. The first measures should be to relieve the pain and combat the shock. For pain, morphine, oxygen, aminophylline or papaverine intravenously are of value. The usual methods of combating shock are used. First in importance is complete and prolonged rest. Moderate dietary, attention to bowels with the least possible exertion on the part of the patient are important. Next in importance is avoidance of over-medication. Then, meet complications if and when they arise. The prognosis is always guarded, but some idea can be obtained from the height and prolongation of fever, leucocytosis and sedimentation rate. The last is important in determining when the patient can be allowed to be out of bed. These patients should never be discouraged. There is a 70 per cent chance for recovery, and an excellent chance that a fair degree of activity can be attained after an adequate period of convalescence Many of these people can be rehabilitated and returned to their former occupation, and this should be the goal in every case.

DISCUSSION

JOSEPH T. PHELPS, M. D.
EL RENO, OKLAHOMA

Since angina pectoris is usually the first indication of coronary sclerosis offering us the earliest opportunity of controlling the progress of the disease, I would like to discuss in a little more detail the treatment of this condition.

The treatment of angina pectoris naturally falls into two parts. First, the treatment of the attack itself and second, the prevention of further attacks.

The treatment of an attack of angina pectoris consists of two important measures, rest and certain vasodilator drugs. Rest is probably the more important. The patient himself soon learns that absolute quiet, either standing or sitting or lying still for a few moments is sufficient to allow the attack to pass. He often finds that the upright position, either sitting or standing, shortens the attack more than lying down, since in the upright position the return flow of blood to the heart is lessened and the work of the heart is thereby decreased. He usually finds that continuing exercise increases the severity and length of the attack. For these reasons, the patient learns, from his own experience, that rest is imperative. Failing to rest surely results in much more severe attacks and may result in death.

Of the drugs used to alleviate an attack, the most common and most effective is some of the nitrites, of which nitroglycerine is the most convenient and dependable, since it is inexpensive and easy for the patient to carry. One tablet of $1/100$ grain placed under the tongue will relieve most attacks in a few minutes. This may be repeated as often as needed as there seems to be no limit to the number of doses that may be safely taken. Other drugs of this same class which may be used in the absence of nitroglycerine are amyl nitrate, sodium nitrate, erythrol tetranitrate, none of which are as generally satisfactory as nitroglycerine and should usually be used only if nitroglycerine is not easily available.

After the immediate symptoms of the attack have been controlled our next problem is to advise the patient as to the proper course to pursue in preventing further attacks. This is not alway easy or even possible but there are certain fundamental principles which, if followed will enable a large number of patients to continue a reasonably active life in comfort. The same treatment in a certain percentage of cases seems to have no effect on the progress of the disease, or the recurrence of attacks.

Rest is the most important of all prophylactic measures. By that is meant relief from mental disturbances and from all exercise which is found to produce an attack. All excesses such as over eating, excessive use of tobacco, coffee or tea, should be avoided. The patient must be advised to avoid long, continued exertion of any kind, loss of sleep, constipation with excessive straining at stool, and mental worries as nearly as possible. It may even be necessary in some cases to advise bed rest until the symptoms are under control. He should be advised that permanent limitation of activities will usually be necessary.

Many patients suffering of angina pectoris are overweight. There is some evidence that disturbances of metabolism also are associated with the disease and for this reason it is often helpful to restrict the intake of food very greatly. The Karell diet, consisting of 200 cc of milk, four times daily and no other food, has been recommended. A little additional water is allowed for thirst. After a few days of this diet a distinct feeling of weakness and hunger develops and it has been observed that attacks of angina pectoris which have occurred frequently then disappear. After a few days of the Karell diet, small amounts of other food should be added to the diet, taking care not to allow over-feeding, even light foods, as attacks often follow a heavy meal. The loss of weight and lowered metabolism resulting from such a diet are reported to lessen the frequency and severity of attacks in many cases.

Certain drugs have been recommended for the prevention of attacks of angina pectoris. Chief among these are the purine derivatives, of which aminophyllin has probably been the most widely used and seems to get the best results. This drug seems to be entirely harmless and so can be administered over long periods of time. It is given with the hope of increasing the lumen of the coronary vessels, thereby increasing the blood supply to the heart muscle. It should be given by mouth in doses of one and one-half to three grains, three or four times daily and should be continued long enough to be certain of the results obtained before other remedies are tried. This drug may profitably be combined with a nerve sedative such as phenobarbital in small doses since most people who have angina pectoris also have an oversensitive nervous system which probably is a factor in the attacks.

It does not seem rational to me to give drugs such as nitrites or alcohol to enable a patient to do a little more work without symptoms. This may mask the symptoms and rob the patient of his only means of determining his exercise tolerance. For this reason, I never advise the use of drugs for this purpose.

In recent years, certain surgical procedures have been tried and found somewhat effective in a limited number of cases. These include sympathectomy, paravertebral in-

jections of alcohol or novocain, total thyroidectomy and implantation of the subpectoral muscles into the paricardial sac in order to establish a collateral circulation. These are all rather radical measures which should be used only as a last resort.

Finally, it would seem that if we see these patients enough and can gain their cooperation in a routine of life consisting of moderate exercise, a cheerful mental attitude, and cultivated poise, and if we can secure for them proper rest, proper diet and give them the advantage of what drug therapy we have, we can feel that we have given them the best chance possible for a reasonably comfortable life.

The Interrelationship of Solid, Liquid and Gas Metabolism*

EDWARD C. MASON, M.D.

Department of Physiology, University of Oklahoma School of Medicine

OKLAHOMA CITY, OKLAHOMA

I hope this ambitious and comprehensive title has not misled you. It is evident that the interpretation of the interaction of the three states of matter, (solid, liquid and gas, within the individual includes the entire field of physiology, and I could add medicine. However, I am going to develop only the fundamental principles that furnish us a working knowledge and an intelligent conception of the numerous problems we may expect to meet. Such problems include the various peripheral vascular diseases; shock, burns, edema of various origins, acid-base-fluid balance, toxemia of pregnancy and, last but not least, abnormal psychological response.

It is quite common to consider the order of importance of these three states of matter to be, *first* solids, *second* liquids and *third* gas. Actually the order of their immediate importance is just the reverse. Urgent need for gas is expressed in terms of seconds, liquids in terms of hours, and solids in terms of days. Therefore, the treatment of an emergency is usually met by aiding gas-

eous exchange or adjusting fluid balance and seldom is an emergency due to insufficient solids. Since faulty gaseous exchange may cause an emergency within a few seconds, I shall begin by discussing this phase of the subject.

THE INTERACTION OF GAS AND SOLID

The inexperienced individual is of the opinion that the more abundantly oxygen is supplied to his tissues, especially his central nervous system, the better he should feel physically and mentally. Actually such is not the case and this is evidenced by the fact that many are willing to pay $5.00 per pint for something that decreases oxidation processes in the brain and thereby gives them the anoxic glow of self-satisfaction.

The opposite personality response may be experienced if the individual increases his rate and depth of breathing. He will then experience doubts, fears, anxieties and lack of self-confidence. We are indebted to Dr. Hinshaw for calling our attention to the fact that hyperventilation is a possible hazard to pilots in both commercial and military aviation.

(*Presented at the monthly staff meeting of the University Hospitals, April 2, 1943.)

While attempting to land his plane in turbulent weather, he became aware that he had certain unwarranted doubts, anxieties, and lack of coordinated skill. Also he became aware that he was hyperventilating and by voluntarily controlling his respiration he quickly regained his normal composure.[1] Following his experiences he and his colleagues made a study of hyperventilation and published their results the latter part of 1941.[2] Most of their subjects, after hyperventilation, showed a markedly diminished ability to perform the coordination test. Hinshaw was of the opinion that the freezing on the controls might be due to the tetany resulting from hyperventilation and he also suggested that stage fright might be a related phenomenon.

We have indicated that the effects of acute anoxia are very similar to those of acute alcoholism. In both, the chief hazard is the absence of physical or mental discomfort or pain which would give the individual a warning of the impending danger. He experiences a sence of comfort and well-being, a feeling of self-satisfaction, and may indulge in outbursts of hilarity or become quarrelsome. His memory is blunted and his judgment and capacity for self-criticism markedly impaired. He is not aware of his shortcomings or inabilities and may feel that he is giving a remarkable performance. He develops a fixity of purpose and will continue whatever task he is engaged in regardless of the consequences. The trapped miner suffering from anoxia, due to the presence of fire damp, may be only a few feet from a passageway which he knows would supply his needed oxygen but he will remain where he is and write death notes. Also, an aviator may realize his need for oxygen but instead of reaching for a valve beside his head he may continue without oxygen and pass out.

The personality change accompanying acute anoxia is probably the cause of numerous aviation accidents and the pilot, in such an accident, is probably not responsible for his error in judgment or his muscle incoordination. There is no doubt that the repeated exposure to reduced oxygen pressure can cause definite and permanent damage to brain tissue. Complete anoxia for 30 to 60 seconds will produce definite histological changes[3]. It is quite possible that the "staleness" which developed during the first World War in aviators who flew at high altitudes without the aid of oxygen, was in reality the result of brain degeneration. Also, the special type of neurosis, the so-called aeroneurosis, described by Armstrong[4] as affecting experienced pilots, may be the cumulative effects of anoxia and resulting brain changes. The symptoms of chronic anoxia experienced by dwellers at high altitudes and aviators are quite the same and include emotional instability, lessened ability to concentrate, decreased patience, constant fatigue, unrefreshing sleep, anxiety and loss of self-confidence.

The above symptoms, resulting from anoxia and so characteristic of the neurotic, may also be produced by a slight alteration in solid metabolism. Recently, Sandler[5] has studied a group of such cases. The individuals experienced headaches, nervousness, dizziness, vasomotor instability, irritability, ill temper, sweats, faintness and syncope. The group had had numerous abdominal operations, some of them having had two operations, however, their distress recurred and they were considered as confirmed neurotics. Following a more careful examination it was determined that they were the victims of chronic hypoglycemia and when given a diet high in fat and protein and low in carbohydrate, they were relieved of their distress. It is to be expected that chronic hypoglycemia should give the same picture as chronic anoxia due to the fact that tissues consume oxygen in proportion as they utilize glucose. This is especially the case in tissues having a respiratory quotient of unity, including the brain. It has been repeatedly demonstrated that during hypoglycemia there is a diminished oxygen consumption by the brain [6,7,8,9]. Fortunately, hypoglycemia and its accompanying symptoms are usually reversible, however, fatal cases have occurred with demonstrable cerebral lesions, especially hemorrhages.[10] Such hemorrhagic lesions are probably related to the observations of Landis,[11] who observed that fluid passes through capillary walls at four times the normal rate after only three minutes lack of oxygen.

While anoxia or hypoglycemia may produce organic and psychological changes, there is a third substance, the deficiency of which may produce changes and symptoms quite similar to those of hypoglycemia. In the course of the induced deficiency of this substance, the subjects who were previously cheerful, happy, vigorous, industrious, young individuals changed and became morose, depressed, fearful, irritable, uncooperative and slovenly in personal appearance. They had neither the strength nor the interest to work. This substance is thiamine and the final proof that Vitamin B1 functioned as an oxidative catalyst was presented by Peters and his collaborators.[12] In the form of its pyrophosphate it is needed for the oxidative removal of pyruvic acid, and indirectly, of lactic acid. Thus it becomes evident why thiamine deficiency gives rise to the various symptoms produced by anoxia or hypoglycemia. *The presence of all three are required to maintain normal metabolism of nerve tissue.*

THE INTERACTION OF GAS AND LIQUID

We will first consider the change in fluid balance resulting from excessive gas exchange. During hyperventilation, two substances leave the blood stream, carbon dioxide and sodium. This blowing off of carbon dioxide soon leads to a reduction of the carbon dioxide capacity (alkaline reserve) of the blood, the average fall in carbon dioxide combining power of venous plasma being 14.3 per cent.[13] Henderson and Haggard were of the opinion that the alkali passed into the tissues and they also noted that when the alveolar carbon dioxide was again raised, the alkaline reserve was restored, due apparently to the passage of alkali from the tissues into the blood. Subsequent work on hyperventilation has revealed the fact that the kidney shares with other body tissues in the passage of sodium from the blood stream. The percentage increase in sodium phosphate excretion during hyperventilation is always greater than the percentage of water increase, e.g., accompanying a five-fold increase in water excretion, there is a six-fold increase in sodium phosphate excretion. The sequence of events indicate that the excessive sodium phosphate excretion is the result of the diuresis and not the cause. During hyperventilation the volume of urine is greatly increased and it becomes alkaline, however, for a period following hyperventilation there is even a greater increase in urine output and it then becomes acid. During this period the alveolar carbon dioxide and consequently, the blood carbon dioxide, returns toward the normal and combines the sodium to build up the plasma bicarbonate, therefore, the urine becomes acid. Hyperventilation for 32 minutes may cause an increase in urinary output from 46 cc per hour to 220 cc per hour.

Summarizing, we find that hyperventilation leads to an acidosis which is due to the loss of carbon dioxide and sodium. Also accompanying the acidosis there is a marked increase in water excretion. The question now arises, "What is the result of reversing the procedure, that is, increasing the body carbon dioxide and sodium?" The effect on fluid balance should be just the reverse of hyperventilation, and such is the case. We have demonstrated that the administration of sodium bicarbonate (4 grams t.i.d. for three days) to 49 normal subjects increased their total body weight 111.75 pounds, the greatest individual gain being 6.5 pounds.[14] These findings support the idea that acidosis promotes loss of body fluid while alkalosis causes fluid accumulation.

Testing the above conceptions still further we may observe the effect of acidosis produced by means other than hyperventilation. Acidosis may be produced by the administration of calcium chloride, ammonium chloride or any salt that has been prepared from a weak base and strong acid. These salts in solution yield an acid reaction and since all are effective in treating edema, it is evident that the cation is not the effective agent. We have administered ammonium chloride (6 grams daily for 3 days) to 31 normal subjects and observed a total weight loss of 61 pounds, the greatest individual loss being 3.75 pounds. Thus we observe that acidosis produced either by hyperventilation or the administration of an acid-forming salt is accompanied by a fluid loss.

THE MECHANISM OF TISSUE HYDRATION

The normal blood plasma contains approximately 7 per cent protein, therefore, this protein is capable of holding somewhat more than 13 times its mass of water. The plasma protein represents complexes of amino acids, a large portion of which are complexes of amino fatty acids. Without the amino group these simple fatty acids may unite with bases to form soaps and a study of the factors producing their hydration and dehydration should yield information concerning the hydration and dehydration of proteins. The sodium soaps of any fatty acid series show a progressive increase in water-holding capacity as we pass from the lower to the higher members of the series, e.g., the gram molecular weight of sodium caprylate holds 200 cc of water while the gram molecular weight of sodium arachidate holds 37,000 cc. The difference in the hydration of these two soaps cannot be due to the osmotic pressure exerted by sodium since the amount of sodium in each is the same.

If any given fatty acid is combined with various bases, the water-holding power of the resulting soap will vary with each base used and follows the order of NH4, K, Na, Mg, Ca, Ba, Hg. This Hofmeister series also holds for proteins, the alkali proteins being the most hydrated, the alkali earths less and the heavy metal protein combinations the least. Again this does not follow the law of osmotic pressure since equal osmotic concentrations should yield equal osmotic pressure.

We have observed that the acidification of body tissues by either the acidosis of hyperventilation or the addition of an acid forming salt results in water loss, and the addition of an alkaline substance such as sodium bicarbonate increases tissue hydration. Soaps also respond to these agents in the same manner; if we add acid to a soap, such as sodium stearate, the soap loses its hydrophilic properties. The hydrogen stearate (stearic acid) formed has a low water-holding power when compared with the original soap and it is evident that no amount of water present will change its hydrophilic properties. This point should be kept in mind when one considers the relative value of water vs. salt restriction in the treatment of edema. If the soap is treated with an alkali, its hydration capacity is not decreased and if any free stearic acid is present it may be converted to sodium stearate and thus increase the hydrophilic properties.

Turning to the plasma proteins we find that, gram for gram, the plasma albumin is much more hydrophilic than the plasma globulin. A one per cent plasma albumin has a water-holding power equal to 7.54 cm of water and a one per cent globulin, 1.95 cm Those favoring the osmotic pressure idea explain this by the fact that the albumin is a smaller particle and, therefore, more particles are present per unit mass. However, the relative size of the two molecules does not support such a conclusion. Also, we have noted that the sodium salt of the large molecules of any fatty acid series holds more water than the lower members of the series. Therefore, everything being equal, the globulin should be more hydrophilic than the albumin. We are forced to explain the difference in the hydrophilic properties of these two substances on some other basis and the difference in their iso-electric point seems to be the answer. The farther the protein is from its iso-electric point, the higher its hydration capacity and at its iso-electric point it has the least hydration. The iso-electric point of plasma albumin is 4.7 and that of the globulin is 5.4 and since both exist in the blood stream with a pH of 7.4, it is evident that the albumin is farther from its iso-electric point. At the iso-electric point, the protein has electrical neutrality, therefore has maximum cohesion, maximum surface tension, smallest mass possible and least hydration capacity.

Considering the other portion of the blood, the red blood cells, we find that the size of the red cells does not remain constant throughout the course of circulation. When the cells give up oxygen they combine with carbon dioxide and this union competes with the hemoglobin for the available base, the resulting combination of tissue, carbon dioxide, and base is more hydrophilic, therefore, the cells swell. Apparently this same order of events occurs in body tissues outside the blood stream, the carbon dioxide combining with the tissue and this union in turn combines with the available base. Is should be remembered that red muscle contains hemoglobin and in addition there is a chromogenic compound, cytochrome, which is found not only in muscle but also in other animal tissues. These hemochromogens are compounds of heme and protein. Also we should consider another possible factor. Roughton

has called attention to the fact that carbon dioxide may combine with the NH2 group of the hemoglobin to form carbamino compounds and probably as much as 20 per cent of the carbon dioxide is carried by this reaction. It is evident that the carbamino reaction could also occur with the cytochromes of the various body tissues, and if carbon dioxide reacts with the NH2 group of hemoglobin, why could it not react with any NH2 group presented by the amino acids forming tissue proteins? This would yield an abundance of carboxyl groups which in turn may be used to combine base. The result would yield increased hydration capacity.

APPLICATION OF THE STATED MECHANISM

Throughout this discussion we have maintained that the accumulation of carbon dioxide in the body tissues leads to the addition of base and the resulting combination becomes more hydrated. This has been illustrated by considering the volume increase of the red blood cell when it is subjected to increased carbon dioxide concentration. The same sequence of events occurs during the activity of skeletal muscle, the muscle increases in weight[15] and this is accompanied by a marked change in the distribution of water and electrolytes[16,17].

Fluid can pass in and out of the body tissues only through the blood. The blood plasma proteins hold approximately 13 times their weight of water and this would represent about three liters in the average man. Contrasted with these figures we find that the body tissues hold only approximately three times their weight of water, however, this still represents about 43 liters. The three liters of available plasma fluid is maintained in delicate equilibrum with the 43 liters of tissue fluid. This equilibrium is disturbed when the hydrophilic capacity of the body tissues is increased or when the hydrophilic capacity of the plasma is decreased. If a marked disturbance in the equilibrium occurs, the result is edema formation.

The object in treating edema is to restore the normal fluid equilibrium between the blood plasma and body tissues. This may be accomplished by either reducing the hydration capacity of the tissues or increasing the hydration capacity of the plasma. Decrease in the hydration capacity of the tissues may be accomplished by removing the carbon dioxide as in hyperventilation or by administering acid forming salts. The water and sodium thus freed are removed by the circulating plasma, provided the hydrophilic colloids of the plasma are in adequate concentration.

Apparently the mopping up of the free water and sodium by the plasma is essentially a mechanical process and may be accomplished by various hydrophilic colloids including gum acacia. The intravenous use of gum acacia in nephrosis will effectively remove both the retained water and salt. [18]

The use of high protein diet in the treatment of edema serves the double role of maintaining the plasma proteins at a high level and maintaining an acid reaction. It is evident why the diet should be such as to yield an acid ash and it may be necessary to augment the acid reaction by adding acid forming salts. The sodium intake should be maintained at the physiological minimum and sodium bicarbonate has no place in the treatment.

Fluid restriction should not be practiced provided the following three conditions are maintained: 1. adequate removal of carbon dioxide, 2. adequate plasma colloids and 3. restricted sodium intake. Actually, increased fluid administration is indicated in most cases and this is due to the fact that such patients are usually required to excrete much more urine than the normal to remove a given amount of solids; a patient with a fixed specific gravity of 1.010 to 1.015 must excrete approximately three times as much urine as the normal. If fluid is restricted in the nonedematous they use their own body fluid to remove the solids; this is evidenced by the fact that they usually maintain a normal blood chemistry. However, fluid restriction in the edematous is not met by the same mechanism and they continue to retain both their body fluid and urinary solids. [19]

BIBLIOGRAPHY

1. Hinshaw, H. C., and Boothby, W. M.: Syndrome of Hyperventilation: Its Importance in Aviation. Proc. Staff Meeting, Mayo Clin., Vol. 16, pages 211-213. 1941.

2. Rushmer, R. F., Boothby, W. M. Hinshaw, H. C.: Some Effects of Hyperventilation with Special Reference to Aviation Medicine. Proc. Staff Meet., Mayo Clin., Vol. 16, pages 801-808. 1941.

3. Thorner, M. W., and Lowry, F. H.: Effect of Repeated Anoxia on the Brain. Jour. A.M.A., Vol. 115, page 1595. 1940.

4. Armstrong, H. G.: Principles and Practice of Aviation Medicine. Page 496. Williams and Wilkins Company, Baltimore. 1939.

5. Sandler, B. P.: Chronic Abdominal Pain Due to Hypoglycemia. Surgery, Vol. 9, page 331. 1941.

6. Himwich, H. E., and Fazekas, J. F.: The Effect of Hypoglycemia on the Metabolism of the Brain. Endocrinology, Vol. 21, page 800. 1937.

7. Holmes, E. G.: Oxidations in Central and Peripheral Nervous Tissues. Biochem., Vol. 24, page 914. 1930.

8. Dickens, F. and Breville, G. D.: Metabolism of Normal and Tumor Tissue. Biochem., Vol. 27, page 832. 1933.

9. Wortis, S. B.: Respiratory Metabolism of Excised Brain Tissue. Amer. Jour Psychiat., Vol. 90, page 725. 1934.

10. Baker, A. B., and Lufkin, N. H.: Cerebral Lesions in Hypoglycemia. Arch. Path., Vol. 23, page 190. 1937.

11. Landis, E. M.: Micro-Injection Studies of Capillary Permeability: III. The Effect of Lack of Oxygen on the Permeability of the Capillary Wall to Fluid and to the Plasma Proteins. Amer. Jour. Physiol., Vol. 83, page 528. 1928.

12. Peters et al: Biochem., Vol. 33, page 1109. 1939.

13. Collip, J. B., and Backus, P. L.: The Effect of Prolonged Hyperpnea on the Carbon Dioxide Combining Power of the Plasma, the Carbon Dioxide Tension of Alveolar Air and the Excretion of Acid and Basic Phosphate and Ammonia by the Kidney. Amer. Jour. Physiol., Vol. 51, pages 568-579. 1920.

14. Mason, E. C., and Hellbaum, A. A.: Acid-Base Water Balance. Annals of Internal Medicine, Vol. 11, page 2206. 1938

15. Bancroft, J. and Kato, T.: The Effect of Functional Activity Upon the Metabolism, Blood Flow and Exudation of Organs. Proc. Roy. Soc., Vol. 88, page 541. 1915.

16. Fenn, W. O.: Changes in Electrolytes After Exercise. Physiol. Rev., Vol. 16, page 478. 1936.

17. Fenn, W. O, and Cobb, D. M.: Electrolyte Changes in Muscle During Activity. Amer. Jour. Physiol., Vol. 113, page 345. 1936.

18. Lehnhoff, H. J., and Binger, M. W.: Nephrosis: Treatment in an Unusual Case. Proc. Staff Meet., Mayo Clin., Vol. 17, page 80. 1942.

19. Newburgh, L. H., and Lashmet, F. H.: The Importance of Dealing Quantitatively with Water in the Study of Disease. Amer. Jour. Med. Scien., Vol. 186, page 461. 1933.

The Control of Syphilis in Oklahoma Industry[*]

DAVID V. HUDSON, M.D.

TULSA, OKLAHOMA

The nationwide program for the control of venereal diseases assumed enormous proportions when the United States entered the war. The blood testing of selectees revealed a large number of individuals with positive and doubtful serologic tests. The examination of these men and the treatment of those found to have syphilis materially increased the work of private physicians and venereal

*Read before the Annual Meeting held in Oklahoma City, May 11-12, 1943.

disease clinics. Many persons with uncomplicated syphilis, at first rejected, have received adequate treatment and are now in the armed services. More recently, selectees with uncomplicated syphilis have been inducted and treatment given them in camp.

Vonderlehr and Usilton,[1] analyzing the reports of clinical examinations and blood tests given to 1,895,778 selectees and volunteers from 21 to 35 years of age through August 31, 1941, report the average syphilis rate of 44 states and the District of Columbia to be 47.7 per cent per thousand. In Oklahoma, the total syphilis rate, white and colored, was 54.7 per cent per thousand, whites, 39.5 per cent and colored, 254.5 per cent per thousand. Further analysis and calculation showed national prevalence rates of 30.1 per cent per thousand for men 21 to 25 years of age, 54.5 per cent for men 26 to 30 and 83.2 per cent for men 31 to 35 years of age. Thus it is apparent that the rate increases with age and it could reasonably be expected that men over 36 years of age would have a higher rate or at least as high as the 26 to 30 year old group. For purposes of classification it is generally accepted by the U.S. Army and the U.S. Public Health Service that, where the duration of infection is not definitely known, it is assumed that persons under 26 have early syphilis (less than 4 years duration), and those 26 years of age or over have late syphilis (over 4 years in duration). It is evident, therefore, that the older men remaining at home in industry will constitute a problem of late, non-infectious and possibly complicated syphilis rather than early infectious or potentially infectious syphilis.

The same preponderance of late syphilis is present in our clinics. In the Tulsa Co-operative Clinic, which is a representative Oklahoma Clinic, the active patient load for the month of December, 1942 consisted of 1026 individuals. Of these patients, 11 per cent had late latent, cardiovascular, neuro, tertiary or late prenatal (congenital) syphilis. In other words, 11 per cent were infectious on admission, 27 per cent potentially infectious and 62 per cent permanently non-infectious. Over half of the clinic population was treated, not to stop or prevent infectiousness, but to prevent, cure or hold in check complications of late, non-infectious syphilis. That diverts time, effort and material from the management of infectious syphilis which is far more of a public health responsibility.

Unfortunately there is a superstition in Oklahoma that only diagnostic test of syphilis worthy of consideration is the blood test or Wassermann. This disease known as syphilis exists in four stages, one plus, two plus, three plus and that most dreaded of all stages, four plus syphilis. How many patients have trembled when their doctor said, "Yes sir, I hate to have to tell you this, but you have four plus syphilis." The man takes a few shots, the chancres clear up and a second Wassermann is negative. That magic word! He goes happily on his way and forgets the admonition to come back in six months for another blood test to see if it has come back on him. He gets married and has

a baby. A breaking out on the child is noticed and a trip is made to a doctor. The doctor finds that the father, mother and the child all have positive blood tests and the treatment starts all over again. Another man, age 45, goes to othe same doctor and he too has four plus. Drug after drug is used and still the blood is four plus. Every time a detail man comes around, the doctor inquires if there is anything new for the Wassermann-fast patient. He did not notice the fixed pupils or absent knee kicks and prescribed aspirin for the rheumatism that shot up and down the man's legs.

The Oklahoma Barber Law excludes all individuals in "any stage of a venereal disease" instead of "any infectious stage of a venereal disease". For years a positive Wassermann has been ruled as grounds for rejection of a barber regardless of other considerations such as duration of the disease, amount of treatment received or negative physical or spinal fluid findings. The cosmetology law is better regulated but the requirement still appears in the regulations that a person must take treatment until the blood test is negative. In other words, the blood test and not the cosmetologist is being treated. If we are not careful, the control of industrial syphilis will follow the same pattern and the Wassermann, not the industrial worker, will be treated.

The objectives of the venereal disease control program in industry as outlined by the Surgeon General's advisory committee[2] are as follows:

"A. Medical and Public Health:

1. To find and refer for proper medical management all cases of venereal diseases among workers in industry.

    a. To prevent the spread of venereal disease through early and adequate treatment.

    b. To prevent the development of late disabling manifestations by arresting progress of the disease through adequate treatment.

    c. To bring contacts of infectious persons under medical observation.

2. To establish equitable policies for the employment of applicants and continuation of services of employees who have venereal diseases.

    a. To assure adequate treatment by requiring that employment be made dependent on the presentation of satisfactory evidence by the employee that he is under proper medical management.

3. To coordinate the community and industrial venereal disease control programs.

B. Employee:

1. To improve the physical condition of employees.

2. To reduce the number of work days lost through illness or injury.

3. To provide job placement in order that the services of individuals having syphilis or gonorrhea may be employed at work which they are physically capable of performing with profit to themselves and to their employer, and without risk to themselves, to fellow workers or to the public.

4. To prolong and increase the earning power of employees by increasing life expectancy.

C. Employer:

1. To reduce compensation costs.

2. To lessen work interruptions and labor turnover.

3. To enhance production by increasing the efficiency of workers.

4. To minimize those personnel problems which arise from syphilis and gonorrhea as causes of ill health and nervous instability."

It is very simple to find a considerable number of positive Wassermanns every time a blood testing jamboree or industrial survey is held, but not so easy to be certain of proper medical management of the individual if found to have syphilis. We all know that early syphilis is infectious or potentially so if not adequately treated and that late syphilis, while not infectious, includes most of the complications found in syphilitic individuals. We also know that individuals with early syphilis, if adequately treated, with the exception of a very small per cent, will become permanently non-infectious and will not develop the complications found in late, untreated syphilis. That we are woefully inadequate in our management of infectious syphilis is obvious from the data of the U.S. Public Health Service Central Tabulating Unit. Miss Usilton[3] states that in the clinics of the United States reporting to this unit, approximately 75 per cent of the patients with early syphilis drifted away before receiving 20 arsenicals and 20 heavy metal treatments. Apparently we are so intent on pouring a barrage of arsenic and bismuth into our patients with late, non-infectious syphilis that the individuals with early syphilis get out of range.

Whether taken from the point of view of the private physician, the industrial physician or health officer, the intelligent management of syphilis is essentially the same and demands first of all a diagnosis. Adequate diagnosis, which includes classification as to the stage of syphilis found, cannot be made without at least a history, repetition of the blood test to rule out false positives, physical examination and darkfield examination if suspicious lesions are present. Spinal fluid examination should be made where indicated and no diagnosis of latent syphilis is really complete unless the spinal fluid is known to be negative. Fluoroscopic examination will reveal a suprising amount of aortic enlargement otherwise overlooked. It is well to question individuals as to lesions when taking the first blood test. Many a man with a chancre will come in ready to show it to an authority on chancres but loses his nerve when he sees a female clerk and merely asks for a blood test. If the report comes back negative, he may think he does not have syphilis and lose an opportunity for an early diagnosis. Any office girl can read a Wassermann report, but it takes a physician to make a diagnosis.

We know that early syphilis should be treated intensively and continuously until at least 30 to 40 arsenicals and about the same number of bismuth treatments are given, excepting intensive therapy, in alternating courses. Spinal fluid examination should be made before releasing the patient unless definitely contraindicated or refused by the patient. If refused by the patient then "spinal refused" should be recorded on his record. He should be told that he is on probation and to report back several times the first year and for yearly observations for five years.

We know that complicated syphilis such as tertiary (skin, bones, viscera), cardiovascular and neurosyphilis take longer and more individualized treatment, usually about two years according to most text books. This may be intensive or symptomatic depending upon previous treatment received. The purpose of treatment here is to keep the individual in the best possible physical condition and not to blast the Wassermann.

We now come to the largest single classification group in private practice, industrial practice or in health department clinics, namely late latent or late uncomplicated syphilis. These are individuals with an infection of more than four years duration with no physical or spinal fluid evidence of damage. Those who have a provisional diagnosis of late latent syphilis but have not had a spinal fluid examination should be designated "late latent syphilis, spinal fluid not examined". Since these individuals with late latent syphilis, spinal fluid negative, run a relatively small chance of developing complications, they may be given a shorter period of treatment. Hudson and Venable[4] showed that routine fluoroscopic examinations in the Tulsa Cooperative Clinic were essential for the consistent diagnosis of early uncomplicated aortitis and with spinal fluid examination screened out a large number of individuals without complications who could be given minimal instead of maximal amounts of treatment. These individuals were given a course of treatment suggested by Dr. J. E. Moore[3] consisting of preliminary bismuth, 12 weekly doses of mapharsen then 12 weekly doses of bismuth. They were then instructed to report once a year during the month of their birthday for physical examination. This series was started about 3 years ago and so far, from the results of the re-examinations, we have found no occasion to regret the reduction in treatment. For those who are dubious as to 12-12 being adequate, a 20-20 schedule would at least meet the requirements for the minimal amount to insure non-infectiousness in case the duration of the infection had been incorrectly estimated. This reduction in required treatment for a large group of patients has noticeably decreased the clinic load and gives the patient more incentive to finish his treatment. A recommended schedule of 40-30 for early syphilis among industrial workers, including barbers, cosmetologists and food handlers with 20-20 or 12-12 for late latent syphilis, spinal fluid negative, would do much to clarify the syphilis in industry problem in Oklahoma. Persons with complicated syphilis will have to be treated as individuals and no rule of thumb can be made. However, infectiousness should not be the motive for treatment when infectiousness does not exist.

If the health officer is sold on the modern treatment of syphilis and is reasonably familiar with its fundamentals, he will have little difficulty in selling it to the employer and employee. When confidence and fairplay exist, there will be cooperation between employer and employee to their mutual advantage. In one of the Tulsa industries the first aid man has the confidence of the men and very few of them contract a venereal disease without reporting it to him. If he could only get their contacts he would be a great help to us indeed. The health department can be of great help to industrial physicians in classifying syphilis in industrial workers especially if they have received treatment in a clinic. It takes but a few minutes to put down the essential data and a 3 x 5 card can be used to record diagnosis with pertinent supporting data, amount of treatment received, etc. The Tulsa Cooperative Clinic has been classifying individuals found to have positive blood tests, lesions or discharge on pre-employment examination for about six industrial physicians and the work has not been too heavy. One company with a very liberal policy have in their employ over 50 patients from the clinic, most of whom are now receiving treatment from private physicians. Companies which arbitrarily refuse to employ persons with positive serology should not be permitted to send blood specimens to any health department laboratory.

CONCLUSIONS

1. The individual and not the blood test should be treated and it is conducive to better therapy to get acquainted with the patient.

2. For industrial workers including barbers, cosmetologists and food handlers, a treatment schedule of 40 arsenical and 30 bismuth treatments is recommended for early syphilis and 12 arsenic and 12 bismuth or 20 arsenic and 20 bismuth for late latent syphilis, spinal fluid negative and late latent syphilis, spinal fluid not examined.

3. The treatment of late complicated syphilis should be individualized.

4. The diagnosis "latent syphilis" should be followed by the words spinal fluid negative or spinal fluid not examined, as the case may be.

BIBLIOGRAPHY

1. Vonderlehr, R. A., and Usilton, Lida J.: Syphilis Among Men of Draft Age. Jour. A.M.A., Vol 120, page 1369, December 26, 1942.
2. Venereal Disease Control Program in Industry. Advisory Committee on the Control of Venereal Diseases, Otis L. Anderson, Chairman. Jour. A.M.A., Vol. 120, page 828, November 14, 1942.
3. Usilton, Lida J.: Personal Communication — not for Indiscriminate Publication.
4. Hudson, David V. and Venable, Sidney C.: A Fluoroscopic Survey of Postnatal Syphilis in a Health Department Clinic. Jour. Okla. State Med. Assoc. October, 1942.
5. Moore, Joseph Earle: Personal Communication.

A physician may possess the science of Harvey and the art of Sydenham, and yet there may be lacking in him those finer qualities of heart and head which count for so much in life.—Sir William Osler.

Army doctors, to an American correspondent in Sicily, on the subject of blood plasma: "Write lots about it; go clear overboard for it; say that plasma is the one outstanding medical discovery of this war."—New York Times.

The County Health Department in Oklahoma*

JOHN W. SHACKELFORD, M.D., M.P.H.
Director, Local Health Service
Oklahoma State Health Department

OKLAHOMA CITY, OKLAHOMA

The full time county health department as we know it today, had its beginning in Yakima County, Washington, in 1911. Dr. L. L. Lumsden of the U.S. Public Health Service had been sent there in response to a request made by the people of the area to investigate the typhoid situation. He made recommendations which led to the organization of a full time county health service designed to cope with the problem. This represented a coordinated Federal, State and Local effort, a pooling of resources to develop a local organization to deal with local health problems.

At first this plan of local health service was slow in its development and acceptance in other areas. It was difficult to convince county appropriating bodies of the worthwhileness of such a program, but in recent years it has become the accepted method of local health administration. On June 30, 1942, 60 per cent of the counties in the United States and 75 per cent of the nation's population were under full time health service.[1] Compared with 1941, this represents a 9.6 per cent increase in the number of counties served and a 5 per cent increase in population served. This plan of health service has the backing of the American Medical Association and at their meeting in June of last year the House of Delegates unanimously voted its approval of extension of such services.[2] In Oklahoma our own State Medical Association, both as an organization and as individuals, has actively supported a sound health program and has been of inestimable assistance in the development of local health departmets throughout the state.

There are two forces which have been outstanding in their contribution to, and promotion of the county health department. One was the Rockefeller Sanitary Commission, particularly interested in the study and control of hookworm disease, and the other was the U.S. Public Health Service, which in this area of its activities was especially concerned with the problem of typhoid fever.

By 1935, the value of health programs had been sufficiently well demonstrated for Con-gress to make available under the Social Security legislation, sizable sums of money for health work. Later, venereal disease funds were added to the sums already available to states. These funds enabled states to increase rapidly the number of county health departments and to improve their quality.

Despite the phenomenal development of the county plan of health administration, difference of opinion still exists with regard to the relative merits of centralized vs local direction.

Applewhite[3] has very ably described these two concepts of administration. "The first and oldest concept has resulted in the establishment of a strong State Health Department designed to render the needed types of public health services directly to the people of the state from the central organization. This concept has resulted in the creation in the central department of quite a large number of bureaus or divisions designed for the solution of some particular and specific problems. Experience has demonstrated that this plan of organization is the easiest to perfect, the most expensive to operate, the less effective in achieving lasting results, and requires less knowledge of public health administration to administer.

"The second and more recent plan of organization is based on the knowledge that most public health problems are of local origin and for that reason require local machinery for their solution. It also calls for local financial participation. This plan of organization calls for a smaller central organization equipped with highly trained specialists, properly integrated, who are capable of rendering expert consultative and technical supervisory services to the local organization."

We believe the latter plan is the sounder of the two and it is the one we have chosen for the development of our program here. Whatever the plan, service must always be performed at the community level.

In agreement with Mountin[4] we do not believe "that local health services can be operated successfully over a period of years by remote control through a corps of circuit riders who make occasional visits to the in-

*Read before the Annual Meeting held in Oklahoma City, May 11-12, 1943.

dividual communities. Such persons have no roots in the community and cannot hope to fully understand or meet its needs."

We now have 37 counties in Oklahoma with full time Health Service, with authority and responsibility resting locally. It is logical that such a plan of local administration would presuppose local support. The plan is considered sound and is the one we have followed of necessity as well as good policy. Federal money must be matched and we feel that is fair to ask counties receiving service to pay a part of its cost. The general policy of asking local governments for one half of the funds for local budgets has been established. In some areas where health problems are great and per capita income is low, more state and federal than local money has gone into the budget; in other areas, less. In the fiscal year 1943, 40 per cent of the funds for county health department budgets came from local sources—county, city and schools. Counties are allowed by State law to appropriate one mill for public health purposes. Cities and schools may supplement county allotments over and above the one mill.

The county health department is regarded as a definite entity and is expected to function as a unit. The medical director is responsible for the entire public health program in the area over which he has supervision subject, of course to the general supervision of those responsible in the State Health Department.

If a program is to be effective under such a plan, it is necessary that trained and qualified full time medical officers be placed in charge. This point is emphasized in a recent editorial[2] in the Journal of the American Medical Association in which is stated in effect that the career of public health is a specialty of medicine requiring graduate university training and practical experience, and that only a full time trained local administrator can be encouraged by the medical profession or be recommended to the local taxpayer as the best his money can buy in public health.

We have realized the need for special training in public health for some time and for several years have been encouraging university training for all professional public health personnel. In the years 1938 to 1942 (the program stopped in 1942 because of the war), nine physicians and one dentist were sent to schools of public health where they received masters degrees. Five other physicians with such degrees have been brought into the program, making a total of fifteen. Of this total, five have been called to the Armed Services, leaving ten with public health degrees at present; which is one

fourth of the medical staff. I do not have figures at hand on nurses and sanitarians, but equal attention has been given to these and other public health workers.

THE LOCAL HEALTH PROGRAM

The appraisal form of the American Public Health Association which has been used as a yard stick for measuring local health services, lists nine activities which are usually included in the program of a county health department. These are:

1. Vital Statistics—supervision of collection and analysis for use in planning the local program.

2. Acute Communicable Disease Control—quarantine and isolation, and epidemiological investigation.

3. Venereal Disease Control—clinics for indigents and search for source and spread contacts.

4. Tuberculosis Control—chest clinics for diagnosis of suspicious cases. The examination of contacts of known cases is always emphasized in the case finding program.

5. Maternity Hygiene — the encouraging of expectant mothers to seek competent medical supervision and care.

6. Infant and Pre-school Hygiene—the encouraging of medical supervision of the child during this age period.

7. School Hygiene—physicial examination of school children and guidance of parents of children with physicial defects in seeking proper professional care.

8. General Sanitation—promotion of protected municipal and private water supplies and safe excreta disposal.

9. Food and Milk Control—supervision of milk supplies and of eating establishments.

Though this program was developed to meet peace time needs, with a little streamlining it is meeting the needs in defense areas satisfactorily. The full time county health department is proving to be the most effective agency for dealing with health problems in war areas, here and over the nation. In fact, several have been organized in these areas as a means of meeting the health problems created by bringing people together for a defense activity.

Significant evidence of the effectiveness of a county health department in a given area is difficult to demonstrate because of the many factors involved and the lack of suitable controls. Nevertheless, there is ample evidence—circumstantial, at least—to convince even the most skeptical that this service is able to reduce the incidence of preventable disease and to raise the health level of the population. As shown in a comparison of the mortality experience in certain preventable diseases during the two preceeding five year periods (Table 1), this reduction is particularly evident in those diseases for which we have had definite control measures.

TABLE 1

Death Rates from Selected Causes in Oklahoma
1933-1937 and 1938-1942

Cause of Death	1933-1937	1938-1942
	Deaths per 100,000 population	
Typhoid fever	7.8	2.7
Scarlet fever	1.0	.4
Whooping cough	3.3	3.8
Diphtheria	6.9	3.2
Tuberculosis, all forms	49.1	45.5
Measles	1.7	2.1
Diarrhea and enteritis under 2 years	15.9	7.9
	Deaths per 1,000 live births	
Infants under 1 year	61.4	48.2
Puerperal causes	5.0	3.7

More specifically, the effect of full time local health service has been brought out by comparing the typhoid death rates in Rutherford County, Tennessee, where a county

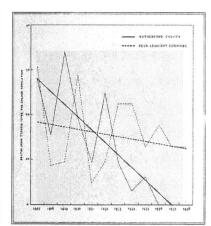

Trends in typhoid fever mortality, Rutherford County, Tennessee, and in four adjacent counties without full-time health service, 1927-1938. In the heavy trend lines annual fluctuations have been smoothed out

health department had been in operation several years, with those in the surrounding counties without full time service. In a study made in 1939 by the Commonwealth Fund[3],

it was shown that in the five year period 1934-1938, Rutherford County had a typhoid death rate of only 1.8 per 100,000 population whereas the four surrounding counties had a rate of 16, yet the two areas had approximately the same rate, 23 per 100,000 population, in 1924-1928 when the health department was organized in Rutherford County. (See Fig. 1.)

The total death rate in Rutherford County in the five years, 1934-1938, was 12 per cent lower than that in the four surrounding counties without organized health service, which is further evidence of the effectiveness of the health department in the county.

Though we have not yet found in Oklahoma such stricking evidence of the value of local health work, we do have programs in the making which are equally as good as the one in Rutherford County and I am confident that in time they will show as good results.

DISCUSSION

MACK I. SHANHOLTZ, M.D., M.P,H.

WEWOKA, OKLAHOMA

Dr. Shackelford's paper on the county health department in Oklahoma is well prepared and certainly nothing of importance can be added. I agree with his statement that the establishment of local health departments with the state health department acting in an advisory capacity is the best means of solving health problems in Oklahoma. It is encouraging to know the Oklahoma Medical Society has approved the extension of such services. To function well any county health department must have the support of the local county medical group or society. Likewise, the local practicing physicians will need a local health department if they are to study, understand and attempt to solve the problems of health existent in their county.

In the first place, the local doctors will need the health department to define the public health problems in their town or community. I am making the following statement not in criticism of the medical profession but simply as an observed fact; the average general practitioner does not know the answers to such questions as (1) what is the incidence or death rate from tuberculosis, typhoid fever, diphtheria, or any other

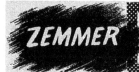

communicable disease, (2) is your town water supply chlorinated, (3) is your milk supply inspected, (4) what kind of sewage disposal does your town have. It is impossible to solve a problem either in mathematics or public health unless you have a clear-cut statement of that problem.

In the second place, a health department will be needed to help educate the public or make them aware of any existing disease or conditions that threaten health. If the public is sufficiently impressed, it will find ways and means to eliminate any health hazard.

In the third place, the medical profession will need material aid from the health department in coping with certain problems of health.

These three points which represent general functions of the health department can be demonstrated from any number of actual problems encountered in Seminole County. To encourage brevity, the simple example of diphtheria in Seminole County will be used. The State of Oklahoma has a rather high prevalence of diphtheria in past years, and Seminole County has been above the state rate. In 1938 we started a county-wide program for the control of diphtheria. Of course our chief control measure was the immunization of children under six years of age. First a survey was made to determine the number of these children already immunized. It was found that less than 5 per cent (2.6 per cent to be exact) had already received diphtheria toxoid. It was estimated that there were some 5,000 children of this age group in the county, and well over 4,000 of these had never been vaccinated. With the establishment of these facts, the problem was fairly well defined.

To persuade large numbers of parents to have their children vaccinated against diphtheria, an "educational barrage" had to be laid down. Parents had all sorts of excuses for not having had their children vaccinated, such as ignorance of the existence of the vaccine, fear of the reaction from the vaccine, lack of funds, lack of interest, the idea that a child should be of school age before being vaccinated, and so forth. The educational program was carried out through newspaper articles, talks to lay groups, distribution of literature and home nursing visits. Even with the program this far along it would have been impossible to immunize any appreciable percentage of these children had the program at this stage been taken over entirely by the practicing physicians. To render them some material aid in the project, free immunization clinics, usually in conjunction with a child health conference or some other service, were established at various points all over the county. An in-

experienced doctor in this type of work might have expected to immunize all of these 4,000 children in one year or less. Our figures do not substantiate this idea. The first year the percentage was raised from 2.6 to 12.6. The second year the percentage was 18.1, the third year 28.3 per cent and the fourth year 42.5 per cent. We are now in our fifth year and even yet only a little better than 50 per cent of the children in this county have been immunized against diphtheria. Of course we have not yet reached our goal in this immunization program. We have had excellent cooperation from the medical profession on this project, as well as an all of our projects in Seminole County. I hope this brief example will impress you with the fact that to solve any public health problem successfully, it takes the combined effort of the local health department, the local practicing physicians and the people of the community.

BIBLIOGRAPHY

1. Kratz, F. W.; Surgeon, U.S. Public Health Service: Status of Full-Time Health Organization at the End of the Fiscal Year 1941-1942. Public Health Reports, page 345. February, 1943.
2. Journal of the American Medical Association: Editorial Page, Extension of Public Health Coverage to the Nation, Vol. 121, No. 14, page 1155. April, 1943.
3. Applewhite, C. C.; Surgeon, U.S. Public Health Serivce. Administrative Features of Public Health in Illinois.
4. Mountin, Joseph W.; Ass't. Surgeon General, U.S. Public Health Service: Responsibility of Local Health Authorities in War Emergency. American Journal of Public Health, Vol. 33, No. 1, page 35. January, 1943.
5. The Commonwealth Fund. Annual Report, pages 13-14. 1939.

A Challenge

'Tis no idle challenge which we physicians throw out to the world when we claim that our mission is of the highest and of the noblest kind, not alone in curing disease but in educating the people in the laws of health, and in preventing the spread of plagues and pestilences; nor can it be gainsaid that of late years our record as a body has been more encouraging in its practical results than those of the other learned professions. Not that we all live up to the highest ideals, far from it—we are only men. But we have ideals, which mean much, and they are realized, which means more. Of course there are Gehazis among us who serve for shekels, whose ears hear only the lowing of oxen and the jingling of the guineas, but these are exceptions. The rank and file labour earnestly for your good, and self-sacrificing devotion to your interests animates our best work.—Aequanimitas with Other Addresses. Sir William Osler. 3rd Edition.

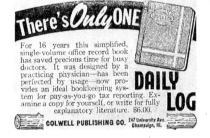

· THE PRESIDENT'S PAGE ·

The Annual County Secretaries Conference recently held was a great success. This is a town meeting, where, while there is a formal program, the subjects presented are then opened for general discussion, and a spirited and lively debate often ensues. The program this year purposely contained some controversial issues on which the profession is divided, in the hope that by focusing attention on them, all of us would give serious thought to them, and thereby arrive at some unanimity of opinion and purpose, and, not like Stephen Leacock's famous horseman, each jump on his horse and ride off in all directions.

Dr. Edward H. Skinner, the able editor of the Kansas City Clinical Society Bulletin, was the guest speaker. His address was frank and was critical of some of our organizational faults. His comments, too, on what the American public seems to expect of the medical profession, as a result of a recent poll, were interesting. This address, and part, at least, of the other proceedings of the meeting will appear in your Journal shortly.

The Post-War Planning Committee presented an admirable set of proposals fitted for Oklahoma use when peace descends upon us and all of our men in the Armed Forces come home. We must be ready for them! It seems obvious that the University of Oklahoma School of Medicine should loom large in the post-war picture . Many of our returning men will want refresher courses to ready them for civilian practice. Some will want to complete internships or residencies—some of them and many of us will want courses in tropical medicine in order to be prepared to cope with strange maladies which the end of war may bring to our State.

In these, and other ways, the School of Medicine can be of great service. It is our duty, as citizens, to keep this school strong—to encourage the teachers who give freely of their time to this institution, with inadequate, or no remuneration—to insist that the State Government allot generously of funds to support it and not have it depend on Federal subsidies. Let us keep it an Oklahoma School of Medicine—not a ward of a paternalistic Federal Government. Only by so doing will its graduates enter the practice of medicine as free men, asking not security, but opportunity!

James Stevenson

President.

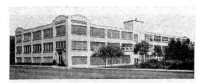

The JOURNAL Of The
OKLAHOMA STATE MEDICAL ASSOCIATION

EDITORIAL BOARD
L. J. MOORMAN, Oklahoma City, Editor-in-Chief

E. EUGENE RICE, Shawnee   NED R. SMITH, Tulsa

MR. R. H. GRAHAM, Oklahoma City, Business Manager

CONTRIBUTIONS: Articles accepted by this Journal for publication including those read at the annual meetings of the State Association are the sole property of this Journal.

The Editorial Department is not responsible for the opinions expressed in the original articles of contributors.

Manuscripts may be withdrawn by authors for publication elsewhere only upon the approval of the Editorial Board.

MANUSCRIPTS: Manuscripts should be typewritten, double-spaced, on white paper 8½ x 11 inches. The original copy, not the carbon copy, should be submitted.

Footnotes, bibliographies and legends for cuts should be typed on separate sheets in double space. Bibliography listing should follow this order: Name of author, title of article, name of periodical with volume, page and date of publication.

Manuscripts are accepted subject to the usual editorial revisions and with the understanding that they have not been published elsewhere.

NEWS: Local news of interest to the medical profession, changes of address, births, deaths and weddings will be gratefully received.

ADVERTISING: Advertising of articles, drugs or compounds unapproved by the Council on Pharmacy of the A.M.A. will not be accepted. Advertising rates will be supplied on application.

It is suggested that members of the State Association patronize our advertisers in preference to others.

SUBSCRIPTIONS: Failure to receive The Journal should call for immediate notification.

REPRINTS: Reprints of original articles will be supplied at actual cost provided request for them is attached to manuscripts or made in sufficient time before publication. Checks for reprints should be made payable to Industrial Printing Company, Oklahoma City.

Address all communications to THE JOURNAL OF THE OKLAHOMA STATE MEDICAL ASSOCIATION, 210 Plaza Court, Oklahoma City. (3)

OFFICIAL PUBLICATION OF THE OKLAHOMA STATE MEDICAL ASSOCIATION
Copyrighted November, 1943

EDITORIALS

MEDICINE'S FOUNDATION

In this issue of the Journal is a review of a timely book on "Psychosomatic Medicine" by Weiss and English. The chief purpose of this work is to revive our lagging interest in the ancient art of medicine. This subject is so important and presents so many angles vital to a people in time of stress and strain that it well deserves successive editorial notices for the duration.

The following qualifications for a writer as laid down by Dr. Samuel Johnson are equally applicable to the doctor who desires to meet the broad demands of his profession:

"Knowledge of nature is only half the task of the writer (doctor) ; he must be acquainted likewise with all the modes of life. His character requires that he estimate the happiness and misery of every condition and trace the changes of the human mind as they are modified by various institutions and accidental influences of climate or custom, from the sprightliness of infancy to the despondence of decreptitude; moreover, he must know many languages and many sciences." This is a large order, but that it was perceived by Hippocrates ceturies ago is implied in the first of his Aphorisius; "Life is short and the art long; the occasion fleeting; experience falacious and judgment difficult."

The developments following Morgagui, Verchow, Louis, Laeunerc, Pasteur and Koch have so advanced the science of medicine that its comprehension necessarily diverts attention from the art of medicine. Yet, in spite of what has happened, human nature remains the same and people throughout the world seek medical attention with minds which are curious and distraught. The wise doctor calmly encompasses the situation, manifests sympathy, tolerance and understanding, inspires confidence and begets a sense of security. Thus, almost immediately, a relationship arises which is genuine, intimate and vital, enabling the doctor to pursue his diagnostic and therapeutic measures with the greatest possible benefit to the patient. But the demands of science leave time for the acquisition of sufficient knowledge, culture and poise to place the art of medicine on a high plain. For many who study medicine these demands begin in high school and continue throughout the educational and professional career.

Those who have sons going into the profession of medicine should insist on a broad foundation which will provide a cultural background. With few exceptions the short cut which has been provided for the student of medicine saves only a little time and money. In the life of every good doctor there comes a day when he wishes he had spent more time in preparation for a career which requires a well buttressed foundation.

The book on Psychosomatic Medicine referred to above, is of special interest to Oklahoma doctors because it is based upon clinical work done under the direction of our own Dr. C. L. Brown, professor of Medicine at Temple University. Dr. Brown graduated from the University of Oklahoma School of Medicine in 1921. We are proud of his career and we profit by his achievements.

WHOOPING COUGH UP IN THE AIR

In the British Medical Journal, December 26, 1942, attention is called to the interesting fact that victims of whooping cough were alleged to be cured, or greatly benefited, by flights of about one hour and thirty minutes, reaching altitudes of 11,000 to 12,000 feet. Infants usually went to sleep after reaching an altitude of 6,000 feet, children and adults experienced some nausea, otherwise there were no untoward symptoms.

Of 250 patients in the paroxysmal stage of whooping cough, 22.8 per cent were promptly cured; 32 per cent were cured within 8 days. No improvements were reported in only 69 cases. No definite relationship to weather conditions could be established but low humidity seemed more favorable than high.

A group of 68 children suffering from whooping cough were placed in low-pressure chambers for 30 minutes. Sudden cure was reported in 31 per cent of the cases; undoubted improvement in 50 per cent; no improvement in 16 per cent and in 3 per cent the disease was made worse. It is apparent that the low-pressure chamber has the advantage of freedom from weather conditions and the psychological effects of flight. There is no explanation as to how these remarkable results come about.

The following questions are raised—"Does exposure to low-pressure have an effect upon H. pertussis?" "Does it break a link in the chain of an ill-conditioned cough reflex?"

Until additional effects are forthcoming, conservative doctors will continue to be skeptical about the results of this method of treatment.

The author recalls that 10 or 15 years ago, upon being called in consultation by a doctor friend in a small town in the state, he was urged to return to Oklahoma City in the doctor's ambulance plane. A laryngitis following an attack of influenza and the damp, foggy weather were advanced as good reasons for not undertaking the hazardous adventure. The doctor, however, insisted, saying, "the high altitude will cure your sore throat." In defense of the above assertion he related the following experience: "A few nights ago I was called to see a child who was choking with croup. Because of the ashy pallor and cyanosis, I brought the patient to the hospital and when we got up about 6,000 feet, she breathed 'just as easy'."

In contemplation, the writer was not breathing so easy and insisted on taking the next train. Unwittingly an opportunity for a therapeutic test which may have had scientific possibilities was turned down.

A. S. A.

This is not the designation of a Government Bureau. In fact, it bears no relation to the numerous administrative alphabetical triads that have swarmed out of Washington like locusts to blight American Liberty. On the contrary, in terms of service to humanity, these three letters represent Promethian gifts which grew out of individual effort and which overshadow the sun of all human beneficence from other sources. These three letters represent Anesthesia, Sanitation and Asepsis.

The genuineness of the benefactious conferred by the medical profession is attested by the fact that, in their application, they are not sectional, not national, but universal, and that they are given without the thought of personal, political or financial gain. Until the United States Government can do what medicine has done for the people of the world, American medicine should not be embarrassed and handicapped by bureaucratic control.

Socialized medicine is incompatible with American freedom, inimical to human welfare and can be conceived only through the union of ignorance and political greed.

Special Article

NAVIGATING THE MEDICAL FUTURE WITH CONFIDENCE*

EDWARD HOLMAN SKINNER, M.D.**

KANSAS CITY, MISSOURI

What with all the cross-currents within the ranks of physicians; with all the global static of alleged social trends; what with the political sabotage of patient-physician relationship; what with national legislation pointing its biggest guns at the very heart of American Medicine as we have cherished it; can anyone still hope to navigate the medical future with confidence?

The answer is YES. While there is still life there is also hope. While the ship still floats there is still an opportunity of rescuing all hands and bringing the ship to any number of safe ports.

We hear much about inevitable social trends. The argument of these planning barnacles upon the magnificent ship of American Medicine include the ultimate absorption of medical practices into the social security program through governmental compulsory health taxation. The amounts of money of geometrical proportions necessary for such social medicine are considered the simplest arithmetic by social planners. It is inconceivable that there is a sane majority willing to agree to such profligate spending upon the advice of social planners.

Social trends are bound to change. There is nothing inevitable about them in the least. The social trends and the political policies that are now in their ascendency or decline have been experienced in other well known historical times. The New Deal in Ancient Rome was described by Henry Haskell with all of its alphabetical connotations. The decline and fall of the Roman Empire proceeded. The bureaucrats of Louis XIV and XV ploughed under grape vines and established national vineyards and wineries, but only to bring on the French Revolution.

History proves that no social trend has been continuous. There is only one thing in nature that I once thought was not to be deflected, reflected or diffracted. That held good for the X-Ray beam for only 25 years until the physicist Bragg discovered that the X-Ray beam could be refracted by quartz crystals. And now the photography of the image on a fluoroscopic screen assures us an indirect reflection. Even the apparent assurances of natural phenomena are inevitably altered by our increasing knowledge. Nature and social processes are never static. Do not be fooled by arguments of inevitable social trends. They are bound to change and it is men who change them. Men with courage and stamina can lick any neuter social planner.

Let us take brief stock of several items in the medical scenery of the moment.

The Wagner-Murray Bill

This may be considered the culmination or peak point of social trends as far as medicine is concerned. At the same time it is the peak point or farthest point yet reached by communistic, totalitarian or fascist elements resident in our American Democracy. It is hardly a democratic document. It is a doctrine of disaster for democratic processes. It would plunge medicine into mediocrity.

Medical Education

With about 15,000 healthy students in uniform and all expenses paid, what will we have to replace the losses of civilian physicians each year? We will have about 1,500 women and cripples. The average yearly mortality of civilian practitioners is 2,500, or more. And these women and cripples are the only medical students allowed to finance their own education independently. They will make fine physicians, but we need more of them. The government intends to absorb about 4,000 physically fit graduates each nine months, which from now on will be a medical year. These medical officers will be indoctrinated in governmental processes and it takes no sage to predict that many will be afraid to undertake the return to individual private practice. Their independence will have been squelched; their ambitions blunted and their freedom will be limited to the air they breathe.

Standards of medical education, internship, residency, independence and individualism are deteriorating. C'est le Guerre!

Medical Meetings

The annual American Medical Association and innumerable state meetings are out for the duration of the war. Fortunately, some regional meetings are being held and with excellent and attentive audiences. When Dr. Frederick W. Rankin was President of the American Medical Association he proposed regional meetings of the AMA as clinical conferences such as the Oklahoma Fall Conference and the Kansas City Fall Clinical Conference. Those to be in the sensible, convenient and accessible geographical centers of the United States. What happened? The Board of Trustees turned President Rankin down flatly and nothing more was heard of such meetings until—

Brigadier General Rankin now finds these medical regional meetings at Army posts and hospitals are favored, promoted and protected by the governmental authorities. The American Medical Association is neatly bi-passed. Again—C'est le guerre !

Women and Children First

The U.S. Children's Bureau, fortified later and implemented by the Shephard-Towner Act, planned successfully to eventually supervise the maternal and childhood problems of millions. The New Maternal and Infant Care Program for wives and children of soldiers amplifies this early beginning to huge and alarming proportions. No physician is going to refuse to take good care of the wives and children of service men. But to do this under this new plan is intolerable, a denial of the rights of a physician as a free man. There is a threat to public welfare and public policy in this program in that it attempts to force citizens to complete professional services below the costs of performance. The emotional reaction is the threat held over physicians. This is really a dastardly use of the emergency plea. But there is little reason to hope that this and other emergency processes will not be continued and maintained. The House of Delegates has agreed to stand by this program officially if the government will contribute reasonable funds to the patients and let the patients make their own arrangements with physician and hospital.

How is the Profession Meeting These Situations

Social Emergency? Military Emergency? What social and governmental crimes are committed thereby. C'est le Guerre!

The Council on Medical Service and Public Relations of the American Medical Association was forced upon the Trustees and Officers by the House of Delegates in

---

*Delivered before the Officers, Secretaries and Editors of the State and County Medical Societies of Oklahoma, Sunday, October 17, 1943.

**Delegate from the Section on Radiology in the House of Delegates of the American Medical Association. Trustee of the National Physicians' Committee for the Extension of Medical Service.

URGENT PUBLIC NOTICE!

THE tremendous gains made against tuberculosis are in danger of being wiped out. Crowded housing, abnormal eating conditions, overwork, and all the other by-products of war can give the dread TB a new lease on life. We found this out in the last war. Your help is needed, *urgently*. To carry on the year's fight against TB, we rely on your purchase of Christmas Seals. Please send in your contribution today, as much as you can give.

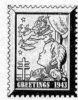

BUY CHRISTMAS SEALS

Because of the importance of the above message, this space has been contributed by

OKLAHOMA STATE MEDICAL ASSOCIATION

June 1943. There have been meetings in August and September. No secretary has been announced. No program has been indicated. No Washington Bureau as yet or ever (?). It would seem logical to fuse the Bureau of Medical Economics and the Bureau of Legislation with this new Council. But it has not been done and it may take further action by the House of Delegates to give the splendid manpower of this new Council a chance to do the job they are capable of doing. It is not a case of C'est le Guerre but La Vue Avec Alarm.

The Committee of Physicians for the Improvement of Medical Care claims to represent 400 physicians of the United States who are largely connected with medical colleges, foundations, state and national health services. Some one has said that the number has dwindled to 28. They are also largely upon a full time salary basis or contractural basis. They are garnished with eminent pasts rather than expanding futures. They have abdicted to what they consider as inevitable social trends. Many have been frustrated in their attempts to engage in the competition of individual private practice of medicine. They now assume an ability at planning the medical future for 150,000 American physicians inasmuch as they are hardly satisfied with their present predicament. It is doubtful if God really intended them to carry such a burden successfully.

This Committee (one should delate the capitals) report that they think Mr. Wagner has done a fine job with his new bill and they hope that they will be called into conference to help work out the details of Dingle-Dangle-Dingle Bill No 7-11. (And they hope they click.)

With more than 90 pages of Governmental printing in this document of disaster, the size of Time Magazine, are there any more details that the authors overlooked?

The forward-looking, aggressive organization, the National Physician's Committee for the Extension of Medical Service, has the backing of the House of Delegates of the American Medical Association by resolution. It has the blessing and cooperation of the new Council upon Medical Service and Public Relations of the American Medical Association. It has had continuous financial support of more than 25,000 physicians of America. It has secured the financial backing of leading pharmaceutical manufacturers. It is in a position of doing things and going places that organized medicine as at present officered and staffed and constituted and taxed cannot or will not agree to complete.

This Committee insists that the Wagner-Murray Senate Bill No. 1161 is a prelude to the centralized control and regimentation of the medical profession and eventually of all professions and eventually industry. The NPC has published a pamphlet entitled Abolishing Private Medical Practice. It has provided an eight page abstract of the pamphlet for wider distribution. If the present speed of distribution continues there will be from 10,000,000 to 15,000,000 in the hands of voters within the next 90 days.

The National Physicians Committee has financed the distribution of 300 word editorials every week to the 12,000 newspapers of the United States with the exception of the metropolitan dailies. We can report about 25 per cent acceptance and publication. This is a tremendous and constant indirect influence upon those who read editorials. We believe that people read them in the smaller newspapers.

Among innumerable projects the National Physicians Committee for the Extension of Medical Service is justifying the second portion of its name by securing at considerable expense the services of the largest research organization in the United States. A Pilot Survey has just been delivered but its results are confidential until these very important findings have been surveyed and appraised and digested by the NPC's Committee upon the Extension of Medical Services, (Dr. Skinner did read from this Pilot Survey to the meeting of secretaries, officers and editors of the Oklahoma State Medical Society and its several county component societies, but not for publication at this time.)

What Can I Do as a Physician to Help Solve this Social Riddle

It is not startling to find that the Pilot Survey, aforementioned, reveals that a majority of the people are security-minded and that they are seeking some means of avoiding the catastrophic expenses of modern medical attention. Therefore, it becomes the responsiblity of organized medicine to develop techniques of practice and payment that will help this situation. Arguments against governmental techniques will not be enough. Such arguments must be capped by programs that are practical.

If sickness benefit insurance, pre-payment plans or budgeting by savings are solutions, then there must be some monumental propaganda erected to sell such processes to the people. But, first, it may be necessary to stimulate, organize, and establish acceptable techniques within the three thousand county societies or among the number that in combination will cover the country.

All social insurance, including medical expense insurance, is unemployment insurance. The present plenty of wages has decreased attendance at clinics and permitted people to pay their way. They are employed now at wages that are sufficient to pay their way all down the line.

Is social insurance by the voluntary process and processed outside of governmental coercion or taxation an impossible hurdle in a democracy? Can we continue to divorce medical insurance from the whole array of social insurances that are now incorporated into the Social Security Act?

The American Medical Association, although officially advocating voluntary processes, cannot be expected to promote successfully such processes by field agents, by printed propaganda or by passing the word down the line through state and county societies. The American Medical Association, as now constituted, could hardly undertake a program that would induce county or state groups of physicians to so organize that they would develop the answers required to satisfy the people who are seeking security and avoidance of high medical costs at unpredictable intervals.

There is no particular propaganda or advertising program which provides national emphasis upon pre-payment medical schemes. There is much local activity in spots—about 10 per cent of the county societies. Whatever emphasis group hospitalization propaganda lends to prepayment medicine is tinctured by their ambitions to include much, if not all, of medical practices in hospitals. Hospitals domination of medical practices would be equally as disastrous to physicians as compulsory health insurance.

Therefore, it seems to me that we must consider the erection of some masterful and nationally distributed technique which will stimulate county medical societies to some action; and if physicians are to stand upon their own feet and conduct their own practice they must learn how to conduct the business side of medicine so that it will be attractive, desirable and so much in demand that the people will agree to pay for it in advance. If the American Medical Association will not or cannot do this, then we may have to depend upon the National Physician's Committee for Extension of Medical Service to fill this gap or develop a new organization.

Up to now there has been no way to gauge the desire or ambition of the medical profession to really tackle solutions. Solutions is plural because local demands and needs are widely different. There can be no question but that a progressive and forward-looking project can be undertaken and successful if we are willing to make the sacrifices and the effort. This must be a broadganged project. It is not one for frightened or timid souls.

In all of our efforts we must keep constantly in mind that our ambitions have no partisan bearing. We must educate the public and the politicians of all persuasions in the standards that we cherish and which must be maintained in the progressive changes that will be necessary to provide good medical care to all the people.

ASSOCIATION ACTIVITIES

FOURTH ANNUAL SECRETARIES CONFERENCE HELD OCTOBER 17

Officers of the County Medical Societies of the State, meeting at the Fourth Annual Secretaries Conference of the Oklahoma State Medical Association at the Biltmore Hotel, Oklahoma City on October 17, heard details of a program of post-war planning for Oklahoma medicine as outlined by Dr. Tom Lowry, Dean of the University of Oklahoma School of Medicine. The program, as outlined by Dr. Tom Lowry, will appear elsewhere in the Journal.

Other features of the meeting included an aggressive analysis of medical problems by Dr. Edward H. Skinner of Kansas City, Missouri; an explanation of the Maternal and Infant Care Program of the Federal Government by Dr. J. .T. Bell of Oklahoma State Health Department; a progress report on the pending surgical care plan of the Oklahoma State Medical Association by Chairman John F. Burton of Oklahoma City; and a description of the role of the Blue Cross Plan in the rural community by Mr. N. D. Helland, director of Group Hospital Service, Tulsa.

Dr. Lowry, opening the program, pointed out the need for a comprehensive program of post-war planning as a means of preventing disturbing upheavals in medical practices at the close of the war. Dr. Lowry's suggestions are embodied in the program which is to be supervised by the Post-War Planning Committee of the Oklahoma State Medical Association.

Dr. J. T. Bell, administrative officer of the Oklahoma State Health Department, informed delegates that the Maternal and Infant Care Program for Wives and Children of Service Men had been resumed after a two-months discontinuation because of protests from civic and social relief agencies. Attempts of the Department to drop participation grew out of a ruling by the state attorney-general to the effect that professional participation in the plan was not limited to medical doctors. The legal interpretation of the act would permit osteopaths, chiropractors, cultists, cooks, midwives, motormen, cowboys, and /or blacksmiths to deliver children for federally granted remuneration.

Dr. Edward N. Smith of Oklahoma City, discussing Dr. Bell's remarks stated that the crux of professional objection to the bill lay not in any individual objection but in the question; "Is medicine doing the right thing in participating in this bill at all?"

Dr. Smith warned that the Maternal and Infant Care Program was a forerunner of state medicine, a wedge for federal bureaucratic regimentation yet to come. He asserted the bill unfair through its indiscriminate distribution of federal funds under the guise of patriotism.

Dr. Grady F. Mattews, director of the Oklahoma State Health Department, expressed the attitude of the Department in saying that its participation in the act was made necessary by the force of public opinion.

The extension of the functions of prepaid hospital care into rural areas was outlined by Mr. N. D. Helland, executive director of Blue Cross, Group Hospital Service, Tulsa. Mr. Helland cited the need of such care as paramount to the successful economic operation of any farm project. By preventing improper medical attention through prepaid hospital care plans, the farmer is enabled to use ready funds for the expenses of the surgeon and doctor. The hospital bill is already provided for, so the idea of doing without needed medical care for lack of funds is averted, Helland said.

The administrator said that such hospitalization insurance plans as the nationwide Blue Cross Plan encouraged the payment of doctor bills since ready funds were not eaten up by hospital expenses. Mr. Helland demonstrated how this worked through references to the group now set up in the Farm Security Administration of Oklahoma.

Dr. John F. Burton, chairman of the Prepaid Medical and Surgical Service Committee of the Oklahoma State Medical Association, Oklahoma City, reported to secretaries that the basic organizational work in establishing a prepaid surgical care plan had been completed. The committee, carrying out the instructions of the House of Delegates of the Oklahoma State Medical Association, has been working for several months in creating a prepaid surgical care plan to be initially tested with selected groups. Administered by Group Hospital Service of Oklahoma, it will be introduced on a statewide basis if operation of trial groups proves successful. Final details are now being ironed out and legal technicalities overcome.

Dr. James Stevenson, President of the Association, in discussion of Dr. Burton's report, pointed out that such a plan was being adopted as a means of combating the growing aggression of the Federal Government in the field of medicine. Successful operation of a prepaid surgical care program would be an excellent weapon against the introduction of a substitute program of state medicine, Dr. Stevenson said.

The conference closed with a dinner at the Biltmore Hotel Mirror Room, at which time Dr. Edward Skinner spoke on the subject, "Navigating The Future With Confidence." Dr. Skinner's address is to be printed in the pages of the Journal and will not be analyzed here.

The following officers were elected for the coming year: Chairman; J. B. Hollis, M.D., Mangum: Vice-Chairman; Clinton Gallaher, M.D., Shawnee: Secretary; D. Evelyn Miller, M.D., Muskogee, (re-elected).

POST-WAR PLANNING WITH REFERENCE TO THE PHYSICIANS RETURNING FROM MILITARY SERVICE

The Committee on Post-War Planning of the Oklahoma State Medical Association first wishes to thank those members of the profession and particularly our President for the suggestion which they have made to the Committee—many of which are incorporated in this report.

This report is made in the hope of making suggestions and plans which might be of some value in maintaining the good health of the people of Oklahoma during and after this war, and to help the doctor who returns to fit himself back into the home service where he will be happiest, where he will have suffered the least loss, and where he will be of greatest service to his community.

First, may we say that we are certainly not unmindful of the tremendous sacrifices which these doctors have made and are leaving their homes and practices to enter the armed services. We owe them our undying gratitude and cooperation.

Therefore, we recommend:

1. That some form of questionnaire be sent to each member of the Oklahoma State Medical Association who is in the armed services at this time and that this questionnaire include such questions as the following:

a. Do you plan to return to Oklahoma after the termination of the war, do you plan on remaining in the armed services, or do you plan on locating elsewhere?

b. Do you expect to return to your original location to practice?

c. Do you want a refresher course in some branch of medicine, do you want an internship, or do you want a residency?

d. Do you want information about other localities of the state in which you might be interested?

e. What do you want American Medicine to be like when you return?

f. What can the Oklahoma State Medical Association or your local County Medical Society do to help you to plan your future and help re-establish your practice?

2. We recommend that every effort be made to preserve, so far as possible, the privileges of the practice of medicine which the doctors enjoyed in this state at the time they entered the service. To this extent we commend the State Board of Medical Examiners and recommend that we support and uphold them in their prevailing laws and rules, realizing that relaxing such laws would encourage an influx of doctors, many of whom would be unqualified, and such would make the re-establishment of our own doctors more difficult.

3. We recommend that the Executive Secretary of the Oklahoma State Medical Association set up an "Information Bureau" or "Clearing House" which would include such information as:

a. Population of towns and centers of the state.

b. Number of doctors including specialists in each community.

c. Health needs of each community.

d. Number of cults in each community.

e. The hospital and diagnostic centers in these communities.

f. Ages of Doctors of Medicine in communities.

g. Commercial, economic and agriculture status of the community.

4. That the Postgraduate Committee of the Oklahoma State Medical Association, the State Commissioner of Health and the University of Oklahoma School of Medicine be giving serious consideration to the feasibility of offering refresher courses in medicine and surgery for the benefit of not only those doctors who have been in the service, but for those who have remained at home and have been deprived of such courses during the same period of time. It is recommended that these courses include tropical medicine and a study of diseased conditions which will be more or less new to most of us who have stayed at home.

5. Every effort should be made by the larger hospitals of the State to meet the requirements for accredited internships and residencies and other postgraduate facilities which returning doctors may want and need.

6. With regard to the care of Rural Communities, we realize that for many years the tendency has been for the majority of doctors to concentrate in larger towns and cities and that the majority of doctors in rural communities are in the upper age group or the age of limited activity. We realize that the chief reasons for this are:

a. Low economic status of some localities.

b. The belief that a larger city offers more social, cultural and educational advantages.

c. The chief reason being that rural communities often do not have the adequate hospital and diagnostic facilities to which the young doctor is accustomed.

We recommend the development and maintenance of hospital diagnostic centers in areas where these facilities are at present inadequate. These hospitals or centers should be located where they are available and open to all qualified physicians serving that community. In many cases, local hospitals could be absorbed, and in other localities the county or city government could be encouraged to supply at least part of the cost of such

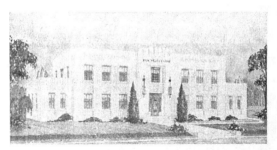

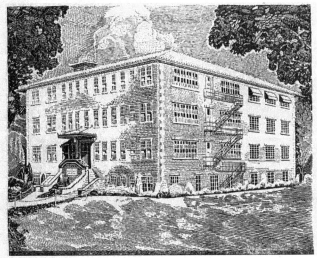

facility. Surely if air transports can parachute hospitals fully equipped which function temporarily in an orchard in Sicily, we should be able, by some means, to provide adequate permanent hospital facilities for every community in this state. We also recommend that, as soon as possible, Blue Cross Hospital Service be made available to the people of small towns and rural communities.

7. We recommend that the teachers of medicine and the doctors of the state take time and care to impress upon the minds of pre-medical and medical students and interns the need for good general practitioners, the advantages of being general practitioners, and the services and other remunerations which accrue therefrom.

8. We recommend that the Oklahoma State Medical Association recommend to the American Medical Association or proper governmental authorities that the doctors in the armed services, who plan to return to civilian practice, be retained on an active status with pay for a period of six months after the war with the privilege of attending any postgraduate school of their choice.

9. We wish to commend the Oklahoma State Health Commission for its splendid cooperation with the Oklahoma State Medical Association and recommend that this cooperation continue. We further recommend the encouragement of the appointment of a five or seven man Board of Health representing the medical profession and allied agencies, which shall determine the general policies of the Oklahoma State Board of Health.

10. Finally, we recommend that County Medical Societies be alert to the proposed changes which are being considered by different agencies which might influence the practice of medicine and the health of the community. In the promulgation of all these plans we owe it to the doctors who are in the service to see that the professional rights, privileges and ethics of the profession shall be preserved.

Tom Lowry, M.D., Chairman
Wann Langston, M.D.
G. E. Stanbro, M.D.

NEW INSTRUCTOR APPOINTED BY POSTGRADUATE COMMITTEE FOR COURSE IN SURGICAL DIAGNOSIS

Announcement has been made by Dr. Gregory E. Stanbro, Chairman, Postgraduate Committee on Medical Teaching, that Dr. A. G. Fletcher of Philadelphia, Pennsylvania, has been employed to teach Surgical Diagnosis in the state of Oklahoma during 1944 and 1945. This is the fourth postgraduate course for physicians to be offered under the auspices of the Oklahoma State Medical Association with financial assistance from The Commonwealth Fund of New York and the Oklahoma State Health Department.

During the past year Doctor Fletcher has been with the Graduate School of Medicine, University of Pennsylvania. Doctor Fletcher has had extensive experience in the past 30 years practicing surgery and teaching.

The present course in Internal Medicine by Dr. L. W. Hunt has been a marked success. Over 1,000 physicians have enrolled and attended the course during the two years Doctor Hunt has been with us in spite of the fact that so many physicians are now serving in the Armed Forces, and those remaining at home are over-burdened with practice. The course in Surgical Diagnosis will open in the Northeastern section of the state in February, 1944. The exact dates and centers will be announced later.

DR. O. C. NEWMAN, SHATTUCK, ENTERS STATE HALL OF FAME

On November 16, Dr. O. C. Newman, Shattuck, pioneer physician of Oklahoma, will be honored by induction into the Hall of Fame at the Oklahoma Historical Society and will also be honored at the annual birthday banquet in the Biltmore Hotel by the Oklahoma Memorial Association.

There have been less than a dozen Oklahoma physicians who, in the past, have had this honor bestowed upon them.

Dr. Newman was born in Peebles, Adams County, Ohio, on December 29, 1876. He was graduated from the University of the South, Sewanee, Tennessee, in 1900, after which he came to Oklahoma to take up the practice of medicine. Dr. Newman first located at Grand, Day County, Oklahoma, and 1907 moved to Shattuck where he is still practicing. Many hardships confronted him and there were many lean years. Out of the struggles and hard work and through self-sacrifice which endeared him to his community, came the Newman Clinic, recognized today as one of the country's finest, a mecca for the sick and suffering of a vast territory. Dr. Newman's three sons have graduated from famous universities as physicians and are connected with him in the Clinic.

Dr. Newman is well deserving of the honor bestowed upon him and the medical profession joins his family and friends in honoring him.

DR. LEWIS J. MOORMAN ATTENDS MEETINGS

Dr. Lewis J. Moorman, Secretary-Treasurer of the Oklahoma State Medical Association and Editor-in-Chief of the State Journal, will attend the Southern Medical Meeting in Cincinnati, November 16, 17 and 18.

Dr. Moorman, President of the National Tuberculosis Association, will then attend a two-day Executive Committee Meeting November 18 and 19. The Association is preparing for its 37th annual Christmas Seal sale drive. On November 20, Dr. Moorman is scheduled to speak in Tulsa at an open meeting of the seal campaign in that city.

COUNCIL ON MEDICAL SERVICE AND PUBLIC RELATIONS OF AMERICAN MEDICAL ASSOCIATION ADOPTS NEW POLICIES

At its September meeting the Council on Medical Service and Public Relations of the American Medical Association adopted a tentative statement of policies. Pursuant to carrying out the duties imposed on it by the House of Delegates, the Council has adopted and perfected the following statement of general policies:

1. The Council on Medical Service and Public Relations recognizes the desirability of widespread distribution of the benefits of medical science; it encourages evolution in the methods of administering medical care, subject to the basic principles necessary to the maintenance of scientific standards and the quality of the service rendered.

It is not in the public interest that the removal of economic barriers to medical science should be utilized as a subterfuge to overturn the whole order of medical practice. Removal of economic barriers should be an object in itself.

It is in the public interest that the standards of medical education be constantly raised, that medical research be constantly increased and that graduate and postgraduate medical education be energetically developed. Curative medicine, preventive medicine, public health medicine, research medicine, and medical education, all are indispensable factors in promoting the health, comfort and happiness of the nation.

2. The Council through its executive committee and secretary shall analyze proposed legislation affecting medical service. Its officers are instructed to provide to the various state medical organizations as well as to legislative committees concerning the efforts of the proposed legislation. It shall likewise be the duty of its officers to offer constructive suggestions to bureaus and legislative committees on the subject of medical service.

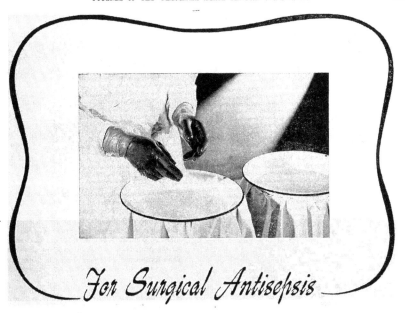
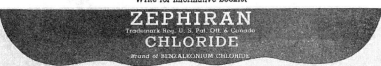

3. The Council approves the principle of voluntary hospital insurance programs but disapproves the inclusion of medical services in those contracts for the reasons adopted by the House of Delegates at the 1943 meeting.

4. The Council approves voluntary prepayment medical service under the control of state and county medical societies in accordance with the principles adopted by the House of Delegates in 1938. The medical profession has always been very much opposed to compulsory health insurance because (1) it does not reach the unemployed class, (2) it results in a bureaucratic control of medicine, and interposes a third party between the physician and the patient, (3) it results in mass medicine which is neither art nor science, (4) it is inordinately expensive, and (5) regulations, red tape and interference render good medical care impossible. Propaganda to the contrary notwithstanding, organized medicine in general, and the American Medical Association in particular have never been opposed to group medicine, prepayment or non-prepayment, as such. The American Medical Association and the medical profession as a whole have opposed any scheme which on the face of it renders good medical care impossible. That group medicine has not been opposed as such is evidenced by the fact that there are many groups operating in the United States which have the approval of the medical profession, and members of these groups are and have been officials in the national and state medical organizations. That group medicine is the Utopia for the whole population, however, is not probable. It may be and possibly is the answer for certain communities and certain industrial groups if the medical groups are so organized and operated as to deliver good medical care.

5. The Council believes that many emergency measures now in force should cease following the end of hostilities.

6. The Council believes that the medical profession should attempt to establish the most cordial relationships possible with allied professions.

7. There is no official affiliation between the American Medical Association and the National Physicians Committee. However, since it is the purpose of the National Physicians Committee to enlighten the public concerning contributions which American medicine has made and is making in behalf of the individual and the nation as a whole, it is the opinion of the Council that the medical profession may well support the activities of the National Physicians Committee and other organizations of like aims.

8. American medicine and this Council owe a responsibility to our colleagues who are making personal sacrifices to answer the call of the armed forces. Therefore, the Council expresses the desire to cooperate with the medical committee on post-war planning in order to assist our colleagues in re-establishing themselves in the practice of medicine, and in the preservation of the American system of medicine.

New Ethicon Eye Sutures Developed by Johnson & Johnson

As a result of several years research a new and complete line of seventeen Eye Sutures has just been announced by the Ethicon Suture Division of Johnson & Johnson.

The new Ethicon Eye Sutures, offered in plain and Type B Mild Chromic Surgical Gut, as well as Twisted Silk, are distinguished by their unusual flexibility.

All Ethicon Eye Stures are equipped with Eyeless Atroloc Cutting Point Needles. These needles, made under a Johnson & Johnson patent, are hand forged and hand sharpened. All materials in Ethicon Eye Sutures are selected to meet the exacting requirements of the Eye surgeon.

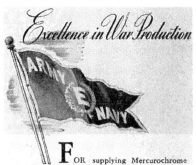
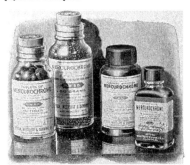

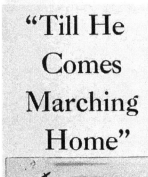

"Till He Comes Marching Home"

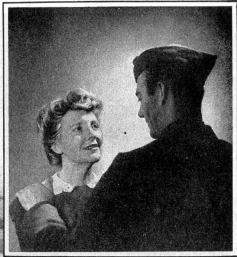

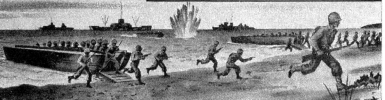

THE lonely lad sleeping in a foxhole remembers Mother as she was when he choked back the lump in his throat to kiss her goodbye for the last time. He does not realize that she may change, physically and psychically. To him she remains the same . . . always.

When he returns a great part of his dream can come true because THEELIN, an estrogen with a brilliant record of effectiveness, gives to many mothers in the climacterium continued relief from menopausal symptoms often intensified by the stress and worry of wartime living. Psychotic manifestations and sometic disturbances associated with ovarian hypofunction usually respond to the governing influence of this pure, crystalline estrogenic substance obtained from pregnancy urine. Its record of therapeutic usefulness and comparative freedom from undesirable side reactions has been proved by millions of doses and hundreds of published papers.

For sustained therapy between injections and for controlling milder menopausal symptoms THEELOL Kapseals* and THEELIN Suppositories are supplied. The latter may also be used in gonorrheal vaginitis in children.

Supplied as: THEELIN AMPOULES—in 1000, 2000, 5000 and 10,000 I. U. in oil, or in 20,000 I. U. in aqueous suspension • THEELOL KAPSEALS—in .12 and .24 mg. of Theelol • THEELIN SUPPOSITORIES—in 2000 I. U. of Theelin.

*Trade-Mark Reg. U. S. Pat. Off.

THEELIN
A product of modern research offered to the medical profession by

PARKE, DAVIS & COMPANY
DETROIT, MICHIGAN

• 25 YEARS AGO •

(Editors Note:)

How true are the statements in this editorial of 25 years ago when the comment is made that the physician is not a good business man!

How often can a careless remark by a physician be the cause of the filing of a suit against a colleague even when there is no basis for a suit.

The Editorial also brings to the attention of the physician that he should never be careless in availing himself with all necessary x-ray and laboratory aid in diagnosis!

JOURNAL, November, 1918

THE PHYSICIAN LOSES

The more we become acquainted with the medical mind, the more we lean to the oft repeated statement and general opinion that the doctor is not a good business man. For seemingly studied disregard of fundamentals where he is vitally concerned, he seems to be the premier in neglecting the simplest formula.

Some months ago the Medical Defense Committee, after much work, bearing in mind the rules and experience of all other state societies having medical defense features, prepared, with the assistance of the Association's attorneys, a concise statement of rules and advices on this most important matter. A copy of the booklet was mailed each member. Across the front was a line indicating its possible importance to the member with the request to preserve it for future reference.

We now have to deny a member defense on his particular suit solely on account of his neglect of the fundamental principles involved. Living in a populous city, with the necessary conveniences at hand for such work, he failed to have a radiograph made of a fractured femur. This alone would operate to lose him defense in nearly all state associations. In addition to that he waited until answering day—three weeks after he was served with summons—to notify the association of his plight.

Our sympathies go out to any physician who is so unfortunate as to be sued. Such suits are nearly always based on meanness on the part of either the plaintiff or possibly some enterprising physician standing on the side lines in the darkness of his own smallness and obscurity, but we simply cannot and will not make exceptions violating the clearly stated rules laid down by the defense committee. Every member has been put on his notice as to these rules, if he fails to observe them he has only himself to blame. The Medical Defense Committee again positively reiterates that it refuses to be held responsible for loss to the individual physician in case he fails to observe the rules. The rules for expenditure of the fund, which is indeed a trust fund in the truest sense, were made long before he was sued and they cannot be set aside to fit the individual demand. Securing defense is such an easy and simple matter that one wonders what the physician is doing to cause him to lose his rights. The only answer is that he neglects the simplest rules of good business and often the well established rules of proper medical practice.

Again members are warned to follow the rule, otherwise they must not try to place the blame on anyone except themselves should they lose.

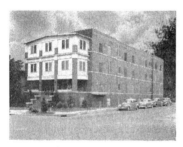
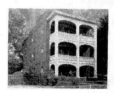

(Editors Note:)

It is interesting to compare the statement of the first World War in relation to the facts concerning membership with the present situation.

Although the membership of our Association is larger than in 1918, there has been a definite loss due to the absence of the members serving in the Armed Forces.

OUR ASSOCIATION AND THE WAR

Contrary to natural expectations the membership of our Association has not been depleted by the war, but has reached the high water mark of history. Never before have we been able to muster as many as fifteen hundred members, although we have run near that number more than once. Now our membership lists run respectably above that figure. It is easy to see the reason for this condition. It is explainable on two grounds: First: Oklahoma has and had for some time prior to the war an unprecedentedly prosperous era; secondly, practically all county societies excepting a few, neglectful of the proprieties involving such a situation, carried the absent member. This latter determination resulted in the absentee receiving his Journal, even though he was overseas in France with the American Expeditionary Forces. In a few counties, noticeably Ottawa, which had a large influx of physicians from other states, an active and widely alert county secretary lost no time in attaching the new-comer to the society membership.

The effort to keep up with the rapidly moving member of the Medical Corps of the Army has been most difficult. In all cases an effort has been made to follow the doctor wherever he goes with his home Journal in order to give him such news as was obtainable of the activities of the doctor he had left at home to look after his community.

In order to keep our mailing lists up-to-date we shall appreciate prompt information of changes of address and status of any of our members.

University of Oklahoma School of Medicine

Dr. H. A. Shoemaker, Assistant Dean of the School of Medicine, will attend the Fifty-fourth Annual Meeting of the Association of American Medical Colleges in Cleveland, Ohio, October 25, 26 and 27, 1943. While in Cleveland, Dr. Shoemaker will also attend the Centennial Celebration of Western Reserve University School of Medicine, representing the University of Oklahoma.

Dr. Arthur A. Hellbaum represented the University of Oklahoma School of Medicine at a meeting of the deans of medical colleges in the Eighth Naval District held in New Orleans, Louisiana, on October 1, 1943. The purpose of this meeting was to work out a plan of procedure for the final selection of medical students who have completed the V-12 Premedical Program of the Navy.

Dr. Ivo A. Nelson, Pathologist, St. John's Hospital, Tulsa, Oklahoma, was recently appointed Visiting Lecturer in Clinical Pathology on the faculty of the medical school and staff of the University Hospital.

Dr. John Walter Barnard has recently become connected with the University of Oklahoma School of Medicine and at the present time is serving as Research Fellow in Anatomy. On January 1, 1944, he will assume the title and duties of Assistant Professor of that Department. Dr. Barnard holds the degree of B.S., M.S., and Ph.D. from the University of Michigan.

Dr. Shoemaker will attend the meeting of the Committee for the Selection of Students, Eighth Naval District, in New Orleans, Louisiana, November 1 and 2.

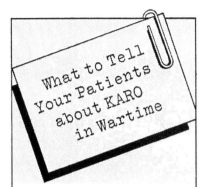
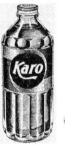

★ FIGHTIN' TALK ★

The War Department has announced that *Lt. Lawrence S. Snell*, Oklahoma City and *Lt. W. F. Bohlman*, Watonga, have been ordered to active duty.

The following Oklahoma physicians have recently been promoted from Lieutenant to Captain: *W. G. McCreight*, Oklahoma City; *Robert K. McIntosh, Jr.*, Tahlequah; *J. M. Bush*, Oklahoma City; *Lloyd N. Gilliland*, Frederick; *Albert J. Love*, Hillcrest Memorial Hospital, Tulsa; *Robert M. Shepard, Jr.*, Tulsa; *P. S. Anderson*, Claremore; *L. A. Munding*, Tulsa.

Pvt. Bill Hemphill, Pawhuska, a student of the University School of Medicine, now a medical corpsman at the Ashburn General Hospital, McKinney, Texas, received a pleasant surprise the other day as he made his rounds of the orthopedic ward. Pvt. Hemphill was talking with a patient who had been wounded in the European theater and during the conversation he showed the patient a picture of his father, *Major Paul H. Hemphill*, Pawhuska, who is a physician with the 45th Division. The patient immediately recognized the picture as the physician who had treated him when he was wounded.

Herbert A. Schubert, M.D., formerly associated with the City Health Department of Chickasha is now a Captain in the Medical Corps and is stationed at Camp Howze, Gainesville, Texas.

Captain William K. Ishmael, Oklahoma City, with his wife and two children, visited for two days recently with Dr. and Mrs. Earl D. McBride. Captain Ishmael was en route from Baton Rouge, Louisiana to Chicago.

Captain John Y. Battenfield, Oklahoma City, who has just returned from several months' service in the Caribbean area, visited relatives in Oklahoma City for two week's before going to his present station.

Lt. S. N. Stone, Jr., U.S.N.R., who practiced in Ardmore prior to entering the service, was recently married to Miss Love Porter of Oklahoma City, daughter of Frank H. Porter. The wedding took place in the First Presbyterian Church of Ardmore. After a brief wedding trip, the couple returned to Hawthorne, Nevada, where Lt. Stone is attached to the Naval Ammunition Depot.

Lt. Stone is the son of the late Dr. S. N. Stone of Edmond, Oklahoma.

Major Moorman Prosser, Norman, is now stationed at Camp Gruber, Oklahoma, where he is chief of the Neuropsychiatric Section. Major Prosser attended the Oklahoma City Clinical Society Meeting that was held in Oklahoma City October 18, 19, 20 and 21.

Lt. Col. S. E. Strader, Oklahoma City, now on duty in the Southwest Pacific, has received one of our first news letters and says that it is the first news or information that he has had from Oklahoma since he has been on his present tour of duty. He writes as follows:

"We are at present in the Southwest Pacific where the winter (if any) comes in July and August. Our day is always one day ahead of that in Oklahoma. After spending a year in the desert where it never rains, we are now where it seldom doesn't rain.

"The spirit of the American Soldier is far superior to that of us who were in the first World War. Their adaptability to the toughest assignment considered in this War is beyond description.

"The Medical Profession must be commended for the fine showing they are displaying here in the jungle. Surgical procedure and alert medical curative measures are being handled in a routine measure as we do in private practice. My outfit has bi-weekly medical meetings in which all the pep is displayed as back home in the states. We are supplied with all the latest texts, our officers are afforded schooling on tropical diseases and with two month old Medical Journals we try to keep abreast of the times, or at least abreast of the situation. Here where we are situated, tropical diseases are the topic. This is quite a contrast for the average doctor in the northern sections of the States.

"For us here in the far away places, news from home is the most cherished. The fortitude and tenacity of our nurses to withstand the hardships of this gosh awful country is worthy of commendation, and this war is just as much theirs as it is ours.

"Have just visited with *Lt. Col. Dan Perry* of Cushing. He is the Assistant Army Surgeon for this area."

Major Edward T. Cook, Jr., Anadarko, writes from his station at ———— and is enthusiastic about receiving news of the Oklahoma physicians.

Comdr. R. G. Jacobs, MC, USNR, Enid, is just now receiving our first and second news letters. He has been outside the continental limits for fifteen months. Cmdr. Jacobs' first assignment was as Executive Officer and Chief of Surgery in a Navy Field Hospital with the Marines. He then became the Commanding Officer and now has command of five Navy Field Hospitals.

Comdr. Jacobs states that the officers and boys in his outfit have done a wonderful job and that he could ask for no better group of men. In closing his letter he states:

"All we want is to finish the war and return to our way of living—then maintain the peace thereafter. Wars are such messy affairs."

Captain F. C. Lattimore, Kingfisher, is located at the Camp Grant, Ill. Replacement Training Center. In his letter to us, Captain Lattimore, sends his regards, indirectly, to *Captain John R. Taylor*, also of Kingfisher. He further states that if Dr. Mason and Dr. Shumacher could hear his lectures on Physiology and Pharmacology, they "would bubble over with pride that I was a former student of theirs and an alumnus of the University of Oklahoma School of Medicine."

Col. Wm. H. Bailey, Oklahoma City, is stationed at the Armed Forces Induction Station in Dallas, Texas, where his is Senior Medical Officer. He finds his work most interesting and states that the doctors' ability in diagnosis is given a good work-out every day. Col. Bailey's letter reads in part:

"You fellows at home are doing a fine job and we ought to appreciate it. You have a difficult assignment to fill and I expect that at times it is hard to show much 'pep'. We ought to give you all the encouragement we can. Everyone is essential in this war.

"I see *Major LeRoy Sadler* every day or so. He is doing a fine job in the office of the Chief Surgeon of the Service Command here. He handles the Personnel Division, so if any of you doctors are coming into the service, just ask him to give you a nice assignment and he will place you where the Army needs you most. He sure is getting 'hard-boiled' but he is very nice and polite about it."

Lt. *Comdr. B. B. Coker*, U.S.N.R., Durant, was the former President of the Bryan County Medical Society at the time of his entrance into the Navy. He is now living in Dallas, Texas. The following News Release concerning Lt. Comdr. Coker was received from the Public Relations Officer, U.S. Naval Air Station, Dallas, Texas.

Lieut. Commander Coker Awarded Flight Surgeon's Wings

Dallas, September 28—*Lieutenant Commander B. B. Coker*, MC-V(S), U.S.N.R., was awarded his flight surgeons wings at the Naval Air Station, Dallas, Texas, Saturday, September 25, 1943, by authority of the Bureau of Naval Personnel, Washington, D. C. His wings were presented to him with congratulations by Commander H. D. Scarney, Senior Medical Officer at the Naval Air Station. Officers and enlisted personnel of the dispensary were mustered, and witnessed the presentation and pinning on of the wings.

The Naval requirements which were met by Lieut. Comdr. Coker to become a flight surgeon, were, that he be a graduate from the Naval School of Aviation Medicine with the designation of Aviation Medical Examiner; complete six months active duty with an operating squadron; and since graduation have logged 60 or more hours of flight time in various types of Naval Aircraft. In addition he must agree not to request change of duty.

Lieut. Comdr. Coker's medical background dates back to 1924 when he received his medical degree at the Vanderbilt University in Nashville, Tennessee. Commissioned as a Lieutenant junior grade, he served his internship at the Naval Hospital, Mare Island, California, and upon completion thereof resigned his commission in 1926 to enter private practice at Durant, Oklahoma.

Entering the Naval Reserve on an inactive duty status in August of 1940, he was commissioned a Lieutenant, and six months later was called to active duty at the Naval Air Station, Corpus Christi, Texas.

In August of 1941 he was assigned to the School of Aviation Medicine at Pensacola, Florida, and upon completion was transferred to the Naval Aviation Cadet Selection Board at Dallas, Texas, reporting there October 1, 1941. After nine months of this duty, he was ordered to report aboard the Naval Air Station, Dallas, Texas, where on October 1, 1942, he was advanced to Lieutenant Commander.

The duties of the flight surgeon may be divided into four general categories. First and foremost he must be a physician. He must never forget that he is a doctor first and a flight surgeon only secondarily. He should be fully qualified not only to diagnose and treat the general run of medical ailments but he should be qualified especially to treat traumatic cases.

The second general type of duty required of flight surgeons involves the selection of candidates for flying training. The physical standards that must be met in these examinations are always regulated by higher authority. The thoroughness of the examinations and the accuracy of the findings, however, are matters for which the flight surgeon is wholly responsible.

The principal duty of flight surgeons is the "care of the flyer." That airplane pilots required special medical supervision first became apparent in 1917 and was a direct cause of the flight surgeon being created. When the American Aviation Medical Mission went to visit Europe in 1917-1918 to study aviation medicine at the Allied Fronts, they were at once struck by the care, or rather the lack of care, of flying personnel. They noted that pilots who were active at the front deteriorated very rapidly and that nothing was being done to investigate this condition or to prevent it. They soon became convinced that pilots in the various air services were being subjected to stresses and deleterious environmental influences which were not properly understood or fully appreciated. They also reached the conclusion that flying personnel were reluctant to seek medical attention for fear of being considered lacking

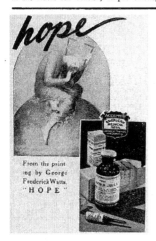

in courage. On returning to the United States, the Mission recommended that selected medical officers be given a course in aviation medicine and assigned to American flying units. These specially trained officers were to study the effect of flight on the pilot, act as his confident and advisor, and also act as an intermediary in medical matters between the flyer, his Commanding Officer, and higher medical authority.

This recommendation was put into practice and immediately became a decided success raising the morale and efficiency of the flying personnel and at the same time markedly reducing the accident rate. Since that time this practice has been continued and is today the essence of aviation medicine.

The fourth duty of the flight surgeon is to continually investigate the effect of flight and to seek remedies for those environmental conditions which may have an adverse influence. Aviation medicine is at best poorly understood in its present state and continues to become relatively more so with each advance in aviation. The increase in size, weight, speed, maneuverability, and technical complications of aircraft each year results in new problems in aviation medicine.

The following Oklahoma physicians, now serving in the Armed Forces, attended the Oklahoma City Clinical Society Meeting which was held in Oklahoma City October 18, 19, 20 and 21: *Captain Gordon Williams*, Weatherford, now stationed at the Army Aircraft School in Amarillo, Texas; *Lt. Frank Joyce*, Chickasha, stationed at Biggs Field, San Antonio, Texas; *Captain Fred Perry*, Tulsa, now at Will Rogers Field, Oklahoma City; *Major M. P. Prosser*, Norman, stationed at Camp Gruber, Oklahoma; *Captain Sanford Matthews*, Oklahoma City, stationed at the Army Aircraft School, Amarillo.

Medicine At War

The foregoing article appeared in the November 6 issue of the American Medical Association.

The following is a copy of a letter sent by Lieut. Gen. Mark W. Clark, commanding General of the Fifth Army, to Major Gen. Norman T. Kirk, Surgeon General of the United States Army, eulogizing the magnificent service rendered by the medical department in the invasion of Salerno Bay. The efficiency of the performance is testimony to the wholehearted, sacrificing effort of the medical profession of the United States. In June 1940 Gen. George Dunham, delegate from the United States Medical Corps to the House of Delegates of the American Medical Association, presented a call to the medical profession to mobilize for the war. Under Surg. Gen. James C. Magee thousands of physicians and Medical Corps men were enrolled and units like the evacuation hospitals, to which special praise is tendered, were established. Under Major Gen. Norman T. Kirk the medical profession continues to respond with courage and self sacrifice. The letter of General Clark is special testimony to the magnificent work of the battalion surgeons who move up with the troops to the front lines and render their aid under enemy fire. General Clark emphasizes particularly the closeness of the medical service to the actual front. As the war intensifies and as our Army drives on to ultimate victory the demand on the medical profession is likely to become greater, the need for its service more imminent . At this time several thousand more doctors are needed and must be enrolled. The letter of General Clark should be an inspiration to every man who can possibly meet the call to come forward and offer his services.

GENERAL CLARK EULOGIZES MEDICAL SERVICES AT SALERNO
Headquarters Fifth Army
Office of the Commanding General
A.P.O. No. 464, U.S. Army

September 25, 1943
In the field

Major General Norman T. Kirk
Surgeon General, U.S. Army,
War Department
Washington, D.C.

Dear General Kirk;

I desire to express the highest commendation for the wonderfully fine work performed by the medical units of this Army. Their devotion to duty under the hazardous and trying circumstances of the landing in Salerno Bay and their skill and efficient administration reflect the best traditions of the Service. Many wounded officers and men, who will eventually be restored to full health, would have died but for the effective work of the Medical Corps. I am especially well pleased with the performance of the Surgeon Fifth Army. He has done a magnificent job.

From the first landing to the date of this letter, 3,335 casualties have been admitted to Fifth Army hospitals. The first hospital opened within 3 to 5 miles of the front lines. The next hospital began to function the following day still closer and under the most difficult conditions. Neither hospital had any nurses when opened. Thus far there have been only 42 deaths in the hospitals. Thirty-two of these cases were those of U.S. personnel who died from wounds. Five were U. S. personnel who died from disease or injuries; 5 were enemy who died of wounds. Many of those who survived would never have reached a hospital alive had the hospitals been located at a normal distance from the front.

Two thousand and sixty-one cases have been evacuated to North Africa by air and sea.

The beach medical service was superior. One medical battalion distinguished itself on the beaches under heavy fire early in the operation. I shall recommend that the unit be cited for its gallant work under terrible conditions.

The medical supply system began to function according to plan with the assault wave, and despite the most difficult conditions it rapidly developed to the highest state of efficiency.

Among the difficulties with which the medical services have had to cope were the loss of the entire equipment of our third evacuation hospital and the bombing of a hospital ship which was bringing the nurses. Fortunately only one nurse was injured, and all are again on their way to Italy to rejoin their units.

The whole performance of the Fifth Army medical services has been most heartening to me and has been of incalculable aid in the operation. I have been so favorably impressed with their performance that I cannot forbear to write you this personal letter to tell you of my gratitude and admiration.

Mark W. Clark,
Lieutenant General, U. S. Army,
Commanding.

New Streamlinined Process of Penicillin Production

A streamline process of Penicillin production, resulting from two years' research in the Parke-Davis Laboratories, promises to substantially cut down the production time required, according to Homer C. Fritsch, General Manager of the Company.

"The present method of producing penicillin requires from $6\frac{1}{2}$ to 3 days without using cumbersome equipment."

This constitutes a significant forward step, since the bottle-neck in the Penicillin situation, to date, has been the fact that the drug has been available only in comparatively small amounts. Parke, Davis & Company is now regularly supplying Penicillin to the government and has recently expanded its facilities for producing the new "miracle" drug.

Bacillary Dysentery
in Adults . . .

SULFAGUANIDINE
Lederle

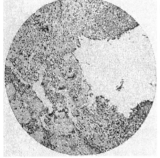

Photomicrograph showing cytological detail in acute lesion of mucosa of colon. Magnification × 650.

THE SERIOUS PATHOLOGY of the colon and rectum, frequently found following severe acute bacillary dysentery in adults, may be averted by the early oral administration of sulfaguanidine.

The use of sulfaguanidine for the treatment of dysentery carriers has been suggested.

REFERENCES:

LYON, G. M.; FOLSOM, T. G.; PARSONS, W. J., and SPROUSE, I: West Virginia M. J. 38:19 (Jan.) 1942.

LYON, G. M.: U. S. Nav. M. Bull. 40:601 (July) 1942.

BREWER, A. K.: Brit. M. J. 1:56 (Jan. 9) 1943.

FAIRLY, N. H., and ROYD, J. S. K.: Brit. M. J. 2:673 (Dec. 5) 1942. (Proc., Royal Society of Tropical Medicine and Hygiene, Nov. 4, 1942).

BULMER, E., and PRIEST, W. M.: J. Roy. Army M. Corps 79:277 (Dec.) 1942.

BANTE, L. A., and KIRBY, W. M. M.: J. A. M. A. 118:1268 (Apr. 11) 1942.

OPPER, L., and HALE, V.: J. A. M. A. 119:1489 (August 29) 1942.

KUHNS, D. M.: South. M. J. 36:593 (June) 1943.

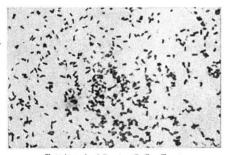

Photomicrograph of Dysentery Bacillus—Flexner— (*Shigella paradysenteriae*) Initial magnification × 1500.

PACKAGES: Bottles of 50, 100, and 1000 tablets, 0.5 Gm. (7.7 grains) each.

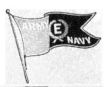

Blue Cross Reports

The one thing to avoid in the matter of hospitalization is government monopoly, the American Protestant Hospital Association was told at its annual banquet September 11, 1943, at Hotel Statler, Buffalo, New York by Rev. John G. Martin, Superintendent of the Hospital of St. Barnabas, Newark, New Jersey and President of the Association for the coming year.

Speaking of the joint committee which has represented the American Protestant Hospital Association, the American Hospital Association and the Catholic Hospital Association at Washington, D.C., Rev. Martin observed that "the subject that engaged most of the time and attention of the committee was the Social Security legislation that is pending in Congress. The committee has witnessed the determined attitude of the technical experts of the Social Security Board in its desire to include hospitalization insurance among the several benefits of its program.

"Notwithstanding the unanimous opinion of the committee, expressed to the technicians, that this coverage should not be included, still it has become an important part of the program. Those who are familiar with the problems that are peculiar to hospitals easily realize the impracticability of applying the hospitalization features of the bill without demoralizing and, in fact, ruining the voluntary hospital system.

"The Federal Government proposes to compel every wage earner to participate in this insurance at a rate far in excess of that charged by the Blue Cross Plans and gives, in return, benefits which are less than those guaranteed by the Blue Cross Plans.

"As a basic principle, widely accepted, the government should not enter the field of private business. After the experience of the wasteful exhibition of W.P.A., in which bureaucracy reigned supreme, the lesson was learned that such procedure is one way not to do things if efficiency and economy are desired.

"Thus, having the experience of the failure of government-managed public works, the administration wisely sought out business men and corporations to produce equipment for the war. What a difference between the two methods. Where would the war effort be now if W.P.A. methods had been followed? So, in the matter of hospitalization, the one thing to avoid is government monopoly.

"The question of federal regimentation of health facilities narrows itself down to the question, 'What kind of life do the American people want.' The attitude of the Social Security Board has always been that any voluntary effort is only ground-breaking for a government plan. The die is cast once the Federal plan is under way—we can't just try it, and then turn back if it doesn't work.

Material Interests Versus Moral Standards

But in the enormous development of material interests there is danger lest we miss altogether the secret of a nation's life, the true test of which is to be found in its intellectual and moral standards. There is no more potent antidote to the corroding influence of mammon than the presence in a community of a body of men devoted to science, living for investigation and caring nothing for the lust of the eyes and the pride of life. We forget that the measure of the value of a nation to the world is neither the bushel nor the barrel, but mind; and that wheat and pork, though useful and necessary, are but dross in comparison with those intellectual products which alone are imperishable. The kindly fruits of the earth are easily grown, the finer fruits of the mind are of slower development and require prolonged culture.—Aequanimitas with Other Addresses. Sir William Osler. 3rd Edition.

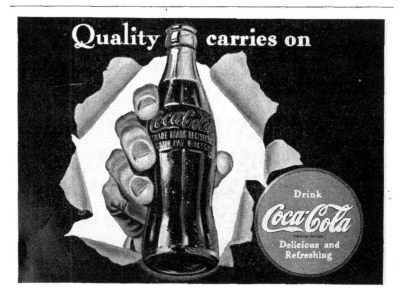

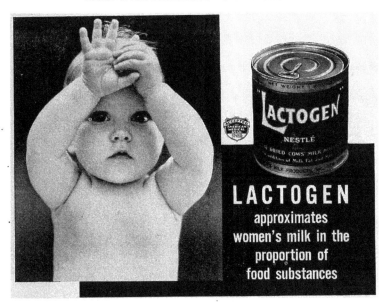
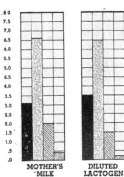

BOOK REVIEWS

"The chief glory of every people arises from its authors."—Dr. Samuel Johnson.

PSYCHOSOMATIC MEDICINE. The Clinical Application of Psychopathology to General Medical Problems. Edward Weiss and O. Spurgeon English. W. B. Saunders Co. 651 pages. $10.00.

There is nothing new about this subject except the term employed to describe it. We have every reason to believe that the well-known Greek physicians looked upon the human organism as a composite whole and directed their therapy to both mind and body. In fact, modern concern about psychosomatic medicine simply suggests the need of a return to the art of medicine. As indicated by the authors, we have permitted cellular pathology, laboratory diagnosis including x-ray and other mechanical diagnosis and therapeutic agents to lead us away from the patient in search of the disease.

This is a timely book in that it represents a comprehensive effort to secure an equable division of the physicians time and effort between mind and body.

Because we have been drifting from the bedside and neglecting the art of medicine for more than half a century, we have to learn not only much that has been forgotten but a goodly sum which is relatively new and now in the hands of the neurophychiatrists greatly augmented by the knowledge which has grown out of the Freudian system.

The authors of this volume in 23 chapters covering approximately 800 pages, have brought this knowledge together in workable form and have made it applicable to the doctors every day diagnostic and therapeutic problems.

The text serves as a genuine stimulus for the consideration of the patient as well as the disease which brings about the patient and doctor relationship, yet it exhibits the balance which has grown out of team work in the wards of the hospital with the cooperation of Dr. C. L. Brown, Professor of Medicine, Temple University. The senior author is Professor of Clinical Medicine and the junior author is Professor of Psychiatry.

Apparently the volume reflects the work of the teaching service at Temple University and the valuable case reports are drawn from this service.—Lewis J. Moorman, M.D.

THE MARCH OF MEDICINE. The New York Academy of Medicine Lectures to the Laity. Columbia University Press. 1943. Price $2.50.

This little volume is a collection of addresses to lay audiences, sponsored and promoted by the New York Academy of Medicine. The addresses are by distinguished physicians, "each an eminent authority in his particular field."

Naturally, education of the laity in medical knowledge is a more desirable goal towards which the vast majority of the members of the medical profession are striving; as witness the changed and changing attitude of the public in the last two decades regarding prophylaxis of diphtheria and typhoid, to mention but two instances; and the present reaction of mothers consenting to, and even demanding hospitalization and the latest treatment for their children with poliomyelitis; but it is the reviewer's belief that this education should be couched in simple terms, avoiding the use of foreign words and phrases and pedantic polysyllabic utterances.

As a criterion, we could assume that the value of a lesson, speech or lecture to an auditor is in direct proportion to what he can carry away with him for future use. Using this as a measuring line, it must be said that the average layman would be able to carry but a few grains home from these lectures, even if he could separate those calculable grains from the chaff of difficult phraseology and strange and unusual words in which they are cleverly hidden.

"Equipotential material type", "egocentricity", "ogtogenetic sequences", "hierarchical continuum", "filiform excrescences", "oxidation rancidity", are among the ponderous combinations found in these lectures.

With the exception of the lecture on tuberculosis, which is worth the price of the book, and the possible exception of that on nutrition, it would seem that these addresses were far over the heads of the hearers: and the reviewer fears that nine-tenths of those in the audiences went home dazed, sleepy and bored.—J. V. Athey, M.D.

CLIMATE MAKES THE MAN. Clarence A. Mills, M.D., Ph.D. Harper and Brothers. New York. 1942. 320 pages. Price, $3.00.

Here is a book which contains an amazing store of knowledge about climate and weather and man's response to their influences throughout the world. The author is well known in the field of experimental medicine and many of the theories advanced are supported by experimental studies.

The historical citations showing the influence of climate upon civilization among various races in different sections of the world are very interesting. On the whole this little volume is well worth a careful perusal by both the professional and the lay reader.

In the opinion of the reviewer the effects of climate are over-estimated and too little attention paid to the human organisms' adaptation to climate influences.

The chapter on "Made-to-Order Indoor Climates" should be read by everyone who is interested in air conditioning. It represents a very sane discussion of the subject, recognizing the disadvantages as well as the advantages of this method of conditioning our environment.

The book is well written and presents a rather fascinating story with appealing continuity.—Lewis J. Moorman, M.D.

SYNOPSIS OF TROPICAL MEDICINE. Sir Phillip Manson-Bahr. Williams and Wilkins Company. Baltimore. Illustrated, 224 pages. Price $2.50.

This book is a synopsis of the standard textbook, "Manson's Tropical Diseases." It was published because of the need for a condensation of the information in this field. The book is intended to serve as a convenient guide to tropical medicine. Its coverage is as broad as that of the original text with the advantage that it has been completely revised and brought up to date. By using small print and expertly condensing the material this book gives a great deal of information in a pocket sized edition. On the other hand, one finds the same faults with this book that he would find in the synopsis of a large, standard textbook in any major branch of medicine.

Chapters include: protozoan diseases, spirochetal diseases, rickettsia diseases, bacterial diseases, virus diseases, climatic diseases, fungous diseases, nutritional diseases, vegetable poisons, animal poisons, worm, insect, etc., infections, and laboratory methods. A few key illustrations are used to assist in laboratory diagnosis. Most of the diseases are discussed under geographic distribution, etiology, pathology, clinical features, diagnosis, treatment and prophylaxis. This book will serve very well for the purpose it was intended and if generally used will be of great assistance to physicians who are meeting these problems in the Armed Forces or in the civilian population.—Donald B. McMullen, ScD.

MEDICAL ABSTRACTS

"THE ABSORPTION, EXCRETION AND DISTRIBUTION OF PENICILLIN." C. H. Rammelkamp and C. S. Keefer. Journal of Clin. Investigation. ..Vol. 22, page 425. May. 1943.

The sodium salt of penicillin, dissolved in distilled water or 0.85 per cent sodium chloride solution, was administered to normal subjects and to patients with various conditions by the following routes; oral, intraduodenal, rectal, intravenous, subcutaneous, intramuscular, intrapleural, intraarticular, and intrabursal. No serious toxic manifestations were noted in the course of study. There were no untoward reactions from intravenous injections of from 5,000 to 40,000 Florey units or from the administration of 102,500 units given to one patient by the intravenous drip method over a period of thirty-eight hours. Intramuscular injection of 10,000 units in distilled water was attended with definite residual soreness; there was no residual soreness if the penicillin was dissolved in saline solution. Subcutaneous injection of 10,000 units in 50 cc of saline solution resulted in soreness and erythemia persisting for from twelve to twenty-four hours. When a somewhat more dilute solution was used, there was no soreness. Oral administration of penicillin solution was unpleasant because of the bitter taste.

The amounts of penicillin in urine, blood, joint fluid, exudates, spinal fluid, etc. were determined by the method of Rammelkamp (Proc. Soc. Exper. Biol. & Med., Vol. 51, page 95. 1942). A table is presented including data on the route of administration, dose, and amounts of penicillin in the blood and urine at various intervals after administration. Graphs illustrate the penicillin concentration in various body fluids according to time. Without repeating the specific concentrations, it may be said that high initial blood concentrations following intravenous administration were succeeded by an abrupt fall, with only traces of penicillin being found after 210 minutes. The sharp fall was associated with increased urinary excretions. The average excretion after intravenous injection was 58 per cent of the injected dose. Penicillin was rapidly absorbed after intramuscular injection, slowly after subcutaneous injection. Excretion in urine was correspondingly rapid or slow. Absorption from body cavities was delayed and this was reflected in slow urinary excretion. Fluid from joint and pleural cavities aspirated thirteen and twenty-two hours after local administration contained appreciable amounts of penicillin. Administration by enteral routes showed that absorption was rapid from the duodenum, whereas oral and rectal doses were poorly absorbed. These findings may be explained by the inactivating effect on penicillin of acid and escherichia coli. After oral, intraduodenal, and rectal administration, the average amount excreted in the urine was extremely small. In the presence of renal failure, as shown in two cases, penicillin was slowly excreted and high blood concentrations were maintained.

Studies on the distribution of penicillin showed that it failed to penetrate the red cells in significant amounts; in general, the concentration in erythrocytes was about 10 per cent of that found in plasma. No penicillin was detected in the spinal fluid, saliva, or tears in subjects receiving the drug intravenously. These studies indicate that the location of the infection is of utmost importance in determining the route of penicillin administration, since it does not diffuse readily and is quickly excreted. It is advisable, therefore, to give penicillin locally rather than intravenously in infections of the pleural and joint cavities. In generalized infections, such as bacteremia, intravenous or intramuscular therapy is indicated.—H.J., M.D.

"MISCONCEPTION ABOUT THE 'SPRINGINESS' OF THE LONGITUDINAL ARCH OF THE FOOT. MECHANICS OF THE ARCH OF THE FOOT." Paul W. Lapidus. Archives of Surgery, Vol. XLVI, No. 410. March, 1943.

The author takes issue with the long-held belief that the longitudinal arch of the foot operates as a spring, functioning by gradually absorbing shock as weight is placed on it, and elastically releasing as weight is removed. The plantar fascis in man is approximately fifteen centimeters long, and has a cross section of at least 0.5 square centimeters. The estimated tensile load of plantar fascia is thirty-five kilograms in a man weighing sixty kilograms, standing on one foot in a relaxed position. Maximum elongation of the fascia is only to 15.21 centimeters, 1.4 per cent of its length, allowing for sagging of the apex of the arch of only 0.1 centimeters. The arch can thus hardly be compared to a "semiellipitic spring."

The arch was really developed in response to functional requirements for increased strength of the foot as a lever. The foot is compared to a simple roof truss. The bottom is under tension; the upper part under compression. The higher the truss, the more it can stand tension and compression; the higher the longitudinal arch of the foot, the greater tension and compression it can bear. The skeletal parts of the foot form struts which are subjected to compression stresses, and the plantar fascia acts as a tie rod taking up all the tensile stresses. Bending stresses are eliminated, and the strength of the foot as a lever is increased.

The integrity of the longitudinal arch is maintained by the ligamentous rather than by the muscle structure. In an anaesthetized subject there is no decrease in the height of the arch, and poliomyelitis cases no flattening of the arch. Protracted standing would be impossible if it were dependent upon the muscles, as they tire easily. Energy must be conserved.

The muscles of the legs further support the longitudinal arch of the foot maintaining balance between the leg and the foot by keeping the weight-bearing line in the plumb line. They help bear weight and assist in locomotion.

Idiopathic "flat foot" is probably congenital or hereditary and not due to faulty muscle function.—E.D.M., M.D.

"LYMPHOMATOID DISEASES INVOLVING THE EYE AND ITS ADNEXA." J. S. McGavic. Archives of Ophthalmology, Vol. 30, No. 2, pages 179-193. Chicago. August, 1943.

The lymphomatoid diseases are exceedingly complex. Little is known about their pathogenesis. The author collected a series of 21 verified cases. Of these, 17 were primary tumors in the region of the eye, while in 4 ocular involvement appeared during the course of already generalized lymphomatoid disease.

Lymphomatoid diseases occur at all ages and in both sexes. They may occur at any site in the body but more frequently occur in the recognized lymphatic tissues. Their diagnosis must be established by histopathology. Incisional biopsies are necessary; aspiration biopsies too often fail to give sufficient information to warrant a diagnosis. Even diagnosis from biopsies is sometimes inconclusive or confusing. Repeated differential blood counts and studies of the bone marrow may be necessary to rule out or demonstrate leukemic changes. In general the outlook for patients with lymphomatoid disease is poor.

Surgical intervention should be limited to biopsy, unless the mass is encapsulated and can be removed without sacrifice of function. Practically all lymphomatoid growths are radiosensitive, but this quality must be differentiated from radiocurability. A given lesion may be treated to complete regression, but this does not preclude the appearance of tumor masses at other sites. Local recurrence after treatment of a primary tumor in the region of the eye has not occurred in the series of 17 cases reported by the author, though a general spread has occurred after such treatment in 6 of these cases.

Immediately successful treatment of a tumor in the region of the eye does not relieve the ophthalmologist or the physician giving the radiation from further care of the patient. Many reports demonstrate the necessity of five to ten years' follow-up. After receiving a report from the pathologist, the clinician should refer the patient to a physician skilled in the application of radiation therapy.

Subconjunctival lymphomas have the same clinical appearance irrespective of the histologic type and clinical course. A primary lymphoma of the iris is reported by the author.

A study of the present series and of the general medical literature suggests that the lymphomatoid diseases represent a great variety of related clinical and histologic responses by lymphoid tissue to currently unknown stimuli. Some of the tumors appear to be neoplastic from their onset, while others may represent transitions from inflammatory to neoplastic lesions.

Despite the generally poor prognosis for patients with localized lymphomatous tumors in the region of the eye, these tumors should be actively treated by radiation, just as one treats carcinoma, with the justified hope that some of the patients will be cured and not have generalized lymphosarcomatosis.

"OSTEOGENESIS IMPERFECTA." William H. Bickel, Ralph K. Ghormley and John D. Camp. Radiology, Vol. XL. page 145. February, 1943.

Called by various names, fragilitas osseum, brittle bones, blue sclera and otosclerosis, etc., these cases are divisible into (1) the hereditary type, which is called an hereditary hypoplasia of the mesenchyme with brittle bones and blue sclera, and (2) the non-hereditary, congenital type comprising two groups; osteogenesis imperfecto congenita and osteogenesis imperfecta tarda. Blue sclerae, while requisite for the first group, may or may not be present in the second.

As to etiology, Knaggs has stated that there is an evolutionary failure of the osteoblasts; Key and others have attributed all the changes to hereditary; the endocrine glands have been implicated, but the evidence is inconclusive. There is probably some inherent defect in the germ plasm, hereditary or non-hereditary, which does not allow the mesenchymal tissue to develop normally.

The present study is of cases seen at the Mayo Clinic from 1920 to 1940. Clinically, it is impossible to distinguish between the hereditary type and the non-hereditary, congenital type. Of the cases studied, 27.5 per cent were of the hereditary type, in one family involving four generations, all presenting brittle bones, blue sclerae, and deafness. Transmissible by either the male or female, the defect follows mendelian characteristics. Once transmission has begun, no generation is without some stigma of the disease. In 72.5 per cent of

the cases, there was no family history of the disease. Few of the non-hereditary, congenital type live to a great age, and many are so badly crippled they do not marry.

There is great variation in the severity of the process, some coming under observation for conditions entirely unrelated to skeletal defect. On the whole, these patients were poorly nourished, short, and presented many deformities.

Multiple fractures occurred in all cases, and, with one exception, were caused by slight trauma and were less painful than usual. Four hundred and thirty-four fractures were recorded in the fourth cases, forty-six being recorded in one case, while in seven they were too numerous to record. The long bones were usually involved, though no bone was exempt. In the non-hereditary type they were more frequent, and occurring earlier and with less trauma than in the hereditary type. Usually of the subperiosteal type, the fractures showed little displacement, but marked angulation. One of the authors (Camp) believes that the majority of the so-called fractures reported in this condition are really pseudofractures or Looser's Zones. The frequency of fractures decreased as puberty was approached, and in some cases fractures ceased after puberty.—E.D.M., M.D.

"ESTIMATION OF PERCENTAGE OF COMPENSABLE HEARING DEFECTS." W. E. Grove. Archives of Otlaryngology. Vol. 38. No. 2, pages 152-155. Chicago. August. 1943.

The percentage estimaton of hearing defects due to accident or occupation is a question which concerns industry, insurance companies, courts of law and compensation boards. The American Medical Association had a special committee to establish some useful procedure for the estimation of hearing defects.

Inasmuch as the loss of ability to hear the human voice was taken as a criterion of traumatic hearing defects by this committee, the "usable hearing" was defined, and what constitutes at total, or 100 per cent, loss of such usable hearing. It was accepted, in agreement with the previous work of other investigators, that all tones or frequencies between 256 and 4096 cycles were of value for the understanding of speech. Also it is believed that the frequencies or bands of frequencies between 1000 and 3500 cycles are relatively more important than the others. Frequencies below 256 and above 4096 cycles have no particular value for the understanding of speech .

On the basis of these assumptions, a number of audiograms were prepared, and a chart produced which is the final weighted audiogram and hearing loss chart.

The method estimates, in a general way, the percentage loss of hearing a person has suffered but does not attempt to evaluate the disability accruing therefrom. Such an estimate of disability is a function of courts, juries and other judicial bodies. When this method is made to apply to persons in specialized occupations, it is the function of these judicial bodies to determine in how far it should apply. This matter of compensable disability is certainly no direct concern of the otologist.—M.D.H., M.D.

KEY TO ABSTRACTIONS

E. D. M. .... Earl D. McBride, M.D.
M. D. H. .... Marvin D. Henley, M.D.
H. J. .... Hugh Jeter, M.D.

I have faith in tomorrow; for I have seen the most wonderful yesterday that ever happened on this planet —William Allen White.

Look to your health; and if you have it, praise God and value it next to a good conscience; for health is the second blessing that money cannot buy.—Izaak Walton.

Do not forget that of all the countless remedies, rest, alone has stood the test of time.—Gerald B. Webb, M.D.

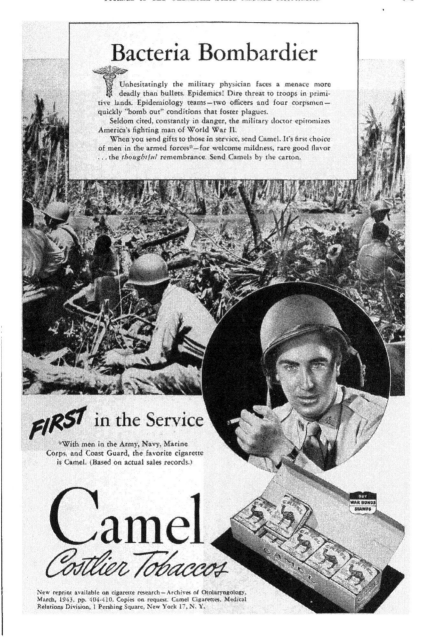

OFFICERS OF COUNTY SOCIETIES, 1943

★

COUNTY	PRESIDENT	SECRETARY	MEETING TIME
Alfalfa	H. E. Huston, Cherokee	L. T. Lancaster, Cherokee	Last Tues. each Second Month
Atoka-Coal	J. D. Clark, Coalgate	J. S. Fulton, Atoka	
Beckham	H. K. Speed, Sayre	E. S. Kilpatrick, Elk City	Second Tuesday
Blaine	Virginia Olson Curtin, Watonga	W. F. Griffin, Watonga	
Bryan	J. T. Colwick, Durant	W. K. Haynie, Durant	Second Tuesday
Caddo	F. L. Patterson, Carnegie	C. B. Sullivan, Carnegie	
Canadian	P. F. Herod, El Reno	A. L. Johnson, El Reno	Subject to call
Carter	Walter Hardy, Ardmore	H. A. Higgins, Ardmore	
Cherokee	P. H. Medearis, Tahlequah	*James K. Gray, Tahlequah	First Tuesday
Choctaw	C. H. Hale, Boswell	E. A. Johnson, Hugo	
Cleveland	J. A. Rieger, Norman	Curtis Berry, Norman	Thursday nights
Comanche	George S. Barber, Lawton	W. F. Lewis, Lawton	
Cotton	A. B. Holstead, Temple	Mollie F. Seism, Walters	Third Friday
Craig	F. M. Adams, Vinita	J. M. McMillan, Vinita	
Creek	H. R. Haas, Sapulpa	C. G. Oakes, Sapulpa	
Custer	F. R. Vieregg, Clinton	C. J. Alexander, Clinton	Third Thursday
Garfield	Paul B. Champlin, Enid	John R. Walker, Enid	Fourth Thursday
Garvin	T. F. Gross, Lindsay	John R. Callaway, Pauls Valley	Wednesday before Third Thursday
Grady	Walter J. Baze, Chickasha	Roy E. Emanuel, Chickasha	Third Thursday
Grant	I. V. Hardy, Medford	E. E. Lawson, Medford	
Greer	G. P. Cherry, Mangum	J. B. Hollis, Mangum	
Harmon	W. G. Husband, Hollis		First Wednesday
Haskell	William Carson, Keota	N. K. Williams, McCurtain	
Hughes	Wm. L. Taylor, Holdenville	Inogene Mayfield, Holdenville	First Friday
Jackson	E. S. Crow, Olustee	E. W. Mabry, Altus	Last Monday
Jefferson	F. M. Edwards, Ringling	L. L. Wade, Ryan	Second Monday
Kay	Philip C. Risser, Blackwell	J. Holland Howe, Ponca City	Second Thursday
Kingfisher	C. M. Hodgson, Kingfisher	H. Violet Sturgeon, Hennessey	
Kiowa	B. H. Watkins, Hobart	J. William Finch, Hobart	
LeFlore	Neeson Rolle, Poteau	Rush L. Wright, Poteau	
Lincoln	H. B. Jenkins, Tryon	Carl H. Bailey, Stroud	First Wednesday
Logan	William C. Miller, Guthrie	J. L. LeHew, Jr., Guthrie	Last Tuesday
Marshall	O. A. Cook, Madill		
Mayes	Ralph V. Smith, Pryor	Paul B. Cameron, Pryor	
McClain	B. W. Slover, Blanchard	R. L. Royster, Purcell	
McCurtain	A. W. Clarkson, Valliant	N. L. Barker, Broken Bow	Fourth Tuesday
McIntosh	James L. Wood, Eufaula	William A. Tolleson, Eufaula	First Thursday
Murray	P. V. Annadown, Sulphur		Second Tuesday
Muskogee-Sequoyah-Wagoner	H. A. Scott, Muskogee	D. Evelyn Miller, Muskogee	First Monday
Noble	C. H. Cooke, Perry	J. W. Francis, Perry	
Okfuskee	L. J. Spickard, Okemah	M. L. Whitney, Okemah	Second Monday
Oklahoma	Walker Morledge, Oklahoma City	E. R. Musick, Oklahoma City	Fourth Tuesday
Okmulgee	A. R. Holmes, Henryetta	J. C. Matheney, Okmulgee	Second Monday
Osage	C. R. Weirich, Pawhuska	George K. Hemphill, Pawhuska	Second Monday
Ottawa	W. B. Sanger, Picher	Matt A. Connell, Picher	Third Thursday
Pawnee	E. T. Robinson, Cleveland	R. L. Browning, Pawnee	
Payne	L. A. Mitchell, Stillwater	C. W. Moore, Stillwater	Third Thursday
Pittsburg	John F. Park, McAlester	William H. Kaeiser, McAlester	Third Friday
Pontotoc	O. H. Miller, Ada	R. H. Mayes, Ada	First Wednesday
Pottawatomie	A. C. McFarling, Shawnee	Clinton Gallaher, Shawnee	First and Third Saturday
Pushmataha	John S. Lawson, Clayton	B. M. Huckabay, Antlers	
Rogers	C. W. Beson, Claremore	C. L. Caldwell, Chelsea	First Monday
Seminole	Max Van Sandt, Wewoka	Mack I. Shanholtz, Wewoka	Third Wednesday
Stephens	W. K. Walker, Marlow	Wallis S. Ivy, Duncan	
Texas	R. G. Obermiller, Texhoma	Morris Smith, Guymon	
Tillman		O. G. Bacon, Frederick	
Tulsa	James C. Peden, Tulsa	E. O. Johnson, Tulsa	Second and Fourth Monday
Washington-Nowata	J. G. Smith, Bartlesville	J. V. Athey, Bartlesville	Second Wednesday
Washita	A. S. Neal, Cordell	James F. McMurry, Sentinel	
Woods	C. A. Traverse, Alva	O. E. Templin, Alva	Last Tuesday Odd Months
Woodward	C. E. Williams, Woodward	C. W. Tedrowe, Woodward	Second Thursday

*(Serving in Armed Forces)

THE JOURNAL
OF THE
OKLAHOMA STATE MEDICAL ASSOCIATION

| VOLUME XXXVI | OKLAHOMA CITY, OKLAHOMA, DECEMBER, 1943 | NUMBER 12 |

The Treatment of Compound Fractures*

M. A. CONNELL, M.D.

PICHER, OKLAHOMA

In the past twenty years, there has been a constant change in the management and treatment of severe lacerations, macerations, and compound fractures. It is not our purpose to advance a new method of treatment, but rather to outline the method that we have been using, and have found to give the most satisfactory results over the past several years.

The basic principle of our method is the one advocated by Dr. Marble of Boston, that is a complete and thorough debridement under constant saline irrigation. To this, we have added the implantation of powdered or crystalline sulfathiazole and the administration orally and subcutaneously of one of the sulfa drugs to obtain maximum concentration post-operatively. The treatment used for compound fractures and severe lacerations and macerations is the same, except for the method of fixation of the fracture.

When the patient is first admitted, the wound is completely filled with powdered sulfa drug, preferable sulfathiazole. No attempt is made to dress or clean the wound, and the foreman and safety men in charge of the mine operation have been advised not to remove clothing or apply dressings other than fixation for comfort, previous to the patient's admission to the hospital. Following the administration of the sulfa drug, preparations for a complete sterile technique are initiated. We do not advocate hurried emergency methods, but feel that these conditions deserve a full operating room set-up with complete sterile technique.

*Read before the Annual Meeting held in Oklahoma City, May 11-12, 1943.

The patient is made comfortable and if signs of shock are present, treatment is immediately instituted. As soon as the operating room preparations have been completed, the clothing about the wound is removed, and the skin and wound itself are washed thoroughly with sterile water and soap. Antiseptic soap has no advantage over an olive oil base soap and is certainly much more irritating to the already badly devitalized tissues. For that reason, a green soap is not used on these wounds.

Following the complete cleansing of the wound and the surrounding tissues, a thorough debridement is performed. A scalpel is preferred to scissors in this procedure. In the set-up, a nurse is delegated to keep a constant stream of normal saline playing upon the wound during the entire operation. A drainage pan has been devised

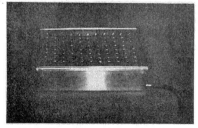

The stainless steel tray with a perforated top and rubber hose connection which is used under the extremity and collects the saline, thus preventing saturation of the sterile dressings and the operating room floor.

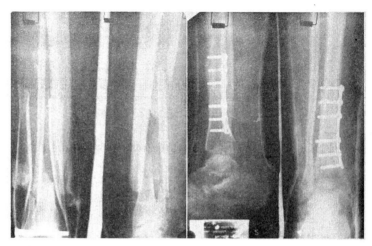

Case 1—Illustration No. 1

Case 1—Illustration No. 2

Case 1. X-Ray on admission to the hospital. This patient was a white male who received a compound comminuted fracture of the tibia and fibula when he attempted to step over a running belt. Upon admission to the hospital the tibia was compounded and was exposed for approximately four inches and was resting on the outside of a short boot which the patient was wearing. In this X-Ray, it is possible to see the tibia outside of the boot. The technique employed followed that recommended in this article. After the thorough de-

bridement under saline, a six-screw Sherman Vitallium plate was used as internal fixation for the tibia. Wound was closed tight following implantation of sulfathiazole and a plaster cast was applied from the center of the thigh to the heads of the metatarsals.

Case 1. X-Ray eight weeks following operation. There is union of fibula and tibia. Patient was placed in a plaster boot with walking iron and in three weeks, patient began using the foot.

for the use with this method, which prevents the soaking of the bedding and the operating room floor. Following the removal of all devitalized tissue, the wound is made as dry as possible and all bleeding points are thoroughly ligated.

In the treatment of compound fracture, any procedure representing a clean operation may be used. Here, if it is necessary for proper fixation, we would not hesitate to do a recognized internal fixation. The use of Vitallium Sherman plates in some cases has been quite satisfactory. All bone fragments which do not appear to be badly contaminated should be left in and around the bone fracture. This, of course, helps to stimulate early healing and callous formation.

Following the fixation of the bone fragments, a sulfa drug is again instilled into the wound. There is no doubt but that the sulfa drugs to some extent are irritating to the tissues and cause edema and induration with a resulting thickening in the scar. Likewise, there is a delayed healing as a result of the use of the drug. For that reason, the drug is not sprayed into the wound in those cases in which we have been able to

perform a thorough debridement. As a matter of fact, the saline and debridement are more important than the sulfa drugs. The patient is given tetanus gas gangrene antitoxin immediately following his operation.

In choosing an anesthetic the local infiltration of tissue is not the desirable method and a general anesthetic is preferable; however, should the patient's condition be such that this may be contraindicated, a nerve block is more satisfactory than local infiltration. A tourniguet often is desirable, but is not used routinely. Sulfanilamide is ordinarily given subcutaneously immediately upon the patient's return to his room, and the administration of the sulfa drug is continued by mouth until a maximum blood concentration is reached. This is continued for approximately one week.

The original cast ordinarily is changed at the end of two weeks. Sutures are removed and a second cast applied and not changed unless there is definite indication due to atrophy of the muscles or to a necessity for beginning manipulative therapy. It is obvious that these patients should not be sent home, but should be hospitalized and kept.

under constant observation for any signs of infection. Should infection result, the cast should be opened and the wound drained. In our experience it has been necessary in one instance to open a cast and drain a superficial abscess, however, this did not involve the bone. The bone healed with good apposition and alignment and there was never any indication of osteomyelitis.

The healing of fractures under this method is somewhat slower than the healing of fractures in which there has been no necessity for an open reduction, but this is consistent with the usual findings in any open reduction, since it is a fact that open reduced fractures do not heal as rapidly, ordinarily, as those that have been reduced by closed method. In fractures of the lower extremities, as soon as it is safe, a walking iron is incorporated in a plaster cast and active motion is encouraged in the extremities.

This treatment eliminates the slow healing which is encouraged in the open wound methods. It has the advantage of fixing the bone fragments in their proper positions at the very onset of treatment, thus, there has been no time lost in fracture healing. The hospital period is definitely reduced, and the man is often returned to work before his healing period is over.

DISCUSSION
LT. COMDR. C. F. FERCIOT
U. S. Naval Hospital—Norman, Oklahoma

First, I would like to express my personal appreciation for the hearty welcome that the Oklahoma medical men have extended to those of us in service who are stationed in this area.

The problems arising in connection with compound fractures are of particular interest to every military surgeon. Dr. Connell has presented in concise form a method for their care and I want to heartily endorse the principle he has outlined.

Probably the greatest advance in traumatic surgery has developed from a more widespread recognition of the importance of the treatment and prevention of shock in every injured person. The value of blood serum and plasma has been proven and with the addition of such effective means of resuscitation to the armamentarium of shock therapy, the surgeon is today being called upon to treat injuries of increasing severity which would previously have resulted in early fatalities.

The primary rules of fracture treatment are applicable to compound fractures as well. They are accurate reduction, adequate immobilization, preservation of blood supply.

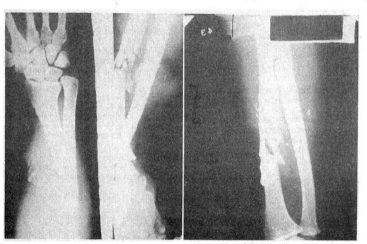

Case 2—Illustration No. 1   Case 2—Illustration No. 2

Case 2. X-Ray made upon admission to the hospital. Patient stated a hoisterman "overshot his mark" and let an empty can fall on the patient's arm, causing maceration with a laceration which lacked about an inch extending around the arm. A Sherman Vitallium bone plate was used. Sulfathiazole was used and the wound closed tight.

Case 2. X-Ray shows the reduction two weeks following operation at which time the skin sutures were removed... There was no evidence of infection and the wound had healed by first intention.

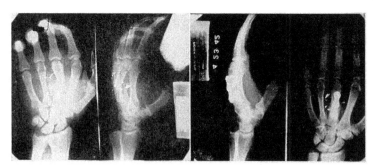

Case 3—Illustration No. 1   Case 3—Illustration No. 2

Case 3. X-Ray made upon admission to the hospital. Patient stated he had been shot through the hand with a twenty-two long rifle about 12 hours previous to his admission to the hospital. Upon admission, usual de-

bridement was performed and a three-screw Sherman plate was applied. No sulfathiazole was administered. Case 3. Final X-Ray of this case several months after his injury, in which the bone plate is still intact.

In compound fractures there are the additional complicating factors of an open wound with severe soft tissue damage, the presence of foreign material in the wound, and the presence of infection.

Dr. Connell has called attention to the limitations of the local use of sulfa drugs in these wounds. Baker of Duke University after a review of 270 cases of fresh compound fractures concluded that "the local use of these drugs is of help in combating infection only when the fundamental rules of wound hygiene have been followed."

On the other hand, recent reports from surgical units near the fighting fronts state that "with the local use of sulfonamides, radical debridement appears unnecessary in many cases actually destructive." It has been my personal impression that it's local use as a first aid measure is of practical importance, making it possible to do a satisfactory debridement of the wound much later than previously although not lessening the desirability of early adequate surgical care.

It would seem that the question of primary closure must be decided upon the merits of the individual case. Certainly in some instances it is possible to use this method to advantage but the general conclusion in the care of war wounds is that in most cases early wound suture is not only unnecessary but is an actual hinderance to eventual wound healing.

The advantages of treatment by the closed plaster method are outstanding and this pro-

cedure received general recognition. In combination with appropriate types of skeletal traction or fixation it affords adequate immobilization of the fracture and support to the soft tissues. By minimizing frequency of dressings it conserves both time and material, adds to the comfort of the patient, and favors eventual rehabilitation.

Recent experimental studies by Thomson of Lincoln and Helwig of Kansas City would indicate the value of the injection of the sympathetic ganglia of an extremity following severe trauma. They found that circulation of an extremity is definitely impaired after trauma by spasm and was markedly improved following sympathetic nerve block. This finding is in accord with the work of Leriche, Oschner, DeBakey and others, and may well make available a new method of combating severe circulatory complications.

In conclusion, let me thank Dr. Connell for his excellent presentation of a method he has found effective in changing a latently infected wound into a relatively clean one.

BIBLIOGRAPHY

1. Allen, H. S., Hoch, S. L.: The Treatment of Patients With Severe Burns. Surg. Gynec. Obstet., LXXIV, 914, 1942.

2. Cloward, R. B.: War Injuries To The Head. Treatment of Penetrating Wounds. Jour. A.M.A., CXVIII, 267, 1942.

3. Duncan, G. W., Blalock, Alfred: The Uniform Production of Experimental Shock by Crush Injury: Possible Relationship to Clinical Crush Syndrome. Ann. Surg., CXV, 684, 1942.

4. Moon, V. H.: Hemoconcentration as Related to Shock. Amer. Jour. Clin. Pathol., XI, 361, 1941.

5. Marble: Lecture-Compound Fractures—Harvard University Medical School, 1939.

6. Scudder: Treatment of Fractures and Sprains, Tenth Edition.

7. Cotton, F. J.: Fractures: Tice Vol. 11, Chap. IV.

8. Davis, A. S., Fortune, C. W.: Journal of Bones and Joints Surgery, Vol. XXV. No. 1, January, 1943.

Problems of Induction*

MONTI L. BELOT, COLONEL, M. C.

Medical Liaison Officer
Headquarters Eighth Service Command

DALLAS, TEXAS

In presenting this subject I hope to give the profession a more comprehensive view of the many problems confronting the military forces in the induction of men for service, and in so doing answer, to the best of my ability, numerous questions that have might arisen regarding this work.

Interesting volumes might be written upon the evolution of methods of inducting manpower at other times and in other countries. William the Conquerer achieved success by the simple method of detailing a mounted bugler to ride through the country and summon the male population. Halie Selassie depended upon verbal summons for all males able to carry a spear and specified in his order that those failing to appear would be subject to the death penalty.

You are all familiar with proceedings used by our country in former wars. Our present system of Selective Service is based upon the legislation of 1921. Induction proceedings during the present emergency are encompassed in Mobilization Regulations 1-9. In setting fourth the objective, I quote from these regulations:

"The objective is the procurement of men who are physically fit for the rigors of general military service or for limited military service, therefore the examining physicians will consider these standards as a guide to their discretion and not construe them too strictly or arbitrarily. The examination will be carried out with the utmost care in order that no individuals who are unfit for service will be accepted only to be discharged within a short time on Certificate of Disability. All minor defects as well as disqualifying defects will be recorded in order to protect the Government in the event of future claims for disability compensation. The likelihood of subsequent claims on account of disability should be borne in mind by the examiners in considering the qualifications of registrants with questionable defects. Whenever a registrant is accepted for general military duty but who nevertheless has a disease or other physical condition which, although

not disqualifying, requires medical treatment, the nature of the condition and the need for treatment will be clearly stated on the report of physicial examination.

Physical classifications are:

a. For general service: Includes those physically qualified for all general military service and registrants in this group will be recommended for assignment to general service if they meet the requirements throughout the entire physical examination.

b. Limited service: Physically unfit for general military service but fit for limited military service. Individuals who fail to qualify for general service but who do not fall below limited service requirements in any phase of the examination will be recommended for assignment to limited service unless because of multiple defects the medical examiners recommend unqualified rejection as non-acceptable.

c. Non-acceptable: Physically unfit for any military service. All individuals who do not meet the physical requirements for general service or limited service will be recommended as non-acceptable."

Based upon Mobilization Regulations of other nations, is is probable that instead of the registrant being classified as being available for limited military service, and at least a part of those registrants being classed as disqualified for any military service in the United States Army, possess health conditions which would be acceptable for general military duty by other governments. United States Army regulations, in setting forth physical standards, describe health conditions that must be attained at the time of physical examination at induction stations. The regulations are predicated on the assumption that registrants qualified for general military service should be physically, mentally, and educationally capable of performing any service that a soldier of the Army may be called upon to do.

Formerly the minimum educational requirements for registrants was the ability

*Read before the Annual Meeting held in Oklahoma City, May 11-12, 1943.

to read and write the English language at the fourth grade level or as well as a student who had satisfactorily completed the fourth grade in grammer school. At the beginning of the present fiscal year, measures were inaugurated at our induction stations for psychological examinations of men heretofore unable to meet previously established educational standards. The objective was to accept registrants who can understand simple orders in English and who are capable of absorbing basic military training. With this in view, professionally qualified psychologists were commissioned in the Army Specialist Corps and assigned with trained enlisted personnel to each of our induction stations. As a part of this test, for those who are illiterates, non-English speaking, or very dull, a Visual Classification Test is made. This is a pictorial, non-language test.

In the beginning of this procedure, registrants who failed to meet the intelligence tests were rejected without complete physical examination. Later is was deemed advisable to complete the entire physical, as illiteracy cannot be considered a permanent disqualification. Regulations authorized the acceptance of 5 per cent of our daily quota of registrants in this low intelligence group. The law of supply and demand covers, to a great extent, induction regulations. One writer has likened the induction process to a huge sieve. As the necessity for manpower increases the regulations relax somewhat so that a greater number may pass through the meshes of the sieve.

In the latter part of 1940 the first selectees were inducted into the service. At this time a rather rigid examination was made by Selective Service Boards and by Army Induction Boards. Rejection rates for all causes ran very close to 50 per cent. After Pearl Harbor and the definite need for military manpower arose, standards were relaxed somewhat, especially dental and visual requirements.

The Eighth Service Command comprises the states of Texas, Louisiana, Arkansas, Oklahoma and New Mexico. This area is served, as shown on the chart, by 14 induction stations and 6 reception centers. Location of our induction stations was made after careful consideration of areas of population, of available transportation facilities so that transportation costs might be kept at a minimum, and that no unnecessary distance be traveled by selectees. The location of available reception centers was considered, the ability to secure suitable buildings for induction purposes, and the facilities for feeding and housing the men reporting for examination. An ideal building for the purpose of induction has been designed by the

Surgeon General. Only two of these buildings are available in the Eighth Service Command. It has been necessary in many instances to remodel buildings leased for induction purposes. The ideal design includes an assembly room for men reporting for examination, and an adjoining room where papers are checked by the administrative department; another adjoining room, which should be large and well-lighted for the use of the psychologists in giving the intelligence test. After this phase of the examination is carried out the selectee passes into the dressing and clothing checking room where his clothing is checked until he completes the physicial examination. He then proceeds to the x-ray department where forty to sixty exposures can be made each hour .

The Genito-Urinary examination is then made and is followed by the laboratory examination. Then pulse rate and blood pressure readings are recorded, followed by the musculo-skeletal and general surgical examination. From here the Eye and Ear, Nose and Throat examination are given, then the dental examination, and in enclosed rooms, the heart and chest, to be followed

Chart No. 2

PERCENTAGE OF REJECTIONS FOR WHITE FOR SIX MONTH PERIOD JULY 1 TO DECEMBER 31, 1942

Selective Service	Eighth Service Command	
Disqualifications	Service Totals	
7-1-42 to 12-31-42	No.	%
Total Reporting	242,116	
Total Qualified	165,400	68.32
Non-Med. Rejections	13,809	5.70
Medical Rejections	62,907	25.98
TOTAL REJECTIONS	76,716	31.68
MENTAL (Illiterates)	11,378	14.83
MORAL	1,235	1.61
OTHER CAUSES (Des., etc.)	1,196	1.56
PHYSICAL:		
Overweight	262	.42
Underweight	1,310	2.08
Eye Abnormalties	4,534	7.21
Ear, Nose and Throat	4,295	6.93
Teeth	959	1.53
Mouth and Gums	764	1.21
Skin	746	1.19
Musculo-Skeletal	5,528	8.79
Feet	895	1.42
Lungs	4,231	6.73
Asthma and Hay Fever	1,475	2.34
Cardio-Vascular	9,485	15.08
Neurocirculatory asthenia	147	.23
Varicose Veins	1,071	1.70
Abdominal Organs and Wall	1,101	1.75
Hernia	6,958	11.06
Syphilis	310	.49
Gonorrhea	424	.67
Other Venereal Disease	97	.15
Albuminuria	613	.97
Glycosuria	357	.57
Mental and Nervous	12,131	19.28
All Others: (Not Listed)	5,214	8.29

by the neuro-psychiatric, and last, the final rechecking by at least three medical officers, one of whom at the present time is a Naval Medical Officer.

More than half of this work is done by civilian physicians employed on a contract basis. Induction is an important phase of the building of an Army that could not have been carried on without the help of the civilian physicians. Universally the profession has made great sacrifice in order to volunteer for this service. During the summer of 1942 it was decided to open an induction station in a centrally located city of about 25,000 inhabitants. I visited this city to consult with medical men regarding available facilities and possible assistance from the profession. I was somewhat discouraged when I found that there were only eight physicians in active practice in this thriving little city with a heavily populated rural district to serve. I know that every physician in the city was carrying a heavy load in his private practice.

Chart No. 3

PERCENTAGE OF REJECTIONS FOR COLORED FOR SIX MONTH PERIOD JULY 1 TO DECEMBER 31, 1942

Selective Service Disqualifications 7-1-42 to 12-31-42	Eighth Service Command Service Command Totals No.	%
Total Reporting	73,208	
Total Qualified	45,407	62.02
Non-Med. Rejections	8,164	11.15
Medical Rejections	19,637	26.82
TOTAL REJECTIONS	27,801	37.97
MENTAL (Illiterates)	7,680	27.62
MORAL	381	1.37
OTHER CAUSES (Des., etc.)	103	.37
PHYSICAL:		
Overweight	41	.21
Underweight	155	.79
Eye Abnormalties	1,999	10.18
Ear, Nose and Throat	339	1.73
Teeth	176	.90
Mouth and Gums	142	.72
Skin	191	.97
Musculo-Skeletal	1,404	7.15
Feet	445	2.27
Lungs	861	4.38
Asthma and Hay Fever	330	1.68
Cardio-Vascular	4,084	20.80
Neurocirculatory Asthenia	31	.16
Varicose Veins	268	1.36
Abdominal Organs and Wall	177	.90
Hernia	1,530	7.79
Syphilis	435	2.22
Gonorrhea	2,170	11.05
Other Veneral Disease	493	2.51
Albuminuria	154	.78
Glycosuria	66	.34
Mental and Nervous	2,603	13.26
All Others: (Not Listed)	1,543	7.86

The president of the county medical society told me that he would call a meeting for that night and we would discuss the problem. I was greatly surprised when I arrived at the meeting to find 26 physicians present; most of them having come from surrounding towns, some as far as 75 miles. Every man present volunteered his services and what is more, they have kept their promise and by rotation of service we have inducted from 150 to 400 men six days out of each week. The medical profession truly realizes that this is everybody's war. Another reason for our appreciation of this service is that the local physicians know the registrant, if not personally, they know his language and his background. The registrant knows them personally or by reputation and he feels that he is in good hands. The community as a whole is better satisfied if the home profession has part in the induction.

A vast amount of clinical material passes through our induction stations. The alert physician has the opportunity of observing many unusual cases. Among others, a number of lepers have reported for induction and in one instance, I regret to state, a leper with quite an insignificant lesion of the ear was inducted, later to be discharged from the Army on Certificate of Disability Discharge.

In all doubtful or borderline cases the medical board is authorized to secure any additional labortaory findings, to consult with other members of the board, many of whom are specialists, and when necessary, the selectee may be held over for further observation and re-examination.

The examining board will consist of at least twelve medical examiners for each 200 registrants. The neuropsychiatric examiners will not examine more than fifty men each during the day. Trained enlisted men act as recorders and assist in certain parts of the examination, such as, weights and measures, color vision tests, preliminary visual tests and auditory acuity tests. Enlisted men are also used as guides. Every effort is made to relieve apprehension and fear of the physical examination. It is realized that the registrants' first contact with military life will make a lasting impression. In stations where space is available some form of amusement or entertainment is arranged in the reception room and every effort is made

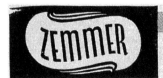

to allay anxiety and fear during the examination.

Malingering of registrants is not one of our most serious problems for the reason that the close and cordial cooperation of selective service and local examining boards where the selectee is well known eliminates many of these cases before they come to us for induction. Many, no doubt, who make elaborate plans to deceive, become doubtful of their plans working when they once get in the induction line and they give up the idea. Some report for examination wearing various kinds of dressings and even plaster casts, and give fantastic histories of injury. In such cases every available diagnostic method is used by the examiner. Some attempts to malinger have been made by the use of drugs to produce tacticardia. This usually occurs in groups from some town or country. Asthma, epilepsy and peptic ulcer are often feigned. In these cases documentary evidence is required and is often furnished by local board examiners. Where doubt exists, the selectee may be held over for observation. Enuresis is often feigned. In this condition documentary evidence is also required. Illiteracy is one of the most frequently feigned conditions and again information from the local board where the registrant is well known is of great assistance to our examiners.

Chart No. 4

COMPARATIVE REJECTIONS

Selective Service	Eighth Service Command	
	Service Command Totals	
Disqualifications	White	Colored
7-1-42 to 12-31-42		
Total Qualified	68.32	62.02
Non-Med. Rejections	5.70	11.15
Medical Rejections	25.98	26.82
TOTAL REJECTIONS	31.68	37.97
MENTAL (Illiterates)	14.83	27.62
MORAL	1.61	1.37
OTHER CAUSES (Des., etc.)	1.56	.37
PHYSICAL:		
Overweight	.42	.21
Underweight	2.08	.79
Eye Abnormalties	7.21	10.18
Ear, Nose and Throat	6.83	1.73
Teeth	1.53	.90
Mouth and Gums	1.21	.72
Skin	1.19	.97
Musculo-Skeletal	8.79	7.15
Feet	1.42	2.27
Lungs	6.73	4.38
Asthma and Hay Fever	2.34	1.68
Cardio-Vascular	15.08	20.80
Neurocirculatory Asthenia	.23	.16
Varicose Veins	1.70	1.36
Abdominal Organs and Wall	1.75	.90
Hernia	11.06	7.79
Syphilis	.49	2.22
Gonorrhea	.67	11.05
Other Venereal Disease	.15	2.51
Albuminuria	.97	.78
Glycosuria	.57	.34
Mental and Nervous	19.28	13.20
ALL OTHERS: (Not Listed)	8.29	7.85

It will be remembered that the colored population comprises approximately 15 per cent of our total population. Non-medical rejections, you will observe, are approximately twice as high in the colored race. This comprises criminal records, aliens, and other administrative causes. Illiteracy is a high cause of rejection for military service in the Eighth Service Command and in other Service Commands as well. You will note that it is approximately twice as high in the colored population. This is true especially in urban districts. It is well known that many illiterates may become useful soldiers and no doubt many of them will eventually find a useful place in the military forces. It must be remembered that we are attempting to build an efficient fighting machine in the shortest possible time and that illiteracy is a great handicap to rapid training.

Moral disqualifications comprise heinous crimes and other moral deficiencies.

In other causes, we have desertion, some of which may be accepted by special permission of the Adjutant General's Office.

Under physical deficiencies, overweight, comprising the small per cent of .42 in white and .21 in colored is a condition, if unaccompanied by pathology, is now often waived. Underweight, with 2.08 per cent rejections of whites and .79 per cent in colored, is often accompanied by other disqualifying cases.

Disqualification for eye abnormalties was, in the early part of induction, one of the highest causes for disqualification. Regulations have been changed from time to time and, at the present time, a vision of 20/200 in each eye without glasses, if correctible to at least 20/40 in each eye, is acceptable for general service. Standard methods are used in the eye examination and refraction is done by a qualified eye man. Other disqualifying eye defects are deformity of eye-lids, such as; inversion or eversion of a degree that forcible closure fails to cover the eyeball, or in which there is a resultant inflammatory process. Disfiguring cicatrices of the eye, pronounced exopthalmos, chronic keratitis, chronic ulcer of the cornea, any active disease of the retina, choroid or optic nerve, detachment of the retina, glaucoma, dystrophia due to paralysis of extrinsic ocular muscles and pterygium if it interferes with vision.

Ear, Nose and Throat disqualifications are 6.83 per cent in whites and 1.73 per cent in colored. Acuity of hearing is made by the whispered voice test at 15 feet. In all of our induction stations we have constructed sound-proof testing tunnels. Hearing acuity must be 8/15 or better in each ear and not less than 5/15 in either ear; deafness in one ear, if acuity is 15/15 in the other ear. Disqualifying defects are perforation of the membrana tympani, acute or chronic mastoiditis, total loss of an external ear, atresia of the external auditory canal or tumors of this part. Standard methods of examination are used by qualified examiners. Sinus infection, chronic laryngitis, perforation of the hard palate, stricture or other organic disease of the esophagus, perforation of the nasal septum associated with interference of function, ulceration or crusting when due to organic disease, are disqualifying defects.

Dental disqualifications, formerly very high in all Service Commands, are now very low, being 1.53 per cent in white and .90 per cent in colored. Disease of the mouth and gums is 1.21 per cent in whites and .72 per cent in colored.

Diseases of the skin are 1.19 per cent in whites and .97 per cent in colored.

Musculo-skeletal defects, 8.79 per cent in colored, comprise a frequently large list of conditions which are correctible or might at one time have been correctible. Many are structural defects of dietary or nutritional etiology. Among the most frequent defects are old injuries of the spine and sacro-iliac joints, limitation of motion due to contractions, loss of parts of extremities, club-feet, flat feet with marked deviation of the foot and bulging of the inner border due to inward rotation of the astragalus. This condition is disqualifying regardless of the absence of symptoms. As an etiological factor in this group of cases, the National Safety Council has compiled statistics of accidents. Following is the list for 1941: 102,500 killed, 9,300,000 injured and 350,000 permanently disabled. No doubt, from the large list of those injured by accident come many of our registrants. Of the structural defects, many are congenital.

It will be seen that lung pathology is less frequent in colored than in whites in this Service Command. A 4 x 5 stereoscopic film of the chest is made in every case. As previously stated, this is made early in the examination so that ample time for the processing of the film may be had. The name, date, address and local board code number is photographed on the film. Army serial numbers

are not given until a man has been accepted for service. Films are a part of the permanent record of every man examined and if a man is rejected for any reason, his film is forwarded to the State Headquarters. These are classified into three groups, i.e., films of individuals recommended for re-examination in six months because of borderline tuberculosis or other chest conditions; films of individuals rejected because of tuberculosis or other chest conditions; films of individuals rejected because of other than chest conditions. In this way the registrant, through his local board, is notified a second time of any pathological condition. The first notification is given him by the chief medical officer at the induction station. If he is accepted, his film is forwarded to the Veteran's Bureau Headquarters, Washington, D. C. Films interpreted as normal are passed without further examination. If, in examination of the films, pathology is seen, or suspected, a plain 14 x 17 chest plate is made or a steroscopic 14 x 17 is made, and consultation is held with one or more qualified chest examiners. Careful histories are taken, blood counts, sputum examinations and sedimentation rates are made. These cases may be hospitalized for a short time for clinical observation. Disqualifying defects are classified residues or lesions of the intra-thoracic lymph nodes, providing any of these lesions exceed an arbitrary limit of 1.5 cms. in diameter and if there is an excess of five such lesions. Calcified lesions of the pulmonary parenchyma, provided there is an excess of 10 in number and provided any of these exceeds 1 cm. in diameter. For acceptance, such calcified lesions should appear isolated in location, circumscribed, homogeneous but dense.

The above arbitrary limits of calcified lesions are set on the assumption that large and numerous lesions are more likely to be partially unhealed and therefore a potential scorce of future recrudescence than small lesions of limited distribution. It is recognized however, that in some individuals, calcified tuberculosis lesions exceeding these limits may be present which are so well healed that the possibility of future reactivation is remote. Further consideration may be given to the acceptability of persons with calcified lesions of this type when the state of health in all other respects thoroughly warrants the opinion that the lesion in question is healed. In such cases the history of the applicant and his age as well as the character of the lesions as seen in x-ray films provide criteria.

If there is no history of active tuberculosis or symptoms which might be interpreted as evidence of this disease and if the applicant is more than 25 years of age and if finally the calcified lesions are dense and discreet in character and not hazy or irregular in outline, such lesions may be considered as not prejudicial to future health. In a review of 10,000 cases by Captain George C. Brown, Chief Medical Officer of one of our stations, this table is presented:

Table No. 2
CHEST REJECTIONS

Cause of Rejection	Number of Cases	Per Cent
Tuberculosis, active	62	.62
Tuberculosis, arrested	30	.30
Non-Tuberculosis Conditions:		
Bronchiectasis	8	
Pleurisy	19	
Pulmonary Fibrosis	3	
Pulmonary Tumor	3	
Mediastinal Tumor	2	
Pneumonia	2	
Cystic Disease of Lung	2	
Pulmonary Emphysema and Fibrosis	2	
Mediastintis, chronic	2	
Pulmonary Atelectasis	2	
Foreign Bodies in Lung	1	
Pneumonoconiosis	1	
Congenital Aplasia of Lung	1	
Pneumothorax	1	
Diaphragmatic Hernia	1	
Aneurysm of Arota	1	
Percarditis	1	
Paralysis of Phrenic Nerve	1	.53
TOTAL	145	1.45

Asthma is difficult to diagnose in our induction stations and a history of Asthma and Hay Fever must be accompanied by documentary evidence.

Of the disqualifications for cardiovascular disease it will be observed that the colored rejection rate is approximately 25 per cent higher than the white. This has been explained by the higher instance of syphilis among colored selectees. Other causes may be environmental and greater neglect of focal infections. Rather startling and unexplainable is the high incidence of cardiovascular disease in certain sections of the Service Command, especially in the north and eastern part. Accepted methods of diagnosis are used, electrocardiac examination is available and every effort has been made to secure qualified cardiologists as examiners in our stations.

Neuro-circulatoriousthenia may not be classed as a clinical syndrome but rather as a condition characterized by a rather definite group of symptoms consisting of dyspnea, palpitation, pre-cardial pains, exhaustion, dizziness, nervousness, tremor, and headache, which symptoms in the soldier often follow excitement or physical or nervous strain.

Varicose veins are cause for rejection if large and ulcerated or, if in the examiner's opinion they are apt to produce disabling affect.

In a small per cent of cases, intra-abdominal tumors, tumors of the wall or weakened abdominal wall may be found. Inguinal, femoral or post-operative or umbilical hernia, if moderately large is not acceptable. However, the diagnosis of hernia is not made upon a moderate impulse produced by cough at the inguinal femoral or umbilical ring or in the site of scars. It must be definitely a viscus within a sac.

At the time of induction of this class of registrants, syphilis was the cause of rejection in .49 per cent of white selectees and 2.22 per cent in colored selectees. Serology reports made by authorized laboratories accompany the selectee's papers at the time he reports for induction. In the latter part of 1942 it was decided to accept syphilis cases exclusive of neuro-syphilis, cardiovascular and visceral syphilis. In all cases at the time, except primary and secondary cases, treatment is begun in our reception centers. Primary and secondary cases are sent immediately to Army hospitals where treatment is instituted. Formerly all cases of gonorrhea were rejected. The rejection rates are .67 per cent in the white selectees and 11.05 per cent in colored. At the present time all uncomplicated cases of gonorrhea are accepted and treatment is instituted by our reception centers. With our modern facilities for treatment of this condition a very high per cent of these are cured within five to ten days time. Other venereal diseases comprise in whites .15 per cent and in colored 2.51 per cent. Albuminuria and glycosuria are evident in a smaller per cent of cases.

In the large number of mental rejectees you will observe that 19.28 per cent are found in the white race and 13.26 per cent in the colored race. This includes those individuals who are found to have any serious mental or neurological disorder such as mental deficiency, phychopathic personality, major abnormalities of mood, psycho-neurotic disorders, pre-psychotic, post-psychotic and Schizophrenic personalties, chronic alcoholism and drug addiction, syphilis of the central nervous system, sexual perversion and stammering to such a degree that the registrant is unable to express himself clearly or to repeat commands.

The neuropsychiatric examiner will interview the selectee outside of hearing of other persons. With this in view, private booths have been arranged in our induction stations. The high percentage of rejections in this group of cases is not understandable to the average layman. I wish to state here that approximately 40 per cent of all the rejections or C.D.D.'s from military service are for neuro-psychiatric cases. The average length of time of service is somewhat less than two months. Approximately 10 per cent of these discharges are insane cases. With figures in mind, greater care in diagnosis is being exercised by our neuro-psychiatric examiners. There are two popular misconceptions of the layman; first, that any person capable of a fair degree of success in civil life can be made into a good soldier; second, that military discipline and environment can make a man of material which in civil life is considered beyond redemption. One's friends and neighbors in general are tolerant of a man's short-comings while the discipline of military life is fairly exacting. In civilian life there is time and opportunity for one to cultivate his hobbies, foibles, and eccentricities. This is everywhere evident and often passes unnoticed or with little comment. In our examination we must consider the possible injustice to the individual who, although he has made a place for himself in the military regime, becomes discouraged, morose and ends by being admitted to the neuro-psychiatric ward of one of our hospitals. If and when he returns to civil life he must carry with him the stigma of failure. Let us assume that every individual has a mental threshold beyond which he will be unable to bear the stress and strain of life without breaking. In civil life adjustment to circumstances may be made gradually. The individual may select his occupation, his place of residence and his friends and is assisted by relatives, friends, and a tolerant community. In the military environment new friends must be made, new and changing environments are encountered and living conditions are more exacting. Among our selectees, 514 occupations are represented. Military life is a new and strange occupation and a man is no longer an individual but a part of a team that must function with mechanical precision. In judging the high rate of rejections for this cause, let us consider the 40 per cent of all C.D.D.'s which break down after less than two months active service. Let us consider also the great number of veterans of World War I, who were hospitalized due to neuro-psychiatric causes and who have remained throughout the years patients in Veteran's Hospitals.

Why cannot more of the limited service men, or men with minor disabilities be used in military service? They can be used and are now being used as rapidly as they can be trained to fill the place of general service men who can be transferred to combat units. Many of you are familiar with an article published recently in one of our leading magazines. In this article, the limited service training school was described quite completely. Very different from past wars, this is a high speed war and it is imperative to get men to the most vulnerable spots in the shortest possible time. Time will solve the limited service problem as it will solve satisfactorily the great problem of this war by victory for our Country.

Observations on the Negro Diabetic*

PAUL B. CAMERON, M.D.

PRYOR, OKLAHOMA

There are presented herewith in brief form some observations on the American Negro who has diabetes mellitus. These are drawn from 200 consecutive cases who were followed by the writer for periods of from one to three years in a clinic devoted solely to the treatment of this disease. For purposes of comparison, 200 cases of diabetes in the white race were analyzed in a similar manner.

The diagnosis was established in the customary fashion, that is by the demonstration of blood sugar in excess of 140 milligrams per 100 cubic centimeters of whole blood in the fasting state, or by a modified glucose tolerance test, in which the blood sugar was determined one hour after investigation of 1.5 grams dextrose per kilogram of body weight. In the event of an equivocal test, the formal three hour test, or Exton's modification was run. All cases not conforming to these criteria were discarded from this series.

*Read before the Annual Meeting held in Oklahoma City, May 11-12, 1943.

The colored female far exceeded the male of the same race in frequency, numbering 173 of the 200 cases, leaving 27 males. There are relatively few obese colored males in relation to the females, and particularly in the South, where these cases were seen. The men are usually employed in arduous manual labor, the women largely in domestic situations and in the culinary departments, which is a favorable environment for the development of obesity. This state and its close association to diabetes requires no elaboration. Thus there are five negro females to one male, whereas the white group showed a preponderance of three to one.

While there were the usual scattering of all ages, it was found that the negro developed at the earlier age than did the whites. As a rule, the age of onset is hard to determine but by careful history one can arrive at the probable date of onset. Many, of course, were without symptoms, and no date of onset could be established. There were too few males to have a concentration at one decade of life. The females were grouped in the 40-49 and 50-59 decade, as most statistics show, but the age of onset was, on the average, 42 years in the negro and 49 in the white. The youngest member of either was a 30 month negro girl, precocious to the extent that she could administer her own insulin, and whose diabetes was discovered at 14 months. Neither parent was diabetic. She was the only patient I have ever seen who developed uriticaria, constantly, on the administration of protamine insulin, and my first to use that drug. She required large doses in proportion to her weight, 25 to 30 units daily, with poor control of the glycosuria in spite of the untiring efforts of her very intelligent mother. The oldest was an ancient patriarch of 80 years, who had a multitude of associated pathologic conditions, and blood sugar was rarely under 320 milligrams per 100 cc of blood. He attended the clinic for, I think, lack of better diversion, as he followed no direction of any kind, nor admitted he was not perfectly well. At 83 he was still active in spite of advanced cataracts, heart block, and adenocarcinoma of the prostate, when we lost sight of him.

The symptoms of the male applicant at this clinic were many and varied, the only constant ones of which were loss of weight and weakness. The younger ones usually had some polyuria, the older ones not necessarily so. The white males followed this general trend. The colored females were admitted to the clinic and out-patient department for a wide range of symptoms. In 89 of the 173 the glycosuria was found on routine urinalysis in other departments. The most frequent chief complaints were pruritis

vulvae in 32, and excessive thirst in 16. In the latter group was one who had combined diabetes mellitus and insipidus. Disbelieving her report on the total quantity of urinary output in 24 hours, we sent the visitor to her home, who corroborated the total quantity of 42 liters, a truly amazing performance. This case was relieved of most of her annoyance by insulin and pituitary extract, and to our regret, she vanished from view. This was an all too common experience in the more interesting cases.

Another unusual symptom was a colored female who had paroxysmal attacks of hyperhidrosis recurring at two hour intervals. She was studied exhaustively in the wards, without definite conclusions as to the cause. She died suddenly in a remote part of the state and no necropsy was possible.

An unusual method of discovery was reported by an unlearned negress who brought her specimen in to the hospital asking if there might be something in it which would cause many ants to gather around her receptacle. She expressed the opinion that sugar might be there, in which idea she was eminently correct, as she was spilling over 100 grams daily. She used this same observation in her dietary management with a good deal of success.

The establishment of hereditary influence in the negro group was quite difficult. In 8.5 per cent of the negro patients we could learn of diabetic forebears, and in 15 per cent of the whites. This is probably not correct as few negroes, and not many more whites, of the class applying at a charity hospital have a very clear idea of the diseases of their parents, and even less so of their grandparents and uncles and aunts. Indeed, in many individuals in the more fortunate social groups, no information of this type is accurate, unless there was close association in the household or community.

Death came to twelve of the negroes in a 30 month period. Gangrene and infection accounted for three, tuberculosis for two, coma one, arteriosclerotic heart disease for four, nephrosis for one, and one died of unknown cause, presumably coronary occlusion. The coma was brought on by a ten day drinking bout, and by omission of insulin for that period.

One would expect to find a large proportion of negroes with positive serological tests for syphilis. Such was not the case in this series. Only 8 per cent of the 200 patients were reported Wassermann positive. In one of the general medical divisions for negroes, one fourth of the patients had positive serology. The white patients in the clinic showed 4 per cent positive serology. It is not clear why there should be such a wide divergence in the diabetic negroes and the general run of clinic patients. Perhaps the older group were able to spontaneously reverse their serological tests if they were ever positive, although this is not a satisfactory reason.

In only one case was there reason to believe that syphilis was instrumental in producing diabetes. A 20 year old negro male contracted syphilis several months before the discovery of diabetes. The glycosuria was very marked on admission, and he was poorly controlled on substantial doses of insulin and a supervised diet. As bismuth and trivalent arsenicals were given, the diabetes grew less and less severe and at the end of several months he was doing very well without insulin, and at the end of a year his glucose tolerance curve was close to normal. On receiving this informaton he stopped coming to the clinic, both diabetic and antiluetic. The writer feels that this was hardly a coincidence, and that there was in all probability a specific reaction near or at the islet tissue, which subsided under proper therapy with restoration of insulinogenic function.

The vascular status was investigated in all diabetics by physical and ophthalmoscopic examination. The greater number of all diabetics, both white and colored, showed arteriosclerosis in some degree. The writer believes, with others, that there are few diabetics of any duration over a few years who do not have thickened and sclerotic arteries, and a widened reflex of the retinal vessels. Nine of the twelve deaths in the negro group were due to vascular disease and its sequelae. Hypertension and arterio-sclerosis are quite common in the negro, and many of the admissions in non diabetics are for these conditions. It is felt, of course, that the diabetic is prone to various vascular disturbances, but it is the writers impression that the diabetic negro does not exceed the non diabetic in the frequency of vascular diseases as much as does the white diabetic.

There was little difference in the incidence of gangrene in the two races but the character of the gangrene in the negro appeared more advanced, possibly due to the notorious procrastination of that race to seek medical aid. In a few cases of peripheral vascular

diseases, with or without claudication, passive vascular exercises with the pressure-suction boot were carried out, with indifferent results. We did not see the marked subjective complaints of pain, burning and the like with the frequency seen in the colder climates. The comparatively mild weather of the Gulf Coast apparently has a beneficial effect on these people. Such individuals were seen, but did not present the problem that is seen even in Oklahoma.

Coronary disease was less common in the negro than the whites. Routine search was not carried out with the electrocardiograph, but only on those whose symptoms or clinical course indicated such need. The whites showed coronary disease three times as often as the negro. In only one patient in the colored clinic was characteristic angina of effort seen, and he had syphilitic aortitis. This does not present the real picture, as coronary disease certainly does appear in the negro, but the percentages were low in this series.

Ocular pathology was more marked in the negro. Cataracts were relatively common. The writer feels that this condition is more frequent in the deep south, but he has no statistics for confirmation. Arcus senilis was common, but scarcely more so than in the non diabetic. Diabetic retinitis paralleled the degree of arteriosclerosis and the state of renal function. We were never able to distinguish accurately between diabetic and albuminuric retinitis.

Surgery in the diabetic was carried out in a number of cases, and for a variety of reasons. I think the diabetic, if acetone free, and the sugar under reasonable control, stands surgery almost as well as the non diabetic. It is essential that measures be taken to establish a glycogen reserve in the liver by carhohydrate and insulin. The most serious procedure was amputation for gangrene, a shocking operation at best. High amputations must be done to secure a level with sufficient blood supply to insure healing. The upper third of the lower leg is best. Amputations above the knee increase the hazard greatly. Spinal anesthesia is very satisfactory.

The diabetic female has always been unsatisfactory when pregnant. The writer is of the opinion that pregnancy aggravates the diabetic condition, and cannot find clinical evidence that the fetal pancreas supplies enough insulin to make much difference in the maternal diabetic. All of our diabetics became worse in pregnancy, in the second trimester or sooner, and required larger doses of insulin to preserve control. In spite of acceptable control, the five full term pregnancies observed in the group under survey terminated unsatisfactorily. Only one of these was delivered of a normal child. To combat hypoglycemia on the first day glucose was administered through the fontanelle, perhaps unwisely, and fatal meningitis resulted. The other women were delivered of large stillborn, macerated fetuses. In view of the economic state of these patients, and other considerations, we had no hesitation in suggesting therapeutic abortion in a severe diabetic, unless religious scruples were held.

Of the complications of pregnancy, one might be mentioned. The single successful delivery was preceded, in the seventh month, by bilateral bronchopneumonia and severe acidosis leading to coma. A marked hydramnios appeared at the height of the disease, which receded under improvement of the pneumonia and control of the acidosis. Possibly the well known chloride imbalance of pneumonia, with the disturbance of water retention in insulin management, is responsible. Since the estrogenic therapy of the pregnant diabetic has been established, it is probable that the number of successful deliveries will increase.

In general, it is found that the negro is just as susceptible to diabetes as the white, and aside from small differences in the relative frequency of age distribution and certain complications he experiences the same course of the disease. I am impressed, however, with the observation that most diabetics handle their disease fairly well, even if poorly treated. Most diabetics of lesser severity are quite negligent of the disease, and I cannot see that they come to much more grief than the comparative few who are meticulous in their self care. I do not know that arteriosclerosis is influenced very much in its pathogenesis and progress by the degree of diabetic control. Such a debate is many sided, of course, but I do not find myself very exacting in treating the mild diabetic. To those of the Joslin and Lemann school these thoughts are probably distressing. Perhaps another generation in the insulin era will afford us more light.

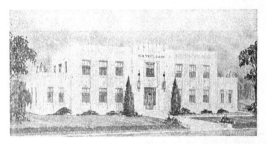

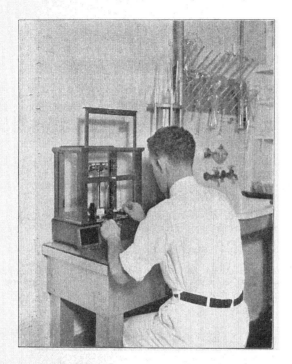

• THE PRESIDENT'S PAGE •

Dr. O. C. Newman of Shattuck was recently elected to the Oklahoma Hall of Fame. This great and good man richly deserves this honor. It is typical of the greatness of this doctor that he regards this as a tribute not to him but to the backbone of American Medicine—the Country Doctor.

Our genial Executive Secretary is now First Lieutenant Graham, and at this writing is at Carlisle Barracks, Pennsylvania. Dick performed a marvelous job for our organization, and he knows he is missed. He is merely "on leave" and will be back with us again when the war is won.

Dick will be pleased to know that Miss Anne Betche, Assistant Secretary, and Miss Jane Firrell, Assistant to the Editor of the Journal, are "carrying on" admirably, and the Officers of the Association are proud of their loyalty and devotion to duty. They do not have "jobs" with us—they are partners with us.

To all members, I extend the Season's Greetings, and to all our members in the Armed Forces—I know you will be back with us in the New Year. Speed the day!

James Stevenson

President.

21 WARREN-TEED Products were accepted by the Council on Pharmacy and Chemistry of the American Medical Association in **1943**

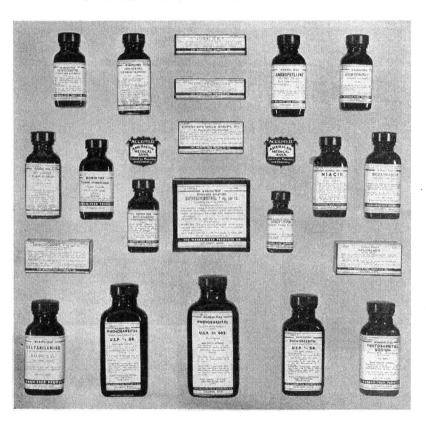

THE WARREN-TEED PRODUCTS CO.
- Columbus 8, Ohio

Medicaments of Exacting Quality Since 1920

The JOURNAL Of The
OKLAHOMA STATE MEDICAL ASSOCIATION

EDITORIAL BOARD

L. J. MOORMAN, Oklahoma City, Editor-in-Chief

E. EUGENE RICE, Shawnee NED R. SMITH, Tulsa

MR. R. H. GRAHAM, Oklahoma City, Business Manager
(Serving in the Armed Forces)

CONTRIBUTIONS: Articles accepted by this Journal for publication including those read at the annual meetings of the State Association are the sole property of this Journal.

The Editorial Department is not responsible for the opinions expressed in the original articles of contributors.

Manuscripts may be withdrawn by authors for publication elsewhere only upon the approval of the Editorial Board.

MANUSCRIPTS: Manuscripts should be typewritten, double-spaced, on white paper 8½ x 11 inches. The original copy, not the carbon copy, should be submitted.

Footnotes, bibliographies and legends for cuts should be typed on separate sheets in double space. Bibliography listing should follow this order: Name of author, title of article, name of periodical with volume, page and date of publication.

Manuscripts are accepted subject to the usual editorial revisions and with the understanding that they have not been published elsewhere.

NEWS: Local news of interest to the medical profession, changes of address, births, deaths and weddings will be gratefully received.

ADVERTISING: Advertising of articles, drugs or compounds unapproved by the Council on Pharmacy of the A.M.A. will not be accepted. Advertising rates will be supplied on application.

It is suggested that members of the State Association patronize our advertisers in preference to others.

SUBSCRIPTIONS: Failure to receive The Journal should call for immediate notification.

REPRINTS: Reprints of original articles will be supplied at actual cost provided request for them is attached to manuscripts or made in sufficient time before publication. Checks for reprints should be made payable to Industrial Printing Company, Oklahoma City.

Address all communications to THE JOURNAL OF THE OKLAHOMA STATE MEDICAL ASSOCIATION, 210 Plaza Court, Oklahoma City. (3)

OFFICIAL PUBLICATION OF THE OKLAHOMA STATE MEDICAL ASSOCIATION
Copyrighted December, 1943

EDITORIALS

INCONSISTENCY ENSCONCED

The Sherman Anti-Trust Act and all subsequent acts related to the same have sought to meet the needs of industrial conditions and secure justice to the people of the United States. Strange to say, the American Medical Association was brought to trial, convicted and fined under these acts. It has been reported that a recent Survey of Current Business conducted by the United States Department of Commerce shows that the so-called great American medical monopoly collected from the people of the United States more than a billion dollars in the year 1941. In return for this huge sum, the medical profession gave only the highest health level, the lowest morbidity and mortality rates and the greatest increase in longevity shown by any comparable nation. Obviously the prosecution of the American Medical Association was based upon alleged injustice to the people. Instead of permitting the doctors to take a billion dollars from all the people for medical service which supplies only the few advantages mentioned above, the powers behind the late prosecution of the medical profession now contemplate a magnanimous plan which will collect three billion dollars from a few employers and withhold three billion more from the pay checks of a few million employees in order to provide the latter with compulsory medical care. What a plum for extramural Trust Busters!

But perhaps we should withhold the ax until we consider the advantages. The proposed plan will provide the services of two laymen for every doctor. This will make it possible for the laymen to tell the doctors what to do and how to do it. The records will be in triplicate so they can be filed in at least three offices for public scrutiny. Whether it be syphilis, suicide, gonorrhea or gout, the public has a right to know. Finally the annoyance and responsibility of personal choice, individual interest and attention, sympathy and sentiment will be eliminated. The study of government bulletins and the execution of the interminable blanks will replace the study of medicine. If the blanks are properly filled out the doctor need not worry about his waning knowledge of medicine or what happens to the patient. Uncle Sam and the lay administrators will be in the practice of medicine and they will see that everybody has the Government's brand of so-called medical service. The Government

Bulletins will suffice. You may rest assured that the service will flow with the cold formality of bureaucracy, wanting in nothing but good medical care.

A CHANCE TO SERVE

Because of the shortage of Nurses for both the Armed Forces and the civilian needs, the Government has provided funds for the training of student nurses with pay during the period of training. These students will wear the official uniform of the U. S. Cadet Nurse Corps.

It is estimated that 65,000 Student Nurses are needed at once to meet the emergency, The doctors of Oklahoma are requested to take this matter under consideration and to do what they can to enlist the interest of young women who are mentally and physically qualified to meet the requirements and who have an ambition to serve their country in time of need.

Applicants should be instructed to address the Nursing School of her choice or the Division of Nurse Education, U. S. Public Health Service, Federal Security Agency, Washington, D. C.

THE CHRISTMAS SEAL AND THE MEDICAL PROFESSION

A list of the doctors who laid the foundation for the National Tuberculosis Association and those who participated in the organization meeting at Atlantic City, June 6, 1904, reads like an American Medical Honor Roll. The following list is inspiring: Edward L. Trudeau, Saranac Lake, N. Y.; William Osler, Baltimore, Md.; William H. Welch, Baltimore, Md.; Theobald Smith, Boston, Mass.; J. G. Adami, Montreal, Canada; Vincent Y. Bowditch, Boston, Mass.; S. A. Knopf, New York City; Mazyck P. Ravenel, Philadelphia, Pa.; Arnold C. Klebs, Chicago, Ill.; Edward G. Janeway, New York City; Henry Barton Jacobs, Baltimore, Md.; Lawrence F. Flick, Philadelphia, Pa.; Hermann M. Biggs, New York City; A. Jacobi, New York City; William S. Thayer, Baltimore, Md.; J. H. Elliott, Ontario, Canada; Robert H. Babcock, Chicago, Ill.; David R. Lyman, New Haven, Conn.; Charles L. Minor, Asheville, N.~C.; Edward O. Otis, Boston, Mass.; John B. Huber, New York City and Thomas Darlington, New York City.

The following were present at the organization meeting: Drs. Edward L. Trudeau, Hermann M. Biggs, Lawrence F. Flick, William H. Welch, and General George M. Sternberg, together with the chairman, Dr. William Osler, and secretary, Dr. Henry Barton Jacobs.

The officers elected at the meeting in Atlantic City were: Dr. Edward L. Trudeau, of Saranac Lake, N. Y., president; Dr. William Osler, of Baltimore, and Dr. Hermann M. Biggs, of New York, vice-presidents; General George M. Sternberg, of Washington, D. C., treasurer; Dr. Henry Barton Jacobs, of Baltimore, secretary.

The first Christmas Seal Sale conducted by Miss Bissell, amounted to $3,000.00. Last year the gross sale was $9,250,000.00. The Sale is now on. The War is letting down our defenses and lowering our resistance. It is clearly our duty to support the work so well begun by the most distinguished clinicians in our profession.

Please push the Christmas Seal Sale.

THE PHYSICALLY UNFIT AND THE WORLD'S WORK

Every time a war comes and mobilization brings our youth under searching medical scrutiny, the government gets excited over the fact that we are not 100 per cent physically fit. Doctors are partly to blame for this unwarranted criticism, not because they have failed to give good medical service, but because they have not taught the people that they are subject to inherited physical defects and that many suffer unfavorable hereditary predispositions both physical and mental. Also because we have not adequately pointed out the evil influences of environment. All of us begin to die as soon as we are born. One of the greatest anatomists the world has ever known often opened his lecture course on regional anatomy by announcing that he could not show the normal in certain organs and tissues because from the time of birth they were subjected to certain changes initiated by the common childhood infections and the ever recurring insults of environment. The doctors, through private practice and public health have done much toward prevention and protection against these insidious evils. But under present conditions perfection is impossible.

If the government agencies were wise they would let the doctors alone and endeavor to improve environment. With the help of the medical profession, they could study environment with a view of improving housing conditions, household hygiene, food values, food distribution, working conditions in and out of industry, controling the evil results of overtime and holiday work. Instead of straddling upon the public an inadequate compulsory medical service, the government might do well to study ways and means by which the people of the United States might be brought into contact with the splendid medical service now available. Much of the present inadequacy and many of the abnormalities discovered by our draft boards could have been avoided if these young people had sought medical and dental advice and if the government had provided a better environment and an adequate knowledge of food values.

Experience in other countries has shown that government medicine is poor medicine. It is impossible to improve the average health level by regimenting doctors who have learned through long years of experience what the needs are. Why not educate the people to the point of creating in them a consciousness of the necessity of seeing a doctor when they are obviously sick and the advisability of periodic health examinations when they are apparently well. Similar cooperation with the dental profession would be of immeasurable value. If regimentation for medical service must come, lets apply it where it will do the least harm. If a well directed educational program should fail, the general health level might be improved by making it obligatory on the part of those who are sick, to seek medical care and to require those who are apparently well to undergo a health examination once or twice a year.

The politicians who would be 100 per centers on health should go back ten generations and fix heredity and then have everybody put on ice at birth to await a better environment which is largely a governmental responsibility. After all, it would be easy to idealize the sick. Much of the world's work is done by sick people, many of whom would have accomplished much less if it were not for the urge of ill health which threatens to rob them of time and opportunity. According to our present standards, Andrew Jackson was totally and permanently disabled when he won the battle of New Orleans.

THE COUNTRY DOCTOR

"There was quite a writeup in the Oklahoman the other day about a beloved country doctor in a western town of this state, whose name has been enrolled in the Hall of Fame for his kindliness, his unswerving loyalty and his sacrificial service to humanity.

"From what we know of country doctors, the honor was deserved. There are few persons more sacrificial of their own health and welfare to aid their fellowmen in their time of greatest need, than are the country doctors. They arise from their beds at all hours of the night, or do not go to bed at all, to drive over the worst roads in the country to isolated rural homes in heat and dust and rain and mud and snow and bitter cold to relieve pain and suffering or to usher babies into the world; and when the hand of death can no longer be stayed by the skill of the doctor, it is he who is the last to give up hope, and it is he whom the sorrowing loved ones want to stand by along with the minister as the heart-beats cease and the soul takes its flight from the mortal body.

"Country doctors, like country editors, are a vanishing species, and all too soon they will be gone.

"Country doctors of Maysville and the world over, we are glad to present each of you a bouquet today."

The above tribute to the Country Doctor recently appeared in The Maysville News. The worthy author, Mr. W. E. Showen, Editor-Publisher, deserves the gratitude of every doctor in the State of Oklahoma. If every newspaper would follow suit and if every doctor deserved the tribute, the people would defeat the Wagner Bill.

University of Oklahoma School of Medicine

Major General James C. Magee, former Surgeon General, United States Army spoke in the auditorium of the Medical School Building Friday evening, November 12, on ''Military Medicine'' with a special reference to tropical diseases.

The basic Sciences Examinations were held at the School of Medicine Building November 29, 1943. The State Board Examinations will be held December 27, 1943.

The Library has added in the past year many new volumes covering practically all the fields of medicine and related sciences. From new editions of such old favorites as DeLee's Obstetrics (8th edition, 1943) and Clendening's Methods of Treatment (8th edition, 1943) to the new Weiss and English's Phychosomatic Medicine (1943) there is a wide variety. In all, 1150 volumes, including bound journals, have been added during the year.

On the four hundredth anniversary of the printing of Vesalius' Fabrica, the Library Staff is particularly proud of a copy of the beautiful edition published by the New York Academy of Medicine, with plates from wood blocks used for the original edition and preserved in the Library of the University of Munich since 1643. Two of the plates are now thought to have been done by the artist Rubens.

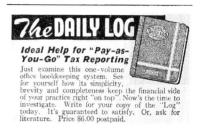

It's Santa's favorite charity!

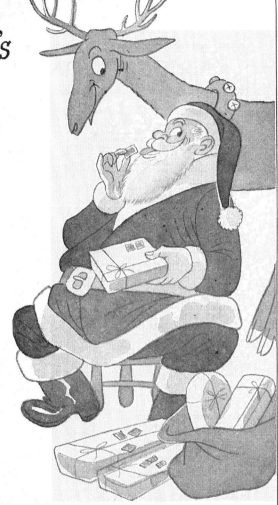

WE'VE never asked Santa Claus what *his* favorite charity is, but we'd bet the old fellow would chuckle: "Why, *Christmas Seals,* of course!"

You see, these little Seals give the greatest gift of all—health, life itself. As long as Santa can remember, the American people have made this a part of their Christmas giving—in depression and prosperity, in peacetime and war.

This year our needs are doubly great—because a wartime rise in tuberculosis must be prevented. So, make sure that every letter and package carried by Santa is stamped with your Christmas gift to mankind—and please send in your contribution *today!*

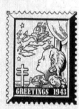

BUY CHRISTMAS SEALS

Because of the importance of the above message, this space has been contributed by

OKLAHOMA STATE MEDICAL ASSOCIATION

ASSOCIATION ACTIVITIES

SUPPLEMENTARY ROSTER 1943

(*Indicates serving in the Armed Forces).

The following is the list of 1943 memberships received in the offices of the Executive Secretary since the publication of the Roster in the July issue and the Supplementary Roster in the August issue.

ALFALFA
*PARSONS, JACK F. ....Cherokee

CANADIAN
*CRADEN, PAUL J. ....El Reno

CARTER
*CARLOCK, J. HOYLE ....Ardmore
*GORDON, J. M. ....Ardmore
JOHNSON, C. A. ....Wilson
MEAD, W. W. ....Ardmore
*MOXLEY, JOE N. ....Ardmore
*PERRY, FRED T. ....Healdton
*STONE, S. N., JR. ....Ardmore

CHEROKEE
*McINTOSH, R. K., JR. ....Tahlequah

CLEVELAND
*HOOD, J. O. ....Norman
*LOY, WILLIAM A. ....Norman
*REICHERT, R. J. ....Moore

GRADY
*BAZE, ROY E. ....Chickasha
*SCHUBERT, H. A. ....Chickasha

HUGHES
*MUNAL, JOHN ....Holdenville
*SHAW, JAMES F. ....Wetumka

JACKSON
ABERNETHEY, E. A. ....Altus
*ALLGOOD, J. M. ....Altus
*FOX, R. H. ....Altus
*HOLT, WILLARD D. ....Altus

JOHNSTON
LOONEY, J. T. ....Tishomingo

KINGFISHER
*LATTIMORE, F. C. ....Kingfisher
*TAYLOR, JOHN R. ....Kingfisher

LOVE
*LAWSON, PAT ....Marietta

MURRAY
WRENN, J. A. ....Sulphur

NOBLE
*EVANS, A. M. ....Perry

OKLAHOMA
BAYLOR, RICHARD A. ....400 N. W. 10th St.,
Okla. City
*HARRISON, LYNN H. ....Okla. City
HASSLER, F. R. ....State Health Dept., Okla. City
RICE, PAUL B. ....801 N. E. 13th St., Okla. City
SHAVER, S. R. ....Medical Arts Bldg., Okla. City
SHELBY, HUDSON ....Hales, Bldg., Okla. City

OSAGE
*DALY, JOHN F. ....Pawhuska
*RAGAN, T. A. ....Fairfax
*SMITH, RAYMOND O. ....Hominy

PITTSBURG
CALLAHAM, J. S. ....Wilburton
ELLIS, H. A. ....Kiowa
*MILLS, C. K. ....McAlester

PONTOTOC
PETERSON, WILLIAM G. ....Ada

ROGERS
*NELSON, C. C. ....Claremore

SEMINOLE
*DEATON, A. N. ....Wewoka
*FELTS, CLIFTON ....Seminole
JONES, W. E. ....Seminole
*KNIGHT, CLAUDE B. ....Wewoka
*LYONS, D. J. ....Seminole
*LYTLE, WM. R. ....Seminole
*RIPPY, O. M. ....Seminole
*TERRY, JOHN B. ....Wewoka

STEPHENS
LINDLEY, E. C. ....Duncan
THOMASSON, E. B. ....Duncan

TEXAS
*BLUE, JOHNNY A. ....Guymon
OBERMILLER, R. G. ....Texhoma

TULSA
BOLTON, FRED J. ....Tulsa
CHARBONNET, P. N. ....Tulsa

WOODWARD
PEARSON, GLENN A. ....Woodward

ANNUAL A. M. A. CONFERENCE OF SECRETARIES AND EDITORS

November 19 and 20 were the dates chosen by the American Medical Association for the Annual Conference of Secretaries and Editors. The meeting, as in the past, was held in Chicago in the American Medical Association Building. Secretaries of the State Associations and Editors of the various State Journals were in attendance, also officials of the state organizations and officers of the Army and Navy. The program covered the wartime policies and various phases of the post-war planning. Also discussed were the problems confronting the profession in regard to Medical Legislation and Public Relations.

The Friday morning meeting was called to order by Dr. Roger I. Lee, Chairman of the Board of Trustees of the American Medical Association. John S. Bouslog, M. D., Constitutional Secretary of the Colorado State Medical Society, was nominated as Chairman and unanimously elected. Dr. Bouslog presided over all sessions throughout the Conference.

Dr. James E. Paullin, President of the American Medical Association made the opening address to the Conference. Dr. Paullin discussed the problems relating to the assignment of duties of Military Surgeons. It was pointed out in the address that the Wartime Medical Training Program should be instituted as a part of the American Medical Association in connection with the American College of Surgeons and the American College of Physicians. The Post-War Planning Committee consists of men appointed by the House of Delegates and their purpose is to take care of the civilian needs of the physicians. There has been a great loss of civilian physicians to the Armed Forces. Some of these men went into the Service immediately after their internship and have never been in practice. Dr. Paullin pointed out the need for an organization to be set up in cooperation with the Committee on Medical Economics, Procurement and Assignment Service and the Committee on Medical Education, to see that information be made available to these men as to locations where they might begin to practice after the war. Committees have been formed to find out from the men in the Service what type of training they wish after they are discharged; whether or not they wish additional internships or residencies; and what they desire in the way

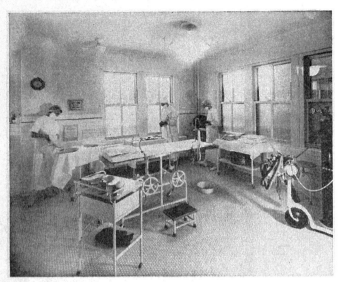

of specialty training. It shall be the principal aim to work out plans for the physicians in the service so that they may easily rehabilitate themselves after they return.

George F. Lull, Deputy Surgeon General of the United States Army, told of the great need of the Armed Forces for physicians. He gave a brief outline of the life of an Army Doctor and cited instances where the profession is making an heroic name for itself in the War. General Lull stressed the fact that more men were needed, although it is realized that the need at home is urgent also. The prospect of obtaining physicians through Volunteer Service is finished—there are no more volunteers. It is vitally important that every man who is able should accept a commission.

Victor Johnson, M.D., Secretary of the Council on Medical Education and Hospitals of the American Medical Association, assured the Conference that the prospects of taking care of the placement of men in the Services as to internships and residencies, and for additional education, are promising. He cited figures showing that the number of hospitals reporting and the number of residencies desired are nearly matched. A total of 37 schools have reported as having facilities available for courses in Basic Science.

The afternoon session on November 19 was opened by an address by Dr. Herman L. Kretschmer, President-Elect of the American Medical Association. Dr. Kretschmer spoke on the Cooperative Relationship of Procurement and Assignment Service and State Medical Associations.

The War Participation Committee as a coordinating Agency was discussed by Walter F. Donaldson, M.D., Chairman of that Committee of the American Medical Association. Dr. Donaldson pointed out that the War Participation Committee could do a great amount of 'leg-work' for the Procurement and Assignment Service, which he feels is hard pressed with work. It is felt that a lot could be accomplished if all states had a special committee of this kind. Physicians for the Armed Forces should be drawn not only from the large cities, but there are many physicians in the smaller cities who, with some adjustments, could be spared. It is the belief that the Committee should be interested in the maintenance of war records of the men in the Services. The Committee can win the admiration of the man in the service by reporting his commission and his services to his country. It is the duty of the Medical Societies at home to keep active in the interests of these men.

Louis H. Bauer, M.D., Chairman of the Council on Medical Service and Public Relations of the American Medical Association, presented a report of the work of the Council. Dr. Bauer stressed the fact that the medical profession had to have something to offer in place of the Wagner-Murry Bill. He further stated that we must not be stampeded into offering any set plans but that we should take time to point out what American medicine has to offer. It was pointed out that every member of the medical profession should keenly feel the magnitude of the problem and not be ultra-conservative or ultra-radical as it is not a situation where miracles can be worked. Group hospitalization has been approved and Voluntary Medical Insurance has been approved although neither are 100 per cent successful. This does not mean that there is anything wrong with the principle. Plans must be elastic as no one set plan is applicable to each and every type of community. The Kaiser Plan and other proposed plans by prominent industrialists were discussed by Dr. Bauer.

On Friday evening the American Medical Association was host to those attending the Conference at a dinner in the Crystal Room of the Palmer House. After the dinner a meeting of the Editors of the State Journals was held with Wingate M. Johnson, M.D., Editor of the North Carolina Medical Journal, presiding. Dr. Austin E. Smith, Secretary of the Council on Pharmacy and Chemistry of the American Medical Association, read an excellent paper on the workings of this council.

The value of the stand of the Council on Pharmacy and Chemistry in regard to advertising in the various State Journals was explained to the Editors.

An open discussion was held after Dr. Smith's paper. Questions were asked by Editors from various sections of the country regarding advertising policies. Dr. Morris Fishbein and Dr. Olin West spoke on the policies of the American Medical Association with reference to the Cooperative Medical Advertising Bureau.

The Saturday morning session was opened by J. W. Holloway, Jr., Director of the Bureau of Legal Medicine and Legislation of the American Medical Association. His address covered Medical Legislation of the American Medical Association. His address covered Medical Legislation in Congress. Mr. Holloway discussed the Chiropractor Bill and the Maternity and Infancy Bill.

The next address was given by L. Fernald Foster, M.D., Secretary of the Michigan State Medical Society, who spoke on Obstetric and Pediatric Care for the Wives and Children of Service Men. Dr. E. F. Daily, representing the Childrens Bureau, made a few remarks. The discussion which followed was animated and showed that the medical profession thoroughly dislikes the program with its arbitrary setting of fees and its payment to all, whether they need it or not. The feeling was universal that the program was merely another entering wedge of the government into the complete Federalization of the practice of medicine.

SCIENTIFIC EXHIBIT OF AMERICAN MEDICAL ASSOCIATION TO BE HELD JUNE 12-16, 1944

The Scientific Exhibit at the Chicago Session of the American Medical Association, June 12-16, 1944, will be held at the Palmer House. Exhibits will cover all phases of medicine and the medical sciences with particular emphasis on graduate medical instruction for the physician in general practice.

Application blanks for space in the Scientific Exhibit are now available and may be obtained by communicating with the Director, Scientific Exhibit, American Medical Association, 535 N. Dearborn Street, Chicago 10, Illinois.

GOVERNOR NAMES COMMITTEEMEN FOR COMMITTEE ON STANDARDIZATION

The Council of the Oklahoma State Medical Association submitted names to the Governor of the State of Oklahoma for appointment to the Committee on Standardization. Governor Kerr named Dr. J. F. Park, McAlester and Dr. V. C. Tisdal, Elk City, to serve on the Committee until July 1, 1946. Dr. Park will succeed himself and Dr. Tisdal was named to succeed Dr. Floyd S. Newman of Shattuck who is now serving with the Armed Forces overseas.

DR. FINIS W. EWING APPOINTED TO STATE BOARD OF MEDICAL EXAMINERS

On October 20 the Council of the Oklahoma State Medical Association submitted the following list of names of doctors to Governor Kerr in compliance with Section 5 of House Bill 222, for his consideration in the appointment to fill the vacancy recently created on the State Board of Medical Examiners by the demise of Dr. C. E. Bradley of Tulsa: E. P. Allen, Oklahoma City; Finis W. Ewing, Muskogee; John A. Haynie, Durant; Hugh Jeter, Oklahoma City; Harold M. McClure, Chickasha; Ralph A. McGill, Tulsa; Lang A. Mitchell, Stillwater; Lewis J. Moorman, Oklahoma City; George R. Osborn, Tulsa; A. W. Pigford, Tulsa; A. S. Risser, Blackwell; W. W. Rucks, Oklahoma City; Oscar White, Oklahoma City; Earl M. Woodson, Poteau.

Governor Kerr has named Dr. Finis W. Ewing of Muskogee to fill the vacancy on the Board.

OFFICERS OF TULSA COUNTY MEDICAL SOCIETY NAMED

Dr. Homer A. Ruprecht, prominent Tulsa heart specialist, has been named President-Elect of the Tulsa County Medical Society. He will serve in 1945, succeeding Dr. Ralph A. McGill, who assumes his presidential duties on January 1.

Other officers named at the annual business meeting of December 13 were: Dr. John C. Perry, vice-president; Dr. E. O. Johnson, secretary-treasurer; and Mr. Jack Spears, executive secretary. Dr. H. B. Stewart and Dr. W. S. Larrabee were named to the House of Delegates, Dr. J. C. Peden and Dr. W. A. Showman to the Board of Trustees, and Dr. Ian MacKensie to the Board of Censors.

The meeting also featured annual reports of eighteen standing and special committees. Dr. James C. Peden, retiring president, was voted a placque in recognition of his services to the Society.

The inaugural banquet will be Monday, January 10, 1944.

DR. NED SMITH RESIGNS FROM BOARD OF TRUSTEES

Dr. Ned R. Smith has resigned from the Board of Trustees of the Tulsa County Medical Society because of ill health. Succeeding him is Dr. James C. Peden.

Woman's Auxiliary

A PROGRAM OF POSTWAR PLANNING FOR THE WOMAN'S AUXILIARY

Morris Fishbein, M.D., Editor
American Medical Association

Postwar planning is engaging the attention of everyone today! I feel quite sure the Woman's Auxiliary has given it some thought. The American Medical Association, on recommendation of Dr. Paullin, has established by action of the House of Delegates a committee on the planning of postwar medical service. There are going to be tremendous changes in the nature of the practice of medicine, despite what many think. The American Medical Association, for many years, has waged warfare to maintain and provide for the American people a high quality of medical service. I have no doubt that the House of Delegates and the Board of Trustees will continue to do their utmost, regardless of what form of medical practice may eventuate in this country, to conserve all the factors that are responsible for maintaining this quality.

There are new social trends, new scientific attitudes and new discoveries developed at a speed greater than has ever previously occurred in the world; all of these are bound to affect the practice of medicine. There is a gradual development of a social trend leading toward "security." In England it is the Beveridge Plan, created to carry man from the cradle to the grave; in the United States it is the National Resource Planning Board, which takes the individual six months before life and carries him twenty years beyond. We are concerned with the prenatal care of the mother and unborn infant, as well as the dependents of those who die and these dependents must be cared for until they reach maturity. Many factors in the scheme in Great Britain will unquestionably affect the lives of those in the United States. Beveridge was asked if the adoption of the "cradle to the grave" plan would mean the end of the private practice of medicine. He replied that he felt that it would.

The National Planning Resources Board here in the United States has many features in its plan that are to be recommended and behind which we should place our best efforts. For instance, during the great depression following the last war there were thousands and thousands of idle ex-service men thrown upon the mercies of charity or given manufactured jobs of no importance; we certainly do not want that to happen again. In this war ten million men and between 50,000 and 60,000 American physicians will be engaged in the war effort. When those men are discharged into civilian life they must be provided with occupations. If they are not, we will see them tramping the streets begging for food, clothing and the necessities of life. We will see some attempt to manufacture work again. A proposal has been made to finance them on their discharge from service to the amount of $8,000 per man.

There are at present 20 million workers in the United States engaged in war work. When the war is terminated new occupations must be found for these men and women. Unless they are made ready, these people will be without work. There are many means of supplying these occupations—living conditions could be improved, a housing expansion program instituted, remodeling of old and building of new hospitals, health center movement for the control of infectious diseases, etc. The health movement is in its infancy and could be extended throughout the United States under the leadership of American medicine and public health. If these steps are to be taken, it is important that somebody begin to plan now where the hospitals and health centers are to be established, who is to run them and how they are to be financed and how managed. An intelligent man would begin planning now and make the necessary study to find out where hospitals are needed, how they should be managed and staffed. All of this is very much in the minds of the Board of Trustees of the American Medical Association.

I am sure if this postwar program develops there will be innumerable places where the Woman's Auxiliary can come to the aid of the medical profession and find new outlets for service. In the growth of the health movement, there are going to be great opportunities for health education. A group such as the Woman's Auxiliary, which has informed itself of the needs in medicine and medical education through Hygeia, can fit themselves well into a program of this kind and render assistance that could not be supplied by any other group. You would also be contributing to the prevention of a world wide depression such as followed World War I and aid in the reconstruction of the United States.

The Board of Trustees is giving special attention to fitting back into civilian life the 40,000 doctors in the armed forces who will be returning, most of them to the United States, to take up the practice of medicine under the conditions that will prevail at the time of their return. It is the greatest opportunity that has ever arisen in this country to meet the challenge of distribution of medical care—the one charge that is made against medicine in the United States. Medical care of this country is distributed primarily according to the economic status of the community in which the medical care happens to be supplied. In other words, in rural areas where the per capita income is low there is a shortage and lowered quality of medical service. In areas where there is a high per capita income, there is an excess and high quality of medical service. To redistribute 40,000 physicians and guide them into the areas where medical service is low, we must begin now and plan for the future creation of conditions that will appeal to those who are returning from service and will be looking for a place to locate. One way is to have available all the necessary clinical, laboratory and scientific diagnostic facilities and aids to enable these men to practice the kind of medicine they were taught in medical schools before they went into the service.

There is at the present moment in Congress new

legislation proposed which would materially change the nature of medical practice in the United States. I refer to the Wagner-Murray-Dingell Bill planned to extend social security to all of the people of the United States.

In all of these movements the Woman's Auxiliary is going to be asked to give to the Board of Trustees every assistance they can. You exercise a tremendous influence not only by your membership in the Auxiliary but by your affiliations with other organizations. It would be the height of folly if the Board of Trustees did not realize that in the Woman's Auxiliary they have a powerful weapon capable of mobilizing vast force in behalf of all that is good in medicine.

Tulsa County News

Committee Chairmen of Tulsa County Medical Auxiliary.

Program and Health Education	....Mrs. D. W. LeMaster
Membership	Mrs. D. L. Garrett
Social	Mrs. G. R. Russell
Philanthropic	Mrs. James C. Peden
Publicity	Mrs. J. W. Rogers
Legislative	Mrs. M. O. Hart
Hygeia	Mrs. Hugh Perry
Courtesy	Mrs. H. W. Ford
Telephone	Mrs. Frank J. Nelson
Public Relations	Mrs. Donald L. Mishler
Year Book	Mrs. Carl J. Hotz
War Aid	Mrs. C. C. Hoke
Advisory Council	Dr. James C. Peden

On October 5 the Auxiliary held a coffee in courtesy to the wives of their Doctors in Service and to Honorary Members.

In November the regular meeting of the Auxiliary was held down town because of the transportation problem. At this meeting a very valuable program on Preparation of Available Meats was given by Mrs. I. J. Nelson.

A team composed of Mrs. H. Lee Farris as Captain, Mrs. J. W. Childs, Mrs. Fred Cronk, Mrs. W. S. Larrabee, Mrs. J. O. Lowe, Mrs. Frank L. Flack, Mrs. D. L. Garrett, Mrs. John C. Perry took the Medical Arts Building on the War Aid Drive.

Mrs. C. S. Summers, sponsored by the Auxiliary showed a picture for recruitment of nurses at Central High School two different times. Mrs. C. H. Haralson gave a talk to the girls on the value of the profession.

The Auxiliary as a group are making Surgical Dressings at the Red Cross every Tuesday.

Pontotoc County

Officers 1943-1944

President	Mrs. E. R. Muntz, 525 S. Highland, Ada
Vice-President	Mrs. Ollie McBride, 1015 E. 9, Ada
Secretary	Mrs. R. H. Mayes, 130 W. 22nd, Ada
Treasurer	Mrs. E. M. Gullalt, Kings Road, Ada

Committee Chairmen

Program	Mrs. O. H. Miller
Membership	Mrs. C. F. Needham
Health and Project	Mrs. R. H. Mayes
Public Relations	Mrs. Ollie McBride
Arrangements	Mrs. T. L. Seaborn
Nominating	Mrs. S. P. Ross

General News

The Fall meeting of the Board of Directors of the Woman's Auxiliary to the American Medical Association met at the Palmer House in Chicago on November 19.

Mrs. Joseph W. Kelso and Mrs. Ray M. Balyeat of Oklahoma City, attended the Woman's Auxiliary meetings at the Southern Medical Association in Cincinnati, November 16 to November 18.

A complete report of all Activities of Oklahoma Auxiliary members for the year 1942-1943 was sent by Mrs. Flack to the Woman's Auxiliary of the Southern Medical Association.

COUNTY SOCIETY NEWS

The regular meeting of the Washington-Nowata County Medical Society on October 13 was made a joint session of the Society and the dentists of the two counties. Physicians and dentists of Osage and Tulsa Counties and of Montgomery County, Kansas, were also invited. The Washington County Memorial Hospital, assisted by the wives of several members, served a dinner to members and guests.

The meeting was devoted to the consideration of "State Medicine," and the evils and objectionable features of the proposed amendment to the Social Security Act and Senate Bill 1161. Two excellent addresses, fully discussing this bill were made by John C. Perry, M. D. and A. L. Walters, D. D. S., both of Tulsa. Free discussion by members and guests followed. Twenty-two guests were present.

The next regular meeting will be held Wednesday, November 10, with the following program: Talk on Harvard Postgraduate Course, J. P. Vansant, M.D.; Poliomyelitis Anterior, E. M. Chamberlin, M.D.; Discussion opened by W. M. Shipman, M.D.

The Carter County Medical Society met on November 1 at Ardmore with five members present. F. W. Boardway, M.D., and T. J. Jackson, M.D., were elected to represent the Society as members of the Blood Plasma Bank.

The Kay County Medical Society met at the Ponca City Hospital, Ponca City, Oklahoma on November 18, 1943, with sixteen members and three guests present. A symposium on the "Rh" Blood Factor was given by Doctors Philip Risser of Blackwell, George Hemphill of Pawhuska and Roy Emanuel of Chickasha. The society thoroughly enjoyed this symposium and expressed a unanimous vote of their appreciation to the speakers.

The next meeting will be held December 16 at Blackwell at which time the annual election of officers will be held.

Dr. V. C. Tisdal of Elk City gave a paper on "Relationship of Tonsils to Lymphatic System" at the November meeting of the Beckham County Medical Society in Sayre, Oklahoma.

The next meeting will be held on December 14 when officers will be elected.

The Okmulgee-Okfuskee County Medical Society met on November 8 at Okemah with twenty-four members and guests present. Dr. Walker Morledge of Oklahoma City spoke on "Malaria" and Dr. H. M. Galbraith, Oklahoma City spoke on "Psychosomatic Disease." The following Medical Officers from Glennan General Hospital, Okmulgee, were present and entered into the discussion: Colonel Work, Neuro-psychiatry; Major Bovenmyer, Internal Medicine; Major Dodge, Ophthalmology and Otology; Major Lubben, Urology; Major Hoyt, Surgery; Major Remesser, Gynecology and Obstetrics. Dr. Clinton Gallaher, Shawnee, Counselor for District No. 7 was present.

A Committee was appointed to consult with Colonel Gandy, Glennan General Hospital Commandant on the effect of working out associate membership for Medical Officers stationed here.

Mr. N. D. Helland, Tulsa, discussed the Blue Cross Plan for Hospitalization at the November meeting of the Pontotoc County Medical Society.

The Oklahoma County Medical Society met on November 23 at the Oklahoma Club in Oklahoma City. The physicians who are in the Armed Forces were invited guests. Dr. Ephraim Goldfain and Dr. D. H. O'Donoghue spoke on the subject of "Metabolic Arthritis."

★ FIGHTIN' TALK ★

The following Oklahoma physicians have been ordered to active duty by the War Department: *Lt. (jg) William L. Tomlinson*, Oklahoma City, who has been commissioned in the U. S. Navy; *Lt. (jg) Lynn H. Harrison*, Oklahoma City, entered the U. S. Navy after serving a residency at the Oklahoma City General Hospital; *Lt. (jg) E. Evans Chambers*, Enid, who has been commissioned in the U. S. Navy; *Lt. E. B. Dunlap, Jr.*, Lawton, entered the Army Air Corps on November 30; *Lt. Forrest M. Swisher*, Oklahoma City, formerly a resident at McBride Clinic; and *Lt. Harold J. Binder*, Oklahoma City.

The following Oklahoma physicians have recently been promoted: From Major to Lt. Colonel: *Alvin Paulson*, Clinton. From Captain to Major: *Thomas J. Hardman*, Tulsa; *Manford S. White*, Blackwell; *Bruce R. Hinson*, Enid; *C. G. Stuard*, Tulsa; *L. G. Neal*, Ponca City; *Louis Kennedy*, Clinton. From Lieutenant to Captain: *Phil L. Salkeld*, Vinita; *W. D. Holt*, Altus; *James T. McInnis*, Public Health Department, Muskogee.

Lt. Dick Graham, former Executive Secretary of the Oklahoma State Medical Association, was commissioned in October and was sent to the Surgeon General's Office in Washington. At the present time, Dick is at Carlisle Barracks, Pa., where he is attending Officer's Training School.

Word has been received that Captain J. O. Akins, Tulsa, was wounded in battle. Dr. Akins was shot in both legs by 30-calibre machine gun bullets and was taken to a North African hospital. It was necessary to amputate his right leg, but he is recovering nicely and is in very good spirits. It is hoped that he will be able to return home soon.

Captain Murray M. Cash, Tulsa, reports from Clewiston, Florida, where he is stationed at Riddle Field. Captain Cash served his internship and then became resident at St. John's Hospital in Tulsa before entering the Army.

Major Paul H. Dube, Shattuck, is now stationed at Fort Logan, Colorado. Major Dube was on the staff of the Newman Clinic at Shattuck as an orthopedist before entering the Army.

Colonel Lee R. Wilhite, formerly of Perkins, called the executive office recently on his way to the old home town on leave to say "hello." Many of those now in service will remember Colonel Wilhite as having been Senior Officer in charge of the Medical Officer Recruiting Board in Oklahoma in 1942 prior to his being transferred to Fort Bragg, North Carolina, to take charge of the 134th Medical Regiment. The Colonel has since reported his new location as being Fort Tyson, Tennessee.

Lt. Edward D. Greenberger, McAlester, reports that he is extremely pleased with his recent change in station. He is now at Camp Carson, Colorado, where he is the Roentgenologist in the Unit. Lt. Greenberger states, "No need to describe to you the majestic beauties of these mountains and vacation spots around Colorado Springs—This is the Army!"

Captain David L. Edwards, Tulsa, reports that he is now stationed at Coral Gables, Florida, and is on Eye Service. He visits occasionally with *Lt. Col. Charles A. Pigford*, Tulsa, who is Post Surgeon at Marianne, Florida.

Major Byron J. Cordonnier, Enid, writes from the Lubbock Army Air Field where he was sent from Randolph Field. He says that he thoroughly enjoys the Army, but will be very happy when the war is over. He, like so many others, is anxiously looking forward to an overseas assignment.

Lt. Comdr. Don W. Branham, Oklahoma City, is serving overseas. In his letter, he says that before leaving he saw *Dr. Wylie Chesnut* of Miami who was on the ship that went into the drive on Kiska.

Major Raymond L. Murdoch, Oklahoma City, writes that he is enjoying our 'news letter.' He is not permitted to reveal his station but states that he is having quite a 'variety.'

Captain James R. Ricks, Oklahoma City, was a junior officer with the 45th Division for a year before he was sent to Panama in 1941. Captain Ricks was then sent to the Southwest Pacific and writes from there. His letter in part, states:

"Have found the training in the States with the 45th Division on maneuvers of 1941 has stood me in good stead. Of course, the year's jungle training and acclimatization has prepared me for this specialized type of field jungle service.

"We are doing general medical service and what Orthopedic and Surgery that we can't get out of doing by passing on to the rear hospitals. Have certainly done a lot of 'Tropical Medicine' and learned to respect the O. U. course in 'Parisitology.'

"We bought a lot of good English Surgical Texts very reasonable in our brief stay in Australia."

Captain L. A. Munding, Tulsa, is taking the course at the School of Aviation Medicine at Randolph Field, Texas. He is enjoying our letters and column and sends the best of luck to those who are still serving on the home front.

Captain Lester P. Smith, Marlow, writes as follows from overseas:

"Have been overseas sometime and have seen lots of country, all of which has been very interesting.

"*Captain Gilbert Tracy* of Cheyenne, *Captain John Daly* of Pawhuska, *Captain Carson Oglesbee*, and *Captain George L. Kaiser* of Muskogee, who are members of our Company and all doctors, send their best regards along with mine."

Comdr. R. G. Jacobs, Enid, writes to us again from his station. He is doing his bit by correspondence concerning the Wagner Act. (Editor's Note: We are pleased by Comdr. Jacob's praise of our letters and want to assure everyone that we will 'keep 'em rollin'.)

Major Charles H. Wilson, Oklahoma City, graduate of Oklahoma University School of Medicine in 1937, is now stationed at Carlisle Barracks, Pa.

Lt. Col. Wayne Starkey, Altus, has been ordered to report to the Surgeon General's office in Washington, where he is to be attached to the training division.

He has been stationed at Camp Barkeley, Texas, with the Officer Candidate School since May, 1942. He entered service as a Captain in the Medical Corps when the National Guard was mobilized in September, 1940.

Word has been received by relatives that *Lt. Donald H. Smith*, Fairview, is a prisoner of the Japanese.

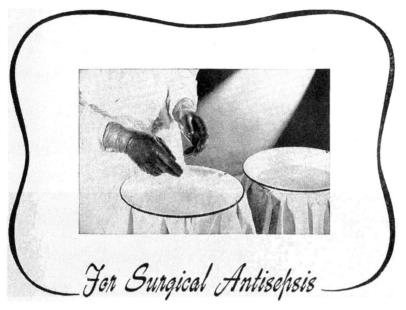

For Surgical Antisepsis

Zephiran Chloride is a germicide of high bactericidal and bacteriostatic potency. In proper dilutions it is nonirritating and relatively nontoxic to tissue cells.

Zephiran Chloride possesses detergent, keratolytic and emulsifying properties, which favor penetration of tissue surfaces, hence removing dirt, skin fats and desquamating skin.

INDICATIONS

Zephiran Chloride is widely employed for skin and mucous membrane antisepsis—for preoperative disinfection of skin, denuded skin and mucous membranes, for vaginal instillation and irrigation, for vesical and urethral irrigation, for wet dressings, for irrigation in eye, ear, nose and throat infections, etc.

HOW SUPPLIED

Zephiran Chloride is available in

TINCTURE 1:1000 Tinted

TINCTURE 1:1000 Stainless

AQUEOUS SOLUTION 1:1000

in 8 ounce and 1 gallon bottles.

Write for informative booklet

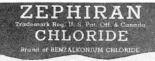

ZEPHIRAN
Trademark Reg. U. S. Pat. Off. & Canada
CHLORIDE
Brand of BENZALKONIUM CHLORIDE

 WINTHROP CHEMICAL COMPANY, INC.

NEW YORK 13, N. Y.   *Pharmaceuticals of merit for the physician*   WINDSOR, ONT.

MEDICINE AT WAR

THE MEDICAL PROFESSION AND FOOD RATIONING

The inauguration of the point system of rationing foods brought forth the problem of special diets for those under the care of the physician and for hospitals in their care of patients requiring special diets. Since point rationing covers a large range of meats, fats and processed foods, it is necessary that extra points be allowed in order to provide these items for diets calling for an increased amount of any special item. In April, 1943, at the request of Mr. Roy Hendrickson, director of the War Food Administration, Dr. Ross G. Harrison, chairman of the National Research Council, appointed a group of nationally known physicians to advice the War Food Administration concerning the extent of these special needs and the best method of meeting them.

There has been much confusion concerning requests for additional points for special diets. In order to clarify this situation the Public Health Committee of the Oklahoma State Medical Association, under the direction of Dr. Carroll Pounders, has, after a careful study, drawn up certain recommendations which are accepted by the Board and which will be followed in issuing additional allotments. The conditions for which additional quantities of food may be needed are mentioned, also the kinds and maximum amounts of foods which will be so allotted for each particular condition. It should be emphasized that the recommendations are for the maximal rather than optimal allowances and consideration in prescribing them must be given to the availability of unrationed foods which may, in part or in full, be substituted for dietetically equivalent rationed foods.

Only certificates issued by persons licensed to practice medicine and surgery in the State of Oklahoma will be honored. The forms will be furnished by the local rationing board and these must be completely and correctly filled out and signed. Varying periods of validity for certification for extra rations are recommended and where none is specified certification should be renewed once a year. The recommendations include milk and eggs because of the possibility that they may be rationed at some future time.

RECOMMENDATIONS FOR SPECIAL DIETS

Diabetes Mellitus

Provisions for patients with diabetes mellitus may need to include per week not more than:

Meat, including fish and poultry	64 ounces
Bacon	8 ounces
Butter or margarine	16 ounces
Other fats and oils	7 ounces
Eggs	7
Milk (adults)	7 pints
Milk (children to age 16)	7 quarts
Fruits and vegetables	72 ounces

This allowance applies only to processed fruits and vegetables and does not indicate total carbohydrate requirements. If these amounts of food are not available to the patients from the rationed foods to which he normally would be entitled, together with commodities obtainable from unrationed sources, supplementary ration points will be allotted to provide them.

To be eligible to receive any supplementary allowances of rationed foods the patient with diabetes mellitus must surrender his sugar ration.

Pregnancy and Tubercular Cases

Meat, including fish and poultry	64 ounces
Fats and oils, including butter and margarine	13½ ounces
Eggs	7
Fruits and vegetables	56 ounces of processed citrus fruits and tomato juice in addition to the ordinary allowance of processed fruits and vegetables.

If the above amounts are not available from rationed foods together with unrationed foods procurable by the patient, sufficient supplementary points will be allotted to provide them.

Peptic Ulcer and Gastritis

Meats, including fish and poultry	22 ounces
Butter	12 ounces
Fruits and vegetables (processed)	72 ounces
Milk	5½ quarts
Cream	5½ quarts

Chronic Suppurative Diseases

Provisions for patients with chronic suppurative processes, especially empyema, osteomyelitis, extensive suppurative lesions of soft parts, subcutaneous tissues or muscles and those infections in which there is profuse pus formation may need to include per week:

Meats, including fish and poultry	64 ounces
Milk	7 quarts
Eggs	7

Certification of patients with chronic suppurative disease must be renewed at 60 day intervals.

Chronic Nephritis, nephrotic type: Cirrhosis of the liver: Severe hepatitis and chronic ulcerative colitis

Patients suffering from any of the above conditions should be allowed a maximum of 7 pounds of meat, including fish and poultry per week.

A diagnosis of chronic ulcerative colitis should not be recognized unless certified to by three physicians and the certification must be renewed every four months and way be authorized by one physician.

Sprue

Meats, including non-fatty fish and poultry	7 pounds
Milk	14 to 21 quarts

A diagnosis of sprue should not be recognized unless certified to by three physicians.

Allergies

These cases will be considered individually. Certificates should be accompanied by statements showing to what foods the patient is clinically sensitive and what foods are needed in extra allotments.

NO ADDITIONAL ALLOTMENTS WILL BE ALLOWED FOR THE FOLLOWING

Anti-constipation	Low salt diet
Children's diets	Diets for hypertension
Obesity	Arthritis diet
High vitamin diet	Diet for debilitation
High protein diet	

It is desirable for each County Society to appoint a Regional Medical Appeals Committee whose duty it is to evaluate and pass on requests for additional food allowances for patients with conditions not specifically provided for in the foregoing recommendations.

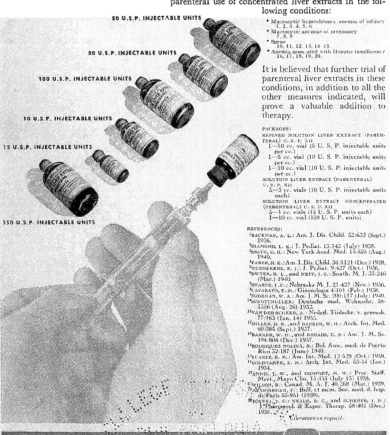

FORM TO BE EXECUTED BY PATIENT

To Ration Board No. .... State of ....
I hereby request an extra allotment of such rationed foods as have been designated for the disease with which I am suffering, namely ....
.... *(name of disease)*
and hereby authorize my attending physician, ...
.... to certify to the existence of such disease for the purpose of obtaining the designated foods.

....
(Signature)

....
(Address)

....
(Date)

....
(Number of Ration Book)

FORM TO BE EXECUTED BY PHYSICIAN

I hereby certify that I have examined ....
.... and that my diagnosis of his (her) condition is ....
.... and that he (she) has been under my care for .... months.
I further certify that he (she) needs the amount of food specified for the disease for 2, 4, 6, 8, 10, 12 months.   *(encircle appropriate No.)*

....
(Signature)   *(Degree)*

....
(Address)

....
(School of graduation)

....
(State and year of licensure)

....
(Date)

Classified Advertisements

FOR SALE: Modern, completely equipped Clinic in prosperous town in Oklahoma. Slight competition. Will lease to responsible party or will hire physician. Hospital Connection. Write in care of Journal.

BOOK REVIEWS

HANDBOOK OF TROPICAL MEDICINE. Alfred C. Reed and J. C. Geiger. Stanford University Press, Stanford University, California. 188 pages. Price $1.50.

The so-called tropical diseases are becoming increasingly important, due to the war and closer contacts with tropical areas. Medical training in this country, covering this field, has been inadequate to meet the present demands. The pocket-sized handbook is an attempt to put essential information on these diseases into a condensed but practical form. The list of topics covering diseases and problems of warm climates is complete in dealing with infections and climatic diseases. It does not cover plant and animal poisons. Each subject is given in proportion to its relative importance, the dysenteries, malarias, and rickettsial diseases receiving the most attention. In the discussion of each disease the essential points on geographic distribution, epidemiology, symptomatology, diagnosis, treatment and control are emphasized.

The material given is up to date but often one feels

the desire for more details. A person already acquainted with the diseases, or one actually confronted with cases would want to consult standard sources frequently. This is freely admitted by the authors and the book is not supposed to take the place of standard works. If a practitioner, seeing these diseases for the first time, wants a brief, inexpensive guide to the field of tropical medicine, this book is of value.—Donald B. McMullen, ScD.

INTERNAL MEDICINE IN GENERAL PRACTICE. Lt. Robert P. McCombs, M.D., Medical Corps, U. S. Naval Reserve. Recently instructor in internal medicine for the State wide Postgraduate Program of the Tennessee State Medical Association. On leave of absence from staffs of Pennsylvania Hospital, Abigton Memorial Hospital and Jefferson Medical College, Philadelphia. Published by W. B. Saunders Company. 694 pages. Foreword and complimentary remarks made by Ross T. McIntire, Surgeon General of the Navy. Price $7.00.

This not very obese but concise tome serves a good purpose in time when medical curricula are shortened or intensified, and the medical student has not the time to absorb the longer texts, which should be in every physicians' library for reference.

The author has had practical experience in the refresher courses which most states are providing for those coming out of retirement, and those not able to visit the medical centers during these hectic times. He thus has tried to cover the ground of the more common disease, and particularly the controversial points which he has encountered in contact with the profession during these courses. He has given an up-to-the-minute conception of the diseases with adequate laboratory procedure when necessary. This is in keeping with the advancement of the basic sciences during the past few years. His differential diagnosis is amply brought out with a teacher's clarity, showing lantern slide accompaniments. He has not tried to be too technical, but very practical in decrying the fact that the drift is away from medicine as an art, whereas bedside observation is most essential in differentiating functional and organic troubles.

He has taken up disorders of the heart in fifty-eight pages, with a physiologic approach, giving history and physical findings before instruments of precision are consulted. He tells of the uses and what the E. K. G. cannot do—and cautions that "it must always be kept in mind that practically all abnormalities of the E. K. G. have been observed to occur on occasions in people with no demonstrable heart disease."

One hundred ten pages are given over to disorders of the gastrointestinal tract, and then with a postscript about nutritional deficiencies. The book is well illustrated, with one hundred fourteen illustrations, and fifteen tables of differential diagnosis which goes to clarify and simply the text.—Lea A. Riely.

DISEASES OF THE LIVER, GALLBLADDER AND BILE DUCTS. S. S. Lichtman, M.D. Lea and Febiger. Philadelphia. 1942. 906 pages. 122 engravings and a colored plate. Price $11.00.

The contents of this textbook cover the diseases of the liver, gallbladder and bile ducts, but they do not stop at a mere clinical presentation of the subject. There is a very fine discussion of the liver lobule from the histological and cytological knowledge. The circulation of the liver are well presented. The relationship of the gallbladder structure and functions are of practical value, for all who have patients with disturbances of this organ.

The discussion on the various tests are up to date and fair. One is particularly conscious of the tests as they relate to special functions and one is guided into the use of several, rather than one. Attention is called to the Hippuric Acid Test, the Cephalin-Cholesterol Flocculation Procedure, the Acetone Modification Icterus Index and the hematological correlations with general liver damage.—I. A. Nelson, M.D.

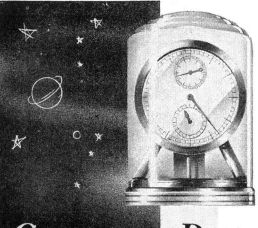

Consistent *Performance*

★ Unchanging, the Naval Observatory clock at Arlington has ticked on for decades. Its unvarying time is the accepted standard throughout the nation. The same consistent performance may be expected from PITOCIN*. Rigid standardization and marked stability assure the same reaction today as yesterday and the day before.

★ PITOCIN'S potent oxytocic principle, negligible amount of pressor factor, low protein content and freedom from impurities assures stimulation of uterine contracture, no appreciable rise in blood pressure and a minimum possibility of reactions—true uniformity.

★ Chief indications for PITOCIN (alphahypophamine) are: medical induction of labor; stimulation of uterus, in properly selected cases, during labor; prevention of postpartum hemorrhage and bleeding following curettage; and treatment of postpartum and late puerperal hemorrhage.

*TRADE-MARK REG. U. S. PAT. OFF.

PITOCIN

A product of modern research offered to the medical profession by
Parke, Davis & Company

PARKE, DAVIS & COMPANY
DETROIT, MICHIGAN

XXXVI   INDEX TO CONTENTS   1943

Copyright, 1943, by Oklahoma State Medical Association,
Oklahoma City, Oklahoma

The use of the index will be greatly facilitated by remembering that articles are often listed under more than one head. Scientific articles may be found under both the name of the author and the subject discussed. Editorials, Book Reviews and Obituaries are listed under the special headings as well as alphabetically.

KEY TO ABBREVIATIONS

(S)—Scientific articles   (br)—Book Review
(A)—Association Activities   (MP)—Medical Preparedness
(E)—Editorials   (abs)—Abstract
(Sp)—Special Article   (o)—Obituary

A

A. S. A. (E) 483
Abdominal Pain in the Female, Lower (S), Lt. Comdr. Clyde M. Longstreth, Norman 330
Absorptioin, Excretion and Distibution of Penicillin, The (abs) 503
Acute Otitis Media and Mastoiditis (abs) 133
Acute Poliomyelitis (E) 292
Administrative Hyperopia (E) 344
Adson, Alfred W., Rochester Minn. (Sp) The Doctor of Medicine and His Responsibility 201
Advances in Internal Medicine (br) 224
Advances in Pediatrics (br) 128
Advances in the Treatment of Chronic Nasal Sinusitis (abs) 456
Air-Borne Infections: Some Observations upon its Decline (br) 407
Akin, Robert H. (S) Verumontanitis—The Application of the Sex Hormones 381
Alien Physicians (E) 111
Allergic Aspect of Vasomotor Rhinitis, The (abs) ..132
Allergy in Otorhinolaryngology, The General Concept of (abs) 227
Alphabet Abused, The (E) 20
Alternates, Delegates and (A) 176
Alumnus, An Illustrious (E) 152
Amaurotic Idiocy, Some Anomalous Forms of, and their Bearing on the Relationship of the Various Types (abs) 272
Amendments to Constitution and By-Laws to be Acted Upon at Annual Meeting (A) 179
American Board of Obstetrics and Gynecology Examinations to be Held (A) 33
American Board of Obstetrics and Gynecology Alters Requirements (A) 348
American College of Surgeons Approves Forty Oklahoma Hospitals (A) 70
American College of Surgeons, Schedules for Twenty War Sessions Announced (A) 116
American Illustrated Medical Dictionary—Nineteenth Edition (br) 128
American Medical Association Annual Meeting (A)..310
American Medical Association Conference of Secretaries and Editors (A) 528
American Medical Association, Council on Medical Service and Public Relations Adopts New Policies (A) 490
American Medical Association House of Delegates Meets June 7, (A) 116
American Medicine, The National Physicians Committee and (E) 66
American Public Health Association Conference Announced (A) 116
Amputation Anesthesia by Freezing (abs) 458
Anderson, Otis L. (Sp) Recommendations for a Venereal Disease Control Program in Industry 289
Angiomatosis Retinae (Von Hippel's Disease): Results Following Irradiation of Three Eyes (abs)..363
Ankle, Internal Fixation in Injuries of the (abs) 412
Annual American Medical Association Conference of Secretaries and Editors (A) 22
Annual Meeting, American Medical Association (A)..310

Annual Meeting, Fifty-First, May 11-12, Oklahoma City (A) 114
Annual Meeting, Thirteenth Annual, Oklahoma City Clinical Society, October 18-19-20 and 21 (A) ..392
Annual Meeting, Program, 1943 (A) 156
Annual Reports
  Reports of Council 250
  Report of District No. 2 252
  Report of District No. 3 254
  Report of District No. 4 254
  Report of District No. 5 254
  Report of District No. 6 254
  Report of District No. 7 256
Annual Meeting, Well Attended, Fifty-First (A)...210
Annual Session, Committee on, Selects Dates for 1943 Meeting (A) 70
Antrum, Technique for Obtaining Bacteriological Specimens From the (abs) 319
Apology (A) 346
Appendicitis, Modern Aids in the Treatment of (S) Forrest M. Lingenfelter, John W. Cavanaugh, Harvey Richey 425
Arch of the Foot, Misconception About the Springiness of the Longitudinal. Mechanics of the Foot (abs) 503
Army Recruiting Program Will Require 6,900 Physicians (MP) 123
Arteriosus, Patent Ductus: A Report of Two Cases (S) Frank T. Joyce 6
Arthritis in Modern Practice (br) 223
Associate Membership to be Acted Upon at Annual Meeting (A) 116
Association to Assist O. P. A. on Food Rationing Program (A) 392
Association to Hold Wartime Industrial Health Institute (A) 70
Audit Report ,Annual (A) 180
Auditory Canal, Osteoma of the External (abs) 88
Auxiliary News, Woman's 31, 80, 120, 214, 314, 356, 402, 442, 532
Aviation Medicine (S) Lt. Col. W. M. Scott, Will Rogers Field, Oklahoma City 93

B

Babies Are Fun (br) 274
Bagby, Louis (o) 124
Barlow, Veneta R., Tulsa Librarian (E) 112
Belot, Colonel Monti L. (S) Problems of Induction ..511
Benevolent Fund, Report of Committee on 172
Bismarck to Beveridge, From, Plus Wagner and Murray (E) 292
Black, Thomas C. (S) Early Diagnosis of Tuberculosis 195
Blood Flow in Extremities Affected by Anterior Poliomyelitis (abs) 411
Blood Transfusions, The Transmission of Diseases by (S) A. Ray Wiley 374
Blue Cross Reports 34, 82, 126, 216, 271, 358, 403, 500
Blue, Johnny A. (S) Hypertension in a Young Athlete Due to Coarctation of Aorta: Report of a Case 143

Bondurant, C. P. (S) A Review of the Management
  of Late Syphilis 382
Bone Cyst, Solitary Unicameral, with Emphasis on
  the Roentgen Picture, the Pathologic Appearance
  and the Pathogenesis (abs) 273
Bone Tumors, Classification of (abs) 136
Book Reviews
  Advances in Internal Medicine, L. W. Hunt 224
  Advances in Pediatrics, George H. Garrison 128
  After Effects of Brain Injuries in War, Harry
    Wilkins 85
  Air Borne Infections: Some Observations upon its
    Decline, Lea A. Riley 407
  American Illustrated Medical Dictionary—19th Edi-
    tion, The, Lewis J. Moorman 128
  Arthritis in Modern Practice, William K. Ishmael 223
  Babies are Fun, Betty S. Moorman 274
  Boy Sex Offender and His Later Career, The,
    Coyne H. Campbell 406
  Chemotherapy of Gonococcic Infections, Robert H.
    Akin 320
  Climate Makes the Man, Lewis J. Moorman 502
  Collected Papers of the Mayo Clinic and the Mayo
    Foundation, Lewis J. Moorman 406
  Condensed Chemical Dictionary, Lewis J. Moorman 320
  Constitution and Disease, Lewis J. Moorman 130
  Disability Evaluation, D. H. O'Donoghue 222
  Diseases of the Breast, Gerald Rogers 224
  Diseases of the Liver, Gallbladder and Bile Ducts,
    I. A. Nelson 538
  Dr. Colwell's Daily Log for Physicians, Lewis J.
    Moorman 37
  Guide to Practical Nutrition, A, A. W. White 366
  Handbook of Tropical Medicine, Donald B. Mc-
    Mullen 538
  Inner Ear, The, L. C. McHenry 365
  Internal Medicine in General Practice, Lea A.
    Riely 538
  March of Medicine, The, J. V. Athey 502
  Medical Parasitology, Hugh Jeter 225

Memoir of Walter Reed: The Yellow Fever Ep-
  isode, Lewis J. Moorman 407
Mental Illness: A Guide for the Family, Ned R.
  Smith 84
Mind and its Disorders, The, Ned R. Smith 130
National Formulary, Lewis J. Moorman 365
Neuro-Anatomy, Harry Wilkins 84
New and Non Official Remedies-1943, L. J. Starry 366
Pathology of Trauma, The, E. Eugene Rice 222
Practical Survey of Chemistry and Metabolism of
  the Skin, C. P. Bondurant 365
Primer on the Prevention of Deformity in Child-
  hood, A, L. Stanley Sell 223
Psychosomatic Medicine, Lewis J. Moorman 502
Rehabilitation of the War Injured—A Symposium,
  L. J. Starry 365
Safe Deliverance, Lewis J. Moorman 223
Shock: Dynamics, Occurence and Management, E.
  Eugene Rice 225
Stedman's Medical Dictionary—Illustrated, Lewis
  J. Moorman 274
Surgical Pathology, Major W. A. Howard 274
Surgical Practices of the Lahey Clinic 406
Synopsis of Clinical Syphilis, A. Brooks Absher ...366
Synopsis of Tropical Medicine, Donald B. Mc-
  Mullen 502
Tables of Food Values, Anne Betche 274
Toxemias, The, of Pregnancy, J. M. Parrish, Jr. ... 37
Tuberculosis Nursing, Golda B. Slief 130
Urine and Urinalysis, W. F. Keller 365
Urology in General Practice, Basil A. Hayes 320
Venture in Public Health Integration, A, Medical
  Staff of Oklahoma State Health Department ..128
War Gases, Their Identification and Decontamina-
  tion, J. F. Messenbaugh 129
War Medicine—A Symposium, Ned. R. Smith 130
When Doctors Are Rationed, Horace Roed 38
Year Book of General Medicine, Bert F. Keltz 84
Year Book on Pediatrics—1942, Bertha Levy 320
Boy Sex Offender and His Later Career, The (br) ..406

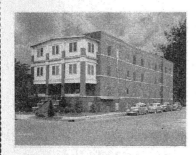
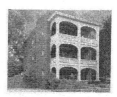

Bowel, The Irritable, (S) Turner Bynum 56
Bradley, Calvin E. (o) 349
Brain Injuries in War, After Effects of, (br) 85
Breast, Diseases of (br) 224
Brice, Marion O. (o) 448
Brights Disease, Diet and (abs) 86
Brown, F. C. (o) 271
Browning, W. M. (o) 124
Buchanan, F. R. (o) 309
Bunn, A. D. (o) 221
Burke, Richard M. (S) Tuberculosis Tracheobronch-
    itis 55
Burn Cases, Treatment of, Off the U.S.S. Wasp (S)
    R. G. Jacobs 235
Burns, Treatment of, (S) John F. Burton 4
Burton, John F. (S) Treatment of Burns 4
Bynum, Turner (S) The Irritable Bowel 56

C

Calcification and Ossification of Vertebral Ligaments
    (Spondylitis Ossificans Ligamentosa): Roentgen
    Study of Pathogenesis and Clinical Significance
    (abs) 39
Cameron, Paul B. (S) Observations on the Negro
    Diabetic 517
Cancer of the Skin, Radium Therapy in the Treat-
    ment of (S) Louis M. Piatt 415
Cancer, Study and Control of, Report of Committee
    on 174
Cardiovascular Origin, The Exigencies of (S) George
    Herrmann 47
Carney, Andie B. (S) Comparative Symptoms in
    Peptic Ulcer and Cholecystitis in 200 Cases 420
Cavanaugh, John W. (S) Modern Aids in the Treat-
    ment of Appendicitis 425
Challenge, The (E) 436
Chance to Serve, A (E) 525
Changes in 1942 Revenue Act (A) 74
Changing Conception of the Management of Chronic
    Progressive Deafness (abs) 43
Chemical Dictionary, The Condensed (br) 320
Chemotherapy of Gonococcic Infections (br) 320
Chemotherapy with Sulfanilamide: Clinical Results
    (abs) 410
Chickasha Physicians Honored (A) 71
Children's Feet, Normal and Presenting Common
    Abnormalities (abs) 364
Cholecystitis in 200 Cases, Comparative Symptoms
    in Peptic Ulcer and (S) Andre B. Carney 420
Chondroysplasia, Hereditary Deforming (abs) 228
Christmas Seal and the Medical Profession, The (E) 525
Civilian Defense, Office of 32, 126
Classified Ads 34, 126, 220, 268, 309, 349, 402, 538
Classification of Bone Tumors (abs) 130
Climate Makes the Man (br) 502
Clinical and Bacteriological Research on the Ton-
    sillar Origin of Focal Infections Assay of A
    Diagnostic Method for Cutaneous Streptococcic
    Allergy and its Results (abs) 411
Clinical Importance of the Lipoid Ring of the Cornea
    (abs) 226
Clinical Society, Oklahoma City, 13th Annual Meeting
    October 18-19-20 and 21 (A) 392
Clinical Society, The Oklahoma City (E) 390
Clinics, Oklahoma City Internists to Conduct Annual-
    Washington Birthday (A) 23
Coachman, E. H. (S) The Role of Medical Short
    Wave Therapy in Otolaryngology 417
Cochlear Response and the Mechanism of the Cochlea,
    The (abs) 362
Cogito Ego Sum (E) 293
Collected Papers of the Mayo Clinic and the Mayo
    Foundation (br) 406
College of Physicians, Regional Meeting of the (E) 154
Colles' Fracture (abs) 86
Color in Protective Night Light (abs) 318
Colwell, Dr., Daily Log for Physician's (br) 37
Combined Operation in Low Back and Sciatic Pain,
    The (abs) 272

Committee on Annual Session Selects Dates for 1943
    Meeting (A) 70
Committee Appointments, Announced by President
    Stevenson (A) 311
Committeemen for Committee on Standardization,
    Governor Names (A) 530
Committee Reports
    Report of Committee on Malpractice Insurance 211
    Report of the Medical Advisory Committee to the
        Department of Public Welfare 211
    Report of Committee on Maternity and Infancy 211
    Report of Committee on Study and Control of
        Cancer 174
    Annual Report of District No. 1 168
    Annual Report of District No. 8 168
    Annual Report of District No. 9 168
    Report of Committee on Medical Education and
        Hospitals 168
    Report of Committtee on Public Policy 170
    Report of Committee on Judicial and Professional
        Relations 170
    Report of Benevolent Fund Committee 172
    Report of Committee on Medical Economics 172
    Report of Committee on Medical Testimony 172
    Report of Committee on Postgraduate Medical
        Teaching 174
    Report of Committee on Public Health 174
    Report of Committee on the Study and Control of
        Cancer 174
    Report of Committee on the Study and Control of
        Tuberculosis 176
    Report of Committee on Venereal Disease Control ..176
Committee Reports Adopted by House of Delegates
    (A) 211
Committee Reports, Medical Advisory (A) 74
Committees, State Officers and xi
Comparative Symptoms in Peptic Ulcer and Choley-
    stitis in 200 Cases (S) Andre B. Carney 420
Compound Fractures, The Treatment of (S) M. A.
    Connell 507
Conference of Secretaries and Editors: Annual
    American Medical Association (A) 22, 528
Connell, M. A. (S) The Treatment of Compound
    Fractures 507
Consideration, A, of the Kenny Treatment of Infan-
    tile Paralysis (S) D. H. O'Donoghue 236
Constitution and By-Laws to be Acted Upon at An-
    nual Meeting, Amendments to (A) 179
Constitution and Disease (br) 130
Contagiousness of Puerperal Fever (Centennial), The
    (E) 207
Control of Syphilis in Oklahoma Industry, The (S)
    David V. Hudson 471
Convulsions Encountered in General Practice (S) T.
    H. McCarley 1
Cordell, U. S. (o) 271
Cornea, Clinical Importance of the Lipoid Ring of
    the (abs) 226
Coronary Sclerosis, Some Clinical Observations on (s)
    Wann Langston 461
Council on Medical Service and Public Relations of
    American Medical Association Adopts New Policies
    (A) 490
Council Reports
    Report of Council 250
    Report of District No. 2 252
    Report of District No. 3 254
    Report of District No. 4 254
    Report of District No. 5 254
    Report of District No. 6 254
    Report of District No. 7 256
Counting the Cost (E) 436
Country Doctor, The (E) 526
County Health Department in Oklahoma, The (S)
    John W. Shackelford 475
County Health Superintendents 453
County Societies, Officers of 46, 92, 138, 184, 276, 322,
                                            368, 414, 506, 552

County Society News 28, 78, 118, 213, 270, 309, 395, 451, 533
Crippled Children Committee Aids in Polio Fright (A) 346
Cullum, John Elwood (o) 221
Cysts of the Floor of the Mouth (abs) 134

D

Darcey, H. J., Chief Engineer of Oklahoma State Health Department (S) Sanitation in War time.423
Dawson, O. O. (o) 221
Dawson, W. D. (o) 82
Deafness, The Changing Conception of the Management of Chronic Progressive (abs) 45
Decompression of Protruded Intervertebral Disks, With a Note on Spinal Exploration (abs) 410
Deformity in Childhood, A Primer on the Prevention of (br) 323
Delegates and Alternates (A) 176
Deliverance, Safe (br) 323
DeMand, F. A. (o) 124
Department of Agriculture Studying Post-War Health Problems (A) 348
Dermatoses, Industrial (S) Everett S. Lain 96
Dermatitis, Occupational (E) 112
Development of Public Health, The (E) 246
Diabetes Insipidus, The Inheritance of (abs) 40
Diabetes Insipidus, Pitressin Tannate in Oil in the Treatment of (abs) 40
Diabetes Mellitus (abs) 412
Diabetes Mellitus, Unusually High Insulin Requirements in (abs) 40
Diabetes, The Relation of Trauma (abs) 412
Diabetic, Observations on the Negro (S) Paul B. Cameron 517
Diagnosis and Treatment of Gall Bladder Disease (S) D. D. Paulus 61
Diagnosis and Treatment of Meniere's Syndrome (abs) 133
Diet and Brights Disease (abs) 86

Dinitrophenol and its Relation to Formation of Cataract (abs) 41
Directory, Physicians xii
Disability Evaluation (br) 222
Diseases of the Breast (br) 224
Diseases of the Liver, Gallbladder and Bile Ducts (br) 538
District Meeting Held at Ft. Supply (A) 22
District No. 1, Annual Report of 168
District No. 8, Annual Report of 168
District No. 9, Annual Report of 168
Doctor of Medicine and His Responsibility, The (Sp) Alfred W. Adson, Rochester, Minnesota 201
Doctor's Reward, The (E) 20
Duncan, John C. (o) 82
Duration, For the (E) 208

E

Early Diagnosis of Tuberculosis (S) Thomas C. Black 195
Economic Committee Meets With Farm Security Administration Officials (A) 114
Editorials
A. S. A. 483
Acute Poliomyelitis 292
Administrative Hyperopia 344
Alien Physicians 111
Alphabet Abused, The 20
Challenge, The 436
Chance to Serve, A, ...525
Christmas Seal and the Medical Profession, The, 525
Cogito Ego Sum 293
Contagiousness of Puerperal Fever (Centennial), The 207
Counting the Cost 437
Country Doctor, The, ...526
Development of Public Health, The 246
Doctor's Reward, The 20

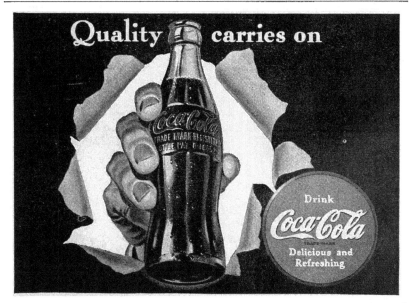

Equality, Life, Liberty and the Pursuit of Happiness 200
For the Duration 208
From Bismarck to Beveridge plus Wagner and Murray 292
Hemoptysis 154
Illustrious Alumnus, An 152
Inconsistency Ensconced 324
Injustice of Justice, The 67
Library of the Tulsa County Medical Society, The 112
Lure of Overtime, The 248
Medical Prescience 389
Medical-Red Cross Relation 110
Medicine's Foundation 482
Milky Way, The 342
Multi-Vitamin Mania 68
National Physicians Committee and American Medicine, The 66
Occupational Dermatitis 112
Oklahoma City Clinical Society, The 300
On The Level 437
On the Move 343
One World 247
Opportunity is Knocking at Your Door 66
Our State Medical Association 19
Physically Unfit and the World's Work 525
Primary Atypical Pneumonias, The 389
Regional Meeting of the College of Physicians 154
Science has Its Limitations 388
Silence and Sunshine 19
State Meeting, The 110
State Meeting, The 152
The Glen Wudna Dae Weel Withoot Wellium MacLure 153
Toxic Effect of Sulfonamide Therapy 67
United States or Appalachiah 247
University of Oklahoma Student Health Service, The 110
Value of Cod Liver Oil and Tomato Juice in the Prevention and Teratment of Intestinal Tuberculosis Complication Pulmonary Tuberculosis, The 18
Veneta R. Barlow, Tulsa, Librarian 112
Voice of the People, The 436
Wagnerites Take Notice 345
Whooping Cough up in the Air 483
Electro-Surgical Excision of Pterygium (abs) 319
Emmetropia (abs) 134
Epidemic Keratoconjunctivitis (S) Victor C. Myers 337
Epidemic Keratoconjunctivitis (Superficial Punctate Keratitis, Keratitis Subepithelialis, Keratitis Maculosa, Keratitis Nummularis.) With a Review of the Literature and a Report of 125 Cases (abs) 42
Epidemic Poliomyelitis (S) Luke W. Hunt 323
Equality, Life, Liberty and the Pursuit of Happiness (E) 206
Estimation of Percentage of Compensable Hearing Defects (abs) 504
Etiology of Malignant Neutropenia (S) Colonel William H. Gordon, M.D., Chickasha, Borden General Hospital 376
Evacuation Unit at Port of Embarkation, University Hospital (A) 395
Ewing, Dr. Finis W., Appointed to State Board of Medical Examiners (A) 530
Exigencies of Cardiovascular Origin, The (S) George Herrmann 47
Eye and its Adnexa, Lymphomatoid Diseases involving the (abs) 503

F

Female, Lower Abdominal Pain in the (S) Lt. Comdr. Clyde M. Longstreth 330
Fever, Haverhill (A Case Report) (S) William K. Ishmael 146
Fever, Rocky Mountain Spotted (S) Paul Sizemore 282
Fifty-First Annual Meeting, May 11-12, Oklahoma City (A) 114

Fightin' Talk 218, 269, 312, 352, 396, 446, 496, 534
First District Meeting Held at Ft. Supply (A) 22
First Member of Association Killed in Action (A)....22
Five-Year Report of University of Oklahoma Student Health Service (S) W. A. Fowler 98
Focal Infections, Clinical and Bacteriological Research on the Tonsillar Origin of: Assay of a Diagnostic Method for Cutaneous Streptococcic Allergy and its Results (abs) 411
Food Rationing, Association to Assist O. P. A. on Program (A) 392
Food Rationing, The Medical Profession and 530
For the Duration (E) 208
Fortson, John L. (o) 448
Fowler, W. A. (S) Five Year Report of University of Oklahoma Student Health Service 98
Fractured Clavicle, A Treatment by Traction (abs)....362
Fractures, Colles (abs) 86
Fractures, Compound, The Treatment of (S) M. A. Connell 507
Fractures of the Olecranon Process (abs) 132
Fractures of the Os Calcis (abs) 132
From Bismarck to Beveridge Plus Wagner and Murray (E) 292

G

Gallaher   Clinton (S) A Study of Trachoma With a Report of 318 Cases, 233 Treated With Sulfanilamide 185
Gallaher, Dr. Clinton, named Chairman of Advisory Committee Public Welfare Department (A) 349
Gallbladder and Biliary Tract, The Medical Management of Diseases of the (S) Fred C. Rewerts ..231
Gallbladder Disease, Diagnosis and Treatment of (S) D. D. Paulus 61
Gasoline Rationing Goes Into Effect (A) 27
General Concept of Allergy in Otorhinolaryngology, The (abs) 227
General Medicine, Year Book of (br) Bert F. Keltz.. 84
General Practice, Convulsions Encountered in (S) T. H. McCarley 1
Gillis, Eugene A, to Texas (A) 116
Glen Wudna Dae Weel Withoot Wellium MacLure, The (E) 153
Gordon, Colonel William., M. D., Chickasha ,Borden General Hospital (S) Etiology of Malignant Neutropenia 376
Greenberger, Edward D. (S) A Radiologists Viewpoint in the Treatment of Some Common Diseases 12
Greer, Major R. E., M. D., Will Rogers Field (S) Treatment of War Gases 139
Guide to Practical Nutrition, A (br) 366

H

Handbook of Tropical Medicine (br) 538
Haverhill Fever (A Case Report) (S) William K. Ishmael 146
Health Feature, Oklahoma City Times Carrying (A) 347
Health Superintendents, County 453
Hearing Defects, Estimation of Percentage of Compensable (abs) 504
Hematology to Otolaryngology, Relation of (abs) ..409
Hemoptysis (E) 154
Hereditary Deforming Chondrodysplasia (abs) 228
Herrmann, George, (S) The Exigencies of Cardiovascular Origin 47
Honorary Membership Applications (A) 179
House of Delegates Meets June 7, American Medical Association (A) 116
House of Delegates, Official Proceedings (A) 250
How Firm the Foundation—How Frail the Superstructure, (Sp) Lewis J. Moorman 431
Hudson, David V. (S) The Control of Syphilis in Oklahoma Industry 471
Hunt, Luke W. (S) Epidemic Poliomyelitis 323
Hypertension in a Young Athlete Due to Coarctation of Aorta: A Report of Case (S) Johnny A. Blue 143

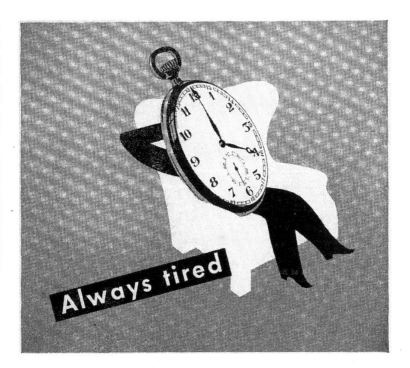

Always tired

"Always tired" is a common enough complaint, but when accompanied by markedly low resistance to infections, low muscular tone and vascular weakness, by mental apathy and depression, the cause may be adrenal cortical insufficiency.

ADRENAL CORTEX EXTRACT (UPJOHN) offers potent replacement therapy with which to combat this syndrome. So carefully are the active steroids extracted to make this *natural* complex, so pure is the final cortical extract, that there is practically no trace of epinephrine, the hormone of the adrenal medulla.

Upjohn pioneering and research have resulted in the potent, reliable preparation many physicians use when a characteristic "syndrome of lowness" points to adrenal cortical insufficiency.

Adrenal Cortex Extract (Upjohn)

Sterile solution in 10 cc. rubber-capped vials for subcutaneous, intramuscular and intravenous therapy

ANOTHER WAY TO SAVE LIVES . . . BUY WAR BONDS FOR VICTORY

I

Illustrious Alumnus, An (E) 152
Impetigo Neonatorium, A Simplified Treatment for
  (S) Charles Ed White 234
Induction, Problems of (S) Colonel Monti L. Belot ..511
Inconsistency Ensconced (E) 524
Industrial Dermatoses (S) Everett S. Lain 96
Industrial Health Institute, Association to Hold War-
  time (A) 70
Infantile Paralysis, A Consideration of the Kenny
  Treatment (S) D. H. O'Donoghue 236
Inheritance, The, of Diabetes Insipidus (abs) 40
Injustice of Justice, The (E) 67
Inner Ear, The (br) 365
Institute on Wartime Industrial Health Held in Tulsa
  March 18, Oklahoma City, March 19 (A) 114
Internal Fixation in Injuries of the Ankle (abs) 412
Internal Medicine, Advances in (br) 224
Internal Medicine in General Practice (br) 538
Internists, Oklahoma City, to Conduct Annual Wash-
  ington Birthday Clinics (A) 23
Interrelationship of Solid, Liquid and Gas Metabo-
  lism (S) Edward C. Mason 467
Intestinal "Decompression"—A Review of Methods
  (S) A. S. Risser 197
Intestinal Tuberculosis Complicating Pulmonary Tu-
  berculosis: The Value of Cod Liver Oil and To-
  mato Juice in the Prevention and Treatment of
  (E) 18
Iron in Nutrition (Requirements for Iron) (abs) 42
Irritable Bowel, The (S) Turner Bynum 56
Ishmael, William K. (S) Haverhill Fever (A Case
  Report) 146

J

Jacobs, R. G. (S) Treatment of Burn Cases Off the
  U.S.S. Wasp 235
Joyce, Frank T. (S) Patient Ductus Arteriosus: A
  Report of Two Cases 6
Judicial and Professional Relations, Report of Com-
  mittee on 170

K

Kenny Treatment of Infantile Paralysis, A Consideration of the (S) D. H. O'Donoghue 236
Keratoconjunctivitis, Epidemic (S) Victor C. Myers.337
Keratoconjunctivitis, Epidemic (Superficial Punctate
  Keratitis, Keratitis Subepithelialis, With a Review of the Literature and a Report of 125 Cases
  (abs) 42
Knee Ligament Strain, A Sequel of: Pellegrini-Stie-
  da's Disease (Metacondylar Traumatic Osteoma
  (abs) 88

L

Laboratory Diagnosis, A Medical Economic Situation
  Regarding (abs) 318
Lahey Clinic, Surgical Practices of the (br) 406
Lain, Everett S. (S) Industrial Dermatoses 96
Langston, Wann (S) Some Clinical Observations on
  Coronary Sclerosis 461
Laryngology and Folk Lore (abs) 362
Laryngotrac Heobronchitis in Children: Classification
  and Differential Diagnosis (abs) 90
Larynx, X-Ray Treatment of Diseases of the (abs)....362
Leg Lengthening Operations: Its Present Status
  (abs) 458
Legislature Convenes (A) 71
Legislature Working to Close, Nineteenth (A) 117
Leonard, Charles E. (S) Recent Advances in Psy-
  chosomatic Medicine 334
Lesions of the Supraspinatus Tendon Degeneration,
  Rupture and Calcification (abs) 409
Library of the Tulsa County Medical Society, The
  (E) 112
Licensed, Physician's Recently (A) 27
Lingenfelter, Forrest M. (S) Modern Aids in the
  Treatment of Appendicitis 425

Lipoid Ring of the Cornea, Clinical Importance of
  the (abs) 226
Lithodelyphopedion (Lithopedion With Calcified
  Membranes) With Some Remarks on Estopic
  Pregnancy in General: Case Report (S) Grider
  Penick 192
Little, Jesse S. (o) 124
Longstreth, Lt. Comdr. Clyde M. (S) Lower Abdom-
  inal Pain in the Female 330
Low Back and Sciatic Pain, The Combined Operation
  (abs) 272
Lower Abdominal Pain in the Female (S) Lt. Comdr.
  Clyde M. Longstreth 330
Lowry, Tom (A) Post-War Planning With Reference
  to the Physicians Returning from Military Ser-
  vice 487
Lure of Overtime, The 248
Lymphomatoid Diseases Involving the Eye and its
  Adnexa (abs) 503

M

Macrae, Donald H. (S) The Private Practitioner and
  the War Industry 239
Malpractice Insurance, Report of Committee on (A)211
Management of Late Syphilis, A Review of the (S)
  C. P. Bondurant 382
Management of Peptic Ulcer (s) Arthur W. White ..104
March of Medicine (br) 502
Marchall, Captain Leslie B., M.S., U.S.N., Norman,
  Commanding Officer U.S. Naval Hospital (S)
  Naval Medicine 369
Mason, Edward C. (S) The Interrelationship of
  Solid, Liquid and Gas Metabolism 467
Mastoid Surgery, The Periosteal Flap in (abs) 226
Maternity and Infancy, Report of Committee on (A)211
Mayo Clinic and the Mayo Foundation, Collected
  Papers of the (br) 406
McCarley, T. H. (S) Convulsions Encountered in
  General Practice 1
Medical Advisory Committee Reports (A) 74
Medical Advisory Committee to the Department of
  Public Welfare, Report of the (A) 211
Medical Dictionary, The American Illustrated Nine-
  teenth Edition (br) 128
Medical Economics 443
Medical Economics, Report of Committee on 172
Medical Economic Situation Regarding Laboratory
  Diagnosis, A (abs) 318
Medical Education and Hospitals, Report of Com-
  mittee on (A) 168
Medical Management of Diseases of the Gallbladder
  and Biliary Tract, The (S) Fred C. Rewets 231
Medical Parasitology (br) 225
Medical Preparedness 30, 83, 122, 417
Medical Prescience (E) 389
Mediesl-Red Cross Relations (E) 110
Medical Testimony, Report of Committee on 172
Medicine, Aviation (S) Lt. Col. W. M. Scott, Will
  Rogers Field, Oklahoma City 93
Medicine's Foundation (E) 482
Medicine, Naval (S) Capt. Leslie B. Marshall, M.S.,
  U.S.N., Norman, Commanding Officer, U.S.
  Naval Hospital 369
Medicine at War 400, 498, 536
Member of Association Killed in Action, The First
  (A) 22
Memoir of Walter Reed: The Yellow Fever Episode
  (br) 407
Meniere's Syndrome, Diagnosis and Treatment of
  (abs) 133
Mental Illness: A Guide for the Family (br) 84
Metabolism, The Interrelationship of Solid, Liquid
  and Gas (S) Edward C. Mason 467
Military Surgeon's Meeting (A) 392
Milk (Sp) 200
Milky Way, The (E) 332
Mind and its Disorders, The (br) 150
Minnesota Congressman Reports (ME) 443

Misconception about the Springiness of the Longitudinal Arch of the Foot. Mechanics of the Arch of the Foot (abs) 503
Modern Aids in the Treatment of Appendicitis (S) Forrest M. Lingenfelter, John W. Cavanaugh, Harvey Richey 425
Modern Treatment of Pneumococcic Pneumonia (abs) 185
Moorman, Floyd J. (S) Spontaneous Pneumothorax in Apparently Healthy Young Adults 277
Moorman, Lewis J., Attends Meetings (A) 490
Myers, Victor C. (S) Epidemic Keratoconjunctivitis..337

N

National Formulary, The (br) 365
National Physician's Committee and American Medicine (E) 66
Naval Medicine (S) Capt. Leslie B. Marshall, M.S., U.S.N., Norman, Commanding Officer, U. S. Naval Hospital 369
Navigating the Medical Future With Confidence (Sp) Edward H. Skinner 484
Neuro-Anatomy (br) 84
Neuropsychiatric Problems Arising in the Civilian Population (S) James Asa Willie 287
Neutropenia, Etiology of Malignant (S) Col. William H. Gordon, M.D., Chickasha, Borden General Hospital 376
New and Non Official Remedies (br) 366
Newman, O. C., Shattuck, Enters Hall of Fame (A)..490
News From County Societies 28, 78, 118, 213, 270, 309, 395, 451
News from State Health Department 34, 81, 220, 316
Nupercain Spinal Anesthesia for Abdominoperineal Resection of the Rectum: A New Technique (abs) 86
Nutrition, A Guide to Practical (br) 366
Nutrition, Iron in (Requirements for Iron) (abs) 42

O

Obituaries
Bagby, Louis 124
Bradley, Calvin E. 349
Brice, Marion O. 448
Brown, F. C. 271
Browning, W. M. 124
Buchanan, F. R. 309
Bunn, A. D. 221
Cordell, U. S. 271
Cullum, John Elwood 221
Dawson, O. O. 221
Dawson, W. D. 82
Duncan, John C. 82
DeMand, F. A. 124
Fortson, John L. 448
Little, Jesse S. 124
Powell, James William 50
Rosenberger, F. E. 124
Sanderson, W. C. 82
Schrader, Charles T. 401
Williamson, Sam H. 448
Wilson, H. B. 349
Observations on the Negro Diabetic (S) Paul B. Cameron 517
Occupational Dermatitis (E) 112
Ocular Pathophysiology, Weather and (abs) 364
Oscular Pathophysiology, Weather and (abs)...........364
Oculoglandular Tularemia (abs) 89
O'Donoghue, D. H. (S) A Consideration of the Kenny Treatment of Infantile Paralysis 236
Office of Civilian Defense 32, 126
Officers of County Societies 46, 92, 138, 184, 270, 322, 368, 414, 368,,506
Official Proceedings of House of Delegates (A) 250
Oklahoma City Clinical Society, The (E) 390
Oklahoma City Clinical Society, 13th Annual Meeting October 18, 19, 20 and 21 (A) 392
Oklahoma City Internists to Conduct Annual Washington Birthday Clinics (A) 23

Oklahoma City Times Carrying Health Feature (A) ..347
Olecranon Process, Fractures of the (abs) 132
On the Level (E) 437
On the Move (E) 343
One World (E) 247
Ophthalmology Examinations Announced, Board of (A) 116
Opportunity is Knocking at Your Door (E) 66
Optic Nerve in Head Injuries, Unilateral Involvement of the (abs) 227
Os Calcis, Fractures of the (abs) 132
Osborn, J. D., Nominated for Place on National Board of Medical Examiners (A) 114
Osborn, J. R., Elected to National Board of Medical Examiners (A) 310
Osteogenesis Imperfecta (abs) 504
Osteoma of the External Auditory Canal (abs) 88
Otitis Media and Mastoiditis, Acute (abs) 133
Otolaryngology, Relation of Hematology to (abs) ..409
Otolaryngology, The Role of Medical Short Wave Therapy in (S) E. H. Coachman 417
Our State Medical Association (E) 19
Overtime, The Lure of (E) 248

P

Parasitology, Medical (br) 225
Patent Ductus Arteriosus: A Report of Two Cases (S) Frank T. Joyce 6
Pathology of Trauma, The (br) 222
Paulus, D. D. (S) Diagnosis and Treatment of Gallbladder Disease 61
Pay-As-You-Go-Tax Procedure, New (A) 311
Pediatrics, Advances in (br) 128
Pediatrics, The Year Book of (br) 320
Pellegrini-Stieda's Disease (Metacondylar Traumatic Osteoma: A Sequel of Knee Ligament Strain) (abs) 88
Penick, Grider (S) Lithodelyphopedion (Lithopedion With Calcified Membrane) With Some Remarks on Estopic Pregnancy in General 192
Penicillin, The Absorption, Excretion and Distribution of (abs) 503
Penicillin, Toxicity and Efficacy of (abs) 458
Peptic Ulcer, Management of (S) Arthur W. White ..104
Periosteal Flap in Mastoid Surgery (abs) 226
Physically Unfit and the World's Work (E) 325
Physicians' Directory xii
Physicians to be Dislocated (MP) 36
Physicians Recently Licensed (A) 27
Piatt, Louis (S) Radium Therapy in the Treatment of Cancer of the Skin 415
Pitressin Tannate in Oil in the Treatment of Diabetes Insipidus (abs) 40
Plan for the Use of Blood Plasma in Rural Communities, A (S) A. Ray Wiley 329
Plasma Bank, The (S) A. Ray Wiley 285
Plasma, Blood, A Plan for the Use of, in Rural Communities (S) A. Ray Wiley 329
Pneumococcic Pneumonia, Modern Treatment of (abs) 185
Pneumonias, The Primary Atypical (E) 389
Pneumothorax, Spontaneous, in Apparently Healthy Young Adults (S) J. Floyd Moorman 277
Polio Fright, Crippled Children's Committee Aids in (A) 346
Poliomyelitis, Acute (E) 292
Poliomyelitis, Blood Flow in Extremities Affected by Anterior (abs) 411
Poliomyelitis, Epidemic (S) Luke W. Hunt 223
Post-War Health Problems, Department of Agriculture Studying (A) 348
Post-War Planning With Reference to the Physicians Returning from Military Service (A) 487
Postgraduate Committee, New Instructor Appointed for Course in Surgical Diagnosis (A) 490
Postgraduate Course Being Formulated, Plans for 1944-45 (A) 210
Postgraduate Medical Teaching, Report of Committee on 174

Pottawatomie County Society Analyses Membership
(A) 116
Pounders, Dr. Carroll, Appointed to Council of
Southern Medical Association (A) 348
Powell, James William (o) 30
Practical Survey of Chemistry and Metabolism of
the Skin (br) 365
Pregnancy, Estopic, Some Remarks in General, Lith-
odelyphopedion (Lithopedion With Calcified
Membranes): Case Report (S) Grider Penick 192
Prepaid Surgical Plan to Attorneys (A) 393
Prepaid Medical and Surgical Service, Report of the
Committee on 210
Prepaid Medical and Surgical Plan, Experimental,
Approved by House of Delegates 210
Prepaid Medical-Surgical Committee Meets (A) 349
President's Page 16, 64, 108, 150, 204, 244, 290,
340, 386, 434, 480, 522
Primary Atypical Pneumonias, The (E) 389
Primer on the Prevention of Deformity in Child-
hood (br) 223
Private Practitioner, The, and the War Industry (S)
Donald H. Macrae 239
Problems of Induction (S) Colonel Monti L. Belot ..511
Procurement and Assignment Classifications for Phy-
sicians in 1943 (MP) 83
Procurement and Assignment Survey to be Made
(MP) 122
Program, 1943 Annual Meeting (A) 156
Psychosomatic Medicine (br) 562
Psychosomatic Medicine, Recent Advances in (S)
Charles E. Leonard 334
Public Health Association, American Conference an-
nounced (A) 116
Public Health Integration, A Venture in; Medical
Staff of Oklahoma State Health Department 128
Public Health, The Development of (E) 246
Public Health, Report of Committee on (A) 174
Public Policy, Report of Committee on (A) 170
Public Welfare Department, Dr. Clinton Gallaher
Named Chairman of Advisory Committee (A) ..349
Puerperal Fever (Centennial), The Contagiousness of
(E) 207

R

Radiologist's, A, Viewpoint in the Treatment of Some
Common Diseases (S) Edward D. Greenberger .. 12
Radium Therapy in the Treatment of Cancer of
the Skin (S) Louis M. Piatt 415
Recent Advances in Psychosomatic Medicine (S)
Charles E. Leonard 334
Recommendations for a Venereal Disease Control Pro-
gram in Industry (Sp) Otis L. Anderson 289
Reed, Walter, Memoir of: The Yellow Fever Ep-
isode (br) 407
Regional Meeting of the College of Physicians (E) ..154
Rehabilitation of the War-Injured (br) 365
Relation of Hematology to Otolaryngology (abs) 409
Relation of Trauma Diabetes, The (abs) 412
Review of the Management of Late Syphilis, A (S)
C. P. Bondurant 382
Rewerts, Fred C. (S) The Medical Management of
Diseases of the Gallbladder and Biliary Tract ..231
Rhinitis, The Allergic Aspect of Vasomotor (abs) ..132
Rhinitis, Value of Fatty Acid Derivatives in Treat-
ment of Chronic Obstructive (abs) 87
Riboflavin: Significance of its Photodynamic Action
and Importance of its Properties for the Visual
Act (abs) 44
Richey, Harvey (S) Modern Aids in the Treatment of
Appendicitis 423
Risser, A. S. (S) Intestinal ''Decompression,'' A
Review of Methods 197
Rocky Mountain Spotted Fever (S) Paul Sizemore 282
Roentgen Study of Pathogenesis and Clinical Signifi-
cance, Calcification and Ossification of Vertebral
Ligaments (Spondylitis Ossifican Ligamentosa)
(abs) 39

Role, The, of Medical Short Wave Therapy in Orolaryn-
gology (S) E. H. Coachman 417
Rosenberger, F. E. (o) 124
Roster, Oklahoma State Medical Association, 1943 296
Roster, Supplementary (A) 346, 528
Rountree, C. R. (A) 74

S

Safe Deliverance (br) 223
Sanderson, W. C. (o) 82
Sanitation in War Time (S) H. J. Darcey, Chief
Engineer of Oklahoma State Health Department 423
Schrader, Charles T. (o) 401
Science Has Its Limitations (E) 388
Scientific Exhibit of American Medical Association
to be Held June 12-16, 1944 (A) 530
Scott, W. M., Lt. Col., Will Rogers Field, Oklahoma
City (S) Aviation Medicine 93
Secretaries Conference Held October 17, Fourth An-
nual (A) 394, 487
Semen and Seminal Stains (abs) 88
Shackelford, John W. (S) The County Health Depart-
ment in Oklahoma 475
Shock: Dynamics, Occurrence and Management
(br) 224
Short Wave Therapy in Otolaryngology, The Role of
Medical (S) E. H. Coachman 417
Silence and Sunshine (E) 19
Sinus Surgery, Some Causes for Failure in Frontal
(abs) 90
Sinusitis, Advances in the Treatment of Chronic Nasal
(abs) 456
Simplified Treatment, A, for Impetigo Neonatorium
(S) Charles Ed White 234
Sizemore, Paul (S) Rocky Mountain Spotted Fever ..282
Skinner, E, H. (Sp) Navigating the Medical Future
With Confidence 484
Smith, James C. (o) 22
Smith, Dr. Ned, Resigns from Board of Trustees (A) 532
Solitary Unicameral Bone Cysts with Emphasis on the
Roentgen Picture, the Pathologic Appearance
and the Pathogenesis (abs) 273
Some Anomalous Forms of Amaurotic Idiocy and
Their Bearing on The Relationship of the Var-
ious Types (abs) 272
Some Clinical Observations on Coronary Sclerosis (S)
Wann Langston 461
Southern Medical Association, Dr. Carroll Pounders
Appointed to Council of (A) 348
Southern Medical Association to Meet in Cincinnati,
Ohio (A) 347
Special Articles
Doctor of Medicine and His Responsibility, The,
Alfred W. Adson, Rochester, Minnesota 201
How Firm the Foundation—How Frail the Super-
structure, Lewis J. Moorman 431
Milk 269
Navigating the Medical Future with Confidence,
E. H. Skinner 484
Recommendations for a Venereal Disease Control
Program in Industry 289
Spinal Anesthesia for Abdominoperineal Resection of
the Rectum: A New Technique (abs) 86
Spinal Exploration, Decompression of Protruded In-
terrvertebral Disks, With a Note on (abs) 410
Spontaneous Pneumothorax in Apparently Healthy
Young Adults (S) J. Floyd Moorman 277
Standardized Technique for Sedimentation Rate (abs) 87
State Health Department News 34, 81, 220, 316, 452
State Medical Association, Our (E) 19
State Meeting, The (E) 110
State Meeting, The (E) 152
State Officers and Committees xi
Stedman's Medical Dictionary-Illustrated (br) 274
Stevenson, President, Announces Committee Appoint-
ments (A) 311
Student Health Service, Five Year Report of Univer-
sity (S) W. A. Fowler 98

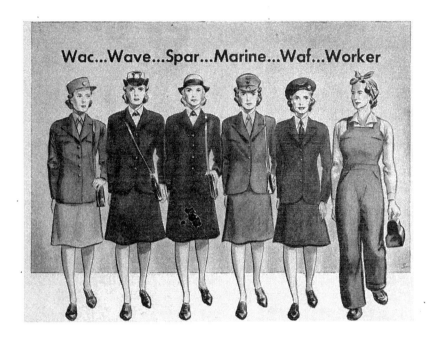

Wac...Wave...Spar...Marine...Waf...Worker

... they still are women

WHATEVER part in the war effort women elect for themselves, they still face certain physiologic upsets peculiar to their sex. Many of these gynecologic disorders are referable to ovarian or hypophyseal dysfunction.

Where estrogenic hormone is indicated, most economical specific therapy is obtained by oral administration of diethylstilbestrol, generally in total daily dosage of one milligram and often less.

For physicians who prefer *natural* estrogenic substance, Amniotin is available in dosage forms for oral, hypodermic and intravaginal administration.

E. R. Squibb & Sons has a most extensive line of Council-Accepted endocrine products. Much that is known of modern endocrine therapy was learned through the cooperative studies with leading independent endocrinologists which the Squibb Laboratories made possible.

When estrogens are needed why not specify Amniotin or Diethylstilbestrol Squibb?

For literature address the Professional Service Dept., 745 Fifth Avenue, New York 22, N. Y.

★ BUY MORE WAR BONDS ★

Student Health Service, The University of Oklahoma (E) 110
Student Nurses Recruitment, Physicians Part in (A) 76
Study and Control of Cancer, Report of Committee on 174
Study and Control of Tuberculosis, Report of Committee on 174
Study of Trachoma With a Report of 318 Cases, 233 Treated With Sulfanilamide (S) Clinton Gallaher 185
Sulfanilamide, Chemotherapy With; Clinical Results (abs) 410
Sulfonamide Therapy, Toxic Effect of (E) 67
Surgical Pathology (br) 274
Surgical Practices of the Lahey Clinic (br) 406
Synopsis of Clinical Syphilis, A (br) 366
Synopsis of Tropical Medicine (br) 502
Syphilis, A Review of the Management of Late (S) C. P. Bondurant 382
Syphilis, A Synopsis of Clinical (br) 366
Syphilis in Oklahoma Industry, The Control of (S) David V. Hudson 471

T

Tables of Food Values (br) 274
Tax Procedure, New Pay-As-You-Go (A) 311
Technique for Obtaining Bacteriological Specimens from the Antrum (abs) 319
Toxemias of Pregnancy, The, (br) 37
Toxic Effect of Sulfonamide Therapy (E) 67
Toxicity and Efficacy of Penicillin (abs) 458
Toxoplasmic Encephalomyelitis, Clinical Diagnosis of Infantile on Congenital Toxoplasmosis: Survival Beyond Infancy (abs) 228
Trachoma Control Report 81
Trachoma, A Study of, With a Report of 318 Cases, 233 Treated With Sulfanilamide (S) Clinton Gallaher 185
Transmission, of Diseases by Blood Transfusions, The (S) A. Ray Wiley 374
Transplants to the Thumb to Restore Function of Opposition: End Results (abs) 39
Trauma Diabetes, The Relation of (abs) 412
Treatment of Burns, (S) John F. Burton 4
Treatment of Burn Cases Off the U. S. S. Wasp (S) R. G. Jacob 233
Treatment of Cancer of the Skin, Radium Therapy in the (S) Louis M. Piatt 415
Treatment of Fractured Clavicle by Traction, (abs) 362
Treatment of Some Common Diseases, A Radiologist's Viewpoint (S) Edward D. Greenberger 12
Treatment of War Gases (S) Major R. E. Greer, M. C. Will Rogers Field, Oklahoma City 139
Trichomonas Vaginalis (S) Kenneth J. Wilson 372
Tropical Medicine, Synopsis of (br) 502
Tuberculosis, Early Diagnosis of (S) Thomas C. Black 195
Tuberculosis of the Greater Trochanter and its Bursa (abs) 363
Tuberculosis, Study and Control of, Report of Committee on 176
Tuberculosis Trachebronchitis (S) 53
Twenty-Five Years Aog 316, 354, 401, 450, 494

U

Unilateral Involvement of the Optic Nerve in Head Injuries, (abs) 227
United States or Appalachian (E) 247
University Hospital Evacuation Unit at Port of Embarkation (A) 395
University of Oklahoma School of Medicine 32, 85, 124, 183, 317, 360, 402, 442, 495, 526

University of Oklahoma Student Health Service, The (E) 110
Unusually High Insulin Requirements in Diabetes Mellitus, (abs) 40
Urine and Urinalysis, (br) 365
Urology in General Practice, (br) 320

V

Value of Fatty Acid Derivatives in Treatment of Chronic Rhinitis, (abs) 87
Value, The, of Cod Liver Oil and Tomato Juice in the Prevention and Treatment of Intestinal Tuberculosis Complicating Pulmonary Tuberculosis (E) 18
Venereal Disease Control, Report of Committee on 176
Venture in Public Health Integration, (A)—Medical Staff of Oklahoma State Health Department, (br) 128
Vertebral Ligaments, Calcification and Ossification of (Spondylitis Ossificans Ligamentosa) Roentgen Study of Pathogenesis and Clinical Significance, (abs) 39
Verumontanitis, The Application of the Sex Hormones (S) Robert H. Akin 381
Victory Tax, The, and the Medical Profession (A) 24
Voice of the People, The (E) 436

W

Wagner and Murray, "From Bismarck to Beveridge Plus" (E) 292
Wagnerites Take Notice (E) 345
War Gases, Treatment of (S) Major R. E. Greer, M. C., Will Rogers Field, Oklahoma City 139
War Gases, Their Identification and Decontamination (br) 129
War Industry, The Private Practitioner and the (S) Donald H. Macrae 239
War-Injured, Rehabilitation of the (br) 365
War Medicine—A Symposium (br) 130
Warning Concerning Government Checks (A) 76
War Sessions Announced by American College of Surgeons (A) 116
Wartime Industrial Health, Institute Held in Tulsa, March 18, Oklahoma City, March 19 114
War Time, Sanitation in (S) H. J. Darcey, Chief Engineer of Oklahoma State Health Department 423
Weather and Ocular Pathophysiology (abs) 364
Western Charity Hospital Superintendent Appointed 116
When Doctors are Rationed (br) 38
White, Arthur W. (S) Management of Peptic Ulcer..104
White, Charles Ed (S) A Simplified Treatment for Impetigo Neonatorium 234
White Coat, The (E) 136
Whooping Cough Up in the Air (E) 483
Wiley, A. Ray (S) The Plasma Bank 285
Wiley, A. Ray (S) A Plan for the Use of Blood Plasma in Rural Communities 329
Wiley, A. Ray (S) The Transmission of Diseases by Blood Transfusion 374
Williamson, Sam H. (o) 448
Willie, James Asa (S) Neuropsychiatric Problems Arising in the Civilian Population 287
Wilson, H. B. (o) 349
Wilson, Kenneth J. (S) Trichomonas Vaginalis 372
Woman's Auxiliary News 31, 80, 120, 214, 268, 314, 356, 402, 442, 532

X

X-Ray Treatment of Disease of the Larynx, (abs) ..362

Y

Year Book of General Medicine (br) 84
Year Book of Pediatrics, The (br) 320

28 WORDS
tell the story...

Clinical tests[*] showed that when smokers changed to PHILIP MORRIS Cigarettes, <u>every</u> case of irritation of the nose and throat due to smoking <u>cleared</u> <u>completely</u> or <u>definitely</u> <u>improved.</u>

[*] *Laryngoscope, Feb. 1935, Vol. XLV, No. 2 — 149-154.*

TO THE PHYSICIAN WHO SMOKES A PIPE: We suggest an unusually fine new blend — COUNTRY DOCTOR PIPE MIXTURE. Made by the same process as used in the manufacture of Philip Morris Cigarettes.

OFFICERS OF COUNTY SOCIETIES, 1943

★

COUNTY	PRESIDENT	SECRETARY	MEETING TIME
Alfalfa	H. E. Huston, Cherokee	L. T. Lancaster, Cherokee	Last Tues. each Second Month
Atoka-Coal	J. B. Clark, Coalgate	J. S. Fulton, Atoka	
Beckham	H. K. Speed, Sayre	E. S. Kilpatrick, Elk City	Second Tuesday
Blaine	Virginia Olson-Curtan, Watonga	W. F. Griffin, Watonga	Second Tuesday
Bryan	J. T. Colwich, Durant	W. K. Haynie, Durant	
Caddo	F. L. Patterson, Carnegie	C. B. Sullivan, Carnegie	
Canadian	P. F. Herod, El Reno	A. L. Johnson, El Reno	Subject to call
Carter	Walter Hardy, Ardmore	H. A. Higgins, Ardmore	
Cherokee	P. H. Medearis, Tahlequah	*James K. Gray, Tahlequah	First Tuesday
Choctaw	C. H. Hale, Boswell	E. A. Johnson, Hugo	
Cleveland	J. A. Rieger, Norman	Curtis Berry, Norman	Thursday nights
Comanche	George S. Barber, Lawton	W. F. Lewis, Lawton	
Cotton	A. B. Holstead, Temple	Mollie F. Sciem, Walters	Third Friday
Craig	F. M. Adams, Vinita	J. M. McMillan, Vinita	
Creek	H. K. Haas, Sapulpa	C. G. Oakes, Sapulpa	
Custer	F. R. Vieregg, Clinton	C. J. Alexander, Clinton	Third Thursday
Garfield	Paul B. Champlin, Enid	John R. Walker, Enid	Fourth Thursday
Garvin	T. F. Gross, Lindsay	John R. Callaway, Pauls Valley	Wednesday before Third Thursday
Grady	Walter J. Baze, Chickasha	Roy E. Emanuel, Chickasha	Third Thursday
Grant	I. V. Hardy, Medford	E. E. Lawson, Medford	
Greer	G. P. Cherry, Mangum	J. B. Hollis, Mangum	
Harmon	W. G. Husband, Hollis		First Wednesday
Haskell	William Carson, Keota	N. K. Williams, McCurtain	
Hughes	Wm. L. Taylor, Holdenville	Imogene Mayfield, Holdenville	First Friday
Jackson	E. S. Crow, Olustee	E. W. Mabry, Altus	Last Monday
Jefferson	F. M. Edwards, Ringling	L. L. Wade, Ryan	Second Monday
Kay	Philip C. Risser, Blackwell	J. Holland Howe, Ponca City	Second Thursday
Kingfisher	C. M. Hodgson, Kingfisher	H. Violet Sturgeon, Hennessey	
Kiowa	B. H. Watkins, Hobart	J. William Finch, Hobart	
LeFlore	Neeson Rolle, Poteau	Rush L. Wright, Poteau	
Lincoln	H. B. Jenkins, Tryon	Carl H. Bailey, Stroud	First Wednesday
Logan	William C. Miller, Guthrie	J. L. LeHew, Jr., Guthrie	Last Tuesday
Marshall	O. A. Cook, Madill		
Mayes	Ralph V. Smith, Pryor	Paul B. Cameron, Pryor	
McClain	B. W. Slover, Blanchard	R. L. Royster, Purcell	
McCurtain	A. W. Clarkson, Valliant	N. L. Barker, Broken Bow	Fourth Tuesday
McIntosh	James L. Wood, Eufaula	William A. Tolleson, Eufaula	First Thursday
Murray	P. V. Annadown, Sulphur		Second Tuesday
Muskogee-Sequoyah-Wagoner	H. A. Scott, Muskogee	D. Evelyn Miller, Muskogee	First Monday
Noble	C. H. Cooke, Perry	J. W. Francis, Perry	
Okfuskee	L. J. Spickard, Okemah	M. L. Whitney, Okemah	Second Monday
Oklahoma	Walker Morledge, Oklahoma City	E. R. Musick, Oklahoma City	Fourth Tuesday
Okmulgee	A. R. Holmes, Henryetta	J. C. Matheney, Okmulgee	Second Monday
Osage	C. R. Weirich, Pawhuska	George K. Hemphill, Pawhuska	Second Monday
Ottawa	W. B. Sanger, Picher	Matt A. Connell, Picher	Third Thursday
Pawnee	E. T. Robinson, Cleveland	R. L. Browning, Pawnee	
Payne	L. A. Mitchell, Stillwater	C. W. Moore, Stillwater	Third Thursday
Pittsburg	John F. Park, McAlester	William H. Kaeiser, McAlester	Third Friday
Pontotoc	O. H. Miller, Ada	R. H. Mayes, Ada	First Wednesday
Pottawatomie	A. C. McFarling, Shawnee	Clinton Gallaher, Shawnee	First and Third Saturday
Pushmataha	John S. Lawson, Clayton	B. M. Huckabay, Antlers	
Rogers	C. W. Beson, Claremore	C. L. Caldwell, Chelsea	First Monday
Seminole	Max Van Sandt, Wewoka	Mack I. Shanholtz, Wewoka	Third Wednesday
Stephens	W. K. Walker, Marlow	Wallis S. Ivy, Duncan	
Texas	R. G. Obernuiller, Texhoma	Morris Smith, Guymon	
Tillman		O. G. Bacon, Frederick	
Tulsa	James C. Peden, Tulsa	E. O. Johnson, Tulsa	Second and Fourth Monday
Washington-Nowata	J. G. Smith, Bartlesville	J. V. Athey, Bartlesville	Second Wednesday
Washita	A. S. Neal, Cordell	James F. McMurry, Sentinel	
Woods	C. A. Traverse, Alva	O. E. Templin, Alva	Last Tuesday Odd Months
Woodward	C. E. Williams, Woodward	C. W. Tedrowe, Woodward	Second Thursday

*(Serving in Armed Forces)

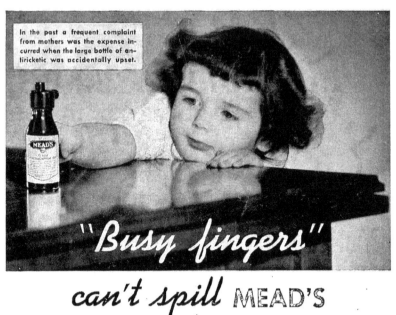

In the past a frequent complaint from mothers was the expense incurred when the large bottle of antiricketic was accidentally upset.

"Busy fingers"

can't spill MEAD'S
OLEUM PERCOMORPHUM

Even if the bottle of Mead's Oleum Percomorphum is accidentally tipped over, there is no loss of precious oil nor damage to clothing and furnishings. The unique Mead's Vacap-Dropper* is a tight seal which remains attached to the bottle, even while the antiricketic is being measured out. Mead's Vacap-Dropper offers these extra advantages also, at no increase in price:

Unbreakable
Mead's Vacap-Dropper will not break even when bottle is tipped over or dropped. No glass dropper to become rough or serrated.

No "messiness"
Mead's Vacap-Dropper protects against dust and rancidity. (Rancidity reduces vitamin potency.) Surface of oil need never be exposed to light and dust. This dropper cannot roll about and collect bacteria.

Accurate
This unique device, after the patient becomes accustomed to using it, delivers drops of uniform size.

No deterioration
Made of bakelite, Mead's Vacap-Dropper is impervious to oil. No chance of oil rising into rubber bulb, as with ordinary droppers, and deteriorating both oil and rubber. No glass or bulb to become separated while in use.

EXIGENCY OF WAR:
Oleum Percomorphum 50% is now known as Oleum Percomorphum 50% With Viosterol. The potency remains the same; namely, 60,000 vitamin A units and 8,500 vitamin D units per gram. It consists of the liver oils of percomorph fishes, viosterol, and fish liver oils, a source of vitamins A and D in which not less than 50% of the vitamin content is derived from the liver oils of percomorph fishes (principally Xiphias gladius, Pneumatophorus diego, Thunnus thynnus, Stereolepis gigas, and closely allied species).

*Supplied only on the 50 c.c. size. the 10 c.c. size is still supplied with the ordinary type of dropper.

MEAD'S OLEUM PERCOMORPHUM
More Economical Now Than Ever

MEAD JOHNSON & COMPANY, EVANSVILLE, INDIANA, U. S. A.

Please enclose professional card when requesting samples of Mead Johnson products to co-operate in preventing their reaching unauthorized persons

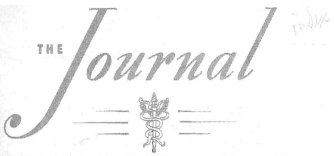

THE Journal

OF THE OKLAHOMA STATE MEDICAL ASSOCIATION

VOLUME XXXVI • OKLAHOMA CITY, OKLAHOMA, DECEMBER, 1943 • NUMBER 12

★ *Published Monthly at Oklahoma City, Oklahoma, Under Direction of the Council*

TABLE OF CONTENTS PAGE IV

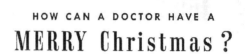

HOW CAN A DOCTOR HAVE A
MERRY Christmas?

You are a healer, a saver of life . . .

Yet, this Christmas you see a world intent on maiming, on killing.

You wish you were out where the wounded and dying are, doing everything in your power for them . . .

But, circumstance holds you and commands, "Stay, do your work here—where the need for it is greater than ever before!"

Because today twice as many people are dependent upon your skill, no hour of day or night is completely and certainly your own . . .

Not even at Christmas.

So, to wish you a merry Christmas at this time would be to wish you the impossible.

However, the House of Wyeth—dedicated, too, to the relief of suffering—does wish that

on Christmas Day you find a moment to yourself . . .

To hope, to believe, that this time the maiming and killing of war are being endured for the last time . . .

To be thankful for the wonderful healers and healing techniques that are coming out of the war to serve the peace . . .

To take pride in the glorious achievements of your professional brothers in uniform . . .

And to feel that your own service, wearying and unheroic though it be, is appreciated—and in the finest traditions of the selflessness of the medical profession.

WYETH
INCORPORATED

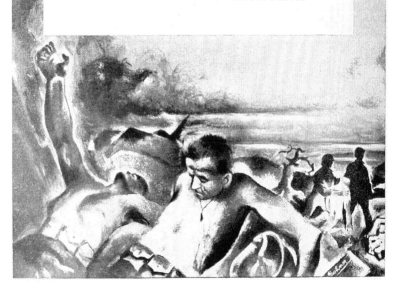

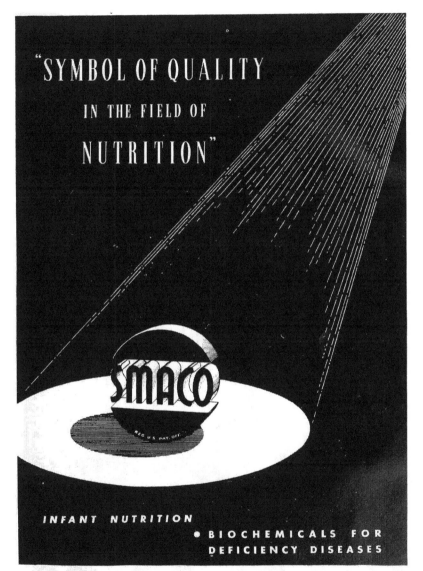

a Poor Scholar . . . because of a Poor Breakfast

MANY a child is scolded for dullness when he should be treated for undernourishment. In hundreds of homes a "continental" breakfast of a roll and coffee is the rule. If, day after day, a child breaks the night's fast of twelve hours on this scant fare, — or less — small wonder that he is listless, nervous, or stupid at school.

Pablum offers a happy solution to the problem of the school-child's breakfast. Mothers who learn about Pablum from their physicians are delighted to serve it, for it needs no cooking and can be prepared in a minute at the table — more quickly than many less nourishing foods. Right now, this feature is especially valuable in homes where the mother is engaged in war work. Pablum not only ends the bane of long cooking of cereals but in addition furnishes a variety of minerals (calcium, phosphorus, and iron) and the vitamin B complex. It is an excellent vehicle for milk.

PABLUM is rich in calcium and iron, minerals likely to be deficient in the school-child's diet yet needed in more than average amounts **during childhood.** Numerous clinical studies have demonstrated that Pablum gives good weight gains and increased hemoglobin values in both normal and sick infants and children. Reprints on request of physicians.

Pablum (Mead's Cereal thoroughly cooked) is a palatable cereal enriched with vitamin- and mineral-containing foods, consisting of wheatmeal, oatmeal, wheat embryo, cornmeal, beef bone, alfalfa leaf, brewers' yeast, sodium chloride and reduced iron. (The oatmeal form of Pablum is called Pabena.) MEAD JOHNSON & COMPANY, EVANSVILLE 21, IND., U.S.A.

6 × 9 - 54

4/19

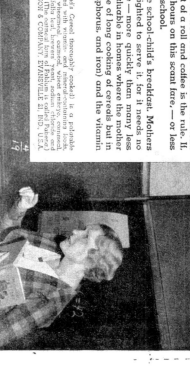

"TOMMY, that's the third time this week you haven't learned your lesson. Why don't you listen to me when I tell you how to work the problems?"

This Book is due on the last date stamped
below.   No further preliminary notice
will be sent.   Requests for renewals must
be made on or before the date of expiration.

DUE	RETURNED
JUN 20 1945	JUN 1 5 1945
APR 3 1963	
MAY 3 1963	

A fine of twenty-five cents will be charged for
each week or fraction of a week the book is
retained without the Library's authorization.

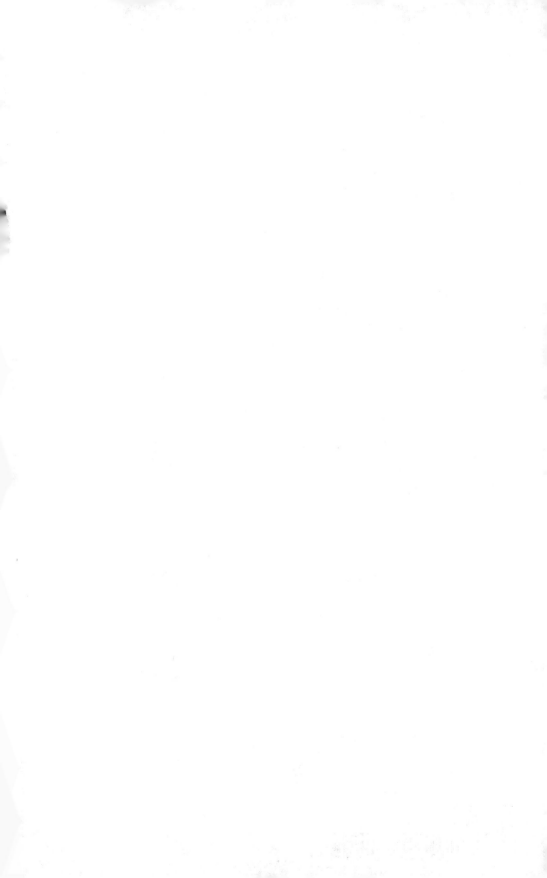

www.ingramcontent.com/pod-product-compliance
Lightning Source LLC
Chambersburg PA
CBHW071354050326

40689CB00010B/1641